TELEMEDICINE TECHNIQUES AND APPLICATIONS

Edited by **Georgi Graschew**
and **Stefan Rakowsky**

Telemedicine Techniques and Applications
Edited by Georgi Graschew and Stefan Rakowsky

Published by InTech
Janeza Trdine 9, 51000 Rijeka, Croatia

Publishing Process Manager Ana Pantar

Technical Editor Teodora Smiljanic

Cover Designer InTech Design Team

Additional hard copies can be obtained from orders@intechopen.com

Telemedicine Techniques and Applications, Edited by Georgi Graschew and Stefan Rakowsky
p. cm.
ISBN 978-953-307-354-5

For EU product safety concerns:
IN TECH d.o.o., Prolaz Marije Krucifikse Kozulić 3, 51000 Rijeka, Croatia,
info@intechopen.com or visit our website at intechopen.com.

Meet the editors

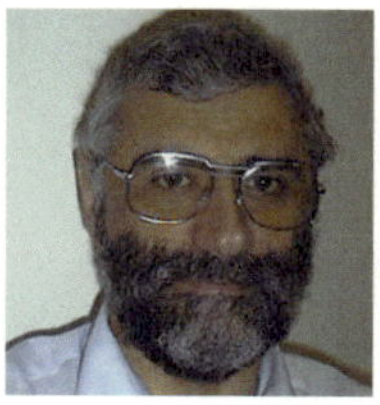

Dr. Georgi Graschew has been a Scientific Coordinator of the Surgical Research Unit OP 2000 at the Max-Delbrück-Center for Molecular Medicine and the Experimental and Clinical Research Center of Charité – University Medicine Berlin (Germany) since 1993. Following his research studies at the Department for Mathematics and Natural Sciences of the Technical University Dresden (Germany) he gained his Ph.D. there in 1974. After research appointments at various international sites, in 1987 he became the co-founder of the Research Unit OP 2000 at the German Cancer Research Center DKFZ in Heidelberg (Germany), where he acted as its Scientific Coordinator until its transfer to Berlin. He made major contribution to numerous leading national and international telemedicine projects: SICONET, PANORAMA, GALENOS, DELTASS, MEDASHIP, EMISPHER. His research interests are telemedicine, laser micro-manipulators, laser diagnostic methods, virtual reality simulations, and high immersive projection systems with tactile feedback. He has co-authored more than 360 scientific publications and presentations and holds 18 patents in Germany, the European Union, Japan and the USA.

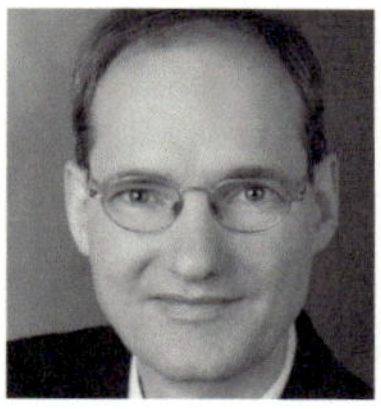

Dr. Stefan Rakowsky studied at the Technische Universität Berlin and received his diploma in physics in 1989. He received his doctoral degree in molecular physics in 1994 at The Pennsylvania State University, USA. From 1994-1996 he was a postdoctoral fellow at the Max-Planck Institut für Strömungsforschung, Göttingen. From 1995 to 2008 he worked as a research assistant at the Surgical Research Unit OP 2000 of the Robert-Rössle-Klinik Berlin in the area of laser induced fluorescence diagnosis, photodynamic therapy and telemedicine. Since 2008 he has coordinated tele-video tumor conferences at the Charité Comprehensive Cancer Center.

Contents

Preface

Telemedicine is not a novelty. The first transmission of patient-relevant data dates back several decades. Respective technologies have been developed rapidly since their introduction and extended application of digital medicine, so today medical data are more and more stored digitally. As we increasingly speak of the paperless hospital, it has become easier to use services such as the Internet and the newly established Web 2.0 as well as Ipv6 to enable the use of applications such as eHealth, ePrescription, and homecare. Several chapters (1-9) in Part I of this book are devoted to practical and theoretical foundations of telemedicine techniques. A number of chapters (10-23) in Part II demonstrate impressive and manifold application examples from practice as well as case studies.

Part I. Theoretical and Practical Foundations of Telemedicine Techniques

The first chapter Innovative Medical Devices for Telemedicine Applications describes several devices which were invented, especially designed, successfully tested and patented by the author. The first applications are remote health monitoring via a wireless (bluetooth/Zigbee and UMTS/GPRS) transmitter of vital parameters acquired by several probes for ECG, Blood Glucose, physical activity, breathing frequency, blood pressure, etc.). The use of a tele-stethoscope for the objectivation of cardio-pulmonary auscultation, a Pain Button / Wireless Pain Button for the provision of extended monitoring of patients with high risk, an RFID-based system allowing doctors easier and quicker access to patient data and PC-based system for remote medical visits allowing the doctor a complete cardio-respiratory control of a remote patient in real-time are important for advanced homecare.

The chapter Pervasive Homecare Monitoring Technologies and Applications gives a comprehensive overview of homecare technology, applications and implementation of wireless technologies which enable pervasive homecare monitoring of elderly, chronically ill (and children). Most existing solutions include a BAN of sensors carried by the patient and environmental sensors forming a PAN connected to the monitoring site by a gateway. The chapter presents detailed analysis of wireless sensor standards (IEEE802.15.4, ZigBee, etc), sensor types including physiological, biokinetic and ambient sensors and signal processing as well as techniques to reduce energy consumption.

A mathematical model for the accuracy and reliability of a communication system for the transmission of vital patient signals in remote health monitoring is given in the chapter Wireless Telemedicine System: An Accurate, Reliable and Secure Real-time Health Care. Transmission errors are analysed based on a WLAN (802.11b) integrated system. The relationships are studied in a simulation of a remote medical diagnosis of typical lung sounds yielding a trade-off between resource consumption and information accuracy. The chapter analyses the security of wireless channels in case of attacks and discusses the enhancement of security.

In Design Criteria for Large eHealth Infrastructure Systems the authors analyse the criteria to be considered before the setup of a nationwide or large eHealth infrastructure. The authors distinguish between the political, institutional, operational and technical level and respective design criteria. On the political level cultural aspects, innovation, healthy growing of the intended system, fears and acceptance by the users and representation in parliament and legislative measures have to be considered. On the institutional level the system acceptance by primary and secondary healthcare centers, health insurance companies, hospitals, pharmacies, nursing homes and patients was analysed. Benefits and costs of the intended system have to be considered against requirements and wishes. On the operational level the actual administration of the eHealth system comes into play through adaptability of the system, accessibility of patient data, maintainability of the network, interoperability of heterogeneous systems and transparency of data transmission.

In the chapter QoS in Telemedicine we learn that Quality of Service (QoS) in IP-based telemedicine systems is required for the delivery of services like tele-consultation, tele-diagnosis, tele-monitoring or tele-education. QoS is determined by delay, jitter, bit rate and packet loss of the network. The author analyses the methods for ensuring quality transmission: traffic differentiation, traffic engineering, error control and data encoding. The emphasis is on traffic differentiation using DiffServ and MPLS and the evaluation of the performance of the proposed solutions.

In the chapter On Redefining Telemedicine Paradigm: An Innovative Integrated Model For Efficient Implementation Of Healthcare Delivery In Developing Countries, by taking into account the healthcare situation in highly populated developing countries such as India and China, the authors redefine the goal of telemedicine as increasing the doctor to patient ratio. It will also be important to reduce the number of patients by introducing preventive healthcare which is also supported by telemedicine. To achieve this, the authors suggest a new approach to keep medical records and start to develop it. They propose a secure and interoperable Electronic Health Record, collecting data in a single file, allowing real time updates, compression of medical data and dynamic transmission of data.

In Novel Prediction Based Technique for Efficient Compression of Medical Imaging Data a predictive model for lossless image compression is described and evaluated. Predictive image coding can be formulated as composed of prediction of a pixel based on surrounding pixels, contextual modeling of the prediction error and entropy coding of the prediction error. The proposed model uses classification and blending of static predictors followed by heuristic contextual error modeling. The description of the predictive coding method is followed by a presentation of experimental results of the two developed complete lossless image codecs. The resulting compression of medical imaging data could be applied for reducing required transmission in telemedical applications and storage of digital image data.

The chapter Clinical Decision Support Systems gives a theoretical background of clinical decision support systems in decision making and qualitative clinical decision analysis. The structure of various clinical decision support systems is characterized well (e.g., according to knowledge-based systems or expert systems and non knowledge-based systems that use machine learning such as in neural networks). The success factors of clinical decision support systems are improved patient safety, quality of care and efficiency of healthcare. The chapter closes with examples of clinical decision support systems in practice and a close look on the example of good practice of clinical decision support system in telemedicine for evaluation of patient health in nursing care.

In the chapter A 2.4 GHz Non-Contact Biosensor System for Continuous Monitoring of Vital-Signs a novel Doppler-radar-based sensor for non-contact detection of respiration and heartbeat rate is presented. The system is composed of off-the-shelf parts and comprises a LabVIEW graphical user interface taking over the discrete Fourier transform of the waveforms. The theoretical background for the chosen method of Doppler radar along with the transceiver architecture and results for the measured vital signs with different generations of the sensor are presented and the data and errors analysed.

Part II. Application Scenarios and Case Studies

In the chapter Mobile Web Application Development to Access to Psychiatric Electronic Health Records a mobile web application (EHR mobile) has been developed based on HL7/CDA and JAVA Servlet and JSP technologies to access electronic health records (EHC) from a PC and with mobile devices. A system overview and detailed data modeling and architecture is given, followed by a description of the user interfaces for different modules of the application which opens new possibilities for information access counselling and cooperation of health professionals. Standards for privacy and confidentiality have been verified.

The chapter Clinical Psychology and Medicine for the Treatment of Obesity in Outpatient Settings: The TECNOB Project presents the TECNOB project designed to determine which features of telemedicine are critical in a cost effective approach. A two step approach is chosen to treat weight loss and maintenance of obese patients consisting of a hospital-based intensive treatment and an out-patient phase supported by telemedicine. In the outpatient phase the patients wear a multisensory armband which monitors their physical activity and have access to the TECNOB web-platform with questionnaires, food record diary, administrative functions and videoconference facility. Through mobile phone the patients can stay in contact with their dietician and in scheduled videoconference sessions with clinicians.

In The Role of Standard 12-lead ECG in a Telecardiology Consultation Service the set up of a telecardiology consultation service and evaluation in a patient study phase is described. A Personal Information Repository document service has been replaced by an internet-based consultation system used for posting consultation requests and storing ECG´s for analysis by the consulting cardiologist. In a real time interactive tele ECG consultation the physician is connected to the consulting expert while the patient is still in the doctor´s office. This technology could make the service more profitable.

In the chapter Tele Oncology for Cancer Care in Rural Australia it is stated that to improve the access to the quality oncological care in rural areas without larger treatment centers, long distance travels to see a medical oncologist are necessary. A tele-oncological network centered in Townsville, Australia is well presented. Medical oncology patients are treated by their local practitioner. Treatment is supported by consultations with specialists in the center via videoconference. In the period from 2007-2010, 150 patients were consulted, resulting in 609 consultations. The model is suitable to provide cancer care to patients closer to their homes. Safety issues, medicolegal aspects and cost-effectiveness are analysed.

Congenital Heart disease is a highly specialized field with great distances between few experts and patients and non-specialist physicians, therefore suited to telemedicine. In the chapter Telemedicine in the Diagnosis and Management of Congenital Heart Disease the authors analyse the situation of pediatric cardiology in UK and discuss hardware, network and personnel requirements for telecardiology. The evidence for application of fetal telecardiology, tele echocardiography in pediatrics both between general hospitals and expert center and in tele-homecare, and the role of a tele-stethoscope in ausculting of pediatric cardiology outpatients is demonstrated well.

Telemedicine in the management of oral anticoagulant therapy improves the interaction between the patients and the medical staff. In their chapter Telemedicine for Managing Patients on Oral Anticoagulant Therapy the authors show that portable coagulometers allow patient self testing and management. The use of this method in Italy is well presented.

In Telemedicine for Chronic Digestive Diseases: A Systematic Qualitative Review a web portal for the home tele-management of the chronic inflammatory bowel disease is used, which allows for patient self-testing and clinicians to customize medication and side effect profiles. A feasibility study for the cognitive behavioural treatment of irritable bowel syndrome and several studies for the telemedicine support of the treatment of chronic hepatitis C infection are reported.

In the chapter Teledermatology: Outcomes and Economic Considerations store-and-forward and live interactive systems are compared as delivery models for teledermatology and the outcome of a number of studies is summarized. Diagnostic accuracy, clinical outcomes and user satisfaction and economic analysis are discussed. Proper application of teledermatology offers a versatile means of providing high quality patient care especially in underserved areas.

Screening for retinopathy of prematurity is an important means to prevent development of a potentially severe retinopathy in premature infants. In Screening for Retinopathy and Prematurity screening criteria, screening protocol and definition of threshold disease signals as well as the gold standard technique of the screening process with an indirect ophthalmoscope are given. RetCam imaging offers the possibility of telemedicine for screening which makes available the expertise of specialists in peripheral hospitals when it comes to improving its accessibility.

The chapter Teleophthalmology in Practice describes novel imaging equipment for retinal care which can be used for different teleopthalmology applications such as diabetic retinopathy screening, screening of retinopathy of prematurity and accident and emergency settings which require ophthalmology. The findings are supported by outcomes in Australia and India. Live video links can help in timely treatment without delay and save transportation of patients from rural areas for retinal examinations in central hospitals. Finally, an outlook on the setup of virtual macular clinics employing optical coherence tomography is given.

In Telemedical Solutions – Practical Approach in Bulgaria standard medical practices contrasted with telemedical solutions are discussed and an overview of telemedicine in Bulgaria is given. Strengths, weaknesses, opportunities and threats of telemedicine are analysed. A review of definitions of telemedicine and a comparison and differentiation of telemetry, telematics and telemedicine is given. The status of Bulgarian telemedicine is compared to the already implemented and more extensive European Health Optimum Project.

The chapter Practical Results of Telemedicine System Between Antarctic Station and Japan gives an impression of the isolation and climatic conditions in a Japanese research station in Antarctica. A team consisting of approximately 40 people is sent there each year over winter and no commutation to the home country is possible during winter. The team of two physicians treat the occurring medical incidents. An overview of possible incidents is given and the need for telemedical consultations by specialists in Japan in some cases is demonstrated. Satellite communication is used for live video communication or offline image transfer.

The high incidence of stroke in patients worldwide and the prevalence of recurrent stroke necessitate the management of risk factors and development of preventive strategies. In Telestroke for the Long Term Management of Risk Factors in Stroke Survivors the authors state that these are especially hampered by the lack of stroke centers in rural areas which can be better served by telemedical services or telestroke. Telestroke makes stroke expertise available to patients living in remote areas and small hospitals. The chapter analyses future developments and provides economic evaluation.

In The Role of Telemedicine in the Management of Acute Trauma Referrals to a Regional Plastic and Hand Surgery Unit in the South East of England the establishment of a store-and-forward telemedicine system at a regional hospital in SE England is reported to assist the referrals of hand and burn injured patients from distant hospitals. The system uses encrypted email transfer of images taken with a compact digital camera. The store-and-forward system was chosen due to easier availability at the referring sites rather than videoconferencing systems and transmission capability. Success factors, evidence of benefit through studies, image quality, legal and security issues, user friendliness, training and support have been demonstrated over the last decade of the use of this system.

Editors

Dr. Georgi Graschew,
Surgical Research Unit OP 2000
Max-Delbrück-Center for Molecular Medicine
and Experimental and Clinical Research Center
Charité - University Medicine, Berlin,
Campus Berlin-Buch,
Germany

Dr. Stefan Rakowsky,
Charité Comprehensive Cancer Center, Tele-Video-Tumorkonferenzen,
Charité Campus Mitte, Berlin,
Germany

Part 1

Theoretical and Practical Foundations of Telemedicine Techniques

1

Innovative Medical Devices for Telemedicine Applications

Agostino Giorgio
Dipartimento di Elettrotecnica ed Elettronica, Politecnico di Bari, Bari
Italy

1. Introduction

Telemedicine is a term generally used to describe a type of patient care which involves monitoring of a patient's condition by a healthcare worker located at a healthcare facility which is remote with respect to the location of the patient. Demand for electronic patient monitoring systems will appreciably grow in next years, bolstered by technological advances. Wireless multi-parameter monitors and stations will place gains in equipment sales.

Although telemedicine systems have been implemented for many years, Ethernet has just begun to be implemented in the last decade. A much more cost-effective solution would be to take advantage of the already existing Internet. Moreover, the spread of wireless technology allows the development of more telemedicine devices with a low or no cost connections, at short or long distance, and also wearable and easily portable.

From this point of view, telemedicine is defined as the delivery of health care and sharing of medical knowledge over distance using telecommunication means. Thus, telemedicine aims to provide expert-based health care to understaffed remote sites and advanced emergency care through modern telecommunication and information technologies. This concept of telemedicine was introduced about 30 years ago through the use of nowadays-common technologies like telephone and facsimile machines. Nowadays, telemedicine integrates network and medical technology, generally comprising remote diagnosis, expert consultation, information service, online checkups, remote communication, etc. Based on computers and network communication, it implements remote transfer, storage, query, comparison, display, and sharing of video and audio information and medical data of a patient.

The availability of prompt and expert medical care can meaningfully improve health care services at understaffed rural or remote areas. Then, telemedicine, if adequately employed, is capable of providing enormous benefits to society. One such benefit is that patients can be examined without having to travel to a healthcare facility. This feature is particularly important for patients who live in remote areas who may not be able to easily travel to the nearest healthcare facility, or who need to be examined by a healthcare worker located far away from the patient, in another State, for example. Another benefit of telemedicine is that it is capable of allowing a patient to be examined more often than would be possible if the patient were required to travel to a healthcare facility due to the ease with which it can be administered.

The only drawback of telemedicine is the risk to dramatically reduce the human contact and the feeling between the patient and the doctor which is the fundamental behind the success of any therapy.
In the chapter are described some of innovative devices invented by the author, patented or patent pending, employing the most advanced information and communication technologies, to show the enormous potential of telemedicine.

2. A remote health monitoring system

The effective and modern health monitoring system as that described in this section, designed and patented by the author (Giorgio, 2009), is a system intended to bring about innovation in remote health monitoring in terms of simplicity, economy and effectiveness in both domestic and hospital applications. It also aims at allowing real-time rescue operations in case of emergency without the necessity for data to be constantly monitored by a practitioner.
Its special management software enables a practitioner or other person authorized to monitor any number of patients simultaneously leaving them free to move, as well as to create and manage an electronic case sheet for each of them.
The system thus conceived meets the needs of both patients and their families. It can be suitably used in hospitals, nursing and care homes, and might be useful not only to GPs but also to sportsmen.

2.1 The concept and the functions

The system is designed for both Bluetooth/Zig Bee (wireless, short-distance) monitoring and UMTS/GPRS (wireless, long-distance) monitoring and data transmission. The Bluetooth-based version also allows to monitor a patient at any distance provided that he/she has a mobile phone with Bluetooth interface.
The system collects data relevant to the health status continuously. These are stored in an on-board flash memory and analysed real-time with an automatic diagnosis program.
Data can be transmitted in the following modes:

a. real time continuously;
b. real time not continuously as follows:
   i. at programmable intervals (for 30 seconds every hour, for example);
   ii. automatically, when a danger is identified by the on board alarm system (explained later);
   iii. on demand, i.e. whenever required by the monitoring centre;
c. offline (not real-time), i.e. by downloading previously recorded (over 24 hours, for example) data to a PC.

In all cases patients do not need to do anything but supply power by simply switching on.
The monitored parameters are: electrocardiogram (and then heart frequency); respiratory frequency; body kinetics (activity of the patient); body temperature; oxygen saturation of haemoglobin (SpO_2); environmental pressure, temperature and humidity; position (by GPS); arterial pressure; blood glucose, not invasively measured.
Each monitored patient is given a case sheet on a Personal Computer (PC) functioning as a server (online doctor). Data can also be downloaded by any other PC, handheld or smartphone equipped with a browser. The system reliability rests on the use of a distributed server environment, which allows its functions non to depend on a single PC and gives

more online doctors the chance to use them simultaneously. Its functioning scheme is presented in Figure 1. The whole system consists of three units:

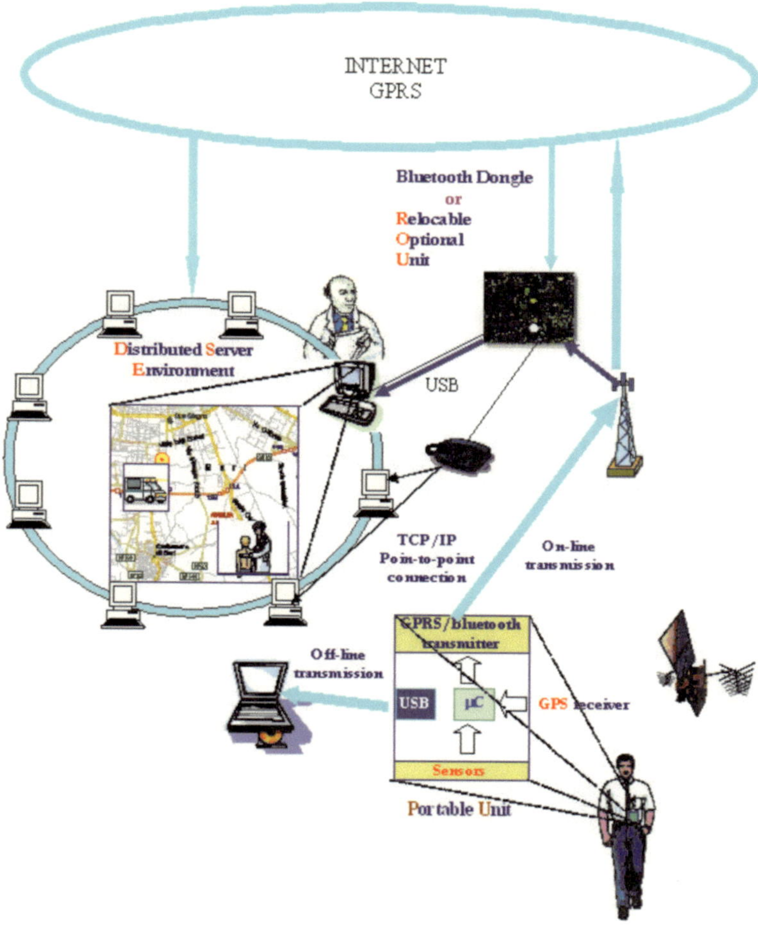

Fig. 1. Functioning scheme of the remote health monitoring system

1. Sensor unit: includes the sensors for the measurement of health parameters and their analog interfaces. The sensors are partly embedded in an elastic band to be round the patient's chest and partly are posed on the patient body;
2. Portable remote transmission unit (PU), miniaturized and wearable. It is designed for both real-time and delayed data transmission (high-speed USB connection to the server) to the patient's case sheet.

The main features of the PU are: 16 analog channels; wireless and wireline transmission capability; GPS location system on-board; automatic real-time diagnostic system; electronic alarm service (automatic sending of warning SMS messages); on-board memory for 24 hours recording and USB port for (offline) data transfer to PC ; rechargeable battery-operated.

3. Relocable Optional Unit, ROU, for local transmission and reception: it ensures system reliability by replacing the PC server when it is out of order. The ROU communicates with the PU by simulation of a point-to-point connection via UMTS/GPRS. It can be

connected via USB to the PC server for on-demand data transmission. This unit is also equipped with an embedded modem which allows a real TCP/IP point-to-point connection to other remote PCs for data transfer when the server is out of order. The unit for Bluetooth transmission simply consists of the Bluetooth dongle.

The whole system is governed by a management software. The main operations it performs are:

GPS real-time location of the patient (city, street, number) and address- and phone-number-searching of the nearest first-aid stations; simultaneous monitoring of many patients; remote (computerized) medical consultation service; creation and management of electronic case sheets accessible on Internet by login and password.

The PU monitors the patient's health status storing data in the on-board memory. Data can be sent to the local receiver, directly to the PC server (online doctor), or to an internet server, which allows anyone to download them by his/her own login and password.

As above mentioned, data transmission can be performed at regular intervals or on the online doctor's demand and because of the detection of any warning sign through the electronic diagnosing system.

The block diagram of the PU is shown in figure 2.

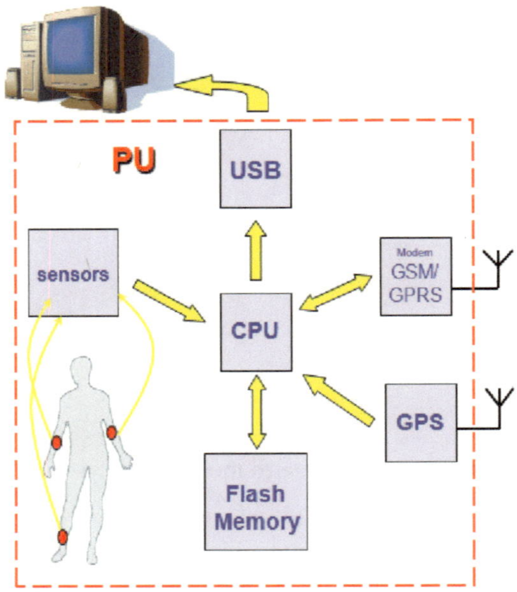

Fig. 2. PU block diagram

In order to ensure the highest levels of security and autonomy, the ROU is also directly connected to the common telephone network: this allows it to keep all its functions even if the server is off or broken down. In fact, a direct call by internal modem allows data transfer to any remote PC.

ROU operates in two modes:

- *Normal mode:* the unit can be used connected to a PC for the transmission on demand.
- *Emergency (alarm) mode*: the unit behaves as a server: it receives the warning signal by the PU and downloads the data transmitted by the PU by GPRS, sending them to the connected PC via USB or to a remote PC by dial-up modem, via telephone cable.

In figure 3 the block diagram of the ROU is shown.

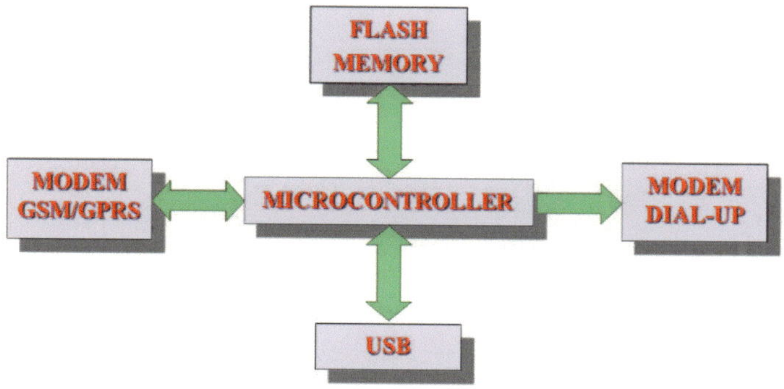

Fig. 3. ROU hardware block diagram

2.2 Example of system operation

The data for the monitoring of the subject's health status are acquired by the remote unit (PU) through sensors which are partly attached to the body, partly to the board. Data are then stored in an embedded flash memory, ready to be transmitted to the ROU or directly to the server PC where the management software has been installed, or to any Internet provider where they can be accessed with permission by login and password.
Data acquisition through the remote PU is immediately followed by an automatic real-time diagnosis performed by the microcontroller of the PU itself.
When a danger is detected the system not only automatically sends a warning SMS message to pre-registered people (doctors, relatives) who are able to arrange for the patient's rescue, but also transmits all data acquired since the detection and the coordinates (GPS mapping) of the subject's position. If the server PC is out of order data are acquired by the ROU or directly sent to a pre-set Internet Provider from which they can be downloaded by any other PC. This accounts for the high system reliability.
The alarm system also includes the automatic GPS location of the patient. Once he/she has been found the management program proceeds to map his/her position thereby indicating the name of the place and the nearest street number as well as the address and telephone number of the nearest hospitals. All these functions do not require any human intervention and are automatically operated only a few seconds after the detection of a danger. Fig.4 shows an example of GPS mapping with the above mentioned informations for a prompt rescue.
The alarm system can be deactivated at any time, whenever the user wishes to stop SMS sending and GPS mapping.
Data can also be transmitted on demand ("ON DEMAND" mode) to the monitoring centre or to any authorized person (i.e. anyone who has been given a login and password). This mode allows the user to fully control the PU through his/her PC. Thereby he/she is not only able to request data transmission at any time, but also to choose the parameters to be transmitted and to deactivate/reset the alarm system.
All "on line" functioning modes enable to set a data acquisition profile peculiar to each patient through the server PC of the monitoring centre.
The management software is also designed to display graphs and maps on handhelds, smartphones and Linux-based PCs.

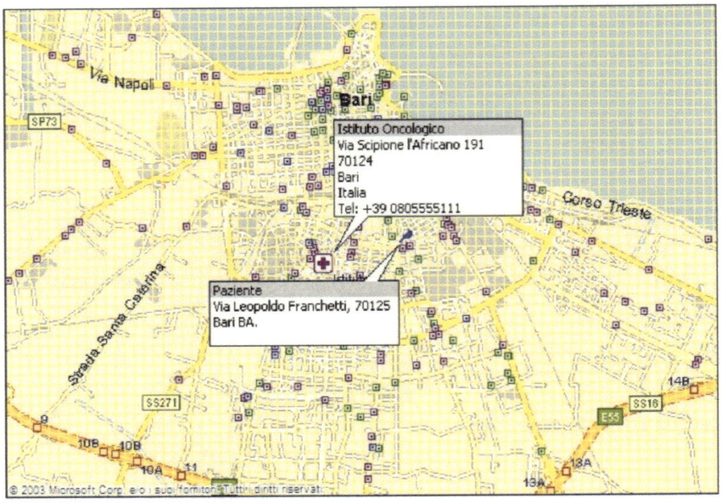

Fig. 4. Location of the patient and the nearest first-aid station

2.3 Diagnostic equipment

2.3.1 ECG and heart frequency monitoring

An electrocardiogram (ECG) is a recording of the electrical activity on the body surface generated by the heart (Carr & Brown, 2001). ECG measurement is performed by skin electrodes properly placed on the body. The ECG signal is characterized by six peaks and valleys labeled with successive letters of the alphabet P, Q, R, S, T, and U (see Figure 5). Each segment between two letters or piece of wave is due to a particular step of the heart cycle and therefore we distinguish among the P wave, the QRS complex, the ST-T segment, the T wave, the QT interval, the U wave. All these waves must have specific characteristics in terms of shape and time extension; different values far from the appropriate ones are symptoms of cardiac diseases.

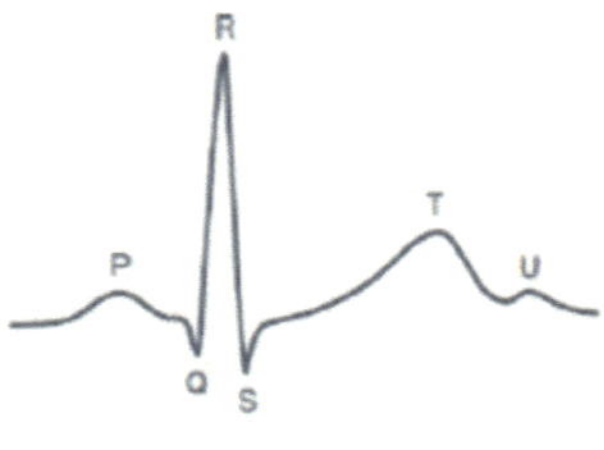

Fig. 5. Typical ECG wave period

The front end of an electrocardiograph must be able to detect extremely weak signals ranging from 0.5 mV to 5.0 mV, combined with a dc component of up to 300 mV—resulting from the electrode-skin contact—plus a common-mode component of up to 1.5 V, resulting from the potential between the electrodes and ground. The useful bandwidth of an ECG signal, depending on the application, can range from 0.5 Hz to 50 Hz—for a monitoring application in intensive care units—up to 1 kHz for late-potential measurements and pacemaker detection. A standard clinical ECG application has a bandwidth of 0.05 Hz to 100 Hz. 10 electrodes needs to detect the 12-lead electrocardiogram. This implies a serious inconvenience for the monitored patient to be free to move.

To solve this problem the remote health monitoring system is equipped with an electrocardiograph that measures body cardiac potentials by using only 5 electrodes placed on the chest (see figure 6) and implements an algorithm able to mathematically reconstruct very accurately all 12 leads. This method is named EASI 12-Leads and was proposed for the first time in 1988 by Gordon Dower (Dower, 1988).
In figure 6 the position of the electrodes is shown to detect the potentials V_I, V_S, V_E, V_A, all referred to the potential V_N. Then, the generic cardiac potential Vi can be calculated by means of the following vectorial relation:

$$\mathbf{V_i = a_i\, V_{ES} + b_i\, V_{AS} + c_i\, V_{AI}} \qquad (1)$$

where ai, bi, ci are constants and V_{xy} denotes the potential difference $V_x - V_y$.
In table 1 are listed the coefficient values allowing to determine each of the 12 derivations:

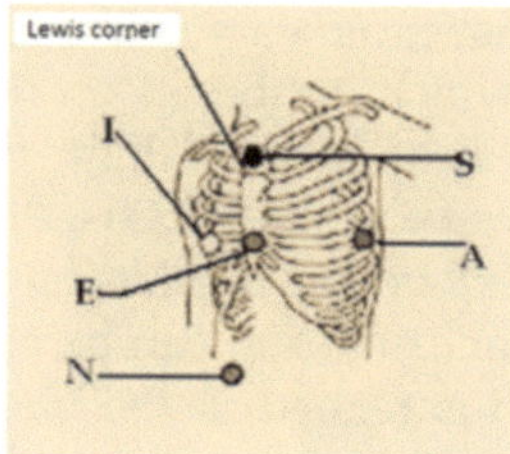

Fig. 6. Position on the chest of the 5 electrodes for the EASI ECG

lead	a_i	b_i	c_i
V_I	0.026	- 0.174	0.701
V_{II}	- 0.002	1.098	- 0.763
V_{III}	- 0.028	1.272	- 1.464
aV_F	- 0.012	- 0.462	0.031
aV_R	0.027	- 0.723	1.082
aV_L	- 0.015	1.185	- 1.114
V_1	0.641	- 0.391	0.080
V_2	1.229	- 1.050	1.021
V_3	0.947	- 0.539	0.987
V_4	0.525	0.004	0.841
V_5	0.179	0.278	0.630
V_6	- 0.043	0.431	0.213

Table 1. Coefficients useful to determine the 12 derivations of the standard ECG by the EASI ECG

The EASI ECG front end consists of an instrumentation amplifier together with an integrator (low frequency - 0.05 hz - noise filter) and an active low pass filter (for limiting the bandwidth - 40 hz - and the amplitude of the signal) that are the building block for each channel of the electrocardiograph. The right led driving circuit is used to remove the common mode voltage.
The heart frequency is calculated from the ECG signal by evaluating the distance between QRS complex.

2.3.2 Blood glucose monitoring

It is well known that high values of blood glucose can indicate serious illnesses, such as diabetes, which in the long-term can produce several complications affecting many body tissues and organs.
Non-invasive glucose monitoring based approaches are very attractive, particularly for patients which require frequent measurements without any inconvenience (Caduff et al, 2003). There are several methods which are based on non invasive approaches. The most interesting technologies are the 1) near infrared light (NIR) spectroscopy, 2) far infrared radiation (FIR) spectroscopy, 3) reverse iontophoresis, 4) optical rotation of polarized light, 5) impedance spectroscopy. Each method has technical problems to overcome.
The measurement of the glucose concentration can be made only indirectly, by measuring the AC conductivity change which is related to the blood's glucose levels (Hayashi et al, 2002). This conductivity variation affects the electric polarization of cell membranes, thus resulting in the skin permittivity change.
In order to not lose the sensitivity to this effect, we must choose a working frequency not greater than 200 MHz. At the same time, the working frequency has not to be too low in order to avoid the electrode polarization.
Then, our approach for monitoring the glucose level changes makes use of an AC analysis of the skin impedance over a wide frequency range, which is scanned until the optimal frequency, corresponding to the best sensitivity, has been reached. The sensor design has been optimized to work in frequency range 1-200MHz, in which the best performances in terms of electrical changes in the blood can be provided.
The general scheme of our sensor is shown in figure 7.
The sensor evaluates the glucose level by comparing a sine signal with the same signal passed through the passive filter constituted by the skin impedance and the resistor R. The skin impedance, which depends on the glucose concentration, is calculated by the following, well known, voltage divider based relationship in equation (2):

$$z = R\frac{V_1}{V_2 - V_1} \qquad (2)$$

The above calculation has to be made for several values of frequency in the range 1-200MHz, in order to evaluate the impedance minimum which provides the best sensor sensitivity. To investigate this wide frequency range a suitable voltage controlled oscillator (VCO) has been employed to provide a sine signal with a high linearity. The output signal, coming from the impedance evaluation block, can be processed by the microcontroller which finds the minimum frequency and stores it in a semiconductor memory. The general scheme is, then, constituted by an analog part, which provides the high frequency sine signal, and a digital section which processes this signal.

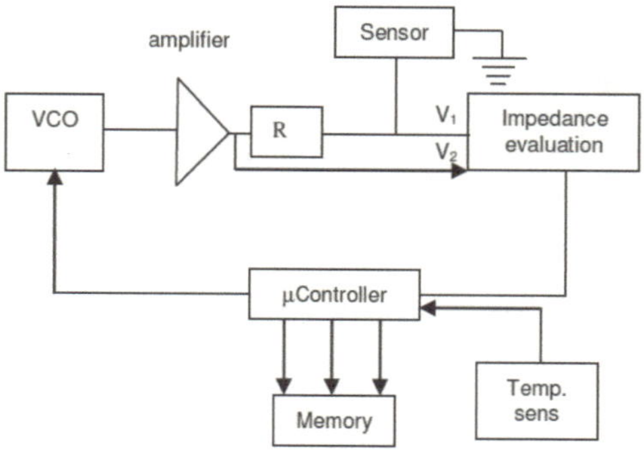

Fig. 7. Block diagram of the impedance spectroscopy based blood glucose sensor

The equation (2) can be easily solved in log forms. To this purpose, the impedance evaluation block is constituted by two differential and two logarithmic amplifiers, as shown in Figure 8:

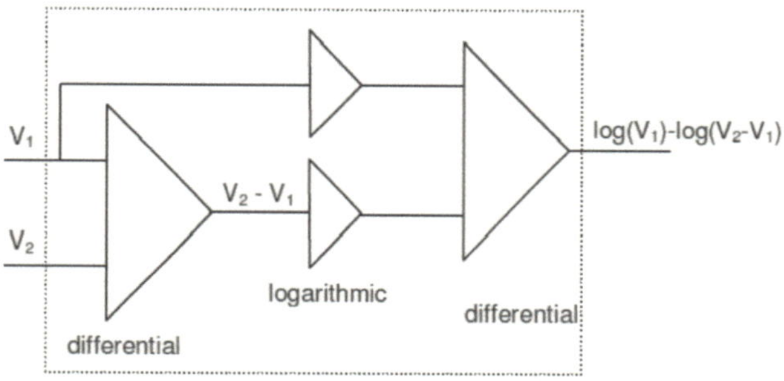

Fig. 8. Block diagram of the impedance evaluation circuit

The VCO has to produce a sine function with a frequency changing in a wide range.
The sensor makes continue noninvasive blood glucose monitoring and is more comfortable than other solutions for patients which require frequent measurements without any pain.
The device is constituted by commercial integrated circuit and is, then, compact, light and easily wearable.

2.3.3 Physical activity (body kinetics) monitoring

In the meanwhile health status is monitored it is very important to know the activities the patient is performing. For example consider how could be different the meaning of an high heart rate whether the subject is running or standing or let's think about how everyday activities such as climbing stairs could "normally" modify heart frequency and/or breathing rate.
For this reason, to make the diagnosis as accurate as possible, the remote health monitoring system includes appropriate sensors for body kinetics monitoring. To this aim we use an accelerometer.
In fact we observed that root mean square (r.m.s.) values of acceleration (passed through a high pass filter) is fully correlated with walking speed. Experimental data show that vertical acceleration on the shoulder of a running patient peaks from -1*g* to 2*g*, while power spectrum spans up to 20Hz. Peaks comes from each impact of foots on ground.

This signal includes a contribute coming from the gravity that is $g\cos\theta$ where θ is the angle between the sense direction of the accelerometer and the gravity. The angle θ is not constant at all when the accelerometer is fixed on the clothes of a patient, and varies widely when a subject bows or stand up. Fortunately the power spectrum of θ is concentrated at frequency below 1Hz (typical), much lower than the frequencies of the acceleration of a walking (running) patient. In conclusion it's necessary and also enough to use a high pass filter to cut off the gravity.
Then, the signal maximum amplitude is +2g (20 m/s^2) and the maximum frequency is 20 Hz. The accelerometer must be high precision (i.e. 0.5mg @ 20hz) and low power (i.e. 700uA @ 5Volt).
The acquisition signal chain is quite simple, it requires a band pass filter to cut off low frequencies at 0.7Hz (related to gravity) and high frequencies at 20Hz to clean unforeseen unwanted signal outside the signal band. Then, the filtered signal pass to a cheap and effective r.m.s. converter. The r.m.s. converter output is filtered to cut off frequencies over 0.1Hz to kill off the residual ripple observed on running patients.
The analog filter signal is clean and spanned voltage range is matched to input span of the ADC of the portable unit.
In figure 9 it is shown the plot of the output of the physical activity monitoring equipment during a running (upper plot) and during a walking (lower plot).

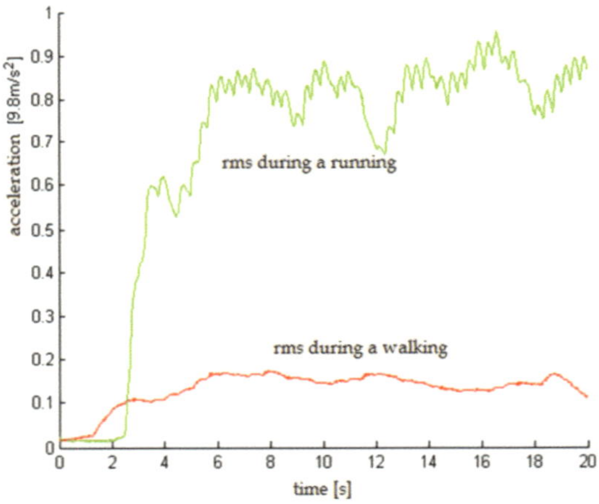

Fig. 9. Plot during a running (the upper one) and during a walking (the lower one)

This kinetic sensor has been tested on several subjects, for each patient it was clearly possible to recognized whether the subject was standing, walking or running.
The observed signal is correlated to the physical activity but also to the weight of the subject, and (we suppose) also the way subject walks. For simple qualitative analysis this is not a problem, if a quantitative analysis were required then a subject by subject calibration would be used, or more simply a statistical parametrization of calibration on some biological parameter (weight, height, sex, age).
With this calibration, we hope that this physical activity measurement would allow a also good quantitative estimator of the energetic expenses to what concern walking and running, and we hope that (using also other biological parameters to evaluate basic metabolism) could be possible to estimate the daily energetic expenses.

This would be very interesting since available method that measure the CO_2 (with mouth and nose tubing,) and the heat production (in a calorimetric box) are not suited for 24 hour measurements and long time monitoring.

2.3.4 Breathing frequency monitoring

For breathing sensing we use an already known method involving a belt to sense the thorax dilatation, but we apply a new kind of belt dilatation sensor on the belt. We sense the resistance changes of the rubber due to stress elongation, the voltage drop on the rubber is amplified (suppressing the DC component).

As much as we know the application of the conductive rubber is new in breathing detection, it is quite cheap and sensitive.

In literature it is possible to find two main methods for breathing monitoring (Webster, 2009). In the first one, the air flow is sensed while in the second one the breast dilatation is sensed.

Air flow monitoring is accurate but is very uncomfortable, since it requires tubing mouth and nose or placing sensors in mouth and in nose. This would rule out 24 hours logging. For remote health monitoring system we are so forced toward the breast dilatation monitoring. This may be quite less accurate, it is sensitive to arms movements but it is much more comfortable.

For breast dilatation monitoring, piezoelectric strain gauge sensor are quite problematic, since the charge generated at typical breathing frequencies (0.25Hz) are difficult to amplify. Accelerometers are not suitable, because the tiny acceleration available (about 0.02g) compares with the gravity acceleration. But the situation is even worse since the accelerometer only sees the vertical component of the gravity, that is $g\cos\theta$ (where θ is inclination angle of the patient), that could vary largely with times comparable with respiration times according to the variations of the angle θ when patient bows. Breast dilatation monitoring is well accomplished using a breast elastic belt, so sensing the belt stress makes it possible to sense breathing.

Aside from several stress sensor we have designed a new, very interesting conductive rubbers sensor, being it also quite cheap and easy tailored. Conductive rubbers are made mixing carbon or iron powder in the chemical reactants used to produce rubbers. They have been applied as flexible conductors and as pressure sensors, but we did not found application as dilatation sensors. Indeed conductivity of these rubbers are sensitive to stress, but among the large kind of conductive rubbers available, not all are suited for this application.

We look for conductive rubber satisfying the following specifications: high sensitivity to the stress; rubber should stand the stress applied to the breast belt, about 10N; moderate conductivity, between 0.1Ωm and 10Ωm.

After performing a great number of tests on various kinds of conductivity rubber we chose a sample of conductive rubber from Xilor, whose resistivity was only $7 \cdot 10^{-5}$Ωm, constituted by an aggregate of small conductive spheroids, about 20μm wide. The conductivity is controlled by the contact surface area between spheroids, this area varies according to the mechanical stress, so that resistivity is high sensitive to the mechanical stress.

We took a sample 120mm long, 20mm large and 0.3mm thick that was fit in the breast belt, at the place of a piece of belt. Since the sample is not capable to stand all the belt stress, it is not feasible a full belt built only with this kind of conductive rubber. To solve this problem, a non conductive rubber was added in a mechanical parallel to our conductive rubber.

Two couples of small iron plates where tightened to each end of the rubbers sandwich to ensure electrical connections.
The resistance of conductive rubber is about 1Ω, measured with the four wires method.
While the breathing rate ranges from about 0.1Hz to 3Hz but the breast movement spectrum has more power in the range from about 0.4Hz to 3Hz, the front end amplifier is connected to the sensor through a capacitor with a low frequency cut off at 0.4Hz, while another capacitor produces upper a cut off at 3Hz.
The dilatation signal after the front end was clear, but it is sensitive to arms movements. After the first amplification stage, signal went through more stages: a peak detection, a pulse shaper and a frequency to voltage converter.
As shown in figure 10, the resulting signal is clear and noiseless; it is also shown the signal from the peak detector which is well behaved.
As already said, the system has been successfully tested on a wide breathing rates interval, but still remain the ageing problem.
Indeed the rubber resistivity raised tenfold after few hour of usage on the belt. While this could be compensated with an automatic gain control at the front end amplifier, much better would be to use the compression method.
A second problem is the sensibility to the arms movements, which could trigger false breathing pulses. This is intrinsic to the belt method, but the effect is not so frequent compared to the breathing rate.
In conclusion, our sensor has been successfully tested, the remaining problems are minor. Anyway, it is recommended to look for other kind of conductive rubbers, cheaper or with better ageing to further improve performances.

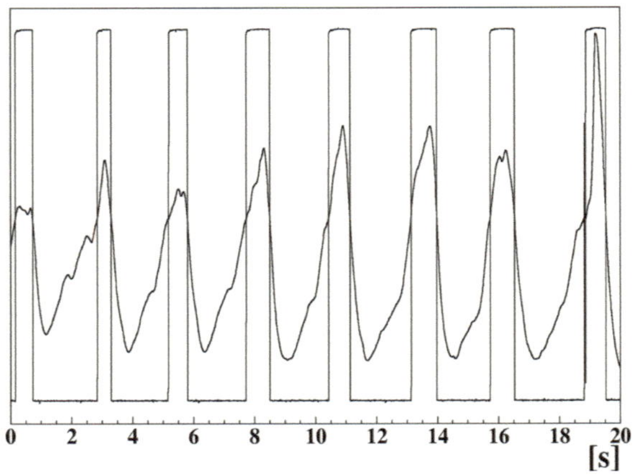

Fig. 10. Sampled signals: the wavy signal is from the sensor while pulses are from peak detector.

2.3.5 Oximetry monitoring

Pulse oximetry provides continuous measurements of blood oxygen saturation, and is from 40 years ago an important medical technique both for emergency and critical care use and for everyday medical checkups (Aoyagi et al, 1974). The theory upon which pulse oximetry operates involves measuring the amount of emitted waves that are transmitted through or absorbed by tissue containing blood. The absorption spectrum of oxygen-rich blood differs from that of oxygen-lacking blood, and oxygen saturation can be measured based on this difference in absorption.

Then, we remember that the coloured substance in blood, haemoglobin, was also its carrier of oxygen. (Haemoglobin is a protein which is bound to the red blood cells.) At the same time, it was noticed that the absorption of visible light by a haemoglobin solution varied with oxygenation. This is because the two common forms of the molecule, oxidized haemoglobin (HbO2) and reduced haemoglobin (Hb), have significantly different optical spectra in the wavelength range from 500nm to 1000nm

The oxygen chemically combined with hemoglobin inside the red blood cells makes up nearly all of the oxygen present in the blood (there is also a very small amount which is dissolved in the plasma). Oxygen saturation, which is often referred to as SaO2 or SpO2, is defined as the ratio of oxyhemoglobin (HbO2) to the total concentration of hemoglobin present in the blood (i.e. oxyhemoglobin + reduced hemoglobin):

Arterial SaO2 is a parameter measured with oximetry and is normally expressed as a percentage. Under normal physiological conditions arterial blood is 97% saturated, whilst venous blood is 75% saturated.

It is possible to use the difference in absorption spectra of HbO2 and Hb for the measurement of arterial oxygen saturation in vivo because the wavelength range between 600 nm and 1000 nm is also the range for which there is least attenuation of light by body tissues. By measuring the light transmitted through the fingertip (or the earlobe) at two different wavelengths, one in the red and the other in the near infra−red frequencies of the spectrum, the oxygen saturation of the arterial blood in the finger (or ear) is measured.

The medical device useful to this aim is the pulse oximeter. Then, a pulse oximeter is integrated in the remote health monitoring system.

The pulse oximeter is interfaced to the human body by a sensor consisting of two LEDs, one emitting red (660 nm) and one that emits infrared (940 nm) light, that flash alternately, controlled by a dedicated circuit and polarization piloting. The light emitted through the tissues undergoing different attenuation for each wavelength. The resulting light intensity or the light radiation that was absorbed by the tissues is received by a photodetector (photodiode or phototransistor) which varies its resistance according to the amount of light incident from a few ohms to hundreds of MΩ.

The signal is then obtained in current and subsequently is converted into a voltage signal, so a transimpedance amplifier needs. The output signal is sampled by two sample and hold (S / H) amplifier (one for each channel) and sent to two parallel and identical sets of filters: bandpass filter for the extraction of a pulsatile component and a low-pass one having a very low cut off frequency (about 0.2 Hz) to extract the DC component for each signal R and IR. The signal such conditioned is managed by the microcontroller of the PU.

2.3.6 Arterial pressure monitoring

Blood pressure systemic (erroneously known only as blood pressure) is the pressure difference per unit area that exists between an artery and the surrounding environment.

We distinguish between systolic blood pressure (or max) and diastolic (or min). The most used method for measuring blood pressure is the auscultatory one which is based on the use of a sphygmomanometer having a cuff, which inflates and deflates, equipped with a pressure sensor well positioned on the arm in correspondence of the brachial artery and a stethoscope to listen to the sounds of Korotkoff heard during the cuff slow deflaction.

This method, although fairly accurate if the dimensions of the cuff are large enough, has some limitations due to the presence of various source of noise and due to acoustic performance of the operator: is the sound of Korotkoff included in a range of frequencies (<200 Hz) where the hearing Human beings are not very sensitive. Moreover, in patients with hypotension, the moment to read the diastolic pressure may be difficult to interpret, as a reduction of blood flow also causes a degradation of Korotkoff sounds.

In place of the auscultatory method, there are other important indirect methods such as the oscillometric method.

This method really provides the mean value of the arterial pressure, but by a numerical algorithm can also provide the systolic and diastolic values. It is based on the measure of the fluctuation of the pressure inside the cuff. In fact, when the blood passes through the artery occlusion caused by inflation of the sphygmomanometer the pressure inside the cuff undergoes small changes. These oscillations are due to the fact that the flow of blood in these conditions appears to be turbulent, so the pressure that the turbulent blood exerts on the walls of the cuff is not constant.

The maximum value of the oscillations occurs at the value average pressure (MAP, mean arterial pressure). Therefore, to assess the values of systolic and diastolic pressure, you should resort to an algorithm mathematician. This algorithm does is to assess the maximum oscillation and calculate the two fractions of correspondence relating to fluctuations in systolic and diastolic pressures. In particular, typical values well correlated with the auscultatory method, are 50% and 80%, respectively for systolic and diastolic pressure. This will involve read the pressure values at these amplitudes of oscillations.

The system designed for arterial pressure monitoring, linked to the portable unit, is based on the oscillometric method and consists of the following main blocks: pressure transducer; band-pass filter for the extrapolation of the oscillations; analog to digital converter (ADC) for signal acquisition output to the transducer and its filtered version; microcontroller for the signal processing: after deflation of the cuff, the microcontroller determines the peak of the pulsatile component and determine the diastolic and systolic pressure as a percentage of that maximum. Figure 11 shows the signals after the filter (oscillating curve) and the output of the sensor (solid curve)

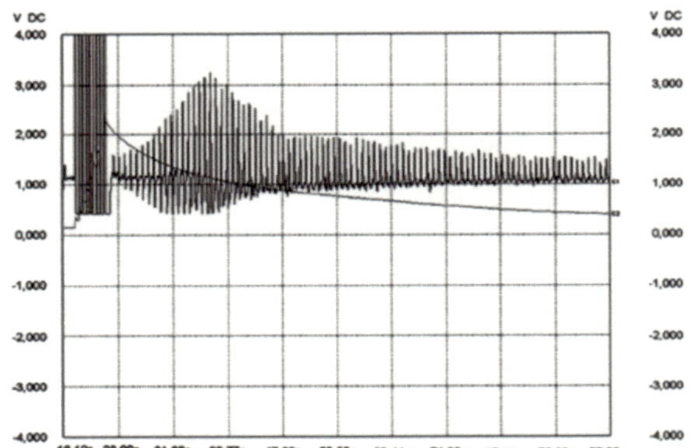

Fig. 11. Arterial pressure monitoring: sensor output (solid curve) and filter output (oscillating curve)

Alternatively the oscillometric method can be implemented the tonometric method that lets you record continuously and non-invasive pulse pressure by compressing superficial artery, usually the radial artery, the underlying bony structures. The registration of the measured pressure values is done through the use of a piezoelectric transducer applied externally over the artery pulse. The main advantages are: absence of a sphygmomanometer; provides a continuous measurement during the entire cardiac cycle; speed and accuracy.

2.3.7 Body temperature

The body temperature monitoring is performed using an NTC (negative temperature coefficient) sensor with the corresponding signal conditioning circuit based on the Wheatstone bridge method, connected to the microcontroller of the portable unit.
The measure of temperature occurs every hour or other time interval to be programmed or on demand.

2.3.8 Environmental parameters

The values of the environmental pressure, temperature and moisture are essentially correlated to the health status of a person. In fact, it is well known that under certain environmental conditions, especially with high temperature and moisture, a person, especially the children and elderly, may have an illness.
For this reason among the parameters monitored by the described system there are also the environmental ones.
To this aim commercial sensors are used, mounted on the portable unit board. These sensors are interfaced with the PU by buffered amplifiers.
Firmware diagnostics correlate environmental parameters with those of health and correctly interpret the situations of real danger if it occurs.

3. The internet tele-stethoscope: The last generation of the electronic stethoscopes

This device aims at solving the problem of objectification in cardio-pulmonary auscultation, currently not objectifiable, and the ability to perform real-time tele-auscultation in order to improve the diagnostic potential of telemedicine, at present mainly limited to the tele-electrocardiography, the tele-consultation and the sending of delayed reports.
In fact, auscultation of lung sounds and heart sounds is one of the classic diagnostic methods commonly used in medical practice, and runs through stethoscope. Although useful, not-invasive and of rapid implementation, it is a diagnostic test particularly sensitive to the physician's subjectivity, both in the reception quality of biological sounds and in their interpretation for the purpose of diagnosis.
From several years by now amplified electronic stethoscopes with noise filtering systems have been developed to improve diagnostic accuracy.
As far as these solutions have allowed a better perception of biological sounds by the physician and even the recording and the archiving of sounds acquired, however there remains the problem of subjectivity by which the interpretation of sounds is conditioned, and the need for the doctor to be close to the patient, since it is currently impossible the real-time remote transmission of sounds, but only deferred, or upon registration.
The device, which represents a technological evolution in comparison to electronic stethoscopes, allows you to transmit sounds at any distance via internet in real time without suffering any distortion or alteration and allows to correlate, in real-time, spectrum of heart

and lung sounds with diseases, thereby allowing an objective diagnosis. In fact there is a deterministic relationship between the spectrum of biological sounds and pathologies.
The device can also store the recorded sounds useful for comparisons over time to monitor the evolution of diseases.
The device was successfully validated for both heart sounds and lung sounds and showed a considerable educational value for physicians in training who need to gain experience in correlating correctly and objectively biological sounds to diseases. In the flowing subsections after just a reminder about the origin of biological sounds in Human beings, necessary to understand the method implemented for objectification, the device is described.

3.1 Origin and spectral properties of respiratory sounds

Organic sounds originate from mechanical vibrations in compressible media and are transmitted through tissues as sound waves. The lung sounds, in particular, are generated in large airways, where high speed and air turbulences induce vibrations along the walls of the breathing tubes. Such vibrations are then transmitted through the tissue of the lungs and the chest walls, up to the surface, where they can easily be perceived with the aid of a stethoscope. The generation of lung sounds is directly related to the speed of airflow and to the architecture of the airways. The velocity of air flow is mainly determined by pulmonary ventilation and cross-section of the airways at every level of the lungs.
Terminal airways or alveoli illnesses are responsible for changes in the lung sounds heard on the surface, because the diseased tissues are responsible for the increase or decrease of the sound transmitted. Differences in intensity and characteristics of perceived sounds are, therefore, of great help in identifying specific diseases of the chest, as changes in tissue density involve acoustic attenuation, reflection and refraction of sound waves. Furthermore, the properties of the sound heard on the surface are determined by factors that affect the sound generation and characteristics of the intermediate tissues: every type of tissue is able to attenuate the sound vibrations of different frequencies and in different quantities, which translates in an alteration of the sound spectrum and a lower amplitude sound in certain frequencies (Jingping et al., 1997). When the acoustic properties of tissues through which the sound propagates differ greatly, as between the air-filled lungs and muscles of the chest wall, much of the sound wave is reflected and sound intensity decreases. Then, the large-spectrum sound, generated in the large airways, it is first filtered by the lung parenchyma (the organic material that constitutes the lungs) and chest wall, then reaches into the skin without the high-frequency spectral components: ultimately the lung-thorax system behaves as low-pass filter for respiratory sounds.
When, due to disease, the spongy and full of air tissue of the lungs is replaced by clusters and liquid and becomes a solid mass, the lung-thorax system is capable of transmitting high tones. Therefore, the presence of high frequency components in lung sounds is a symptom of respiratory diseases. The frequency range of the lung sounds in healthy people extends up to 1000 Hz, although the greatest concentration of power is observed between 60 Hz and 600 Hz. With increasing age there is a small increase in power in the band between 330 Hz and 600 Hz. Spectral differences exist between women and men in general, women have tones of breath sounds higher than men.
The best frequency band to obtain the average power is the band between 100 Hz and 600 Hz, because here we have a probability of error less than the band between 100 Hz and 800 Hz, and the information that is lost is negligible because the power is almost entirely concentrated in the first band.

In addition to the chest, another common position to auscultate breath sounds with a stethoscope is on the neck in the hollow above the breastbone to the extrathoracic trachea. The sounds recorded here are called tracheal sounds. These sounds have an amplitude large enough, on average, greater than about 20 dB at low frequencies, and have a frequency range wider than the sounds listened from the chest.

The intensity of breath sounds is greater during expiration than during inspiration. Their spectral power density does not show a peak at low frequency, rather it extends nearly flat in amplitude between 100 Hz and 700Hz, where the first peak appears, then decreases down to the second peak at about 1500 Hz.

However, the spectral characteristic of tracheal sounds varies considerably among patients, and also depends on the width of the trachea and physiology and physique of the patient. It has been shown that patients with tracheal stenosis have a spectrum with a significant increase both in power, with a peak at about 1 KHz, and in bandwidth, with spectral power that extends from 600 Hz to 1300 Hz.

3.2 Origin and spectral properties of heart sounds

Heart sounds are produced by the movement of the valves and the turbulent flow of blood. The normal heart sounds consist of two parts: a first pulse due to the closure of the atrio-ventricular valves, which denotes the complete passage of blood in the ventricle, a second pulse due to the closing of the valves between ventricles and great vessels, which denotes the complete passage of blood from the ventricles to the aorta and pulmonary arteries.

The blood is pushed through the arteries by the mechanical movement of the heart, but if the arteries are partially occluded blood flow is disturbed, and this creates turbulence in the arterial. Following this pressure variations are produced and heart sounds called murmurs due to blockage of his arteries, can be heard on the surface of the chest, matching the outbreaks of auscultation. The murmurs are high frequency sounds that cover a range between 250 Hz and 1000 Hz. They become appreciable when the occluded area of the arteries reaches 75% of the total. Several studies confirm that the frequency range between 400 and 800 Hz is associated with coronary artery stenosis.

The spectrum of non-pathological heart frequencies extends between 10 and 400 Hz, but the range that provides more info is between 20 and 150 Hz. The lung sounds and the muscle noise contained within the bandwidth of 100 Hz interfere with the heart sounds and this makes difficult the distinction necessary for diagnosis. With the use of electronic devices and appropriate numerical algorithms (Yang-Sheng et al, 1998) it is possible to distinguish the heart sounds and lung sounds by filtering out noise.

3.3 Description of the internet tele-stethoscope

The device permits the acquisition of lung sounds and heart sounds, the real time spectral analysis and transmission via internet to a remote PC, both for sounds and for its spectrum. The device is PC-based being connected to a PC to function, and has a hardware component consisting of a sensor and a filter-amplifier and a software driver.

The hardware side, respiratory and cardiac sounds are picked up by the microphone capsule, housed in a bell stethoscope to be affixed to the patient's chest. The transduced signal is amplified and filtered. The user can select the type of filtering to be applied to the signal, so as to enhance the cardiac and respiratory components. The conditioned signal is then sampled and quantized by a form of A/D conversion.

The system is powered by a rechargeable battery in the device itself using a special charger.

It has not been allowed the use of any compression algorithm, so as to preserve the quality of the transmitted signal.
The connection to a PC is possible as with a cable to the sound card of the PC as via Bluetooth. A microcontroller is necessary to oversee the management of the device functioning.
The prototype of the internet tele-stethoscope has the same chassis of the typical well known electronic stethoscope but it can also be redesigned assuming the appearance similar to that of a normal PC mouse, as shown in figure 12.

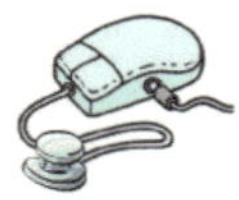

Fig. 12. Possible new mechanical design of the internet tele-stethoscope, alternatively to the classical chassis

The software allows the acquisition of sound through a PC and real-time transmission of audio streams, via web, to another PC; the software implements, moreover, all the digital filtering necessary to optimize the auscultation including the osculation, the Fourier transform to perform spectral analysis, environmental and muscle noise filtering, heart sounds from lung sounds filtering (Paris et al, 2000). The interface, shown in figure 13, allows archiving of sounds, playback, deferred analysis, spectrum printing, zoom, sending audio files.

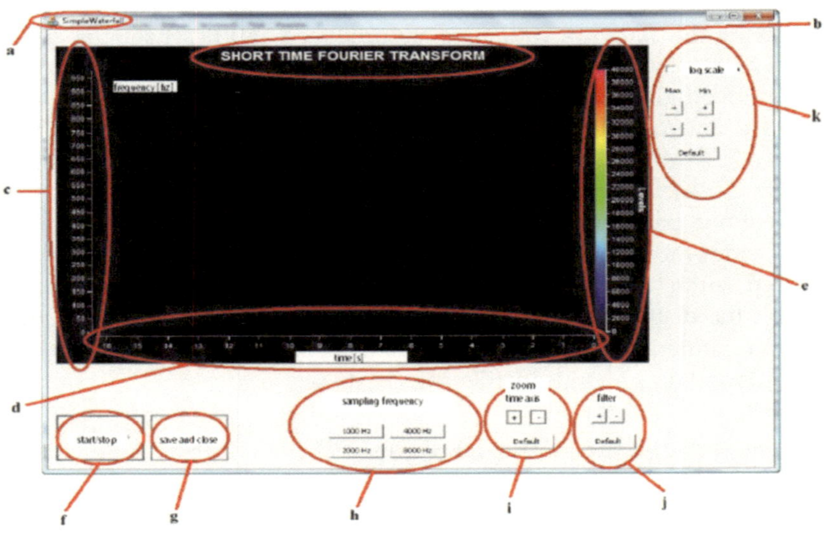

Fig. 13. Software User Interface: (a) Program name. (b) Title. (c) Frequency axis. (d) Time axis. (e) Intensity scale. (f) Start button: to start the program, pause it and restart it. (g) Quit button. (h) Sampling rate selection buttons: 1 - 2 - 4 to 8 kHz. (i) Zoom of the times. (j) Filter: allows you to increase or decrease the application of the video filter; if the limit is decreased, the filter is not applied. (k) Management of the intensity scale: allows you to switch between linear and logarithmic scale, and vice versa, and to vary the range of the scale. Move your mouse over the image appear zoom options, files, etc...

3.4. Validation

Several acquisitions of lung sounds and heart sounds have been made and compared, both with the new device and with a reference electronic stethoscope of the best commercially available. The comparable results indicate the reliability of the new diagnostic device. A few pictures are shown as examples of the sound spectrum. Figure 14 shows the sound spectrum of a tracheal sound acquired and recorded by the reference stethoscope (a) and by the new device (b).

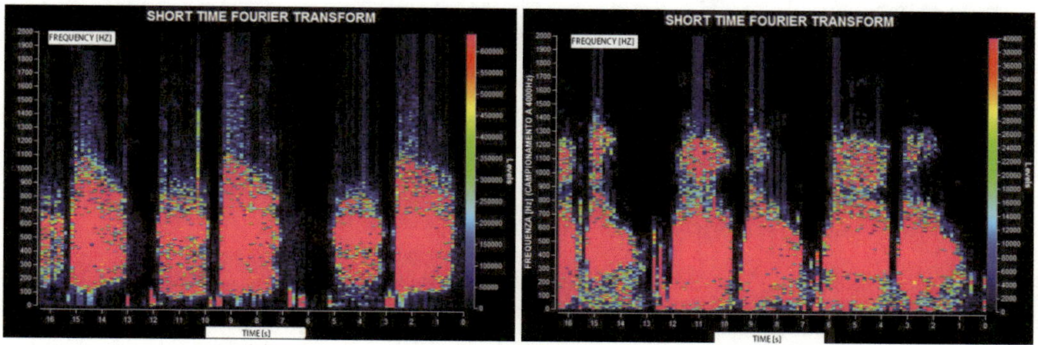

(a) (b)

Fig. 14. Spectrum of a tracheal sound acquired by the reference electronic stethoscope (a) and by the new device (b)

Figure 15 shows the sound spectrum of a heart sound concerning the aortic acquired using the reference electronic stethoscope (a) and by the new device (b), respectively.

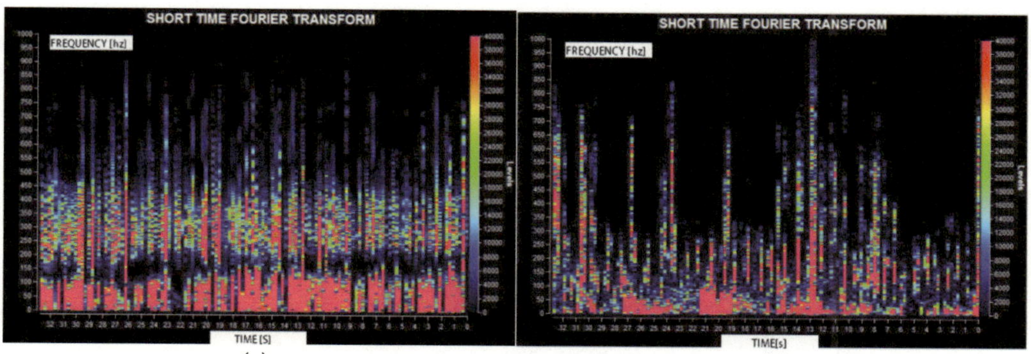

(a) (b)

Fig. 15. Spectrum of the heart sound in aortic area by electronic stethoscope (a) and by the new device (b)

Figure 16 shows the sound spectrum of a heart sound concerning the tricuspid outbreak acquired and recorded by the reference electronic stethoscope (a) and by the new device (b). In all cases, the diagnosis obtained via the new device and by reference stethoscope is the same.

Remote transmission test were also performed to assess the feasibility and accuracy of Web-based Heart and Lung sounds Auscultation (W) HLA in comparison to Traditional (T) HLA. For this purpose have been studied 21 patients in a routine setting of the Cardiomyopathy Unit of Policlinico di Bari. Each patient was assessed by two expert cardiologists (Obs1-2) in two consecutive steps (W-HLA and T-HLA) using a cross-over study design. W-HLA was performed by using the internet tele-stethoscope. The high-quality audio signal was transmitted over the Internet by standard ADSL connection from the internet tele-stethoscope to a remote personal computer where the observer was able to hear and record HLA audio for W-HLA

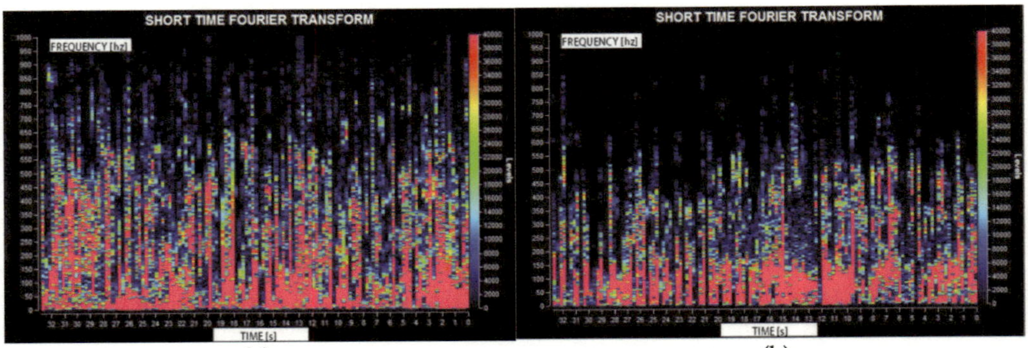

(a) (b)

Fig. 16. Spectrum of the heart sound in tricuspid area by the electronic stethoscope (a) and by the new device (b)

A trained nurse positioned the stethoscope on topographical areas under webcam-assisted audiovisual guidance. T-HLA was performed by traditional binaural stethoscopes. Auscultatory findings were assessed by pre-classified values. Data were analyzed for concordance and tested by Fisher's exact test ($p<0.05$) and kappa-test.

The results are summarized in table 2 in terms of intraobserver concordance of W- vs T-HLA (No. of concordant findings, (%)) for Obs1 and Obs2 for the overall findings, for heart sounds, and for pulmonary findings; and in terms of interobserver concordance of Obs1 vs Obs2 for the same findings.

FINDINGS	INTRA WEB versus ACOUSTIC		INTER OBS 1 versus OBS 2	
	OBS 1	OBS 2	WEB	ACOUSTIC
Overall	217/231 (93.9%)	214/231 (92.7%)	224/231 (96.8%)	219/231 (94.8%)
Heart sounds	81/84 (95.2%)	79/84 (94.1%)	79/84 (94.0%)	83/84 (98.8%)
Pulmonary	60/63 (95.2%)	59/63 (93.6%)	59/63 (93.6%)	62/63 (98.4%)
Systolic heart murmur chronology	19/21 (90.5%) κ=0.82	18/21 (85.7%)	17/21 (80.1%)	19/21 (90.5%) κ=0.82
Pulmonary rales	20/21 (95.2%) κ=0.64	19/21 (90.4%)	20/21 (95.2%)	21/21 (100%) κ=0.47

Table 2. Validation statistics for the internet tele-sthetoscope

Therefore, heart and lung auscultation, as assessed by concordance analysis in our patient series, yielded high concordance of auscultatory findings for the traditional and web approach. Intra- and interobserver concordance were not different for the two observers in the two settings. Thus, web heart and lung auscultation is a promising method for telemonitoring of patients affected by heart failure and the designed internet tele-stethoscope is reliable.

4. A pain button for real-time rescue of patients having heart failure and high risk of life

The purpose of the pain button device described in this section is the provision of extended monitoring for patients under therapy after infarction, data collection in some particular cases, remote consultation, and low-cost ECG monitoring for the elderlies that are unable to announce their failure condition. So the system allows real-time rescue of patients having heart failure and high risk of life. The pain button is based on the SMTP (Simple Mail Transport Protocol) and SMS (Short Message Service). The device will be described in to two different configurations:

i. Pain Button (PB), that features GSM/GPRS technology for data transmission. It is suitable for outdoor use.
ii. Wireless Pain Button (WiPB), that features Wi-Fi 802.11g technology (over and above GSM/GPRS) for data transmission. It is suitable for indoor and outdoor use.

Communication between PB (or WiPB) and a remote PC (or portable phone) server is achieved through programming the device by an user-friendly web server interface. Through the use of Wi-Fi connection is possible to configure the device while the patient wear it remaining free to move (without using wired connections).

Access to web interface to configuring the device is granted only to users that have right permissions by a login/password access form.

The device can send automatic and manual alarm status reports. In case of illness the patient presses the Pain Button. Otherwise, PB acquires and processes ECG signal and reports automatically abnormal cardiac behaviour (automatic status report). The system performs analog-to-digital conversion and analyzes in real-time any variation in shape, duration, amplitude and frequency of ECG. So it is able to examine and identify a disease from its symptoms identifying: tachycardia, bradycardia, arrhythmia, sinoatrial node block and ventricular extra systole, ischemia and infarct.

Digital data are stored into internal flash memory or in external memory card MMC/SD. The system embodies a GPS (Global Positioning System) receiver to acquire the real-time patient position.

To ensure the resilience of system, PB uses three different transmission technology: GSM to send SMS (Short Message Service), GPRS and Wi-Fi 802.11g to send verbose alarm report (ECG signal and GPS coordinate) to PC. The remote observer can monitor the patient ECG and his position, simply by typing the connection parameter.

4.1 Concept and design

As we have stated, the device purpose is the provision of extended monitoring for patients under therapy after health disease (especially after infarction), health status data collection, remote consultation and low-cost ECG monitoring for the elderlies that are unable to announce their failure condition. So the system allows also real-time rescue.

The device has been designed and prototyped into two configurations.

The former configuration, named Pain Button (PB), features GSM/GPRS wireless technology for data transmission. It is suitable for outdoor use. The block diagram is shown in figure 17.

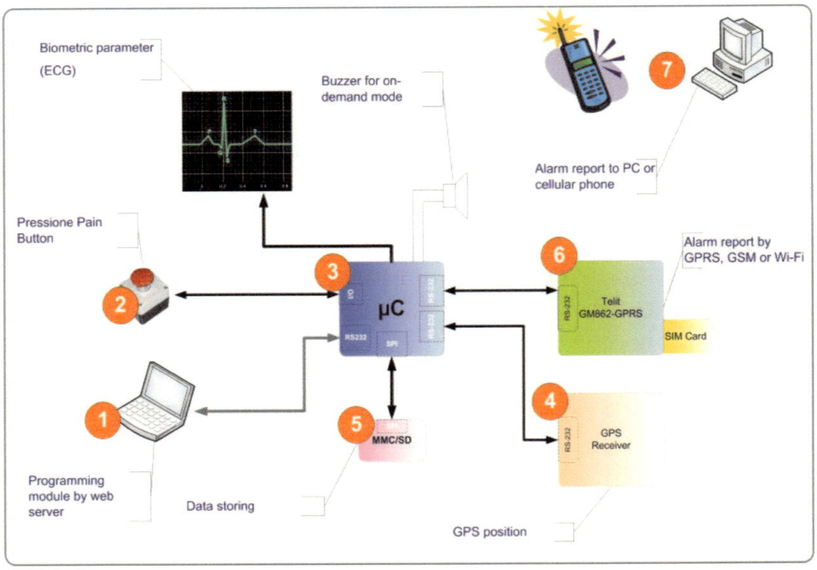

Fig. 17. Pain Button (PB) block diagram

The latter configuration, named Wireless Pain Button (WiPB), features Wi-Fi 802.11g wireless technology (over and above GSM/GPRS) for data transmission. It is suitable for indoor and outdoor use. Its block diagram is shown in figure 18.

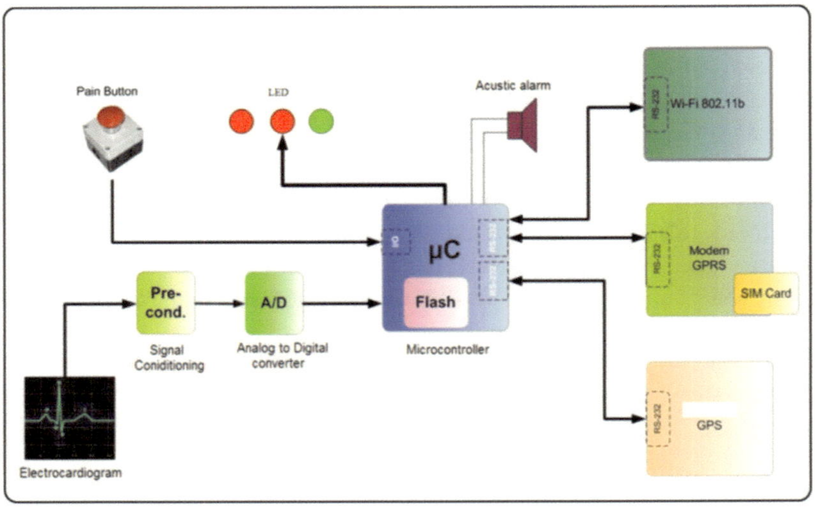

Fig. 18. Wireless Pain Button (WiPB) block diagram

Both configurations are equipped with a GPS receiver to signalling the exact patient position. It is a basic requirement for a telemedicine system, since it is necessary to allow an immediate assistance in case of disease.

Both configurations are equipped with an analog-to-digital front-end to convert data and transmit them to the central unit. An external sensor port is provided in patient home communication interface device.

The ECG device is integrated in PB and WiPB. It is because ECG parameter is the main factor to determine the patient condition and possible risk of life.
In the following paragraph the method implemented in PB/WiPB to automatically determine heart disease will be described.

4.2 ECG automatic interpretation and the algorithm for heart disease detection

As already reminded in section 2. electrocardiography is a transthoracic interpretation of the electrical activity of the heart over time captured and externally recorded by skin electrodes by an electrocardiographic device.
A typical ECG tracing of a normal heartbeat (or cardiac cycle) consists of a P wave, a QRS complex and a T wave. A small U wave is normally visible in 50 to 75% of ECGs. The baseline voltage of the electrocardiogram is known as the isoelectric line. Typically the isoelectric line is measured as the portion of the tracing following the T wave and preceding the next P wave. Figure 19 shows the model a typical ECG waveform (which real shape is shown in figure 5) .

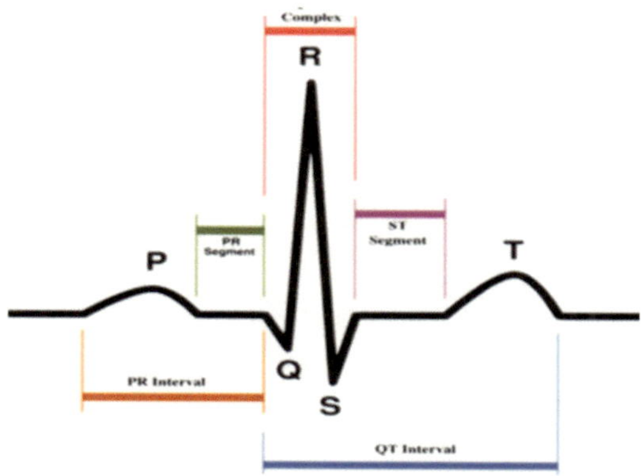

Fig. 19. Electrocardiogram waveform model

The shape, length and amplitude of ECG allows to determine the heart condition and possible heart disease. To reveal all ECG parameters, the system uses a QRS detection algorithms based on threshold method. Since the QRS is the wave complex with higher amplitude, it is a simpler method to calculate the heart beat. The problem associated with this method is right threshold choice.
To this aim, according to (Evans, 1998), the equation (3) has been used:

$$U_{TH} = \frac{A}{2} + \frac{N}{A} \cdot \ln\left(\frac{P_0}{P_1}\right) \tag{3}$$

where P_1 and P_0 are respectively the probability to have and not to have a QRS complex, A is the ECG signal amplitude and N is noise variance. So, assuming typical value for this parameter (according to AAMI - Association for the Advancement of Medical Instrumentation), it results a threshold of 70%. This value was the starting point for microprocessor data processing to calculate the heart beat (HB). In fact, when HB is found it is simple to identify various heart disease like tachycardia ($HB > HB_{tach}$[bpm]) or bradycardia ($HB < HB_{brady}$[bpm]).

The parameter HB_{tach} and HB_{brady} could change from patient to patient. So the system implements a simply web interface to change these reference parameter.
Moreover, the algorithm implemented in the device (as PB as WiPB) allows to automatically identify arrhythmia, beyond tachicardia and bradycardia. In this case, we defined an arrhythmia factor α as in equation (4):

$$\alpha = \frac{\Delta T_1}{\Delta T_2} \tag{4}$$

where ΔT_1 and ΔT_2 are respectively the time between three consecutive QRS complex, like Figure 20 shows. In an ideal case, we will have an arrhythmic complex when $\alpha \neq 1$, while in the real case, we define the following range by equation (5):

$$\Delta T_1 < (\Delta T_1 + \Delta T_2) \cdot 40\% \tag{5}$$

that is,

$$(\alpha < 0.25) \text{ and } (\alpha > 4) \tag{6}$$

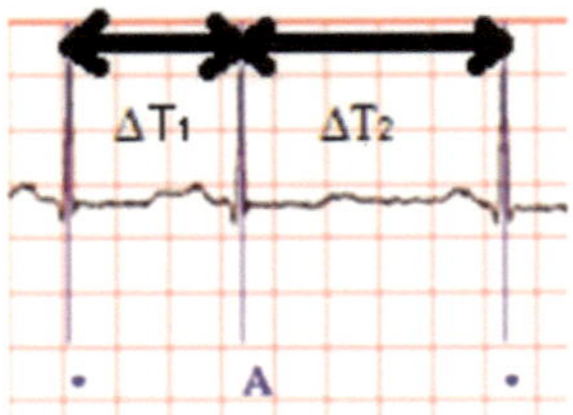

Fig. 20. arrhythmia factor α and detection method

4.3 Operation example: Wireless alarm and data transmission

The device can send automatic and manual alarm status reports. In case of illness the patient presses Pain Button to signalling his condition (manual status report). Otherwise, PB/WiPB acquires and processes ECG signal and reports automatically abnormal cardiac behaviour (automatic status report). The system performs analog-to-digital conversion and analyzes any variation in shape, duration, amplitude and frequency of ECG in real-time accordingly to the previous described algorithm.
Digital data are stored into internal flash memory or in an external memory card MMC/SD, based on overall data.
In order to ensure the resilience of the system, PB/WiPB uses three different transmission technology: GSM to send SMS, GPRS and Wi-Fi 802.11g to send verbose alarm report (ECG signal and GPS coordinate) to PC. Figure 21 shows all possible transmission method implemented in PB/WiPB.
Thanks to Wi-Fi 802.11g interface, it is possible to configure the system without using any cable and while the patient wears it, even directly by clinic. Moreover, the system integrates a web server to make simpler the configuration step. Simply connecting trough a web browser (like Internet Explore, Firefox or Safari) and inserting the IP address of device, is possible to enter the ECG parameter, phone number to send the alarm report or email address of PB-Client, like shown in Figure 22.

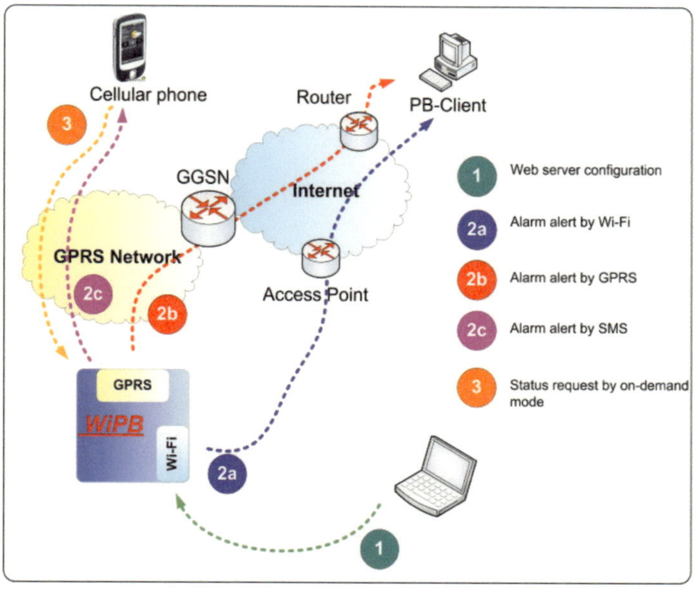

Fig. 21. Data transmission from PB to PC and cellular phone

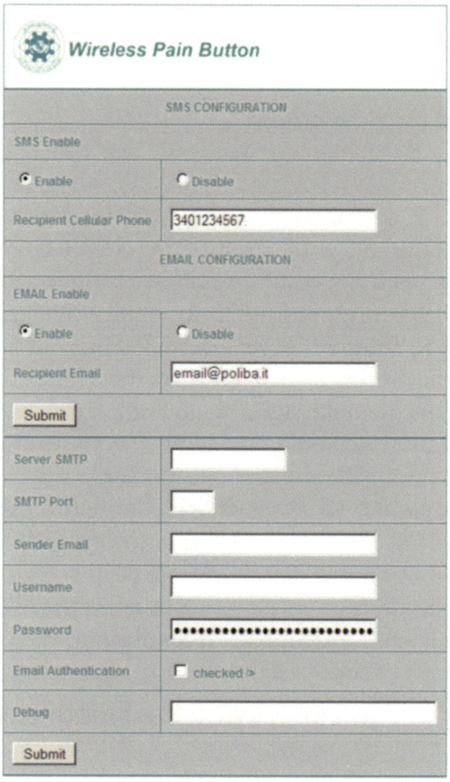

Fig. 22. Web Interface to programming WiPB by Wi-Fi

To allow the security access to the system, all web pages access has been protected with username and password.
In this project data transmission by GPRS or Wi-Fi 802.11g uses application layer protocol (SMTP) based on reliable TCP protocol as it offers permanent connection channels and data integrity.

4.4 Management software

To be useful, a telemedicine system have to be supervised by an integrated client software. The software for PB/WiPB (named PB-Client) was developed using Delphi language. It is capable to supervising more than one PB/WiPB, showing for each PB/WiPB alarm status and type, ECG trace and geographical position.

4.5 GPS

A reliable telemedicine system have to automatically notify an illness. Beyond this main requirement, it is necessary, for example in case of heart failure or high risk of life, to know exactly where the patient is. In this way it's possible to reduce the rescue time. So the PB/WiPB device embodies a GPS receiver to acquire the real-time patient position. It has been also developed the client-side software with a Graphical User Interface (GUI), able to capture alarm status report, showing exact patient position by interaction with software for geographical visualization and analysis, like Microsoft Mappoint and Google Maps (however it is possible to integrate with other software for geographical visualization). So the remote observer can monitor the patient ECG and his position, simply by typing the connection parameter.

4.6 Features and future of the pain button

A working prototype of PB/WiPB has been realized. The dimensions are 9.5x5.5 cm^2, so it is easily wearable.
PB and WiPB consists of a set of WiFi/GPRS-enabled instruments that communicate wirelessly over Internet. Equipped with a miniature circuit board, devices such as a ECG monitor or other external sensors can communicate with clinic until they are within range of an access point (only in WiPB configuration); if no access points are found, the device uses a GPRS connection to access to Internet; even if no GPRS signal is detected, the device uses the GSM network. It sends the encrypted data to the clinic, which consists of multiple redundant servers and makes the data available to authorized specialist via web server. The same advanced communication technologies allow the transmission of data dealing with implantable devices such as defibrillators and pacemaker.
The PB/WiPB is easy to operate, so patients with limited abilities or patient with heart disease can use it without difficulty: they only have to press the pain button if needed, but even if they can't press this button, the device automatically sends data.
Due to its features the PB should be a very nice solution in the future to improve the quality of life and the life expectancy of diseased, high risk subjects.

5. RFID technology application improving the health-care quality and efficiency

The effect of information and automation technology is manifesting more and more widely in medical procedures, bringing substantial benefits to the health and welfare of all patients.

We can think about already existing applications as the ability to book a medical examination via internet, or use sophisticated diagnostic techniques (CT, MRI, PET), or the possibility to perform minimally invasive endoscopic techniques, or telemedicine.
Among these, data processing certainly is a crucial aspect for patient care. Health management and control, indeed, are based on using, transmitting and comparing a large amount of data, information and heterogeneous knowledge. However, in recent years the need to exchange data has increased dramatically, both within a health facility (among different subjects and specialized units.), and among geographically distant facilities. Amongst other things, with the rising organization cost and complexity, we can't think to disregard an adequate information system consisting of management software and complex databases which ensure organization control and optimization (Mori et al, 2001).
Although computerization drastically increases the efficiency and effectiveness of data processing procedures, has less impact in terms of increasing the care quality or the patients' quality of life, especially for elderly, chronically ill, accident-prone patients. Nevertheless, these benefits not always improve patient's health directly. For example, in the case of an emergency relief to an injured or sick person, it is essential to obtain timely patient's past medical history , in order to prevent the supply of incorrect treatments which could further aggravate the situation.
Then, the computerization of health services through the use of complex software and data base, allows a more efficient organization of service and care but doesn't usually have a significant impact in terms of improving the care or patients' life quality, especially for elderly, chronically ill, accident-prone patients and in need of urgent assistance. In order to address this shortage, it is useful a system invented by the author based on RFID (Radio Frequency Identification) technology, consisting of both hardware and software part, described in this section.
It wants to demonstrate how to dramatically improve medical history acquisition procedures and face the most serious situations, using RFID technology; not forgetting, among others, further important advantages as integration into an existing computer system, or the economic factor.

5.1 A quick reminder about RFID Technology

RFID is a wireless technology that represents an innovative solution in the field of processes automation. Although its origin is not recent, it will provoke a veritable revolution in every productive sector in the coming years. The reason why only in recent years RFID has spread, is because its use has changed over times and, if until recently, RFID could be considered as a still evolving technology, currently is moving towards a stage of expression maturity.
The very acronym definition is very clear in specifying and limiting the technology involved:

- Is a technology that allows the identification (i.e. the unique recognition) of an object or living being.
- Is a technology that uses radio frequency.

At the basis of its operation there is an intuitive idea of being able to identify, through an intelligent label (called "tag", "transponder" or "data-carrier device") without any need for physical connection, any object such as products, animal or people. These transponders, unlike their predecessors bar codes, have the ability to store on a chip an information that

can be transmitted via radio waves to the appropriate reading devices (readers or interrogators). Then data is sent to a central computer to be interpreted and processed.
To understand the significance of this mechanism is enough to think that on a single chip you can put several pieces of information (from the serial identification code, name, last name, etc.) and that the readers, depending on applications, are able to capture tags information at a distance ranging from a few centimeters to several meters.
The best RFID transponder package matching the described project criteria is compliant to the ISO 7816 standard, where we find credit cards, personal identification cards and especially smart cards. In fact, these are often used when transactions must be processed quickly or hands-free, such as on mass transit systems, where a smart card can be used without even removing it from a wallet.
RFID technology has a very large presence in the smart cards field.
There are standards like ISO/IEC 14443 or ISO/IEC 15693 that allow for communications at distance ranging from a few centimeters up to a meter at operative frequency of 13,56 Mhz, or also ISO/IEC 11784 ISO/IEC 11785 allow for communication at 134,2 Khz frequency and the just mentioned distance.
Smart cards are advertised as suitable for personal identification tasks, because they are engineered to be tamper resistant.
The embedded chip of several smart card models usually implements some cryptographic algorithm.
Last but not least, the amount of embedded memory varies from a few bits up to a megabyte and allows us to insert all necessary personal and clinical data.

5.2 The advantages of RFID technology applied to the health-care services

The RFID-based system we are describing, allows to improve the health care quality because it allows doctors a very quick consulting of the clinical data of a patient; moreover, the system is perfectly integrated into any local/national or international health information system and data base.
The importance of having promptly the patient's medical history is also crucial to speed up healing process and reduce risk likelihood. Consider, for example, a patient must be urgently admitted to hospital and does not know or cannot report all the critical information needed before surgery, he should be first subjected to a series of investigations and then undergo surgery, or suffer intervention without collecting the above information with high risk of mortality.
Therefore, by equipping any person of an RFID smart card and by equipping any hospital of an RFID wireless smart card reader for patient identification connected to a computer, we have implemented the instantaneous and automatic access to all patient's clinical/medical history information stored in a personal folder of files into database containing one folder for each patient.
The database should be world wide and everywhere located, not necessarily on the hospital computer, if the hospital computer is internet connected.
The designed system meets requirements and benefits ranging from simple procedures streamlining for acquisition of individual's clinical data, to the access to all clinical / history data for patients unable to exhibit them (because they are unconscious, or because don't remember, etc.), to the automatic creation of a database in compliance with health service computerization requirements.

In the flowing subsections will be discussed the support technologies and the system characteristics in particular.

5.3 RFID-based system technical and operation features

The hardware part of the device consists of RFID smart card (tags) and a receiver (reader). As already stated, their radio frequency interaction allows the unambiguous recognition of people, objects or animals at distance.
In the patient tag are stored the main patient's data (i.e. name, surname, age, address, main pathologies, eventual allergies, etc, depending on the integrated memory available).
The software, however, is composed primarily of a relational data base which is a health facility database with patient's information and clinical details inside, and secondly of a very intuitive graphic interface to manage both the RFID device and the data base. The data base is self-creating, as will be explained later.
Any health facility user is delivered with an RFID tag card, which stores his data (and clinical details). By equipping any person of an RFID smart card, and by equipping any hospital of an RFID wireless smart card reader for patient identification connected to a computer, the system allows the instantaneous and automatic access to all patient's clinical/medical history information stored in a personal folder of files into data base containing one folder for each patient. The data base should be world wide and everywhere located, not necessarily on the hospital computer, if the hospital computer is internet connected.
Assuming the use of the system in the hospital or nursing home reception, if the user comes with wearing the tag within the detection distance (less than a meter), the system automatically recognizes the individual and searches his data within the central data base, which then are also printed on the screen of an operator.
If a detected tag contains invalid reference data in the database, or if the patient is inserted for the first time in the database, it is quite automatically updated by the system by creating, without any human intervention, a new record that contains the data taken directly from the tag and possibly displaying the new acquired information. Then, for the new patient, the system provides the automatic creation of the personal folder as the patient has been identified by the RFID reader, and the automatic transfer of the main data from the personal smart card (self-creating data base).
Therefore, the system allows you to create a dynamic database that updates itself without the aid of any employee and that makes immediately available to health professionals (doctors, paramedics, etc..) all information relating to patient data stored in the its own RFID smart card, such as medical history including current therapies, diseases, examinations reports, specialist reports and all that is deemed useful to include in the data base. The remarkable feature is that the access to the patient's folder occurs suddenly and automatically on a computer connected to the RFID reader, as the patient has been identified. In this way is not needed for any description by the same patient about its own clinical history thus reducing drastically the misunderstanding and the forgetfulness.
To fulfill these tasks, the system was modeled according to the block diagram in figure 23.
From the left, we have the presence of the RFID tag assigned to each patient which interfaces to the reader through the appropriate antenna; the reader, in turn, is connected via serial cable to the port available on the PC and controlled by a dedicated software class. The data flow goes directly into the main form, which provides data management and visualization through the dedicated forms. Finally, the same core module provides the graphical interface for input / output with the healthcare professional.

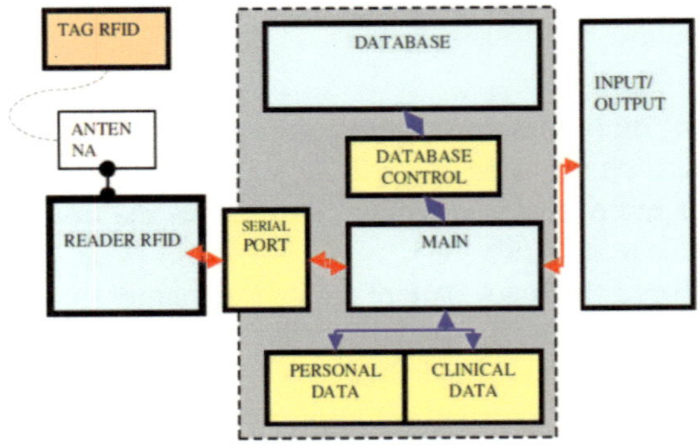

Fig. 23. Block diagram of the hardware part of the designed RFID-based system

The software part of the system, developed in Visual Studio environment, consists primarily of a relational database simulating a health facility database with patients' clinical data inside, and secondly of a very intuitive graphic interface to manage both the RFID device and the data base.

The software interface is designed to provide maximum ease of use and maximum usability of the information by using a rational approach that privileges the automatic rather than total control of the instrument but without sacrificing functionality.

In the main window of the software, shown in figure 24, are condensed all necessary controls to access software features as the data table and controls for managing records and information related to them. These controls reproduce features like search, delete, edit, create new record, regardless of the particular format of the database connected to the system (Access, SQLServer, MySQL). Indeed, designing the database control class through ADO.NET methods and the SQL language, allows a certain independence from the data source, which, in this context, translates into a great ease of integration with existing databases.

In addition there are buttons for connecting and disconnecting the RFID device from database.

Buttons for RFID reader are only two, allowing the connection and disconnection from the device. The procedures for reading the tags, recognizing and displaying information, are autonomously managed by the software, which requires the reader to make cyclical readings every two seconds. The device responds in three main ways:

- Tag not found
- Tag found
- Tag is invalid o not recognized

An answer like "tag not found" occurs in the absence of a transponder within the operative range. A message such as "tag detected", however, starts procedures for the recognition and eventual data drawing, which takes about one second of operation. The third message ("Invalid tag or not recognized") involves the display of warning messages in circumstances of incorrectly coded or partially damaged tags.

Even if reader detects a valid tag that does not match any reference in the database, or if the patient is included for the first time in the database, he is quite automatically updated by the system by creating, without any human intervention, a new record that contains the data taken directly from the tag and possibly displaying the new acquired information. Then, for the new patient, the designed system provides the automatic creation of the personal folder as the patient has been identified by the RFID reader, and the automatic transfer of the main data from the personal smart card. This important feature allows you to create a dynamic database that updates itself without the aid of any employee Moreover, the speed of data exchange with the effectiveness of a good RFID system spares the transponder owner to show his card, and linger near the recognition point, in the interest of timely intervention in urgent cases.

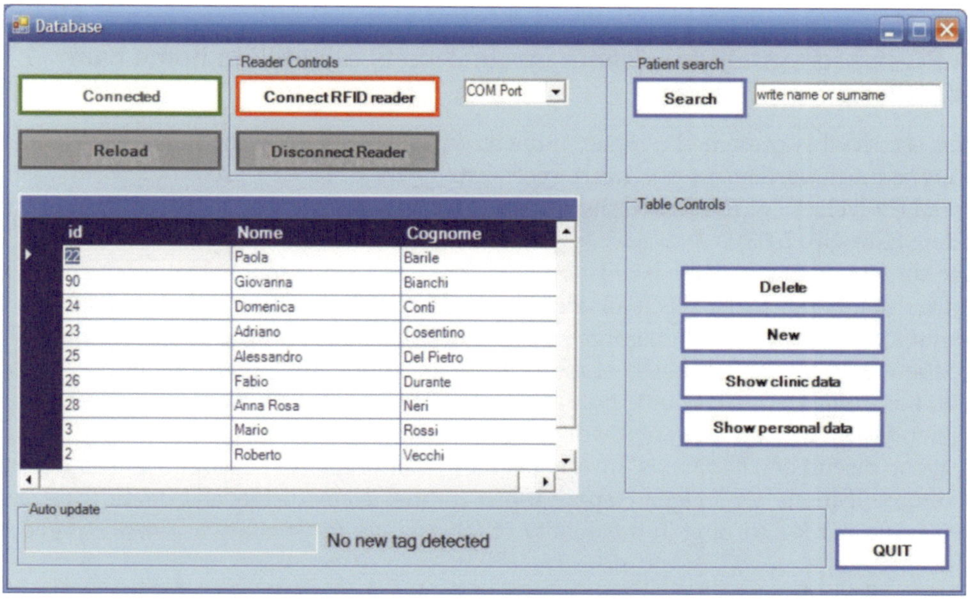

Fig. 24. Main menu of the software part of the RFID-based system

Finally, we should highlight that the system also has the possibility of writing information on transponder, so any new intervention, examination or, a more general clinical and medical history data updating can be always recorded on the patient smart card.

5.4 System usefulness

The use of well designed system actually allows a drastic reduction in recognition time and the immediate availability of patients' generic and clinical data. For example, in the case of manual recognition and data acquisition, the time ranges from a minimum of a few minutes to a maximum of about 40 minutes, while exploiting the automation of our system, we need about one or two seconds. It's obvious that in a urgency situation, the immediate availability of the subject's medical history provides the choice of an effective and especially timely cure.
Another remarkable feature is that the access to the patient's folder or the creation of it occurs suddenly and automatically on a computer connected to the RFID reader, as the patient has been identified. In this way is not needed for any description by the same patient about its own clinical history thus reducing drastically the misunderstanding and the forgetfulness.
Furthermore, the particular system architecture with the extreme simplicity and high automation, do not steal time to health personnel to assimilate new procedures, contributing to an effective integration in any existing health facility information systems.

Also the economic sphere should not be underestimated, in fact the cost of RFID devices for such applications is, after all, quite low; just think that now transponders price varies from a few cents to a few dollars depending on the amount of memory or the complexity of the integrated circuit. Thus, a system conceived in this way is capable to combine an information procedures streamlining with a cost containment policy.

Ultimately, the system can operate in a simple and efficient data flow (medical records, personal data) that is immediately available and always updated, providing a definite advantage for both the medical staff and patients.

6. A PC-based system for remote medical visits oriented to home care applications

In this section it is presented a highly innovative system aimed at the home tele-assistance, prototyped and verified by the heart specialists of the U.O. of Cardiology in the general hospital (Polyclinic) of the University of Bari. The system, invented by the author, is patent pending (Giorgio, 2008).

In the context of telemedicine it must be considered as a really innovative product in which all the most advanced technologies of biomedical engineering, information and communication converge to guarantee an efficient and reliable home assistance that allows the patient a highly better quality of life in terms of prophylaxis, treatment and reduction of discomfort connected to periodic out - patient controls and/or hospitalization, and allows considerable savings on the sanitary expenses.

The most recent developments in the field of electronics (technology), informatics and telecommunications let imagine applications in the telemedicine and home care sector which could mark a turning in the quality of the services for sanitary assistance prevention and care.

It above all deals with home care services of chronic patients or patients afflicted by pathologies (such as cardiac decompensation or obstructive chronic bronchopathy), for which the home monitoring, as sketched in figure 25, can often substitute the hospitalization with significant advantages in terms of the patient's quality of life and of sanitary expense saving.

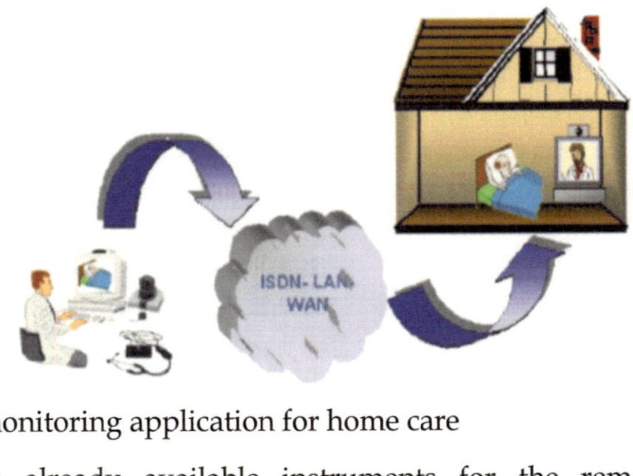

Fig. 25. Typical telemonitoring application for home care

Although there are already available instruments for the remote detection of the electrocardiogram, the cardiac and pulmonary tele-auscultating is not carried out yet.

Moreover, the known tele-electrocardiographs are able to transfer the electrocardiograms only after the acquisition, not in real time and are mostly and strongly orientated towards

the sanitary emergencies. In fact they are typically installed on ambulances and need experienced staff for the utilization.
On the other hand it is essential to observe that, through the electrocardiogram is extremely important, it is not the only source of information useful to evaluate the patient's health.
It is obvious, therefore, that there is a rather limited offer of the current market with regard to the requirements which a health service should meet, if it is in the lead with regard to the effective potentialities offered by the present technology.
Particularly we recognize deficiency or total absence of reliable and valid telemedicine platforms which allow the follow up of patients with cardiac decomposition or of chronic ones or which allow the execution of medical examinations with a doctor in a different place regard to the patient but the doctor must be able to execute a complete and meticulous control of all the main vital parameters presently measurable: electrocardiograms, spirometry, oximetry cardiac tones, pulmonary sounds. The described system aims to compensate for these shortcomings.

6.1. Main features and diagnostic capabilities of the remote medical visits system

As previously stated, the remote medical visits system is a medical electronic and informational platform for diagnostic use, which permits the doctor to carry out a complete cardio-respiratory control on remote patients in real time.
The system consists of two parts: a patient station and a doctor position, both compact and light easily transportable both the positions are composed of committed laptop, hardware and software.
The patient position is equipped with miniaturized PC-based diagnostic instruments and is suitable for pediatric use. It is possible to get also many patient positions for only one doctor position.
The diagnostic instruments are connected to the host PC via USB or via Bluetooth or zig bee.
Then, the system is made up of the following basis items:

a. Server placing (posting) (used by the patient) or rather PC/notebook equipped with:

- Diagnostic instruments (electrocardiograph, electronic stethoscope, pulse oxymeter, etc.)
- Software tool put in beforehand and used for the transmission of the data in real time and filing of the data acquired also by different patients
- Kit for the audio/video communication and the remote transmission of the sounds.

b. Remote client posting (used by the doctor) or PC/notebook equipped with:

- Software tool put in beforehand and used for the acquisition of the data in real time and for the filing of the data coming also from different patients
- Kit for the audio/video communication.

Although there are many diagnostic tools, the system is contained in a small suitcase, as shown in figure 26, easy to move and carry. This is because miniaturized and PC-based diagnostic tools, are used.
As if the doctor is present personally near the patient, the system allows him to receive, the data simultaneously at the acquisition (in real time):

- auscultation of cardiac tones and broncho-pulmonary sounds;
- oximetry;
- arterial blood pressure;
- electrocardiogram and heart frequency;
- phonocardiography;

- spirometry;
- image and audio of the patient, of professional quality.

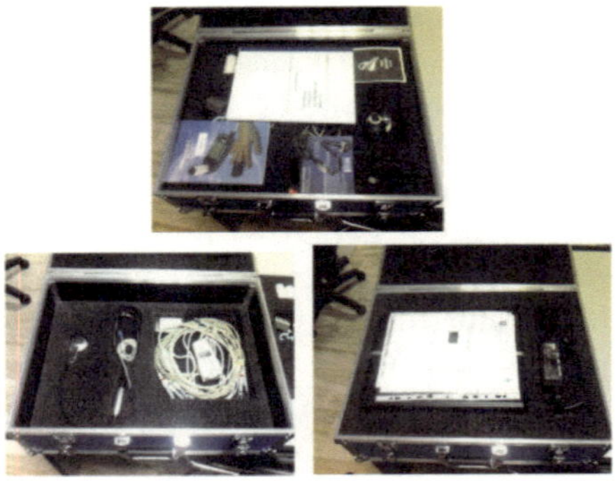

Fig. 26. The remote medical visit system, prototyped for experimental validation, assembled in a small suitcase

6.2 Electrocardiograph

The electrocardiogram can be registered by the remote medical visit system up to 12 derivations and is interpretative, or automatically carries out the reading and the diagnosis of the tracing which the doctor must reaffirm.

It is possible to carry out monitoring without time limits and always in real time. This makes possible the capture of uneven heartbeats or also intermittent ones of other nature. The acquire tracing is registered and filed.

The ECG is PC-based and high resolution (HRECG), very useful to find the late potentials in the heart potentials. They are potentials of very very small amplitude (uV) at high frequencies (300 Hz typically, up to 500 hz), localized in the ST-T segment of the ECG (see figure 27), arising in people with heart deseases and having high risk of life. They are because of a delayed ventricular activation which happens in case of ischemia as a result of a disturbance of the electrical conductance of the heart and then they announce that serious heart fatal failures probably are incoming, especially arrhythmias and sustained ventricular tachycardia. Then, the early detection of late potentials allows to undertake promptly therapies able to reduce the risk of death.

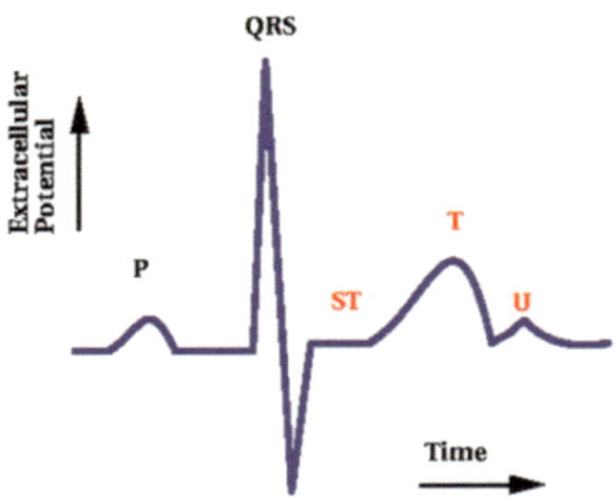

Fig. 27. Typical ECG wave period

Late potentials characteristics detected by the ECG are the following (see table 3):

Parameter	Description	Value if late potentials occur
QRSD	QRS cycle	>114 ms
RMS40	Mean value of the last 40 ms of the QRS cycle	<20 uV
LAS40	Duration of the signal with amplitude < 40 uV at the end of the QRS cycle	>38 ms

Table 3. Features of the ECG wave (one period) in presence of late potentials

The PC-based HRECG has been designed according to the specifications for late potentials detection: the bandwidth ranges from 0.03 hz to 500 hz due to the expected value of the maximum frequency of late potentials; the ADC resolution is 24 bit due to the very very small amplitude of late potentials. The connection with PC is possible as via USB as via Bluetooth.

The device has an hardware part and a software part (the driver of the hardware). The use of a PC allows to perform a lot of functions (i.e. filtering, real time elaboration, storage, printing, etc.) via software thus making very light the hardware part. This makes the electrocardiograph miniaturized and easy to use.

One of the most interesting functions implemented in the HRECG software is the spectral analysis of the ECG waveform (which is measured in the time domain, obviously). This analysis allows a more accurate and deep diagnosis than the only time domain analysis. In figure 28 is shown as an example the spectral analysis of the ECG of an healthy subject.

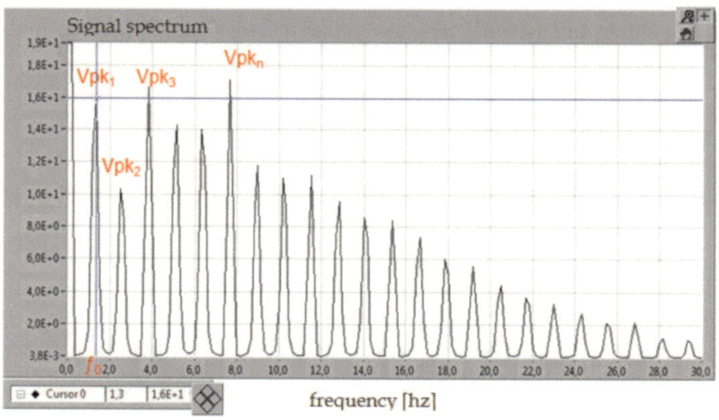

Fig. 28. Spectral analysis of the ECG of an healthy subject

Experimental results have shown us that there is a correlation between the frequencies and the amplitudes of the peaks of the ECG spectrum and cardiac diseases. These results are summarized in table 4 where:

fo is the fundamental frequency of the spectrum, corresponding to the hearth frequency; Vpkn the amplitude of the n-th peak in the spectrum; f_{taglio} is the frequency of the harmonic which peak is 1/10 of that of the fundamental harmonic.

Pathology	Spectrum features
Tachycardia	fo>1.66 hz
Bradycardia	fo<1hz
Ischemia	$Vpk_1 < Vpk_2$ and $Vpk_3 < Vpk_2$
Miocardial infarction	$Vpk_3 < Vpk_2$ and $Vpk_{n-1} / Vpk_n > 1.8$ e $Vpk_{n+1} / Vpk_n > 1.9$ in 66.7% of examined cases n=4
Left bundle branch block	$f_{taglio} / f_0 < 16.5$ in V5 and V6
Right bundle branch block	$f_{taglio} / f_0 < 16.5$ in V1 and V2

Table 4. Correspondence between spectrum features of the ECG signal and cardiac pathologies

Then, the remote health monitoring system uses a very advanced electrocardiograph, that goes beyond the nowdays clinical practice.

The joint use of the electrocardiograph and of the stethoscope lets you perform also phonocardiograph.

6.3 Stethoscope

The tele-stethoscope is of electronic kind (as described in section 3) and obtains biological sounds in the 20 Hz - 2 kHz band and can be used in three modes in order to improve the cardiac and pulmonary auscultation: membrane modality, bell modality and extensive one. Moreover, it allows the 75% (seventy-five percent) abatement of the external noise. It is equipped with software for the spectrum analysis in real time and it automatically starts at the beginning of the auscultation procedure.

The positioning of the stethoscope is led by a remote doctor thanks to the full time audio/video communication and the biological sounds can be simultaneously heard either by the patient (or by an operator helping the patient in the completion of the examination) or by the doctor in remote.

The biological sounds are also registered during the acquisition with significant advantages in accuracy terms of the diagnosis and possibility of carrying out diagnostic comparisons in the course of time.

The technical specifications for audio acquisition and transmission are the following:

Audio band from about 0 Hz to 4 KHz

Sampling frequency (transmission) 16 KHz

A/V Codec 16 KHz; H323-based

Sampling frequency (record) 8 KHz

6.4 Oximeter and spirometer

The tele-spirometer is of USB kind and it allows to carry out the FVC, VC, MVV tests and to determine the respiratory frequency and is autodiagnostic. The system is compatible with any commercial USB or Bluetooth spirometer.

The finger (optic) tele-saturimeter allows to carry out the monitoring of the SpO_2 value as it is equipped with plug-in which permits the tracing of a curve of blood oxygen saturation and of heart frequency values in time function, the curve will be knowledgeable in real time and visualized by the practitioner. The PC-based spirometer is often equipped with the saturimeter.

6.5 Arterial pressure measurement

The arterial pressure measurement is performed by a PC-based sphigmomanometer which consists of a classical cuff with a pump and having a valve for inflating and deflating the cuff, as shown in figure 29.

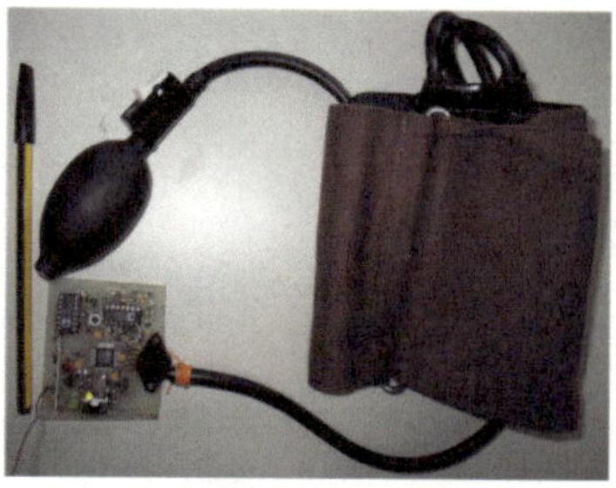

Fig. 29. Prototype of the arterial pressure measurement instrument, PC-based and wi fi connected to PC

The measure is performed by a stethoscope placed under the cuff that hear the Korotkovv sounds. The instrument is connected to a PC by a wireless short distance connection. A software properly developed calculates the min and max values of arterial pressure. These values are sent real time to the remote practitioner and are stored on the patient's station.
Alternatively, the instruments based on the oscillometric method can be plugged-in to the system. The PC connectivity is in this case via bluetooth or via USB interface.

6.6 Other capabilities

The filing of the data concerning the carried out examination occurs in a dynamic data base both on the patient post and the doctor post; the data will be filed by ordering them for each patient.
Thus to each patient a clinical record will be associated with all the reports as regards him. This kind of filing is very useful to carry out diagnostic comparisons on the evolution of a disease or on the outcome of a therapy, and it eases him of the burden of having the record documentation regarding him personally. In the patient data base there is also a filed schedule containing the personal details of the patient, the case history in addition to various notes, values of blood tests, the outcome of other diagnostic tests, treatments undertaken during the time, therapy in course, etc.
The system also makes possible the transmission of echograms, X-rays radiograms/other tests in digital form to the doctor and also the filing in the patient data base.
The doctor can also prescribe other subsequent clinical tests advised and/or treatments to undertake and he can subscribe with electronic signature using a smart card.
The patient data can be transferred by RFID smart card, as described in section 5.
The system doesn't present connectivity limits of any kind find and requires a 320 Kb/s minimum band or a UMTS mobile telephone is able to allow the execution of a medical examination.
The system has a user-friendly software interface of very simple employment, which implements the one touch philosophy, and requires extremely reduced operating costs. In figure 30 a draft is shown of the interface, by the patient side (part "a") and by the doctor side (part "b").

The patient can ask for a medical examination and the doctor can accept or refuse to examine him under the availability of the moment. As a result of the doctor's availability the medical examination can start and the doctor can ask for the necessary tests through a simple "click".

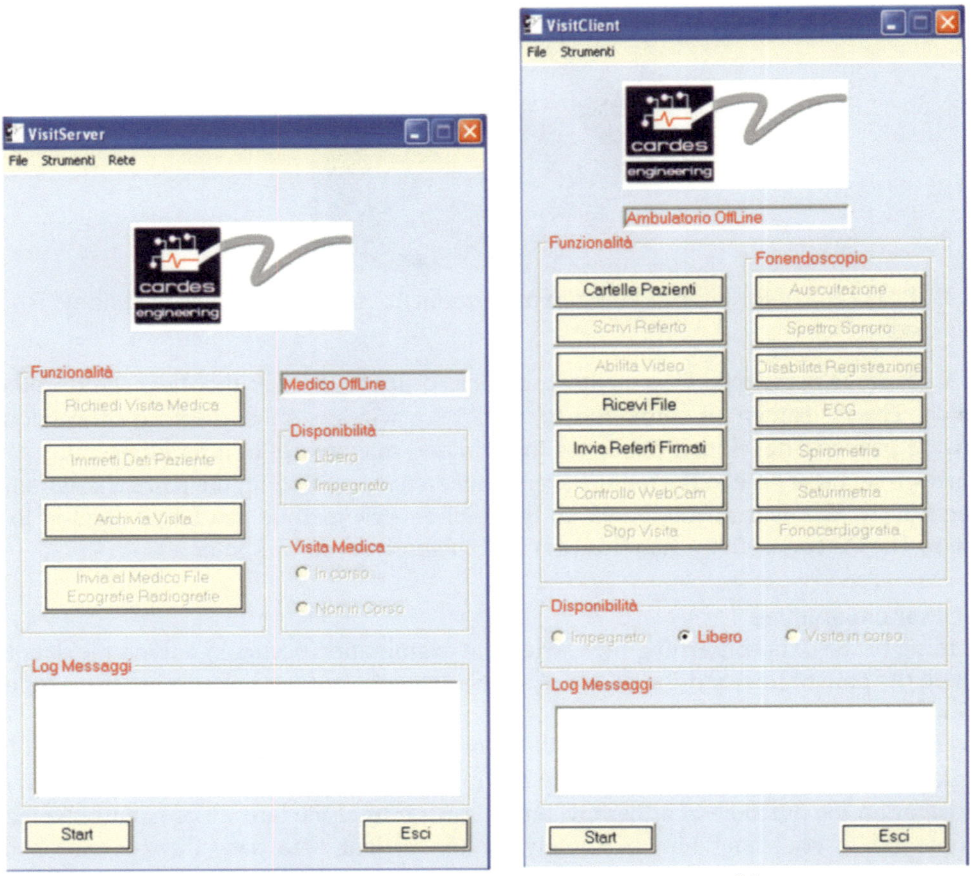

(a) (b)

Fig. 30. Software interface: patient side (a) and doctor side (b)

The system has been planned/designed in the observance of the current regulations in the order of medical devices and of computer security and privacy:
Audio-Video Communication: AES - 256 bit (Advanced Encryption Standard)
Login and password for user ID
Data acquired unchangeable
Asynchronous transmission: SSL connection
Virtual LAN: AES - 256 C-B-C in Tx; 96-bit version of HMAC - SHA1 for user ID
Possible implementation of the electronic signature.
It is possible to conclude that the system is marked by three distinct and basic fundamental characteristics:

1. the transmission of data in real time, by assuring the remote doctor the simultaneous control of the data at the acquisition of the same ones;

2. the possibility to carry out a complete telematic medical examination, including the teleauscultation, or all the operations the doctor performs when he examines the patient directly at home or at the surgery and even more as the system is equipped with typically diagnostic instruments not available at the family doctor's but at hospital units;
3. the possibility to establish a continuous audio/video communication during the examination, in order that the same doctor can intervene with the patient, verify the correct positioning of the sensors and of the tele-stethoscope and he can also have a very high quality image of the patient, image of ten useful for diagnostic aims.

Among the most evident and important applications we can indicate the following ones:

- home teleassistance of cardiac patients in decompensation or of chronic sufferers with pathologies attributed to the cardio-circulatory or respiratory apparatus;
- mass prophylaxis with complete cardio-respiratory control which is frequent and at low cost;
- teleconsultation;
- follow-up of patients discharged early (precociously) and in need of teleprotection;
- closed-circuit monitoring of the health of patients waiting for hospitalization.
- opportunity of a complete cardio-respiratory check up in real time at home (much more complete than a classic visit at home or at surgery) but also at a chemist's or in other equipped centres of services;
- To cut down the number of calls to emergency services (118, first aid, etc.) and the number or/and the times of admission to hospital;
- To carry out specialistic check up frequently and at low cost;
- To give the prescription of the suggested therapy or of the possible further specialistic suggested examinations at the visit result;
- To have (get) mass prevention not only at cardiac level but also at respiratory one.

7. Conclusions

In this chapter 5 examples of innovative telemedicine devices have been described.

First of all, the remote health monitoring system has been described, which is patented and each its part has been designed, prototyped and successfully tested. Currently a process of design optimization is in progress; the next step is the validation and system certification. The system is useful especially to improve the quality of life of patients who require continuous monitoring in order to prevent sudden serious damages without long stays in hospital. The system is wearable and allows the patient to be free to move.

Secondly, the internet tele-stethoscope, able to objectify and to send biological sounds in real-time via web, has been described. It seems to be of great interest both to improve the diagnostic potential of one of the most simple, fast, and completely devoid of drawbacks medical examination such auscultation, and for telemedicine applications that now seems a fixed course for reducing healthcare costs and improve quality of life of chronically ill patients through the implementation of treatment protocols in home care. The device is also very useful for monitoring patients during therapy and to evaluate through accurate comparisons of auscultation reports the evolution of a disease. This type of monitoring, being objective, is to be shared with other doctors. For the academic point of view, the internet tele-stethoscope could be a great training tool.

Third, the pain button and the Wi-Fi pain button (PB/WiPB) have been described. They are a somesort of electronic cargiver very useful to allow a prompt rescue in case of illness. The best of the well known GPS, internet and wireless transmission technologies are employed in the design of these devices. The interpretative algorithm implemented on board, able to detect in real time cardiac diseases, makes the PB/WiPB more than a warning source when the disease has occurred because incoming pathologies are promptly detected thus appearing very useful to prevent damages.

Fourth, the RFID based system for automatic identification of a patient and his clinical history has been described: the requirements to which the system meets, therefore the benefits and innovations from it, range from simple procedures streamlining for acquisition of individual's clinical data, to the access to all clinical/history data for patients unable to exhibit them (because they are unconscious, or because don't remember, etc..), the automatic creation of a data base in compliance with health service computerization requirements. Moreover, the system allows a drastic reduction in recognition time and the immediate availability of patients' generic and clinical data. In a urgency situation, the immediate availability of the subject's medical history provides the choice of an effective and especially timely cure.

Finally, the remote medical visits system has been described: the system is patent pending.

The system aims at offering home care services for chronic patients or people afflicted with pathologies (for example, some forms of cardiac decompensation or chronic obstructive bronchopathy) for which the domestic monitoring can quietly avoid the admission to hospital with significant advantages in terms of quality of the patient's life and of cutting down the sanitary expenses. The described system allows to carry out remote complete medical examinations, or rather with a doctor placed in another place as to the patient but able to effect a check-up more complete and precise than that one effected with the current available means if the doctor goes the patient's house or even if he examines the patient at his own surgery. Then, the system could permit a significant saving of the health care expenses and an improvement of the quality of chronic patient's life by offering them frequent and easy check-up in the privacy of the home and by avoiding expensive hospitalization.

Among the developments of the system we expect the use of pocket PC (palmar) as base element of the doctor station.

The reduction of hospitalization time, because of home teleprotection, and the possibility to avoid the hospitalization of patients in decompensation monitored from home imply an economic assured saving.

It is also manifest that we can reduce the waiting lists in a remarkable way.

By the applications described it results that wireless transmission technology, at short or long distance, is the best way to realize a remote patient control. It results that it is necessary to transmit, beyond patient health status data, also video and audio signal to have a complete patient diagnose and a mean for a human interaction between the doctor and the patient. So the amount of the information to be transmitted is more and more high. This move the development of telemedicine systems towards those technology, like Wi-Fi and Wimax, that assure more bandwidth.

Telemedicine systems can severely reduce health certificate expense, but to do this it is necessary a centralized monitoring system, based on a database engine to which each hospital can connect and download the information. In such a way the patient is free to move away from hospital and even from his home. In fact, the trend of this system is to use GPS to track patient's position.

We conclude by saying that the success of those systems also depends on their wearability: if it is small enough the patient wears it. So the biggest challenge is to integrate more and more the dimension of microcontroller and sensors embedded.

8. References

[1] Aoyagi, T., Kishi, M., Yamaguchi, K., Watanabe, S., (1974), Improvement of the earpiece oximeter, *Proceedings of 13-th Annual Meeting of the Japan Society of Medical Electronic and Biological Engineering*, Osaka, April, 1974, pp. 90–91.

[2] Caduff, A., Hirt, E., Feldman, Y., Ali, Z. & Heinemann, L., (2003) First human experiments with a novel non-invasive, non-optical continuous glucose monitoring system, *Journal of Biosensensors and Bioelectronics*, Vol. 19, issue 3, pp. 209-217, ISSN: 0956 - 5663

[3] Carr, J. J. & Brown J. M., (2001). *Introduction to biomedical equipment technology*, 4/E, Prentice Hall, ISBN: 0-13-010492-2, Upper Saddle River - New Jersey.

[4] Dower, G. E., Yakush, A., Nazzal, S. B., Jutzi, R. V. & Ruiz, C. E., (1988). Deriving the 12-lead Electrocardiogram from four (EASI) electrodes. *Journal of Electrocardiology*, Vol. 21, supplement 1, pp. S182- S187, ISSN 0022-0736

[5] Evans, T., (1998), Cardiac Arrests Outside Hospital, *British Medical Journal*, Vol. 316, No. 7137, (1998), pp. 1031-1032, ISSN: 0959-8138

[6] Giorgio, A. (2008). Sistema per visite mediche in remoto, *Italian Patent Pending* N. BA2008A000054

[7] Giorgio, A. (2009). Sistema Universale di Monitoraggio delle Attività Vitali Umane e Dispositivi Dedicati, *Italian Patent* N. 0001354840

[8] Hayashi, Y., Livshits, L., Caduff, A. & Feldman, Y., (2003) Dielectric spectroscopy study of specific glucose influence on human erythrocyte membranes, *Journal of Physics D: Applied Physivs*, Vol. 36, N. 4., pp. 369-375, ISSN: 022 - 3727

[9] Jingping, X., Cheng, J. & Yanjun, W., (1998), A Cepstral Method for Analysis of Acoustic Transmission Characteristics of Respiratory System. *IEEE Transactions On Biomedical Engineering, Vol. 45, No. 5, (May 1998), pp. 660-663, ISSN: 0018-9294*

[10] Paris, D., Mastrorocostas, A., Tolias, Y. A., Theocharis, J. B., Hadjilentiadis, L. J. & Panas, S. M., (2000), An Orthogonal Least Squares-Based Fuzzy Filter for Real-Time Analysis of Lung Sounds, *IEEE Transactions On Biomedical Engineering, Vol. 47, No. 9, (September 2000), pp. 1165-1176, ISSN: 0018-9294*

[11] Rossi Mori A., Ricci, F. & Maceratini, R., (March 2001). *Il Medico on Line: Manuale di informatica medica*. Verduci editore, ISBN: 9788876205750.

[12] Yang-Sheng Lu, Wen-Hui Liu & Guang-Xia Quin, (1988). Removal of The Heart Sound Noise From The Breath Sound. *Proceedings of the 10-th Annual International Conference of the IEEE Engineering In Medicine And Biology Society*, ISBN 0-7803-0785-2, New Orleans, LA, USA, November 1988, pp. 175-176.

[13] Webster, J. G., ed., (2009) *Medical instrumentation, Application and design*, J. Wiley, ISBN: 978-0-471-67600-3

2

Pervasive Homecare Monitoring Technologies and Applications

Demosthenes Vouyioukas[1] and Alexandros Karagiannis[2]
[1]University of the Aegean, Department of Information and Communication Systems Engineering
[2]National Technical University of Athens, School of Electrical and Computer Engineering
Greece

1. Introduction

Research studies and population statistics records indicate that elderly population increases in the developed countries whilst forecasts reveal that 65 and over age group will be nearly 20% of the overall population. One of the major challenges related to this observation is the delivery of homecare and the reduction of healthcare cost without compromising the quality of services provided. Pervasive homecare systems provide information and mechanisms to alert when pathological situations are identified. The implementation of technological solutions for homecare applications minimizes the time to provide help in abnormal situations and improve quality of life in elderly and chronically ills. Pervasive homecare networks provide continuous medical monitoring, control of home appliances, medical data storage and processing and emergency situations awareness. Constant monitoring provides early detection of emergency conditions and assists in optimum scheduling of a wide range of healthcare services for people with various degrees of cognitive and physical disabilities.

Researchers continuously explore technological solutions in order to provide homecare and healthcare services for the elderly, chronically ill and children. The amount of proposals reveal a rapidly growing scientific area of high impact on sensitive groups that significantly improve quality of life and prevent or deal with life threatening situations. However, the use of this wireless sensor technology in medical practice not only allows a supreme level of complexity in patient monitoring with regards to existing parameters (such as vital signs), but also offers the prospect of identifying new ways of diagnosing and preventing disease.

Although wired communication technologies, such us ATM (Asynchronous Transfer Mode) and optical communication, are widely used, the key aspects for pervasive healthcare communication is the transfer of high-speed and ubiquitous health data in every place in earth securely and promptly. Wireless technology came to encompass the e-health monitoring everywhere from any given location, providing the so-called m-health services. Research and development advances in the e-health community include data gathering and transfer of vital information, integration of human machine interface technology into handheld devices, data interoperability and integration with hospital legacy systems and electronic patient records.

However, several major challenges still need to be clarified so as to expand the implementation and use of mobile health devices and services and reinforce the market development. In recent years, there has been increased research on commercial mobile health systems based on WLAN (Wireless Local Area Networks), WiMAX, GPRS (General Packet Radio Service) and 3G UMTS (3rd Generation Universal Mobile Telecommunications System) networking technologies, in conjunction with the improvement of the radio frequency identification (RFID) and wireless sensor technology. These technologies have been utilized in the deployment of emerging healthcare and homecare systems. The introduction of high speed data rate, wide bandwidth, digital and encrypted communication technology, makes possible the delivery of audio, video, health status and waveform data to wherever and whenever needed. It is hoped that the current miniaturization of wireless sensor devices, context-aware and intelligent applications and the deployment 3G-based systems with global operational morphologies will improve some of the limitations of the existing wireless technologies and will provide a well-organized platform for homecare services.

The mission of this book chapter is to provide a comprehensive analysis of the homecare technology, applications and implementation of wireless technologies in the healthcare sector by using in addition case studies to highlight the successes and concerns of homecare projects. There are a variety of applications, devices, and communication technologies emerging in the homecare arena, which can be combined to create a pervasive mobile health system. This study highlights the key areas of concern and describes the various types of applications. An inclusive overview of some of these homecare health applications and research is presented.

The rest of the study is organized as follows; the recent advances in homecare enabling technologies using wireless body sensors and body and personal area networks technologies are discussed in Section 2. The classification of the wireless technologies is illustrated according to their total throughput within the relevant applications following the end-users view. Section 3 aims to describe, review and categorize the wireless sensors depending on the sensor principle, which detects the measurable quantity, the signal processing algorithms of the perceived information, their energy efficiency and categories of health status information. Section 4 describes various applied homecare platforms and case studies, along with their applications and services. A classification of these platforms is prepared in terms of the main focus categories such as fall detection, ambient assisted living, aging and rehabilitation, location tracking and continuous healthcare monitoring, in conjunction with some results and suggestive extensions. A brief discussion and concluding remarks will also be given in Section 5 in succession to the future trends for pervasive homecare delivery.

2. Enabling homecare technologies

Various wireless telecommunication technologies are employed in order to integrate medical applications and networking in unified fields of smart homecare services. Coexistence and cooperation of personal area technologies such as radio frequency identification (RFID), bluetooth, ZiBee and wireless sensor networks with large scale wireless networks such as 3G, Wi-Fi, WiMAX provide complete context-aware homecare applications if high quality services. Several issues concerning the integration of these technologies are open and need to be addressed as the technologies mature. There are various applications and prototypes developed, some of them devoted to continuous monitoring for cognitive disorders like Alzheimer's, Parkinson's or similar cognitive diseases. The trend of homecare and healthcare services moves from the large scale technologies that provide the medium of data transfer and processing to the small scale devices attached to or even implanted to subjects in order to monitor physiological parameters and provide actuators capabilities in dealing with an acute and life-threatening situation. Some focus on fall detection, posture detection and location tracking and others make use of ambient information to identify patients' health status.

The development of wireless sensor networks (WSN) to monitor patient' s physical and biochemical parameters continuously establish a health monitoring system and the specific application of them, the body sensor network (BSN), provides a low cost homecare health monitoring system capable to detect and analyze abnormal situations and even enable the delivery of immediate health services. Focusing on a specific example, BSN homecare health monitoring system is appreciated in heart rhythm abnormalities. A trial fibrillation is encountered in nearly 4% of the population over the age of 60, high blood pressure (hypertension) is one of the most widespread cardiovascular diseases affecting millions of people in the developed countries and heart failure is responsible for hundreds of thousands deaths annually. BSNs offer the chance to diagnose cardiac disorders earlier in risk groups such as elderly as well as the ability to monitor the disease progress and the response to any treatment delivered.

Context information is necessary in homecare monitoring networks because it enables the understanding of the special conditions and provides the framework in which monitored parameters are interpreted in an optimum way. If for example sensors placed in the chest of the subject detect an increased heart rate then the initiation of immediate actions in order to prevent the progress of a tachycardia is controlled by context information gathered by sensing systems that incorporate more than one type of sensing capabilities. The initiation of immediate actions is then decided from the output of a processing stage that uses as input several sensor streams in order to form a clear understanding of the context. The context information enhances the identification of the unusual patterns and making more precise inferences about the situation.

Most of the existing solutions include one or more types of sensors carried by the patient, forming a Body Area Network (BAN), and one or more types of sensors deployed in the environment forming a Personal Area Network (PAN). Data from BAN and PAN are connected via gateway nodes to large-scale networks. A common characteristic in commercially available products or prototypes is the categorization of possible homecare services users (children, elderly and chronically ill, caregivers, healthcare professionals). These groups interact with the BAN and PAN.

One essential issue concerning BAN is the power consumption. There are various proposals for energy efficient MAC protocols but only a few of them are applicable in real situations and can be implemented. The other part of energy consumption problem is related to the energy efficient sensor devices, which is addressed mainly from the development of microelectronics and the implementation of low power consumption devices. Technologies used to form BANs exclude Bluetooth and Wi-Fi since these technologies offer only a few weeks runtime if energy efficient protocols are implemented. Some of the issues addressed in this chapter are the technologies used to implement BANs, some case studies with sensor nodes sampling biosignals such as electrocardiogram and respiration signal and the energy consumption problem where theoretical, simulation and measurements are provided in order to establish a basis for optimum radio transmission use since the radio subpart of the BAN nodes is considered to be the most energy consumable part.

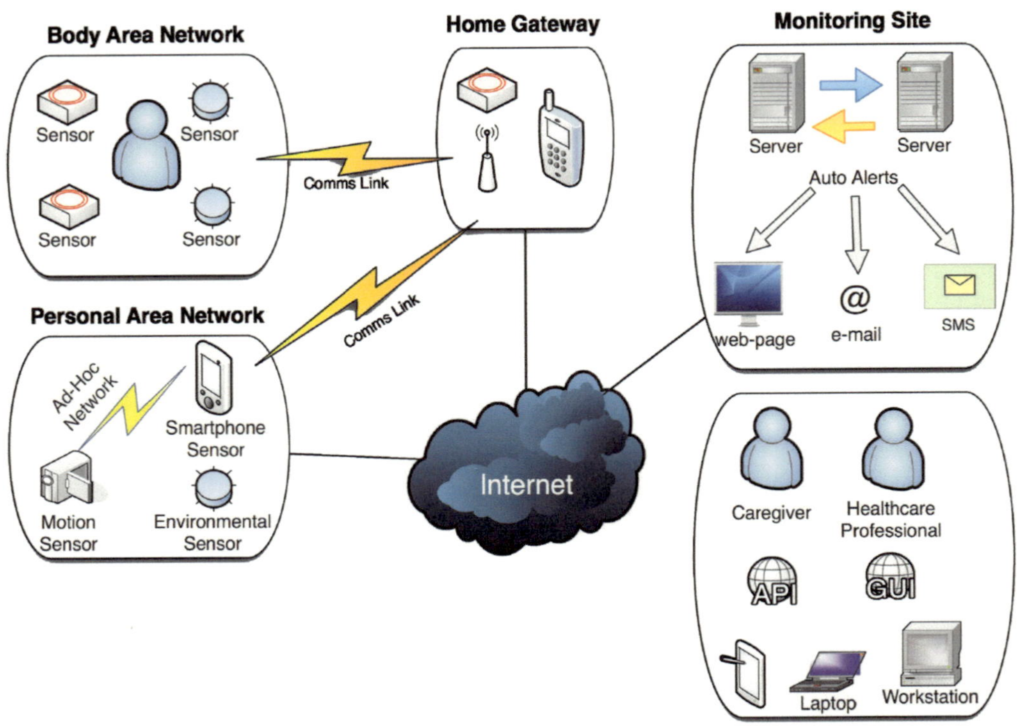

Fig. 1. Simple BSN - PAN application scenario for homecare monitoring application

Personal area networks are composed of environmental sensors deployed around and mobile or nomadic devices. Environmental sensors like RFIDs, video cameras, sound sensors, temperature and humidity sensors provide contextual information. Location information is possible to be provided by this category of sensors.

The gateway subsystems connect BAN and PAN subsystems to the Wide Area Networks (WAN) and mobile devices carried by the user or sensor nodes with WAN interfaces implement it. Local processing capabilities at the BAN and PAN subsystems have a significant effect on network congestion in the gateway. Therefore the processing of information gathered by the BAN and PAN is proved to be necessary (as it is stated in numerous research papers) before transmitted in the WAN. The gateway can relay information to one or more network systems depending on the application. Wide area networks can be cellular networks, ordinary telephone network, satellite networks or even internet.

3. Wireless sensor standards and homecare concerns

A basic issue concerning communication is the choice between the transmissions of real time multimedia, electronic health record and biosignals data and the "Store and Forward" method with implies asynchronous communication. In this section, a detailed description of the available wireless sensor standards is prepared and the related homecare technology considerations for the design and implementation of such systems are presented.

3.1 Sensor standards

One of the critical requirements in wireless sensor networks is the low power consumption, which sets the constraints in the wireless sensors standard development and provides the interfaces to other network technologies. Some of these standards include IEEE 802.15.4 [1], ZigBee [2], WirelessHART [3] ISA100.11 [4], IETF 6LoWPAN [5][6] IEEE 802.15.3 [7], Wibree [8], IEEE 802.15.1, Medical Implant Communications Service (MICS) [18], Wireless Medical Telemetry Service (WMTS) [19].

3.1.1 IEEE 802.15.4

The main standard for low rates WPAN is IEEE 802.15.4 with the main characteristics of low complexity, low cost deployment and low power consumption. Battery lifetime is maximized in wireless sensor networks compliant with IEEE 802.15.4. Topologies supported are star and peer-to-peer between devices either via a network controller or via adhoc links.
IEEE 802.25.4 defines the two lower layers, namely the physical and MAC layer. In the physical layer 868/915 MHz bands are supported as well as 2.4GHz band whilst in MAC layer access is controlled using the CSMA/CA mechanism. In MAC layer network synchronization, device association and frame validation and delivery are implemented.
The physical layer (PHY) ultimately provides the data transmission service, as well as the interface to the physical layer management entity. PHY manages the physical RF transceiver and performs channel selection and energy and signal management functions. It operates on one of three possible unlicensed frequency bands (Table 1):

- 868.0-868.6 MHz: Europe, allows one communication channel (2003, 2006)
- 902-928 MHz: North America, up to ten channels (2003), extended to thirty (2006)
- 2400-2483.5 MHz: worldwide use, up to sixteen channels (2003, 2006)

The original 2003 version of the standard specifies two physical layers based on direct sequence spread spectrum (DSSS) techniques: one working in the 868/915 MHz bands with transfer rates of 20 and 40 kbit/s, and one in the 2450 MHz band with a rate of 250 Kbit/s. The 2006 revision improves the maximum data rates of the 868/915 MHz bands, bringing them up to support 100 and 250 Kbit/s as well.
Beyond these three bands, the IEEE802.15.4c study group is considering the opened bands 314-316 MHz, 430-434 MHz, and 779-787 MHz bands in China, while the IEEE 802.15 Task Group 4d is defining an amendment to the existing standard 802.15.4-2006 to support the new 950 MHz-956 MHz band in Japan. First standard amendments by these groups were released in April 2009. In August 2007, IEEE 802.15.4a was released expanding the four PHYs available in the earlier 2006 version to six, including one PHY using Direct Sequence Ultra-wideband (UWB) and another using Chirp Spread Spectrum (CSS). The UWB PHY is allocated frequencies in three ranges: below 1 GHz, between 3 and 5 GHz, and between 6 and 10 GHz. The CSS PHY is allocated spectrum in the 2450 MHz ISM band [9]. In April 2009 IEEE 802.15.4c and IEEE 802.15.4d were released expanding the available PHYs with several additional PHYs: one for 780 MHz band using O-QPSK or MPSK [10], another for 950 MHz using GFSK or BPSK [11].
It is the basis for the ZigBee, WirelessHART specification, each of which further attempts to offer a complete networking solution by developing the upper layers which are not covered by the standard. Alternatively, it can be used with 6LoWPAN and standard Internet protocols to build a Wireless Embedded Internet. The basic framework conceives a small distance communications range with a transfer rate of 250 Kbit/s.

For low cost and low complexity purposes, IEEE 802.15.4 defines Reduced Function Devices (RFD) and Full Function Devices (FFD). RFDs implement a subset of IEEE 802.15.4 and cannot act as coordinator. FFDs have a full implementation of the standard. Any IEEE 802.15.4 compliant radio is capable of performing three different signal power measurements, Link Quality Indication (LQI), Energy Detection (ED), Clear Channel Assessment (CCA).

Frequency Bands	Coverage	Channels	Data Rate	Data Modulation	Chip Modulation
2.4 GHz	Worldwide	16	250 kbit/s	16-ary orthogonal	OQPSK, 2 Mchips/s
868 MHz	Europe	1	20 kbit/s	BPSK	BPSK, 300 kchips/s
915 MHz	Americas	10	40 kbit/s	BPSK	BPSK, 600 kchips/s

Table 1. IEEE 802.15.4 Frequency Bands, Data Rates and Modulation Techniques

3.1.2 ZigBee

ZigBee defines the higher layers of communication protocols on top of IEEE 802.15.4 standard for low rate personal area networks. It was developed by the ZigBee Alliance with the ambition of enabling reliable, cost-effective, low power and wirelessly networked monitoring. Primal targets of ZigBee are long battery life, advanced networking capabilities, reliability and low cost.

ZigBee devices can form mesh networks connecting high number of devices together. There are three types of ZigBee devices: ZigBee Coordinator, ZigBee router, and ZigBee end device. The ZigBee Coordinator is the IEEE 802.15.4 PAN coordinator. ZigBee router is a IEEE 802.15.4 Full Function Device (FDD) that participates in a ZigBee network and is not the ZigBee coordinator but may act as a coordinator if needed. A ZigBee router is capable of routing massages between devices and supporting device associations. ZigBee end device is a IEEE 802.15.4 Reduced (RFD) or FFD that participates in a ZigBee network and is neither the ZigBee coordinator nor a ZigBee router. The end device consists of the sensors, actuators, and controllers that collects data and communicates only with the router or the coordinator.

ZigBee builds a Network Layer and an Application Layer on the IEEE 802.15.4 defined layers. The PHY layer provides the basic communication capabilities of the physical radio, while the medium access control layer provides services to enable reliable single hop communication links between devices. The network layer provides routing and multi hop functions for different network topologies. The application layer includes an Application Support (APS) sub-layer, the ZigBee Device Object (ZDO) and the ZigBee applications defined by the user or designer. ZDO is responsible for overall device management and APS provides servicing to both ZDO and ZigBee applications.

3.1.3 IEEE 802.15.1

The Bluetooth SIG, as a medium-rate standard used for short-range wireless communications worldwide, developed IEEE 802.15.1. IEEE adopted and converted

Bluetooth V1.1 specifications into an IEEE Standard, which was officially released in June 2002 [12]. In addition an IEEE 802 Logical Link Control interface was included in order to make Bluetooth a real member of the IEEE 802 family of communication standards as well as the addition of SDL (Specification and Description Language) material.

Bluetooth supports up to seven simultaneous wireless links at a peak data rate of 720 kbit/s over a maximum distance of some decades of meters. Link layer security is supported. All the properties mentioned in IEEE 802.15.1 Bluetooth protocol stack are defined by the specification.

Bluetooth operates in the 2.45GHz ISM frequency band. This band is split into 79 (USA, Europe) or 23 (Japan) RF channels of 1MHz each, in which a Gaussian Frequency Shift Keying (GFSK) modulation scheme is used. It is achieved maximum raw bit rate of 1 Mbit/s per RF channel. Bluetooth devices can be classified into three different power classes: Class 1 with a maximum transmitted power of 20 dBm; Class 2 with a maximum transmitted power of 4 dBm (nominal 0dBm); Class 3 with a maximum output power of 0dBm. Accordingly it varies the effective range of communication. Relevant regulatory rules are set forth in FCC 15.247 (US) and ETSI 300.328 (EU).

IEEE 802.15.1 functions with a spectrum-spreading technique called Frequency Hopping (FH). A Bluetooth radio transmits in the whole 2.45 GHz ISM band, but at a certain instant only one of the available 1-MHz RF channels is used. When a frequency hop occurs, the centre transmission frequency switches to that of another channel.

3.1.4 IEEE P802.15.3

The scope of IEEE 802.15.3 development was to enable quick high load data transfers within a WPAN, e.g. the transmission of multimedia files, and even high-definition video transmission (around 20 Mbit/s) by means of a low-power and low-cost wireless system. Therefore, new MAC and PHY specifications aiming at high data rates for fixed, portable and moving devices within a personal operating space were created [13].

IEEE 802.15.3 MAC and PHY features [14] are: data rates of 11, 22, 33, 44, and 55 Mbit/s over a 2.4 GHz ISM radio link, a MAC protocol that supports asynchronous and Quality-of-Service (QoS) isochronous data transfers and that is partially based on HiperLAN/2, a security suite and ad-hoc peer-to-peer networking, where wireless devices dynamically become master (Piconet Controller) or slave (Device) according to the existing network structure. The IEEE 802.15.3 MAC layer supports secure and non-secure data frames.

The current IEEE 802.15.3 PHY layer operates in the 2.4 GHz band, occupying 15 MHz of RF bandwidth per channel. Hence, three or four non-overlapping channels can be accommodated within the available 83 MHz of the 2.4 GHz band. Relevant regulatory rules are set forth in FCC 15.249 (US) and ETSI 300.328 (EU).

High-rate WPAN chooses a single-carrier PHY in an effort to reduce complexity and power drain. Rather than employing spread-spectrum techniques, the original IEEE P802.15.3 PHY uses Trellis-Coded Modulation (TCM) with multi-bit symbols at 11 MBaud and achieves 11 to 55 Mbit/s peak data rate over a range of some decades of meters.

An alternate IEEE 802.15.3 PHY layer was developed leading to the inception of IEEE P802.15.3a. Ultra wide band became an emerging technology and Multiband-OFDM proposed by the MultiBand OFDM Alliance appeared leaving IEEE 802.15.3a behind with an unclear future.

3.1.5 WirelessHART

The WirelessHART [15] standard provides a wireless network communication protocol for process measurement and control applications. It uses IEEE 802.15.4 compatible radios operating in the 2.4 GHz Industrial, Scientific, and Medical radio band (ISM). The radios employ DSSS technology and channel hopping. It is TDMA synchronized and provides latency-controlled communications between devices on the network.

Power management options enable the wireless devices to be more energy efficient. WirelessHART is designed to support mesh, star, and combined network topologies. A WirelessHART network consists of wireless field devices, gateways, process automation controller, host applications, and network manager. Each device in the mesh network can serve as a router for messages from other devices. This extends the range of the network and provides redundant communication routes to increase reliability.

The process automation controller serves as a single controller for continuous process. The network manager configures the network and schedule communication between devices. It also manages the routing and network traffic. The network manager can be integrated into the gateway, host application, or process automation controller.

3.1.6 ISA100.11a

ISA100.11a supports low data rates wireless monitoring and process automation applications. It is an open wireless networking technology standard developed by the International Society of Automation (ISA). It defines the specifications for the OSI layer, security, and system management. The standard focuses on low energy consumption, scalability, infrastructure, robustness, and interoperability with other wireless devices. ISA100.11a operates in 2.4 GHz radio band; it supports channel hoping and takes care for interference minimization.

3.1.7 6LoWPAN

6lowpan is an acronym of IPv6 over Low power Wireless Personal Area Networks. It enables IPv6 packets communication over an IEEE 802.15.4 based network. Low power device can communicate directly with IP devices using IP-based protocols. 6lowpan is the name of a working group in the internet area of the IETF. The 6lowpan group has defined encapsulation and header compression mechanisms that allow IPv6 packets to be sent to and received from over IEEE 802.15.4 based networks.

Address management mechanism handles the forming of device addresses for communication. 6LoWPAN is designed for applications with low data rate devices that require Internet communication.

3.1.8 Wibree

Wibree, also called "Baby Bluetooth," is a low-power wireless local area network (WLAN) technology that facilitates interoperability among mobile and portable consumer devices such as pagers, personal digital assistants (PDAs), wireless computer peripherals, entertainment devices and medical equipment. Wibree is a wireless communication technology designed for low power consumption, short-range communication, and low cost devices.

Wibree operates on 2.4 GHz and has a data rate of 1 Mbit/s. The linking distance between the devices is 5–10 m. Bluetooth–Wibree utilizes the existing Bluetooth RF and enables ultra-low power consumption. Wibree was released publicly in October 2006.

	Bluetooth	Wibree	ZigBee
Band	2.4 GHz	2.4 GHz	2.4 GHz, 868 MHz, 915 MHz
Antenna/HW	Shared		Independent
Power	100 mW	~10 mW	30 mW
Target Battery Life	days - months	1-2 years	6 months - 2 years
Range	10-30 m	10 m	10-75 m
Data Rate	1-3 Mbit/s	1 Mbit/s	25-250 kbit/s
Component Cost	$3	Bluetooth + 20¢	$2
Network Topologies	Ad-hoc, point-to-point, star	Ad-hoc, point-to-point, star	Mesh, ad-hoc, star
Security	128-bit encryption	128-bit encryption	128-bit encryption
Time to Wake and Transmit	3 s	TBA	15 ms

Table 2. Feature comparison of Bluetooth, Wibree and ZigBee [16]

3.1.9 Medical Implant Communications Service (MICS)

The MICS is an ultra-low power, unlicensed, radio service available worldwide for implanted medical devices, such as cardiac pacemakers and defibrillators. Licensing is not required. Maximum radiated power in the frequency band from 402-405 MHz is 25 µW, with 25 kHz channel spacing. Therefore, the coverage of MICS is approximately 1-2 meters.

3.1.10 Wireless Medical Telemetry Service (WMTS)

The MICS is an ultra-low power, unlicensed, radio service available worldwide for implanted medical devices, such as cardiac pacemakers and defibrillators. Licensing is not required. Maximum radiated power in the frequency band from 402-405 MHz is 25 µW, with 25 kHz channel spacing. Therefore, the coverage of MICS is approximately 1-2 meters.

3.2 Sensors measurement range

Sensors are the front-end of sensor networks nodes that collect signals. They fall into three main categories. Physiological sensors measure ambulatory blood pressure, continuous glucose monitoring, core body temperature, blood oxygen, and signals related to respiratory inductive plethysmography, electrocardiography (ECG), electroencephalography (EEG), and electromyography (EMG). Biokinetic sensors measure acceleration and rotation caused by human activity. Ambient sensors measure environmental phenomena such as humidity, temperature and provide the context along with biokinetic sensors for captured data interpretation.

Particularly in wireless sensor networks designed for homecare and healthcare applications, sensors are few, heterogeneous and require specific placement. Ineffective placement may lead to serious degradation of captured data interpretation.

Commercial sensors exhibit a wide range of power supply requirements, calibration parameters, output interfaces, and data rates. In typical healthcare or homecare sensor application scenarios, the energy consumption of wireless sensor networks nodes is dependent on sampling and type of signal acquired. Fig. 2. presents energy consumption and data rates across a sampling of commercial systems for continuous monitoring application.

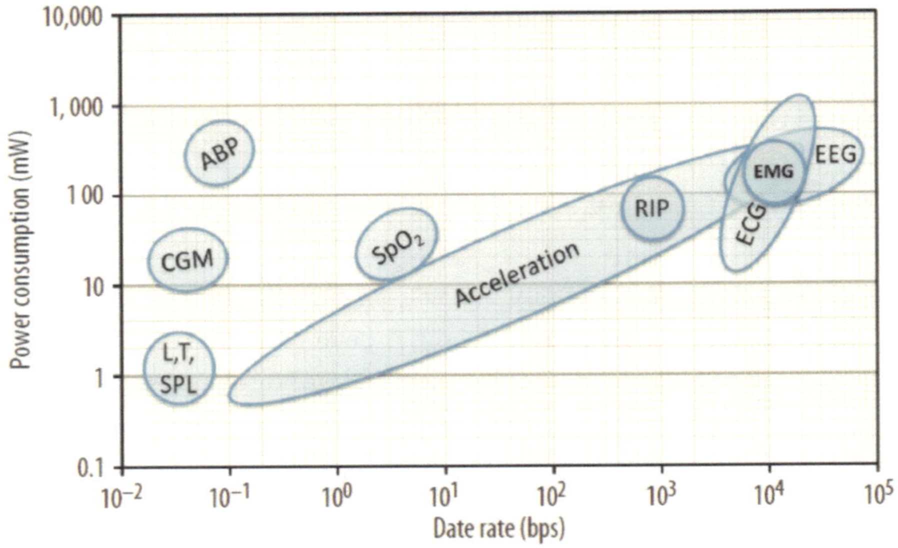

Fig. 2. Average Power Consumption of continuous monitoring applications [17]

3.3 Signal processing

Signal processing is needed to extract valuable information from captured data related with transient signals or events, such as biosignals. It is desirable to rely on sensors with redundant or complementary data to maximize the information content and reduce both systematic and random errors. Additionally the combination of information facilitates the processing and signal analysis stage to extract necessary information from a wide variety of captured data representing time series related to the physical processes monitored.

Whilst the use of multiple identical sensors for error minimization is easily understood, different sensors employment in terms of both sensing type and location requires pattern recognition techniques and machine learning. In practice, the use of multiple sensors with information fusion many advantages compared to single sensor systems, such as improved signal to noise ratio (SNR), robustness and reliability, extended parameter coverage.

The integration of information from heterogeneous networks and sensors reveal the need for multi sensor fusion. In general, the nature of information interaction involved in sensor fusion can be classified as competitive, complementary, and cooperative fusion [20][21].

In competitive fusion, each sensor provides equivalent information about the physical process. It typically involves the handling of redundant, but sometimes inconsistent, measurements. In complementary fusion, on the other hand, sensors do not depend on each other directly as each sensor captures different aspects of the physical process. The measured information is merged to form a more complete picture of the phenomenon. In cooperative fusion, sensors work together to provide information that is not obtainable by any of the sensors alone [22].

Processing data at a given rate consumes less power on average than transmitting same data wirelessly, and data rate reduction reduces power consumption for both wireless transceivers and microprocessors [17][23]. Results indicate a significant reduction of energy consumption at applications, which implement RF transceiver management, and on board signal processing, verifying the well-established belief of trading off radio communication with signal processing. The limited resources of wireless sensor network nodes especially in processing power define the constraint of this trade off. On-node signal processing will consume power to extract information, but it will also reduce in-network data rate and power consumption. Fig. 3 shows the power consumption of wireless transceivers and microprocessors in popular BASN and WSN platforms.

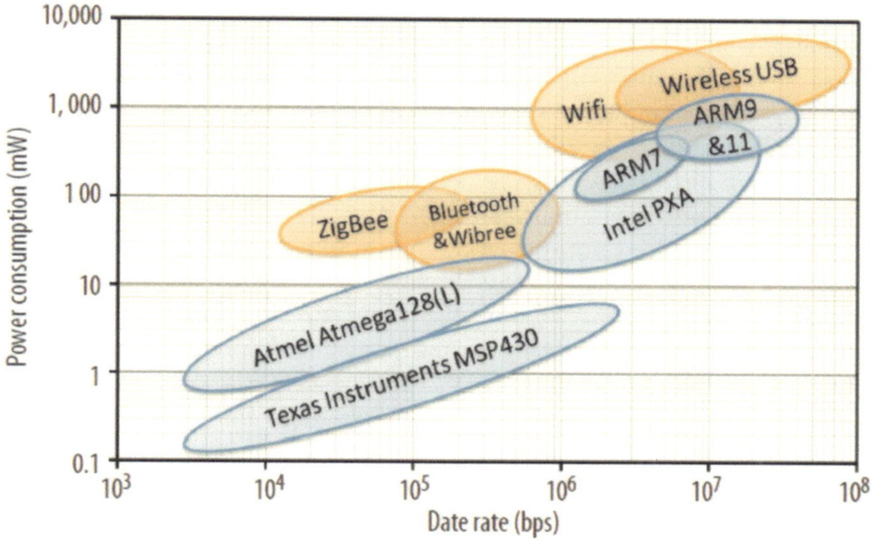

Fig. 3. Average power consumption of wireless transceivers and microcontrollers in Wireless Sensor Networks [22]

3.4 Energy efficiency

As sensor nodes are generally battery-powered devices, the critical aspects to face concern how to reduce the energy consumption of nodes, so that the network lifetime can be extended. The energy breakdown heavily depends on the features of specific nodes. Despite the fact that node's subsystems may differ significantly there are some remarks that generally hold and have well documented in literature as well.

The communication subsystem has energy consumption much higher than the computation subsystem. It has been shown that transmitting one bit may consume as much as executing a few thousands instructions [24]. The radio energy consumption in transmitting, listening mode, idle state is much higher than in sleep state mode of the radio transceiver. Therefore the radio should be put to sleep when possible. Sensory subsystem is another significant source of energy consumption.

Several approaches are employed in order to reduce energy consumption. At a very general level, they are identified in three main categories, namely, duty cycling, data-driven approaches, and mobility.

Duty cycling is mainly focused on the networking subsystem. The most effective energy-conserving operation is putting the radio transceiver in the (low-power) sleep mode whenever communication is not required. Ideally, the radio should be switched off as soon as there is no more data to send/receive, and should be resumed as soon as a new data packet becomes ready [25].

Data-driven approaches impact on sensor nodes' energy consumption in two ways. In the first way sampled data generally have strong spatial and/or temporal correlations, so there is no need to communicate the redundant information to the sink. In the second way the energy consumption is focused on the sensing subsystem. If it is energy consumable then the reduction of radio communication subsystem usage is not enough.

In case some of the sensor nodes are mobile, mobility can finally be used as a way to reduce energy consumption. In a static sensor network packets coming from sensor nodes follow a multi-hop path towards the sink(s). Thus, a few paths can be more loaded than others, and nodes closer to the sink have to relay more packets so that they are more subject to premature energy depletion [26]. If some nodes are mobile then ordinary stationary nodes can save energy because path length, contention and forwarding overheads are reduced. In addition, the mobile device can visit the network in order to spread more uniformly the energy consumption due to communications.

Batteries are currently used for powering most wireless devices. Where the power requirements are modest, primary batteries are usually chosen for their higher energy densities, lower leakage rates and low cost. A lifetime of one year with a few μW as a likely power requirement corresponds to 32 J per μW of average power. Lithium based primary batteries typically provide 1400–3600 J/cc [27], so, in principle, a lifetime of several years is achievable for a battery well below 1 cc. Thus, although the finite lifetime remains a disadvantage other additional issues (such as operating temperature range and toxicity) may reduce their practicality for homecare and healthcare network applications, primary batteries remain a very attractive source for sensor nodes.

Energy sources available in the sensor nodes' environment have been investigated to some degree for energy scavenging applications. The main categories include motion and vibration, airflow, temperature differences, ambient electromagnetic fields and light and infrared radiation. Solar cells provide an excellent solution.

If scavenging methods are successfully exploited, they are likely to be supplementary to, rather than a replacement for, battery technologies. The need for integrated power conditioning circuits with energy scavenging also encourages a trend towards intelligent energy modules, possible incorporating several forms of scavenging as well as storage, power conditioning, and power management electronics.

3.5 Health status information

Homecare and healthcare applications of wireless sensor networks improve the existing monitoring capabilities especially for the elderly, children and chronically ill. Such pervasive systems allow the monitoring of daily living activities, fall and movement detection, location tracking, medication intake monitoring and medical status monitoring.

In the first category the applications with the appropriate equipment identify the status of patients and particularly to distinguish the type of activity taking place (sleeping, walking, running, etc). In the second category the applications are focused on the identification of posture and possible fall detection and alarm for further actions. Location tracking and the medication intake reminder and monitoring systems can help cognitively impaired people to survive independently. Medical care applications make use of medical and environmental sensors in order to obtain comprehensive health status information of the patients, including ECG, heart rate, blood pressure, skin temperature, and oxygen saturation.

4. Homecare platform systems and case studies

In the literature several prototypes and commercial applications exist for pervasive homecare monitoring purposes Medical care applications make use of medical and environmental sensors in order to obtain comprehensive health status information of the patients, including ECG, heart rate, blood pressure, skin temperature, blood glucose and oxygen saturation. Hereinafter, the main categories include (i) fall detection, (ii) complete ambient assisted living, (iii) aging and rehabilitation, (iv) location-based health monitoring, and (v) continuous homecare monitoring.

4.1 Fall detection

Fall detection concept for pervasive healthcare monitoring is quite new employed method for elderly, children and chronically ill people. Movement detection applications give attention to physiological conditions for the people who need special care in case of sudden fall. Information regarding the human movement and activity in assisted environments is frequently acquired through visual tracking of the patient's position, body posture and walk analysis. In the literature, regarding fall detection applications, the researchers are making use of accelerometers, gyroscopes, and tilt sensors for movement tracking, as well as image or video recognition for patient fall incident detection.

There are significant related research endeavor in the field regarding formulas, applications, integrated systems, which may be retrieved from the literature; selected research work of them can be found in [28][29][30]. The most typical applications consider the placement of the patient along with the time of his/her occupation in rooms can be detected from the collected data of the accelerometers. These data can be used in order to verify and detect abrupt movement that could be associated with the fall or other normal and abnormal events. Detection is performed using predefined thresholds and association between current position, movement and acceleration. These systems generally use a 3-axis accelerometer to identify the human placement and movement. Also, base stations can gather the information from the accelerometer and the relayed sensors, and the data can be further processed using signal processing techniques identifying unusual behavior. The most important parameter in such techniques is the discrimination between the actual fall and fall-like situations like lying down, jumping, sitting quickly down on a chair and going up or down the stairs. Advanced algorithms have been introduced so as to distinguish falls and daily living activities [31].

For indoor environment homecare monitoring there are several kinds of sensors that integrate devices like accelerometers, gyroscopes, contact sensors and microphones. These sensors are small, lightweight and embed wireless transceivers, allowing patients and especially elderly people to move freely in the rooms and transmit collected movement and audio information to monitoring units, like access points, wirelessly. An additional sensor category is area sensors that have been used in order to track and analyze patient movement. Particularly, in [32] a system is described utilizing vibration-based detector that can detect falls based on the vibration caused on the floor. Also, in [33], infrared sensors are used in order to provide thermal information regarding the patient's location and movement. The last two approaches depend less on issues like patient physiology and more on environmental information and can be used for a variety of techniques enabling user activity recognition.

On body sensors can also be used in combination with image sensors and video capture equipment. Image sensors detect the position of the patient and a sudden fall can be verified through image processing analysis [34]. Monitoring methods that need special equipment to be installed on site are, among others, are the overhead tracking of the patient through cameras in indoor locations, which provides the movement trajectory and gives information about the user activity on predetermined monitored areas. Unusual inactivity (e.g., continuous tracking of the patient on the floor) is interpreted as a fall. Correspondingly, omni-camera images are used in order to determine the horizontal placement of the patient's body on the floor in case of fall. For the latter work, the fall detection gives accurate results at 81%.

An alternative method for homecare monitoring of falls and body movement is sound processing. In previous works [35], advanced classification techniques and Kalman filtering for producing more accurate results are presented for a patient fall detection system based on such body sensors. Most of the related work in this context focuses on collecting and analyzing sound data captured from the patient's close environment. Authors in [36] present a sound analysis system enabling the detection of special sounds and their association with events related to specific activities or situations where first aid is needed (e.g., falls, glass breaking, call for help, etc). The examined sounds are categorized into classes according to their corresponding average magnitude levels in order to detect a variety of sound signatures of both distressful and normal events. The aforementioned methods are based on acquisition and processing of sound data that originates from user's monitored environment. A different method has been proposed [37] for detecting patient suffering situations utilizing sounds captured by microphones attached on body sensors and spectrogram analysis sound processing. This technique has provided satisfying accuracy in detecting body fall sounds and distress speech expressions, while it was proved more tolerant to background noise and sounds not originating from the patient.

A configuration of an integrated system for fall detection is illustrated in Fig. 4 [38]. The system comprises of on-body sensors, microphones, accelerometers, video cameras, wireless nodes and wireless pulse oxymeter. The on-body sensors collect specific physiological data (e.g., ECG and blood oxygen saturation) accelerometer and sound data that are transmitted wirelessly to the monitoring node. At the same time, camera devices record video frames from the user's site and provide feed to the video tracker. The latter, tracks the movement of the patient's body and generates body shape features. Based on a predefined classification model, like a train model, the patient status is detected (i.e. emergency status when fall detected, normal status otherwise). Arterial pressure and blood oxygen saturation level are wirelessly transmitted to the monitoring unit from the device. The device has an embedded sound alarm mechanism that can notify caregivers in case predefined thresholds for arterial pressure and oxygen levels are exceeded.

Apart from the indication of a fall incident, an important scope is the estimation of the severity of the incident, which can be extracted by the patient's behavior after the fall. Therefore, ontologies have been used to model the patient's status and context, while proper rules evaluation provides the severity estimation. Both sensor and normal visual activity can indicate that patient has recovered from fall, and no activity at all can indicate higher severity of the incident. One method called body video tracker and is able to provide across time the frame regions occupied by human bodies. The tracker is built around a dynamic foreground segmentation algorithm [39] that utilizes adaptive background modeling. One step ahead, is the Incident Severity Estimation. This can be accomplish by introducing Semantic Representation and Rule-based Evaluation. An emergency incident can be characterized by its severity (e.g., high or low) based on fall estimation and more precisely if high or low visual and motion activity is identified after the fall, respectively. The patient movement ability level can also provide important information regarding the patient's ability to recover from falls. The assessment of heart rate and blood oxygen levels is also very informational; according to studies [40], low oxygen levels and in conjunction to sudden drop of heart rate can indicate a potential unconscious state of human body.

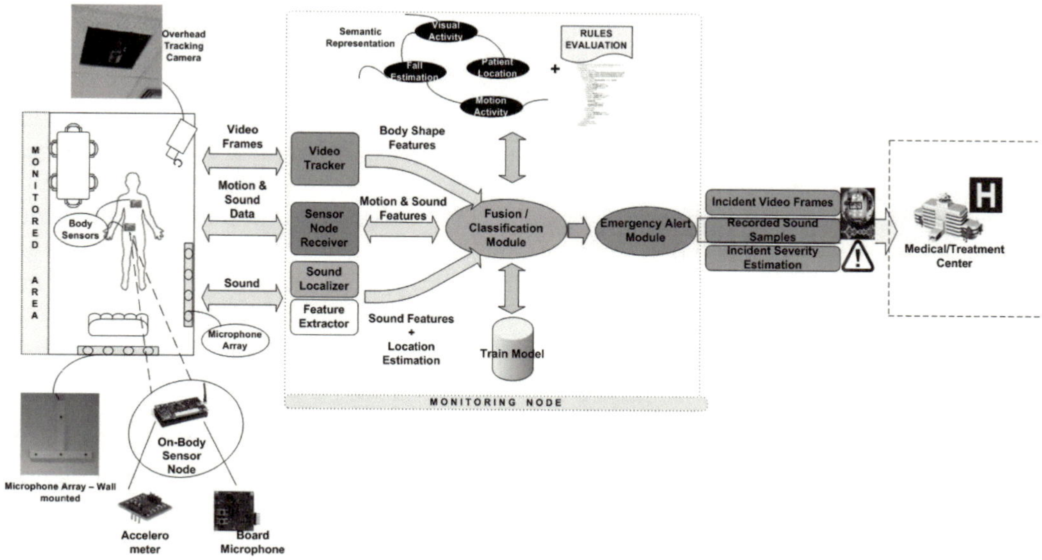

Fig. 4. System Architecture and Data interaction between the movement capturing tools and monitoring node

The aforementioned methods for fall detection concerning the characterization of falls against other movement types (i.e., walking and running) are very promising, especially when compared next to results in related work. Accuracy of 81% fall detection is accomplished using cameras and 91.58% using sound information.

4.2 Complete ambient assisted living

Assisted living facilities provide supervision and assistance with activities of daily living (ADL). In the literature one can find numerous applications and systems dealing with ambient assisted lining environments and homecare monitoring. These applications are trying to monitor, coordinate and differentiate the everyday resident activities by outside healthcare providers and trying to ensure their health, safety, and well being. The continuous monitoring of the elderly' s health is a very important issue in view of the fact that the majority of the elderly inhabitants need special care because of chronic diseases and chronic health-related conditions and scheduled office visits are infrequent. Medical services target at a number of medical parameters, which are monitored by specific devices and the measurements are assessed, analyzed and controlled by the specifically designed devices and by the responsible physicians. Arterial blood pressure, heart rate, capillary oxygen saturation, as well as body weight, are some of the most important medical parameters that may be supported in an at-home environment. Homecare patients take advantage from improved health as a result of faster diagnosis and treatment of diseases.

The user's management is strongly bound with the composition and deployment of service personalization [41]. The integrated services involve the user and a service synthesis environment interacting for the production of a personalized service specification. Based on the user, the system maintains a profile that specifies the user information, retrieves personal data from the medical devices and stores the information, monitors the status of the sensors, defines the rules for the medical data and appliances measurements, and executes actions based on the rules defined by the user for each service and the related measurements that were collected.

CAALYX [43] is an EU funded project that aims at increasing older people's autonomy and self-confidence by developing a wearable light device capable of measuring specific vital signs of the elderly, detecting falls and location, and communicating automatically in real time with his/her care provider in case of an emergency, wherever the older person happens to be, at home or outside. The project aims at developing a Wearable Light Device (WLD) to measure specific vital signs of the elderly, detect falls, and communicate automatically in real time via a mobile computer-phone (a Nokia N95 in the current prototype) with his/her caregiver in case of an emergency, wherever the person happens to be, at home or outside. The emergency information includes the geographic position alongside the health information of the elderly to enable the caretaker or emergency service to direct an appropriate response in a timely manner.

One of the recent research projects in assisted living environment is INHOME project [42], which the main goal is to provide the means for improving the quality of life of elderly people at home, by developing generic technologies for managing their domestic ambient environment, comprised of white goods, entertainment equipment and home automation systems with the aim to increase their autonomy and safety. In order to meet an individual's specific needs, a thorough and comprehensive analysis of the user requirements is one of the most important factors to be considered for the design and implementation of a similar project. User choices and preferences are also necessary so as to design interventions at the living environment. In order to define better and arrange the various medical user requirements of the elderly and also incorporate them in the distinguished non-medical requirements, a classification according to the possible most common disease-related profiles of the elderly people has been formulated. The results of the homecare related services could be categorized suitably in a mixture of goals and targets aiming primarily at early detection of a recorded event and intervention, analysis and interpretation of the clinical data, independence from caregivers while receiving healthcare in their own home, independence from physician visits and affordability instead of patients' transport and accommodation.

In order the daily homecare activities to run efficiently, careful planning of the different patients' needs so as to become easier and flexible to continuous changing of scheduling, a complete care solution by STT Condigi [44] is upon an optimum solution. There is a high risk of mistakes in case of bad reporting system, and the patient could not receive what he or she is entitled to. The activity reporting of all visits and current status of the patient is essential and reduces the risk of mistakes and also confirms the actual workload. The platform offers several different functions and products, which the patient can select what he or she actually needs. The platform optimizes the planning of homecare services in a manner that the available staff resources are according to the home visits. The behavior of the patient is recorded in real time and the data are updated so as the homecare services are efficiently comprehended and reliably performed. There are a range of tools that the patient can use to the activities undertaken, such as an easy-to-use handheld unit for staff with no experience of computers or with limited language skills, mobile phone where the activity reports are transferred directly via the GSM network to the platform, digital pen where nursing staff reports directly in predefined easy to learn forms, and PDA where the whole report is displayed on the screen and is tranferred via GSM directly to the platform. There are also particular alarm systems that are activated for the authorized staff in case of an emergency.

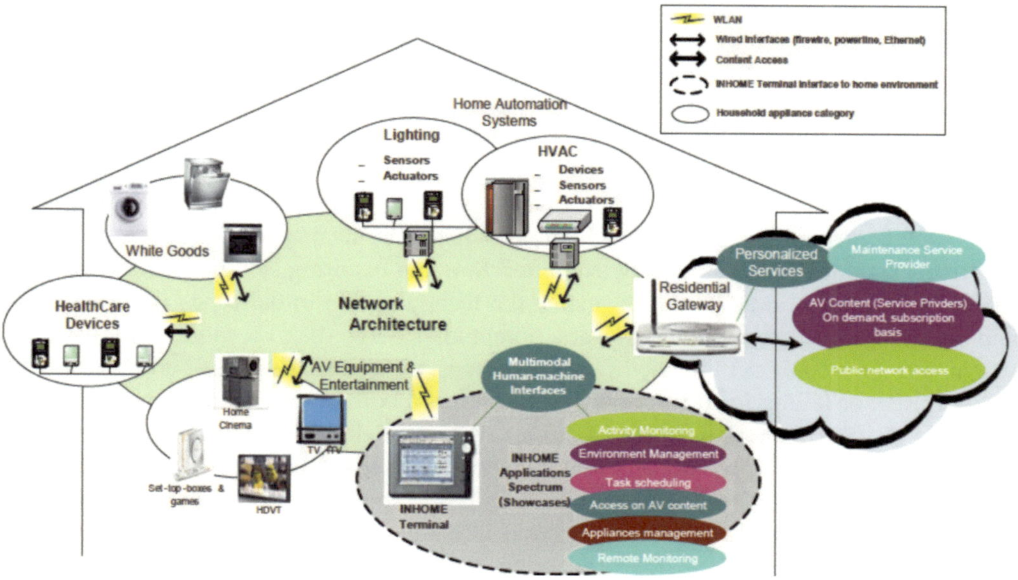

Fig. 5. The INHOME network architecture

4.3 Aging and rehabilitation

We all want the best for our aging parents or grandparents. Fortunately, there are products available that help to ease the concerns of friends and family members of the elderly or infirm aided. Medical alert services are perhaps one of the foremost humanitarian developments of our time. These services can be a saving grace when a patient is not in a frame of mind or physically able to handle a medical emergency. Help can be called for within minutes or even seconds. Experience has shown that the patient feels more confident and less anxious with a medical alert system in place, because friends and loved ones of an elderly or infirm individual can rest easy knowing that there is an extra measure of security.
A nursing home [46] is an alternative way to provide skilled nursing care and rehabilitation services to the people with are chronically ill, injured or with functional disabilities. Most of the applied facilities are applied for the treatment of the elderly people. However, some facilities provide services to younger individuals with special needs, such as developmentally disabled, mentally ill, and those requiring drug and alcohol rehabilitation. Nursing constitutes of independent facilities, however some of those are operated within a hospital or retirement community. Most of the patients and especially elderly people do not want to be in a nursing home or an institute as well as the most relatives of them. But a mixture of circumstances makes institutionalizing a necessity and not a choice.

A variety of different aids for dispersed alarms in home environment are available depending of the safety solution and requirement procedure [47]. The alarm equipment can be classified in two significant categories: the manual alarm equipment and the equipment for automatic alarms. Depending on the patient's situation and the monitoring capability, the suitably alarm equipment can be selected. Most of the alarm equipment is wireless and easy to install sensors. In the case of manual equipment, the alarm transmitters can specify or not the position of the patient, for patients with weak finger or who are permanently confined in bed there are wireless drawstring with and without shut-off, and there also alarm transmitter with fall sensors in case the person is an horizontal position for a pre-programmed period of time. In the special cases for people who have motor disabilities, there exist customized transmitters, which are comprised of pressure, finger and cheek contact, as well as breath-activated sensors, sound-activated alarm and light pressure holder.

An interesting task for homecare monitoring concerns the evaluation of the eNeighbor resident monitoring system [48]. This system can prevent the serious complications that often result from elderly people who experience incidents, such as falls, to receive assistance in a timely manner. This case study examined how the resulting savings in hospitalization and skilled nursing home costs can enable the technology to initially pay for itself in less than one year - and, in subsequent years, potentially in less than six months, by using this system. The time to detect the need for assistance is a major factor in the seriousness of the incident. Risk of falling is an important issue between both older adults in the community and those residing in long-term care facilities. When an elderly person falls in their home and cannot get to a telephone, he or she is dependent upon being found by someone who visits them regularly. These visitors can help detect problems and perhaps reduce the severity of an incident if the person is found in a timely manner. This valuable response time to an incident is critical for preventing complications, and the remote monitoring system tends to be beneficial. The eNeighbor remote monitoring system uses a series of small, unobtrusive sensors that work together to monitor a resident's daily routine. Sensors are placed strategically throughout the residence to detect general activity, or "Activities of Daily Living". The system looks for basic activities, such as movement in the living room or bedroom or the opening and closing of the refrigerator or front door, and establishes a normal range for these activities. If a resident were to fall in the shower or wake up one morning and not be able to get out of bed, the system would not see the expected level of daily activity and would trigger a call to a designated list of contacts that could check on the resident.

4.4 Location-based health monitoring

Recent advances in mobile positioning systems and telecommunications are providing the technology needed for the development of location-aware telecare applications. The positioning system is the perfect solution to create a safer environment for people at risk of wandering. Both indoor and outdoor positioning systems are available in the market. In an indoor situation, the location system can be incorporated for increasing the context-awareness of the systems and for better efficiency. In an outdoor scenario, it can assist people with cognitive disabilities or people suffering from the Alzheimer disease to locate themselves by pressing a button and expect the arrival of help. Given that GPS is the commonly available outdoor location system, and do not function properly indoor, the development of an indoor location-based health monitoring system is among the most encouraging and beneficial procedure.

In case of nurse houses, the positioning system helps the staff to locate a wanderer either inside or outside the care home. The position givers consist of wireless equipment, such as door opening sensors and indoor or outdoor loop antennas. Wireless positioning givers offer a fairly accurate localization of the patient. In addition to the location, the staff members have also the ability to receive an ID of the wanderer. A mini alarm positional transmitter store the last registered location, that is the signal picked up from the positioning givers, and sends the information wirelessly to the management central station. The staff members can receive the alarm on any displays (screen, DECT phones, pagers). An alarm is automatically sent when the resident enters an unauthorized area. The resident can also activate the alarm manually by pressing the button on the alarm positional transmitter. In both cases, the transmitter sends the last position/location registered to the central station. The system can be customized according to the resident and the authorized and unauthorized areas have to be defined for each resident. The positioning system increases the security for the resident. The positioning components give a real peace of mind not only to the caregivers and residents but also to the relatives.

An additional location-based system for emergency purposes is the EmerLoc [49]. The authors used existing technologies of wireless networks (Bluetooth, WLAN/802.11, GPRS), location-based services (Nibble, GPS), middleware and network application standards (HTTP, OSA/Parlay, WAP, RMI, Jini), in order to assemble an integrated system. EmerLoc incorporates patient-carried equipment comprised of wireless sensors and his/her portable device that continuously monitors the user's biosignals, a micro-computing unit, which is responsible for processing sensor readings and a central monitoring unit (CMU), which transmits the information to the medical personnel. The primary configuration of the system is depicted in Fig. 6 comprising our architecture are the patient and his portable equipment, the attending doctor and his portable equipment and the controlling infrastructure hosted in a hospital or independent telemonitoring service organization. The patient's device (PD) communicates with the CMU to relay critical biosignal and report its present location. Thus, a crisis situation is detected by the PD and communicated to the CMU. Since the CMU is completely aware of the present context of the patient (i.e., physical status and location), it is capable of alerting the attending doctor (or any doctor in proximity to the patient) on the situation and advice him to handle the incident. This platform is making use of heterogeneous network infrastructures (e.g., WLAN, PAN, GSM/UMTS) and the exploitation of the position fixing technologies that such networks offer. In case of an emergency, the transmitted messages contain an overall estimation of the patient's status determined by the deviated biosignals (e.g., serious, very serious), the justification for the estimation and the most recent biosignal readings acquired by the sensors. The CMU has a module of patient's record archive that contains all the medical records of the monitored patients and a module of location-based services (LBS) middleware and provisioning platform handling all different kinds of positioning technologies, i.e. terrestrial position fixing in GSM/UMTS networks, WLAN positioning in 802.11 networks and GPS-based location estimation. A routing algorithm is implemented so as to navigate the doctor via the shortest path to the emergency situation, both in indoor and outdoor scenarios.

In [50] the authors have developed an intelligent, multimodal tracking and observation solution for Assisted Living Facilities (ALFs) incorporating RFID technology and make use of video analysis algorithms for patient tracking and monitoring. The healthcare environment for the elder people consists of a wireless wearable unit along with an attached

RFID tag for the transmission of the patient's vital data and location, wireless transceivers located in the facility communicating with the RFID tags and the wearable unit in order to track and locate the patients, video cameras, which continuously monitor the patients and alarm the staff when an emergency may occur, a PC for video recording and a PDA carried by the staff for receiving alarms, video clips, and vital signs of the patient. The location of the patient can be determined by the relative signal strength of the RF signal received by the RFID tag along with the visual contact of the patient provided by the video cameras. If an emergency situation has arrived from the video analysis, for instance the patient has left the authorized area or the patient lies on the floor for an extended period of time, an alert will arise and the associated video clips will be transferred to the related staff, so as to execute proper commands.

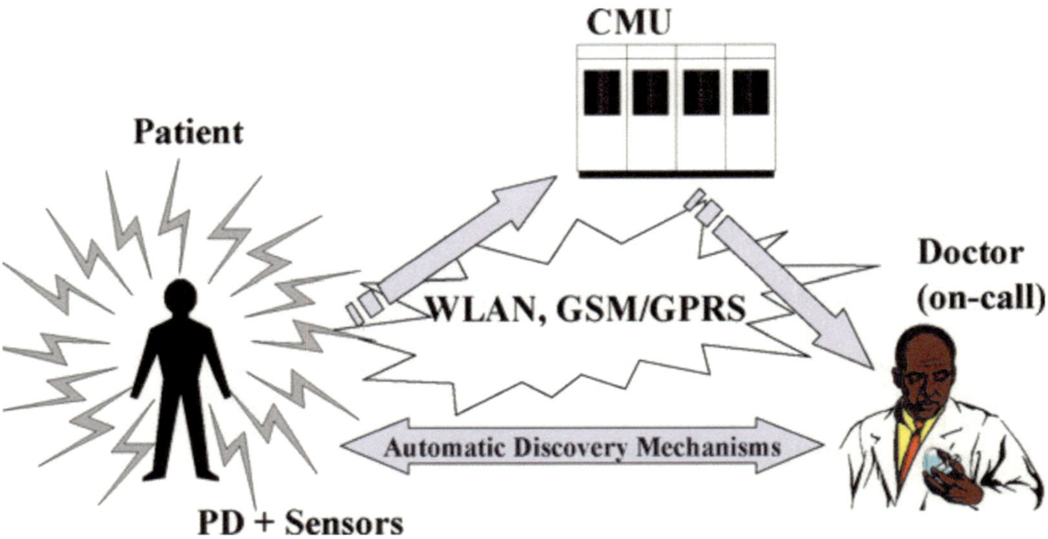

Fig. 6. EmerLoc overall system architecture

4.5 Continuous homecare monitoring

The medical status in homecare of the patients is extensively studied and in the market there a numerous of different pervasive healthcare systems depending on the monitored vital signals. Mobile and wireless concepts in healthcare (e.g., wireless and mobile networks, wireless sensors) are typically related to homecare monitoring. Homecare monitoring using mobile networks includes physiological monitoring of parameters such as heart rate, electrocardiogram (ECG), electroencephalogram, (EEG) monitoring, blood pressure, blood oximetry, and other physiological signals, physical activity monitoring of parameters such as movement, gastrointestinal telemetry fall detection, and location tracking. Using mobile technology, patient records can be accessed by healthcare professionals from any given location by connection to the institution's internal network. Physicians now have ubiquitous access to patient history, laboratory results, pharmaceutical data, insurance information, and medical resources. Handheld devices can also be used in home healthcare, for example, to fight diabetes through effective monitoring.

ZyXEL [51] introduces the Smart Home Gateway (SHG) for health monitoring applications, which is a rugged, pocket-sized, battery powered wireless router. In addition to providing wireless Internet connectivity through fixed broadband (ADSL/Cable) and 3G/4G broadband, it also enables multiple applications including state-of-the-art, real-time health monitoring through home networks. Via one of its two USB ports, it can connect to IEEE11073 USB, Bluetooth and Zigbee-compliant medical sensors to send real-time data from heath monitoring devices or smart home sensors such as blood sugar or heart rate readings to remote healthcare providers. Health care providers are under regulatory pressure to reduce costs through early detection and prevention and millions of baby boomers are entering the phase that requires greater healthcare support. This has opened up market potential and new revenue opportunities and solutions providers who can use the SHG to offer remote health monitoring services to healthcare providers. Health monitoring services are grouped into three main types - vital sign monitoring like blood pressure etc., disease management like diabetes and hypertension and aging independently that includes bed pressure and other emergency sensors.

A platform that integrates wireless and cellular technologies along with web-based applications is MedApps Remote Health Monitoring Solution [52]. It provides professional care to chronic disease patients in their own residence, by means of sending valuable and timely biometric data to the therapists. This ability can help to improve patient compliance and stabilize patient's conditions, which in turn drives down related care costs. Some of the biosignals that the system use are glucose meters, blood pressure monitors, scales and pulse oximeters. This platform transmits readings from retail health monitors to Electronic Health Records automatically and can be effectively associate patients with chronic conditions with their care providers and family. A remote unit called HealthPAL uses a combination of embedded cellular and bluetooth technologies to automatically transmit readings from compatible monitors to a secure central server. The readings of this unit can be tracked by individuals through an electronic health record (EHR) or an online medical records service, such as Microsoft HealthVault or Google Health. Consequently, healthcare providers can review patient data via enterprise level EHR or by accessing MedApps' full-featured, web-based patient management portal for care professionals.

Another major issue of home monitoring is about the babies. Intelligent Clothing [53] was founded ten years ago to pursue an idea that ordinary washable undergarments could provide an intensive care standard of wireless healthcare monitoring. Continuous evolution of both the industry and the research has produced a manufacturable SmartPatch™ with internet connectivity, suitable for Special Care Baby Units and the home. It is small and least invasive ambulatory monitoring system that weights approximately 9 grams, continuously monitors the heart, respiration and temperature and radios the data to a Bedside Display Unit for onward transmission to doctors via the company's web server. SmartPatch™ enhances collision avoidance integrity suitable for both the home and hospital environment. Each SmartPatch™ will run for 24 hours continuously, on a small inductively rechargeable cell battery. The product is developed for Special Care Baby Units, birthing hospitals, for doctors to monitor their home-based patients remotely and to improve the cost-efficiency of multi-centre clinical trials. The Internet connectivity software monitors respiratory, pulmonary, oximetry and temperature waveforms in real-time. Intelligent Clothing's wireless technology uses ultra low power low frequency radio, an order of magnitude lower than Bluetooth or mobile phone frequencies. Flashing lights in the teddy bear's eyes advice the user that the system is working and, during the recharge cycle, which the battery is fully charged. Data is transmitted to a nearby Bedside Display Unit for onward transmission via

802.11b to a Nurse's Central Station computer in the hospital region or in the home environment via wireless broadband access point.

5. Conclusions and future trends

In this chapter book we analyzed the impact of wireless technology networks and sensors in the homecare environments. Wireless technologies can serve as a new generation technology for mobile health systems providing immediate and ubiquitous health care in a range of different circumstances, as it may handle a variety of homecare needs. We illustrated the different wireless sensor standards that they are making use of, showing their corresponding energy consumption in terms of the biosignals' data rate. Moreover, the measurement range of the sensors is depicted along with the power supply requirements, calibration parameters, output interfaces, and data rates. Signal processing mechanisms are crucial for the extraction of valuable information from the captured biosignals and are closely coupled with the energy consumption. By virtue of that rationale, the taxonomy of approaches to energy saving in sensor networks is also depicted.

We described a number of different systems and case studies of the existing pervasive homecare systems, showing great performance and the biosensors that will mark swift growth in the future and will become integral part of our life. There are appliances easy in their use, precious and very important for the patient, contributing to the improvement and in the prevention of the patient's health. We have provided the confrontations to overcome in different healthcare circumstances, like fall detection, complete ambient assisted living, aging and rehabilitation, location-based health monitoring, and continuous homecare monitoring.

The use of new technologies for the applications of the homecare system appears today as an essential solution. The wireless sensor devices and wireless network systems have become a standardized infrastructure for access in the complex applications for the provision of pervasive homecare for the elderly, chronically ill and children. Such standardized platforms of communication guarantee the advantages of possibility of access and utilization both in the customers (patients) and in the suppliers (caregivers). In other words, we can declare that making use of these technologies offer to the patients who typically live at home, high quality and efficient health services, outweighing the provisional cost and energy consumption.

There are still a few obstacles and open issues in the wireless sensor networks that should be stated and the healthcare research community ought to take into consideration. Selected obstacles can be summarized at the reliability of short-range communication, the changes of policy and organizational flaw to regulate payments and reimbursements of physicians for monitoring or/and consultation, the insufficient battery life, the sensitivity to sensor placements, lack of seamless integration with infrastructure network, privacy and security considerations along with standardization and interoperability. In particular, certain challenges have to be declared and further studied so as the wireless sensor networks to play an important role in enabling ubiquitous communications. The aforementioned challenges can be categorized in hardware issues, in all the layers of the TCP/IP model, and in layer-independent challenges.

As far as hardware issues are concerned and despite the major challenge of energy saving, the unobtrusive design, development and integration of the devices carried by the patients is the main concern since inhabitants must not appear in poor health. The size, form factor, and physical compatibility to human tissues are crucial, while the sensitivity and the calibration of the sensors transmitting vital signals, particularly in harsh environments, is an additional research challenge, in combination with the real-time data acquisition effectiveness.

With reference to the physical, MAC and network layer, the transmission and routing of the signals is of prior importance. The miniaturization of the devices due to low power energy and small antennas causes higher transmission errors, low bandwidth efficiency and mutual interference when operating in the unlicensed Industrial, Scientific and Medical (ISM) band, allowing the interoperability of the sensors and the systems. Insignificant latency and delay, as well as high Quality of Service (QoS) requirements when vital real-time data are transmitted, are the key issues to provide efficient and best possible delivery of the signal in a fair manner, especially under emergency conditions. Power management and context-aware network configuration of the networks need to be revisited as well. In addition, dynamic management of resources including sensor functionalities is also essential to be compromised. Transport layer should be reliable for medical data delivery ensuring adequate congestion and flow control mechanisms, while application layer is responsible to organize, store and forward medical data securely, intelligently and in a user-friendly context-aware approach, as already discussed in this study.

Different levels of security should be identified, and appropriate mechanisms shall be developed to distinguish life-threatening requests from other applications with various security priorities and appropriate privacy protection measures. The privacy sector requires successful and efficient authentication techniques in wireless sensor networks. Multimodal authentication schemes based on human faces, hand features, and biosignals are actively being developed in both academia and industry. Complex but distinguishable human body characteristics provide an ideal way of authenticating users, but they also create other challenges in protecting their privacy. Software as a service method could be exploited for increasing the scalability and improvement of software deployment.

The technologies of today are tools for a high-quality coordination procedure. Their capabilities are improving rapidly from time to time and their cost decreases exponentially with their use. What is needed is coordination of relevant concepts, attitudes and best practices, so that we can seize the great opportunities that they provide.

6. References

[1] Howitt, I. & Gutierrez, J.A. (2003). IEEE 802.15.4 low rate-wireless personal area network coexistence issues. *Proceedings of WCNC 2003 Wireless Communications and Networking,* pp. 1481-1486, Vol.3, ISBN 0-7803-7700-1, New Orleans, LA, USA, March 16-20, 2003

[2] ZigBee: wireless control that simply works, Available from http://www.zigbeeresourceguide.com / images /ZigBee_RG_2008.pdf

[3] HART - The Logical Wireless Solution, Available from http://www.hartcomm2.org/hart_protocol/wireless_hart/hart_the_logical_solution.html

[4] ISA100.11a, Available from http://www.isa.org/MSTemplate.cfm?MicrositeID=1134&CommitteeID=6891

[5] 6LoWPAN, Available from http://6lowpan.net

[6] Mulligan, G. & Group, L.W. (2007). The 6LoWPAN architecture. *Proceedings of the EmNets 2007 4th workshop on Embedded networked sensors*, ISBN 978-1-59593-694-3, Cork, Ireland, June 25-26, 2007

[7] IEEE Standard 802.15.3, Wireless medium access control (MAC) and physical layer (PHY) specifications for high rate wireless person area networks (WPANs), September 2003.

[8] Wibree, Available from http://www.wibree.com

[9] IEEE Computer Society, (August 31, 2007). IEEE Standard 802.15.4a-2007

[10] IEEE Computer Society, (April 17, 2009). IEEE Standard 802.15.4c-2009

[11] IEEE Computer Society, (April 17, 2009). IEEE Standard 802.15.4d-2009

[12] IEEE 802.15.1™, (2002). IEEE standard for information technology - Telecommunications and information exchange between systems - Local and metropolitan area networks - Specific requirements - Part 15.1: wireless medium access control and physical layer specifications for wireless personal area networks, Available from http://standards.ieee.org/getieee802/download/802.15.1-2002.pdf

[13] IEEE P802.15.3™, Project Authorization Request (PAR), (2000). Available from http://grouper.ieee.org/board/nescom/802-15-3.pdf

[14] IEEE P802.15.3™, (2003). Draft IEEE standard for information technology - Telecommunications and information exchange between systems - Local and metropolitan area networks - Specific requirements - Part 15.3: wireless medium access control and physical layer specifications for high-rate wireless personal area networks, Available from http://standards.ieee.org/getieee802/download/802.15.3-2003.pdf

[15] Available from http://www.hartcomm.org

[16] Available from http://johnkooker.Com/blog/wpcontent/uploads/2009/05/jkooker_BTZigBeeWibree. pdf

[17] Hanson, M.A.; Powell, H.C.; Barth, A.T.; Ringgenberg, K.; Calhoun, B.H.; Aylor; J.H. & Lach, J. (2009). Body Area Sensor Networks: Challenges and Opportunities. *Computer*, Vol.42, No.1, Jan. 2009, pp. 58-65, ISSN 0018-9162

[18] Medical implant communications, Available from http://wireless.fcc.gov/services/index.htm?job=service_home&id=medical_implant

[19] Wireless medical telemetry service, Available from http://wireless.fcc.gov/services/personal/medtelemetry

[20] Sadjadi, F.A. (1996). *Selected papers on sensor and data fusion*. SPIE Milestone, SPIE, Optical Engineering Press, ISBN 978-0819422651

[21] Brooks, R.R. & Iyengar, S.S. (1998). *Multi-sensor fusion: fundamentals and applications with software*. Upper Saddle River, Prentice Hall, New Jersey, USA

[22] Yang, G.Z. (2006). *Body Sensor Networks*, Springer

[23] Karagiannis, A.; Kokkorikos, S. & Constantinou, P. (2009). Energy consumption analysis and optimization techniques for Wireless Sensor Networks, *Proceedings of ISCC 2009 IEEE Symposium on Computers and Communications*, pp. 8-14, Sousse, Tunisia, July 5-8, 2009

[24] Pottie, G. & Kaiser, W. (2000). Wireless integrated network sensors, *Communications of the ACM*, Vol.43, No.5, pp. 51–58

[25] Anastasi, G.; Conti, M.; Francesco, M. & Passarella, A. (2009). Energy conservation in wireless sensor networks: A survey, *Ad Hoc Networks*, Vol.7, No.3, (May 2009), pp. 537-568, ISSN 1570-8705
[26] Li, J. & Mohapatra, P. (2007). Analytical modeling and mitigation techniques for the energy hole problem in sensor networks, *Pervasive Mobile Computing*, Vol.3, No.3, pp. 233–254
[27] Brodd, R.J.; Bullock, K.R.; Leising, R.A.; Middaugh, R.L.; Miller, J.R. & Takeuchi, E. (2004). Batteries, 1977 to 2002. *Journal of the Electrochemical Society*, Vol.151, No.3, (January 2004), pp. K1-K11.
[28] Noury N. (2002). A smart sensor for the remote follow up of activity and fall detection of the elderly, *Proceedings of 2nd Annual International Conference on Microtechnologies in Medicine and Biology*, pp. 314-317, ISBN 0-7803-7480-0, Madison, WI, USA, May 2-4, 2002
[29] Miaou, S.G.; Sung, P.H. & Huang, C.Y. (2006). A Customized Human Fall Detection System Using Omni-Camera Images and Personal Information, *Proceedings of 1st Transdisciplinary conference on Distributed Diagnosis and Home Healthcare*, pp. 39-42, ISBN 1-4244-0058-9, Arlington, VA, USA, April 2-4, 2006
[30] Allen, F.R.; Ambikairajah, E.; Lovell, N.H. & Celler, B.G. (2006). An Adapted Gaussian Mixture Model Approach to Accelerometry-Based Movement Classification Using Time-Domain Features, *Proceedings of 28th Annual International Conference of the IEEE Engineering in Medicine and Biology Society*, pp. 3600-3603, New York City, New York, USA, Aug. 30–Sep. 3, 2006
[31] Wang, C.C.; Chiang, C.Y.; Lin, P.Y.; Chou, Y.C.; Kuo, I.T.; Huang, C.N. & Chan, C.T. (2008). Development of a fall detecting system for the elderly residents, *Proceedings of 2nd IEEE International Conference on Bioinformatics and Biomedical Engineering*, pp. 1359–1362, Shanghai, China, May 16-18, 2008
[32] Alwan, M.; Rajendran, P.J.; Kell, S.; Mack, D.; Dalal, S.; Wolfe, M. & Felder, R. (2006). A smart and passive floor-vibration based fall detector for elderly. *Proceedings of 2nd Information and Communication Technologies Conference, ICTTA 06*, pp. 1003–1007, ISBN 0-7803-9521-2, Damascus, Syria, April 24-28, 2006
[33] Sixsmith, A. & Johnson, N. (2004). A smart sensor to detect the falls of the elderly, *IEEE Pervasive Computing*, Vol.3, No.2, (April-June 2004), pp. 42–47, ISSN 1536-1268.
[34] Tabar, A.M. & Aghajan, H. (2006). Smart home care network using sensor fusion and distributed vision-based reasoning, *Proceedings of 4th ACM International Workshop on Video Surveillance and Sensor Networks*, pp. 145–154, Santa Barbara, CA, USA, Oct. 27, 2006
[35] Doukas, C. & Maglogiannis, I. (2008). Advanced Patient or Elder Fall Detection based on Movement and Sound Data, *Proceedings of 2nd International Conference on Pervasive Computing Technologies for Healthcare*, pp. 103 - 107 ISBN 978-963-9799-15-8, Tampere, Finland, Jan. 30-Feb. 1 2008
[36] Istrate D.; Castelli E.; Vacher M.; Besacier L. & Serignat J.F. (2006). Information extraction from sound for medical telemonitoring, *IEEE Transaction on Information Theory in Biomedicine*, Vol.10, No.2, (April 2006), pp. 264-274, ISSN 1089-7771
[37] Doukas, C. & Maglogiannis, I. (2008). Human Distress Sound Analysis and Characterization using Advanced Classification Techniques, *Proceedings of 5th*

Hellenic Conference in Artificial Intelligence: Theories, Models and Applications, SETN 08, ISBN 978-3-540-87880-3, Syros, Greece, October 2-4, 2008.

[38] Doukas, C. & Maglogiannis, I. (2011). Emergency Fall Incidents Detection in Assisted Living Environments Utilizing Motion, Sound and Visual Perceptual Components, *IEEE Trans. on Information Technology on Biomedicine*, Vol.15, No.2, pp. 277–289, (March 2011), ISSN 1089-7771.

[39] Pnevmatikakis, A. & Polymenakos, L. (2006). Robust Estimation of Background for Fixed Cameras, *Proceedings of CIC 2006 15th International Conference on Computing*, ISBN 0-7695-2708-6, Mexico City, Mexico, 2006.

[40] Kelly, J. (2001). Loss of Consciousness: Pathophysiology and Implications in Grading and Safe Return to Play, *Journal of Athletic Training*, Vol.36, No.3, (July-September 2001), pp. 249–252.

[41] Vergados, D.D. (2008). Service personalisation for assisted living of elderly people at home. *Proceedings of SMAP'08 3rd international workshop on semantic media adaptation and personalization*, pp. 135–140, ISBN 978-0-7695-3444-2, Prague, Czech Republic, December 15–16, 2008

[42] INHOME Deliverable D-5.1.2 Integration and evaluation report

[43] Available from http://www.caalyx.eu

[44] Available from http://www.sttcondigi.com/uk

[45] Available from http://www.wellawaresystems.com

[46] Nikolidakis, S.; Vergados, D.D. & Anagnostopoulos, I. (2008.) Health Care Information Systems and Personalized Services for Assisting Living of Elderly People at Nursing Home, *Proceedings of SMAP'08 3rd international workshop on semantic media adaptation and personalization*, pp. 135–140, ISBN 978-0-7695-3444-2, Prague, Czech Republic, December 15–16, 2008

[47] Newell, A. & Gregor, P. (2002). Design for older and disabled people-where do we go from here?, *Universal Access in the Information Society, Springer*, Vol.2, No.1, (November 2002), pp. 3-7, ISSN 1615-5289

[48] Available from http://www.healthsense.com

[49] Maglogiannis, I. & Hadjiefthymiades, S. (2007). EmerLoc: Location-based services for emergency medical incidents, *International Journal of Medical Informatics, Elsevier*, Vol.76, No.10, (October 2007), pp. 747-759, ISSN 1386-5056

[50] Bowser, S. & Woodworth, J. (2004). Wireless multimedia technologies for assisted living, *Proceedings of 2nd LACCEI International Latin American and Caribbean Conference for Engineering and Technology*, Miami, FL, USA, June 2-4, 2004

[51] Available from http://us.zyxel.com

[52] Available from http://public.medapps.net/Products.html

[53] Available from http://www.intelligentclothing.com

3

Wireless Telemedicine System: An Accurate, Reliable and Secure Real-time Health Care

Huyu Qu[1], Le Yi Wang[2], Christopher M. Klaus[3], Qiang Cheng[4], Ece Yaprak[5] and Hong Wang[6]

[1]*Scanning and Mobility Division, Honeywell International Inc., Cupertino*
[2]*Department of Electrical and Computer Engineering, Wayne State University, Detroit*
[3]*Drighten Research Inc., DeKalb*
[4]*CS Department, Southern Illinois University, Carbondale*
[5]*Division of Engineering Technology, Wayne State University, Detroit*
[6]*Department of Anesthesiology, Wayne State University, Detroit*
USA

1. Introduction

Rapid development in telecommunication technologies, especially wireless communications, has made remote monitoring of patient vital signs feasible. When a signal is transmitted through a communication channel, accuracy of information transmission at the receiver is one of the most significant issues. For medical diagnosis, errors in signal processing and communications introduce substantial artifacts, making pattern recognition and diagnosis less reliable, leading potentially to an erroneous diagnosis. Consequently, when system resources are limited, such as transmission bandwidths, appropriate utility of available resources becomes imperative to ensure accuracy of information.

For a given communication bandwidth, the communication system can first process original medical signals by waveform transformation, data compression, and quantization to reduce the data size, which will result in a reduced rate of data transmission through communication channels, but introduce more information processing errors. This chapter analyzes fundamental relationships between accuracy of information exchange and available resources on a platform of wireless local area network (WLAN) systems that involve typical function blocks of discrete cosine transform, data compression, magnitude quantization, stochastic WLAN channels, and inverse discrete cosine transform. The main complexity relationships developed in this chapter provide a trade-off between resource consumptions and information processing errors, and a strategy for optimal allocation of resources.

An example of these relationships is simulated in a typical medical diagnosis problem using lung sounds. Respiratory sounds contain a rich reservoir of vital physiological and pathological information that is of critical importance for clinical diagnosis and patient management in operating rooms (OR). Several research groups have investigated potential computer-assisted sound analysis and classifications for asthma, cystic fibrosis, pneumonia, etc. (17; 19; 24). This chapter evaluates the impact of communication channels on diagnostic accuracy and the benefits of studying signal processing and communications in an integrated framework. The main findings of this chapter indicate that effective utility of communication resources is essential for tele-monitoring and telemedicine when the communication bandwidth is shared by many users, and hence is very limited for each connection.

There are extensive efforts in studying integrated information processing and communication systems, especially in feedback control. For example Firoozbakhsh et al. (7) provided a versatile framework for incorporation of sensing, monitoring, information processing and wireless communication devices. Sayeed (22) proposed a signal modeling framework for sensor networks that interact between space-time signal sampling, distributed signal processing, and communications. This chapter is focused on a stochastic analysis and simulation of complexity relationships among typical components on integrated medical information processing and communication systems. A stochastic optimization problem is formulated that explicitly relates communication resources to information transmission accuracy. Solutions to the optimization problem leads to a strategy of communication resource allocation. A typical medical diagnostic problem on lung sounds is used, in combination with a standard IEEE 802.11b WLAN network simulation model, to show the utility of this strategy by finding the optimal resource allocation between compression ratios (and/or quantization levels) and transmission rates.

WLAN standards allow freedom for laptops, computers on wheels, medical sensor nodes and other medical equipment to efficiently roam through hospitals, but encounter potential vulnerabilities of wireless beds, wireless medication robots, wireless I.V.s, wireless heart monitoring & medication devices, and various other wireless medical technologies. There are several common security threats to WLAN networks, such as eavesdropping, denial of service, theft of service, etc., revealing weakness of the current security methods (RADIUS servers, MAC filtering, etc.). Even proprietary systems have been shown to quickly succumb to attacks. Control systems, which are the basis for medical equipment, also have weaknesses that allow unauthorized control via these WLAN networks. As such, transmitting and receiving a medical signal via an open medium like Wi-Fi is a critical concern. Interference with these systems from congestion to outright manipulation of medical information can not only put private medical information (PMI) at risk but also patients' lives in peril. WiFi-based telemedicine systems need to be immune from deny of service attacks, and provide service all the time. Any kind of congestion is intolerable. Moreover, the privacy medical data should not be intercepted and eavesdropped. As such, it is essential to have a multi-layered defense starting with conventional security tactics to the implementation of more in-depth methods like wireless covert channel signaling and wireless self protection systems. By increasing wireless network security in this way, vulnerabilities of medical equipment and sensor nodes can be significantly reduced to help ensure medical services are secure and available when needed.

The remainder of the chapter is organized as follows. Section 2 introduces the basic system settings for an integrated wireless-based medical information system. The main mathematics models of the system modules are described. The trade-offs of compression errors and compression ratios, quantization errors and quantization levels, transmission errors and transmission rate as well as power levels are established in a stochastic framework. An optimization problem for resource allocations to achieve overall error reduction is presented. A standard IEEE 802.11b WLAN is used as a communication channel to illustrate the usefulness of optimal resource allocations. An example of uniformly distributed signals through a 1Mbps WLAN channel is employed to show the optimal choice of quantization levels. Section 3 focuses on the integrated medical systems for diagnosis. A lung sound signal is transmitted through a simulation model of WLAN-based medical information systems in three different scenarios. The trade-offs among compression ratios, quantization levels, transmission rates, and signal-to-noise ratios are demonstrated in a stochastic framework. The overall error reduction can be achieved by optimizing information and resource allocations. The impact of information processing and transmission errors on medical pattern recognition and diagnosis accuracy is discussed. Session 4 discusses security weakness and security enhancement methods in WLAN-based telemedicine system, and talks about the secure roaming among different access points. Session 5 briefly summarizes the findings of the chapter.

2. Integrated and wireless-based medical information systems

2.1 Mathematics models and error analysis of communication systems

A typical integrated system of information processing and wireless communications is shown in Figure 1. The input sequence $u = \{u_k : k = 1, \ldots, L_0\}$ belongs to an input ensemble U. For system analysis, the length L_0 of $u \in$ U is assumed to be fixed and known. This represents the size of a signal or the number of samples in a fixed time interval T. Hence, $f = L_0/T$ will be the data sampling rate. The probability of occurrence of a specific sequence $u \in$ U will be denoted by $P\{u\}$. The following typical components of communications will be considered in this chapter, and their accuracy and complexity will be analyzed.

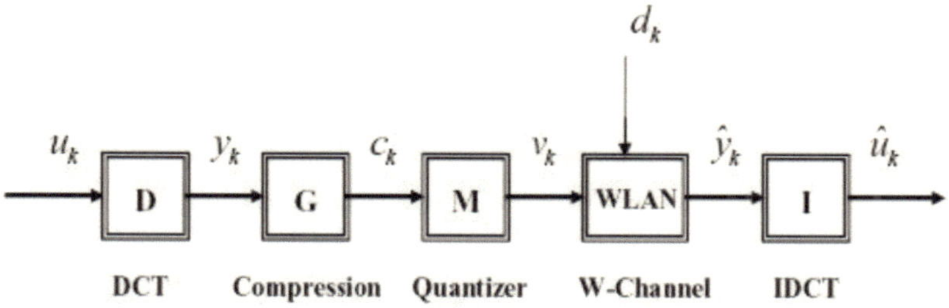

Fig. 1. System blocks

Discrete Cosine Transform

Several algorithms of transform data compression (TDC), such as fast Fourier transform (FFT), discrete sine transform (DST), discrete cosine transform (DCT), 2D discrete cosine transform (DCT2), etc., were compared in (29), showing that DCT has least compression errors in most cases for medical signals. As a result, the DCT algorithm is used in our system modeling.
The input data block $u = \{u_k : k = 1, \ldots, L_0\}$ of medical signals passes a DCT block to generate a coefficient sequence $y = \{y_k : k = 1, \ldots, L_0\}$.

$$y_k = D(u) = 2 \sum_{n=0}^{L_0-1} a_n u_n \cos\left(\frac{\pi k n}{L_0 - 1}\right), \quad 0 \leq k \leq L_0 - 1, \tag{1}$$

where $a_n = \begin{cases} 1/2, & n = 1 \text{ and } L_0 - 1; \\ 2, & 2 \leq n \leq L_0 - 2. \end{cases}$

The DCT coefficient sequence $y = \{y_k, k = 0, \ldots, L_0 - 1\}$ belongs to an ensemble $\mathbb{Y}$, and $\mathbb{Y}$ is uniformly bounded by $\sup_{y \in \mathbb{Y}} \max_{k=0,\ldots,L_0-1} |y_k| \leq y_{max}$. The length of $y \in \mathbb{Y}$ is same as the input sequence u.

Data Compression

To reduce data sizes, y is first compressed. In this chapter, we will use the following scheme of truncation in data compression for concreteness of analysis, although the main tools of analysis can be readily extended to other data compression schemes. For a given threshold ε,

$$c_k = G(y_k) = \begin{cases} y_k, & \text{if } |y_k| > \varepsilon \\ 0, & \text{if } |y_k| \leq \varepsilon \end{cases} \tag{2}$$

The length N of c depends on y with $N \leq L_0$, and hence is a random variable. The average data compression ratio is defined as the expected value of N/L_0

$$\mu = E\left(\frac{N}{L_0}\right) = \sum_{y \in \mathbb{Y}} \frac{N}{L_0} P(y).$$

Observe that for any given $y \in \mathbb{Y}$, N is a monotone non-increasing function of ε. Namely, the larger the threshold ε, the shorter the compressed sequence. As a result, μ is a monotone non-increasing function of ε. This function will be denoted by $\mu = h(\varepsilon)$. $h(\varepsilon)$ represents the *compressability function* of the input ensemble $\mathbb{Y}$. The main information we need for subsequent complexity analysis, in terms of data compression, is this compressability function. Typical compressability functions are shown in Figure 2.

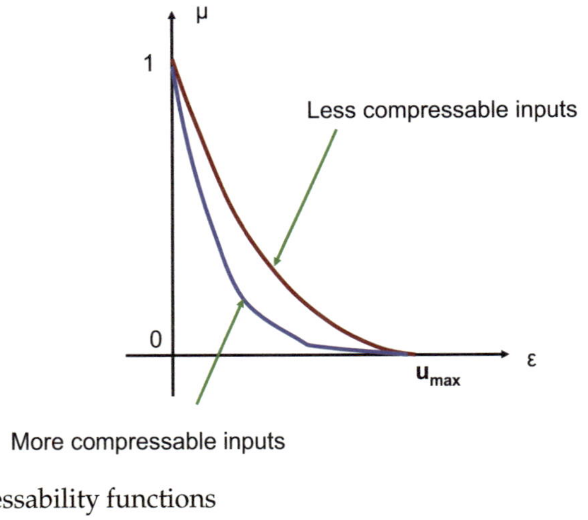

Fig. 2. Typical compressability functions

Data Quantization

Before transmission, c_k is first quantized. Suppose that the signal range $[-y_{max}, y_{max}]$ is divided into m equally spaced intervals of length $\delta = 2y_{max}/m$. Quantization output sequences take m possible values $Q = \{q_j : j = 1, \ldots, m\}$, defined by

$$q_j = -y_{max} + (j - 0.5)\delta, j = 1, \ldots, m. \tag{3}$$

The quantization maps $c_k \in [-y_{max}, y_{max}]$ into its nearest element in Q. The complexity of quantization is characterized by the size m of Q, or $l = \log_2 m$ in bits. The quantization errors are bounded by $\delta/2 = y_{max}/m = y_{max}/2^l$, hence is inversely proportional to m.

Data Transmission

The output of the quantization process is $v_k = M(c_k)$, which will be transmitted through a WLAN channel, whose output sequence will be denoted by w_k. At a system level, a DMC (discrete memoryless channel) channel can be modeled by its transmission conditional probability matrix:

$$\Phi = \begin{bmatrix} p_{11} & p_{12} & \cdots & p_{1m} \\ p_{21} & p_{22} & \cdots & p_{2m} \\ \vdots & \cdots & & \vdots \\ p_{m1} & p_{m2} & \cdots & p_{mm} \end{bmatrix}. \tag{4}$$

where $p_{ij} = P\{y_k = q_i | v_k = q_j\}$, that is, the conditional probability of receiving q_i when q_j is transmitted.

It should be emphasized that this is a system-level representation of the communication channel. The physical-level channel may vary. For instance, if the underlying modulation scheme is a BPSK (bi-phase shift keying) modulation, then a binary memoryless channel model may be used in representing the physical-level channel, with a probability matrix

$$\Phi_0 = \begin{bmatrix} p^0_{11} & p^0_{12} \\ p^0_{21} & p^0_{22} \end{bmatrix}. \tag{5}$$

In this case, v_k, that takes m possible values, will be represented by a binary sequence of length $l = \log_2 m$ for transmission. The matrix Φ in (4) can be derived from Φ_0 as the l-tuple Cartesian product $\Phi = \Phi_0 \otimes \cdots \otimes \Phi_0$. Similar discussions (26) can be made for DBPSK (differential bi-phase shift keying), DQPSK (differential quandary phase shift keying) modulation, or other modulation schemes which are used in IEEE 802.11b WLAN.

Inverse Discrete Cosine Transform

The received sequence $w = \{w_k : k = 0, \ldots, N-1\}$ of the wireless channel are processed through the inverse cosine transform block to recover the original time-domain signal sequence $\widetilde{u} = \{\widetilde{u}_k : k = 0, \ldots, N-1\}$.

$$\widetilde{u}_k = I(\widetilde{y}) = \frac{1}{N-1} \sum_{n=0}^{N-1} a_n \widetilde{y}_n \cos\left(\frac{\pi k n}{N-1}\right), \quad 0 \le k \le N-1, \tag{6}$$

where $a_n = \begin{cases} 1/2, & n = 0 \text{ and } N-1; \\ 2, & 2 \le n \le N-2. \end{cases}$

2.2 Relations between errors and complexity: Analysis and optimization

2.2.1 Information accuracy and complexity

Assumption A: DCT and IDCT do not involve errors.

Under assumption A, only data compression, quantization, and communications introduce errors in information representation and transmission. The sizes of the errors depend on certain complexity measures of the operations. In particular, data compression introduces compression errors that increase when the compression ratio μ decreases. Quantization errors increase when the quantization complexity m decreases. Communication errors increase when the signal/noise ratio decreases, or the transmission rate increases, or the assigned bandwidth decreases. We shall start with a more precise description of these errors.

- **Compression Errors and Compression Ratios**

  Assume that y_k takes values in $[-y_{max}, y_{max}]$ with a probability density $f_c(x)$ that is an even function and the sequence $\{y_k\}$ is independent and identically distributed (i.i.d.). The compression error $e_k^c = y_k - c_k = y_k - G(y_k)$ has mean

$$Ee_k^c = \int_{-y_{max}}^{y_{max}} (x - G(x))f_c(x)dx = \int_{-\varepsilon}^{\varepsilon} xf_c(x)dx = 0,$$

  and variance

$$\sigma_c^2 = E(e_k^c)^2 = \int_{-y_{max}}^{y_{max}} (x - G(x))^2 f_c(x)dx = \int_{-\varepsilon}^{\varepsilon} x^2 f_c(x)dx = S_c(\varepsilon).$$

  It follows that the variance is

$$\sigma_c^2 = E(e_k^c)^2 = \int_{-y_{max}}^{y_{max}} (x - G(x))^2 \frac{1}{2y_{max}} dx = \int_{-\varepsilon}^{\varepsilon} x^2 \frac{1}{2y_{max}} dx = \frac{2\varepsilon^3}{3} \frac{1}{2y_{max}} = \frac{\varepsilon^3}{3y_{max}}.$$

  Combining the relationship between σ_c^2 and ε with the compressability function $\mu = h(\varepsilon)$, assuming $h(\cdot)$ is invertible in the range $[0, y_{max}]$, we have a complexity relationship

$$\sigma_c^2 = S_c(\varepsilon) = S_c(h^{-1}(\mu)) := \lambda_c(\mu). \tag{7}$$

- **Quantization Errors and Complexity**

  The quantization error $e_k^q = c_k - M(c_k)$ is bounded by $|e_k^q| \le \delta/2$. Suppose that e_k^q is i.i.d. with a density function $f_q(x)$ that is an even function on $[-\delta/2, \delta/2]$ (31). Then the mean and variance of e_k^q can be derived as $E(e_k^q) = 0$ and

$$\sigma_q^2 = E(e_k^q)^2 = \int_{-\delta/2}^{\delta/2} x^2 f_q(x)dx = S_q(\delta) = S_q(2y_{max}/m) := \lambda_q(m), \tag{8}$$

  noting that $\delta = 2y_{max}/m$. The function $\sigma_q^2 = \lambda_q(m)$ defines the complexity relationship for quantization. For example, if e_k^q is uniformly distributed, then $f_q(x) = 1/\delta$ and

$$\sigma_q^2 = \int_{-\delta/2}^{\delta/2} \frac{x^2}{\delta} dx = \frac{\delta^2}{12} = \frac{y_{max}^2}{3m^2} = \frac{y_{max}^2}{3} 2^{-2l}.$$

- **Transmission Errors and Communication Power and Bandwidth**

  The impact of signal power and bandwidth on the transmission channels is typically summarized in the normalized signal-to-noise ratio E_s/N_0, where E_s is energy per symbol and N_0 is average noise power per unit bandwidth. This parameter defines the communication complexity or resource requirements since signal power and bandwidth are the key resources in a communication system. For a given physical level modulation, the transmission matrix Φ defined in (4) depends on E_s/N_0 and may be expressed as

$\Phi(E_s/N_0)$. Intuitively, the larger the signal-to-noise ratio E_s/N_0 is, the closer the matrix Φ is to the identity matrix.

To understand the transmission errors, we note that if $v_k = q_j$ occurs with probability $p_j = P\{q_j\}$ and q_j is transmitted, then the output $\widehat{y}_k$ may take any values in Q with probability $P\{\widehat{y}_k = q_i | v_k = q_j\} = p_{ij}$ and error $e_k^t = q_j - q_i$. It follows that the conditional mean squares error $E[(e_k^t)^2 | q_j] = \sum_{i=1}^m (q_j - q_i)^2 p_{ij}$. Consequently, the overall mean squares error is $E[(e_k^t)^2] = \sum_{j=1}^m \sum_{i=1}^m (q_j - q_i)^2 p_{ij} p_j$. The last quantity depends on the input probability distribution $p = \{p_1, \ldots, p_m : p_j \geq 0 \text{ and } p_1 + \cdots + p_m = 1\}$. A characterizing quantity for the transmission error is the worst-case mean squares error

$$\sup_p E[(e_k^t)^2] = \sup_p \sum_{j=1}^m \sum_{i=1}^m (q_j - q_i)^2 p_{ij} p_j \leq \max_{j=1,2,..m} \sum_{i=1}^m (q_j - q_i)^2 p_{ij} := \sigma_t^2. \tag{9}$$

It is noted that since Φ is a function of signal-to-noise ratio E_s/N_0 and transmission rate which is determined by compression ratio μ and quantization level m, so is σ_t^2. This dependence will be denoted by

$$\sigma_t^2 = \lambda_t(E_s/N_0, \mu, m). \tag{10}$$

For some typical communication modulation schemes, we will derive explicit expressions for $\lambda_t(E_s/N_0, \mu, m)$ in subsequent sections.

2.2.2 Optimal resource allocations

Assumption B: Compression errors, quantization errors and transmission errors are independent.

Under assumption B, the overall errors in the integrated information processing and communication system can be derived as follows:

$$e_k = y_k - \widehat{y}_k = y_k - c_k + c_k - v_k + v_k - \widehat{y}_k = e_k^c + e_k^q + e_k^t,$$

where e_k^c is compression error, e_k^q is quantization error (31), and e_k^t is transmission error. Hence, under assumption B, and under the worst-case input distributions, the mean squares error is

$$\sigma^2 = \sup_p Ee_k^2 = E(e_k^c)^2 + E(e_k^q)^2 + E(e_k^t)^2 = \sigma_c^2 + \sigma_q^2 + \sigma_t^2. \tag{11}$$

where σ_c^2, σ_q^2, and σ_t^2 is mean square errors for compression, quantization and transmission respectively. By substituting the complexity relationships (7), (8), and (10) into this expression, we obtain an overall complexity function

$$\sigma^2 = \lambda\left(\mu, m, \frac{E_s}{N_0}\right) = \lambda_c(\mu) + \lambda_q(m) + \lambda_t\left(\frac{E_s}{N_0}, \mu, m\right). \tag{12}$$

For a given communication resource, compression ratio μ and quantization level in bits $\log_2^m$ are inversely proportional to each other for a particular transmission rate, namely $\mu * \log_2^m = C$, and C is determined by the assigned channel bandwidth and the selected modulation method. In order to minimize the overall mean squares error, we shall minimize the following performance index:

$$\min_{\mu,m}\left[\lambda\left(\mu,m,\frac{E_s}{N_0}\right)\right]=\min_{m}\left[\lambda_c\left(\frac{C}{\log_2^m}\right)+\lambda_q(m)+\lambda_t\left(\frac{E_s}{N_0},\frac{C}{\log_2^m},m\right)\right]. \tag{13}$$

2.3 Mathematical analysis of WLAN-based medical information systems

2.3.1 Typical modulation schemes and channel models

In digital communication systems, popular modulation schemes include phase shift keying (PSK), frequency shift keying (FSK), amplitude shift keying (ASK), continuous phase modulation (CPM), and some hybrid combinations such as quadrature amplitude modulation (QAM). For every modulation scheme there are several sub-modulation methods, for example, PSK includes bi-phase shift keying (BPSK), quadri-phase shift keying (QPSK), multiple phase shift keying (MPSK), differential PSK (DPSK), etc.

Suppose that a memoryless symmetric binary channel transmits $x_k = a > 0$ for the bit $v_k = 1$ and $x_k = -a$ for the bit $v_k = 0$. The output of the channel is $w_k = x_k + d_k$, where d_k is the additive channel noise. The decoding scheme is that $\widehat{y}_k = 1$ if $w_k \geq 0$, and $\widehat{y}_k = 0$ if $w_k < 0$. d_k is assumed to be i.i.d., zero mean, and has finite second moments. The probability density function of d_1 is $f_d(x)$, which is symmetric to the origin. The accumulative probability distribution is denoted by $F(x)$. Consequently, the probabilities of transmission errors can be derived as

$$P\{\widehat{y}_k = 0|v_k = 1\}= P\{w_k < 0|x_k = a\} = P\{d_k < -a\} = \int_{-\infty}^{-a} f_d(x)dx = F(-a) := p_e.$$

$$P\{\widehat{y}_k = 1|v_k = 0\}= P\{w_k \geq 0|x_k = -a\} = P\{d_k \geq a\} = \int_{a}^{\infty} f_d(x)dx = F(a) := p_e.$$

since $f_d(x)$ is symmetric.

For example, if the disturbance is Gaussian distributed with variance σ^2, its probability density function is

$$f_d(x) = \frac{1}{\sqrt{2\pi}\sigma}e^{-x^2/\sigma^2}. \tag{14}$$

It follows that $p_e = \int_a^\infty f_d(x)dx = Q(a/\sigma)$ where $Q(x) = \frac{1}{\sqrt{2\pi}}\int_x^\infty e^{-\tau^2/2}d\tau$ is called the complementary error function.

In a typical BPSK modulation (11), $\sigma = \sqrt{\frac{N_0}{2T_b}}$, where $T_b = \frac{1}{R}$ and R is the transmission rate. In this case,

$$p_e = Q(a/\sigma) = Q\left(a/\sqrt{\frac{N_0}{2T_b}}\right).$$

For BPSK energy per symbol $E_s = a^2 T_b$, and symbol error probability is

$$p_e = Q\left(\sqrt{\frac{2E_s}{N_0}}\right). \tag{15}$$

Consequently, the probability transition matrix Φ in (5) under BPSK modulation is $\Phi = \begin{bmatrix} 1-p_e & p_e \\ p_e & 1-p_e \end{bmatrix}$.

Similarly, the symbol error probability for differential binary PSK (DBPSK) modulation is (23)

$$p_e = \frac{1}{2}exp\left(-\frac{E_s}{N_0}\right). \tag{16}$$

The symbol error probability for M-ary PSK (MPSK) modulation is

$$p_e \approx 2Q\left(\sqrt{\frac{2E_s}{N_o}}sin\left(\frac{\pi}{M}\right)\right), \tag{17}$$

and the symbol error probability for M-ary DPSK (DMPSK) modulation is (15)

$$p_e \approx 2Q\left(\sqrt{\frac{2E_s}{N_o}}sin\left(\frac{\pi}{\sqrt{2}M}\right)\right), \tag{18}$$

where M is is the size of symbol set.

2.3.2 Transmission errors of WLAN(802.11b) integrated systems

To simplify our analysis we use IEEE 802.11b WLAN as a typical communication environment (802.11a, 802.11g or 802.11n will have similar results). There are four transmission rates, 1Mbps, 2Mbps, 5.5Mbps and 11Mbps, in IEEE 802.11b WLAN. Different transmission rates use different modulation methods (38). When the transmission rate equals 1Mbps, DBPSK modulation and DSSS (direct-sequence spread spectrum) are used. When the transmission rate equals 2Mbps, DQPSK (differential quandary PSK) modulation and DSSS are used. When the transmission rate equals 5.5Mbps and 11Mbps, combined PSK and CCK (complementary code keying) are used. Precise evaluation of symbol errors of each transmission rate is a complex problem. Here we analyze the transmission errors of DBPSK and DQPSK modulations as examples.

1. **System Analysis under DBPSK Modulation**

   The probability transition matrix Φ_0 in (5) under DBPSK modulation is similar to that under BPSK modulation, and p_e is given in (16), then

$$\Phi_0 = \begin{bmatrix} 1-p_e & p_e \\ p_e & 1-p_e \end{bmatrix}.$$

   If inputs have only two possible values, i.e. the quantization level m is 2, then matrices Φ and Φ_0 are equal, and by (9)

$$\sigma_t^2 = \sup_{\substack{p_1,p_2\geq 0\\ p_1+p_2=1}} \sum_{j=1}^{2}\sum_{i=1}^{2}(q_j-q_i)^2 p_{ij}p_j = (q_2-q_1)^2 p_e(p_1+p_2) = (q_2-q_1)^2 p_e.$$

   Since $p_{12} = p_{21} = p_e$ and $p_1+p_2 = 1$, by (3), $\sigma_t^2 = (q_2-q_1)^2 p_e = \delta^2 p_e$. In general, the corresponding elements of the probability transition matrix Φ in (4) under DBPSK modulation is $p_{ij} = (p_e)^{\alpha}(1-p_e)^{(l-\alpha)}, i,j = 1,2,..,m$, where l is the number of bits per code, and α is the number of error bits. As a result, the mean squares errors of transmission

(9) is

$$\begin{aligned}\sigma_t^2 &= \sup_{\substack{p_1,\dots,p_m \geq 0 \\ p_1+\dots+p_m=1}} \sum_{j=1}^{m}\sum_{i=1}^{m}(q_j - q_i)^2 p_{ij} p_j \\ &= \sup_{\substack{p_1,\dots,p_m \geq 0 \\ p_1+\dots+p_m=1}} \sum_{j=1}^{m}\sum_{i=1}^{m}(q_j - q_i)^2 (p_e)^{\alpha}(1-p_e)^{(l-\alpha)} p_j \\ &= \max_{j=1,\dots,m} \sum_{i=1}^{m}(q_j - q_i)^2 (p_e)^{\alpha}(1-p_e)^{(l-\alpha)}.\end{aligned}$$

2. **System Analysis under DQPSK Modulation**

The probability transition matrix Φ_0 in (5) under DQPSK modulation now becomes a 4 $\times$ 4 matrix. We have

$$\Phi_0 = \begin{bmatrix} 1-2p_e-p_e' & p_e & p_e' & p_e \\ p_e & 1-2p_e-p_e' & p_e & p_e' \\ p_e' & p_e & 1-2p_e-p_e' & p_e \\ p_e & p_e' & p_e & 1-2p_e-p_e' \end{bmatrix}.$$

By equation (18)

$$p_e \approx 2Q\left(\sqrt{\frac{2E_s}{N_o}} sin\left(\frac{\pi}{4\sqrt{2}}\right)\right).$$

For DQPSK modulation $p_e' \approx p_e^2$, and the transmission error σ_t^2 in equation (9) is

$$\begin{aligned}\sigma_t^2 &= \sup_{\substack{p_1,\dots,p_4 \geq 0 \\ p_1+\dots+p_4=1}} \sum_{j=1}^{4}\sum_{i=1}^{4}(q_j - q_i)^2 p_{ij} p_j \\ &= \max_{j=1,\dots,4} \sum_{i=1}^{4}(q_j - q_i)^2 p_{ij} \\ &= (q_2-q_1)^2 p_e + (q_3-q_1)^2 p_e' + (q_4-q_1)^2 p_e \\ &= 10\delta^2 p_e + 4\delta^2 p_e'.\end{aligned}$$

3. **An Illustrative Example: Uniformly Distributed Signals through 1Mbps Rate WLAN Channel (DBPSK Modulation)**

Suppose a signal is transmitted through a WLAN channel using 1Mbps transmission rate (DBPSK modulation). Assume the input signal v_k is uniformly distributed from 1 to m, where m is quantization level. Then we have $p_j = \frac{1}{m}$, for $j = 1, ..., m$. A quantized value needs $l = log_2 m$ bits to represent, and transmission probability matrix Φ of the WLAN channel is same as matrix (4) with $p_{ij} = P\{y_k = q_i | v_k = q_j\} = (p_e)^{\alpha}(1-p_e)^{(l-\alpha)}$ where α is the number of error bits. If no error occurs after passing through a wireless channel, then $y_k = v_k$, $p_{ij} = (1-p_e)^l$, and $\sum_{i=1}^{m} p_{ij} = 1$. Normally when a quantized value is transmitted through the WLAN channel, the possibility of error transmission is much less than the possibility of error-free transmission, namely, $p_e << 1 - p_e$. Hence, for simplicity we assume that all error possibility for a particular input is $p_{ij} = \frac{1-(1-p_e)^l}{m-1}$ for any $i \neq j$.

When quantization level is m or bits per value are l in our case, p_{ij} is

$$p_{ij} = \begin{cases} (1-p_e)^l & \text{if } q_i = q_j; \\ \frac{1-(1-p_e)^l}{m-1} & \text{if } q_i \neq q_j. \end{cases}$$

The probability matrix (4) becomes

$$\Phi = \begin{bmatrix} (1-p_e)^l & \frac{1-(1-p_e)^l}{m-1} & \cdots & \frac{1-(1-p_e)^l}{m-1} & \frac{1-(1-p_e)^l}{m-1} \\ \frac{1-(1-p_e)^l}{m-1} & (1-p_e)^l & \cdots & \frac{1-(1-p_e)^l}{m-1} & \frac{1-(1-p_e)^l}{m-1} \\ \vdots & & \cdots & & \vdots \\ \frac{1-(1-p_e)^l}{m-1} & \frac{1-(1-p_e)^l}{m-1} & \cdots & \frac{1-(1-p_e)^l}{m-1} & (1-p_e)^l \end{bmatrix}.$$

The transmission error σ_t^2 of (9) is

$$\begin{aligned} \sigma_t^2 &= \sup_{\substack{p_1,\ldots,p_m \geq 0 \\ p_1+\ldots+p_m=1}} \sum_{j=1}^{m}\sum_{i=1}^{m}(q_j-q_i)^2 p_{ij}p_j \\ &= \frac{1-(1-p_e)^l}{(m-1)m}\sum_{j=1}^{m}\sum_{i=1}^{m}(q_j-q_i)^2 \\ &= \left[\frac{1-(1-p_e)^l}{(m-1)m}\right]\delta^2\sum_{j=1}^{m}\sum_{i=1}^{m}(j-i)^2 \\ &= \left[\frac{1-(1-p_e)^l}{(m-1)m}\delta^2\right]\left[2L\sum_{i=1}^{m}i^2 - 2\left(\sum_{i=1}^{m}i\right)^2\right] \\ &= \left[\frac{1-(1-p_e)^l}{(m-1)}\delta^2\right]\left[\frac{m(m+1)(2m+1)}{3} - \frac{m(m+1)^2}{2}\right] \\ &= \delta^2\left[1-(1-p_e)^l\right]\left[\frac{2^l(2^l+1)}{6}\right], \end{aligned}$$

where p_e equals $\frac{1}{2}exp\left(-\frac{E_s}{N_0}\right)$ by equation (16).

To get a general equation of overall error in the studied system, we do not compress the signal here, since as shown in Figure 2, compression ratio μ and compression error σ_c^2 are highly specific to the input signals. The compression ratio will vary greatly for different signals with a given threshold ε. Consequently, the overall error in equation (11) for signal y_k is:

$$\sigma^2 = E[e_k - E(e_k)]^2 = \sigma_q^2 + \sigma_t^2 = \frac{y_{max}^2}{2^{2l}}\left[\frac{1}{3} + 4\left(1-(1-p_e)^l\right)\left(\frac{2^l(2^l+1)}{6}\right)\right].$$

Figure 3 shows the mathematic results for a signal with $y_{max} = 1$. For a given uniformly distributed signal y_k there is an optimized value l to minimize the overall error when

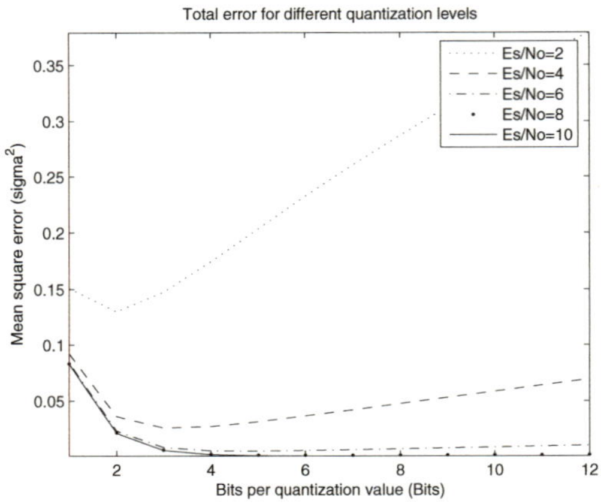

Fig. 3. Optimized quantization levels for Es/No=2, 4, 6, 8, 10

the signals are transmitted through a wireless channel. The optimized values vary with different signal-to-noise ratios.

3. Wireless-based medical information processing: Information accuracy and diagnosis reliability

3.1 WLAN-based medical information system simulation model

An integrated medical information processing and WLAN system is simulated in a MATLAB environment. Similar to the mathematical model in Figure 1, it includes six blocks: DCT block, data compression block, transmitter block (quantizer is included inside) (18), WLAN channel block, receiver block (18), and IDCT block.

The compressed DCT coefficients is embedded into IEEE 802.11b WLAN physical layer frames by adding PLCP (physical layer convergence protocol) preamble and header, modulation and spreading, upsampling and pulse shaping, etc. Packet sizes (1 to 8191 bytes) and preambles can be selected manually. The thermal noise characteristics (additive,white,and Gaussian) are used to model the noise in most wireless systems (13; 23). We simulated the WLAN channel using a memoryless symmetric binary AWGN (add white Gaussian noise) channel. Different channel (1 to 11), different signal-to-noise ratio (-10db to 20 db) and different transmission rates (1Mbps, 2Mbps, 5.5Mbps, and 11Mbps) can be selected. At receiver side, the 802.11b physical layer frames are processed by demodulation and despreading, deframing, removing PLCP preamble and header, etc., to recover the input DCT coefficients from the transmitter, and further through the IDCT block to retrieve the original time-domain medical signals.

1. **Simulation Scenario 1**

   Compression ratios and compression errors are highly specific to the input medical signals. As a result, it is difficult to get a general mathematics equation of compression errors. However, we can study compression effects using our simulation models. For simulation parameters, we select the signal-to-noise ratios to be sufficiently large to avoid errors involved with the WLAN channel. Figure 4 shows simulation results with compression ratio $\mu = 0.2$ (threshold $\varepsilon = 0.0141$). It compares the original time-domain signal and DCT coefficients with the received DCT coefficients and recovered signals, and shows the absolute errors in the fifth sub-figure. The errors in this scenario are mainly introduced through compression (note: in this scenario we set the quantization level to 2^{16}, and the resulting quantization errors are much smaller than the compression errors). We use the percentage RMS difference (PRD), which is calculated as in (19), to evaluate signal distortion. The PRD for the simulated lung sound signal is 2.59% when the compression ratio equals 0.2.

$$PRD(\%) = \sqrt{\frac{\sum_{i=1}^{n}[x_{org}(i) - x_{rec}(i)]^2}{\sum_{i=1}^{n}[x_{org}(i)]^2}} \times 100. \qquad (19)$$

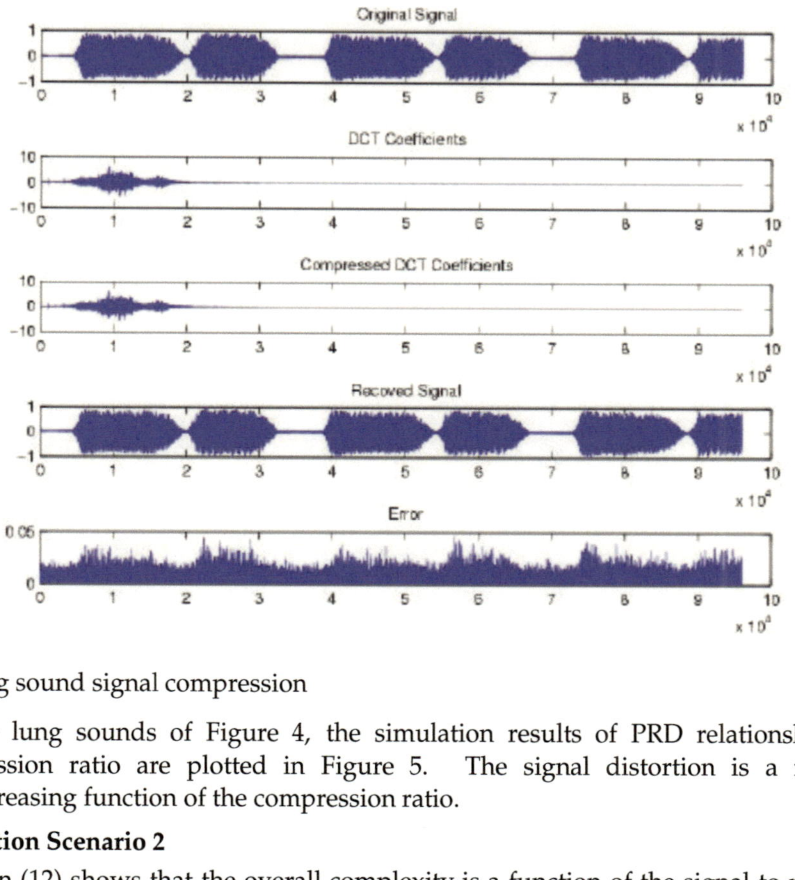

Fig. 4. Lung sound signal compression

For the lung sounds of Figure 4, the simulation results of PRD relationship to the compression ratio are plotted in Figure 5. The signal distortion is a monotone, non-increasing function of the compression ratio.

2. **Simulation Scenario 2**

   Equation (12) shows that the overall complexity is a function of the signal-to-noise ratio. To find the relationship of PRD to E_s/N_o, we transmit the lung sound signal through four WLAN channels (1Mbps, 2Mbps, 5.5Mbps, 11Mbps) with different signal-to-noise ratios. Figure 6 shows the results. In general, the larger the signal-to-noise ratio is, the less the transmission error is. If E_s/N_0 is larger than 12 dB, there is no transmission error on any WLAN channel. If Es/N_0 is smaller than 2 dB, 1Mbps becomes the only reasonable transmission rate. When the environment is noisy, to keep the same PRD value, we must increase the signal strength or transmit the signal at a low transmission rate. This involves an optimization problem between transmission power and transmission rate.

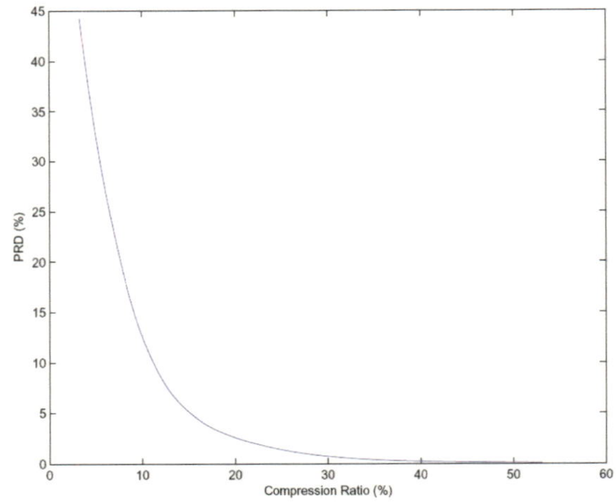

Fig. 5. PRD to compression ratio

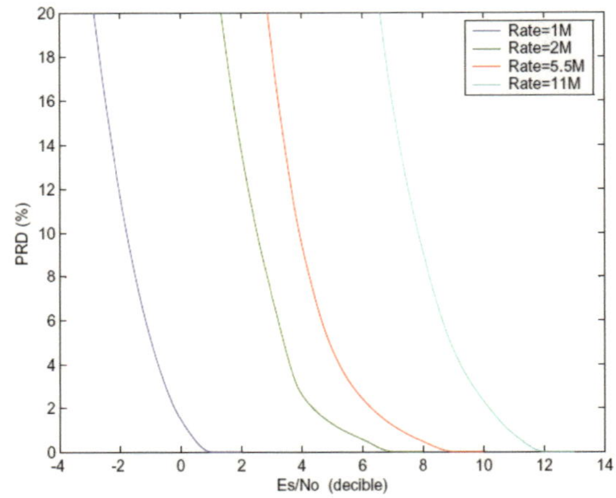

Fig. 6. PRD to Es/No using different WLAN transmission rate

3. **Simulation Scenario 3**

   In this scenario, we study the trade-off between compression ratios (and/or quantization levels) and transmission rates in WLAN under different signal-to-noise ratios.

   The more the compression ratio is (and/or the less the quantization levels are), the less the data size becomes. So the medical signal can be transmitted at a slower transmission rate with a higher compression error (and/or higher quantization error) and lower transmission error. There is an optimal point to minimize the overall error. Figure 7 shows the simulation results in different signal-to-noise ratios with a fixed quantization level (2^{16}). There is an optimized compression rate for a given signal-to-noise ratio with a fixed quantization level. For example, when E_s/N_o is 10db, the optimal compression ratio is about 40% with very small PRD. When E_s/N_o is 2db, the optimal compression ratio is about 10% with PRD around 16%. Optimizing medical data and wireless resources is important for an integrated medical information processing and

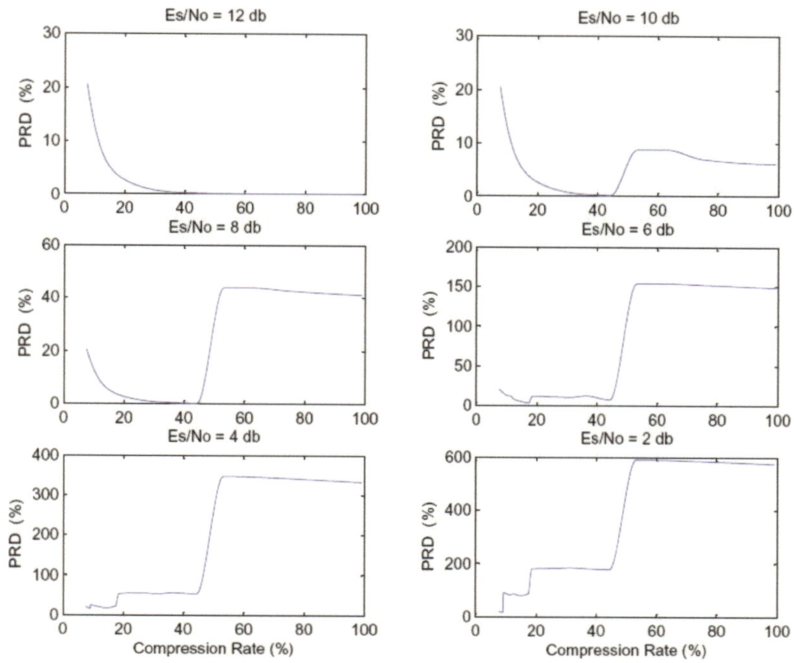

Fig. 7. PRD to compression ratio in different Es/No environment

communication system. From the figures, we notice that a small difference in compression ratio for a fix quantization level can result in a large difference in overall errors.

3.2 Medical pattern recognition and diagnosis reliability

3.2.1 Impact of information processing and transmission errors on lung sound diagnosis

Shown in the previous section, wireless transferred lung sound may be contaminated by data processing errors and/or transmission errors. If the overall errors are so severe as to alter the lung sound waveforms and patterns significantly, the lung sounds may no longer be suitable for diagnosis. Here we use an example of wheeze detection to illustrate the impact of overall errors on lung sound pattern recognition and diagnosis. Lung sounds were collected from a sophisticated human patient simulator under normal and wheeze conditions. Low, medium and high random noises were added to lung sounds to generate three sets of simulated overall errors. Several essential lung sound parameters were derived from lung sound data, such as FC_e (exhale peaking frequency), PS_e (exhale frequency bandwidth, i.e., exhale 90% frequency bandwidth that contains 90% of total power,), P_e (exhale total power), T_i (inhale length), S_i (inhale strength: RMS values), T_e (exhale length), S_e (exhale strength: RMS values), T (breath cycle length), etc., and diagnosis regions were designated from one or several parameters. Figure 8 illustrates the lung sound frequency domain parameter points (X-axle: exhale peaking frequency; Y-axle: exhale frequency bandwidth) under low, medium and high levels of overall error conditions respectively. Under the low error level, parameter points are clustered for both normal breath and wheeze, indicating a potential in achieving a high level of confidence in distinguishing wheeze from normal patterns. When the lung sound is corrupted by medium level errors, the parameter patterns are intervened, leading to a difficult pattern recognition problem. When errors are further increased to a high level,

the problem becomes even worse, and the parameter points of wheeze start to drift out of the wheeze region towards the normal region. This pattern shifting by noise artifacts significantly reduces diagnosis accuracy.
From the figure we can see that when lung sound is interfered by errors to some levels, the lung sound patterns have larger deviations and have a pattern shifting as well. Reduction of noise artifacts and signal processing errors is of essential relevance in medical diagnosis and highlights the issues of optimal utility of communication resources in medical diagnosis problems.

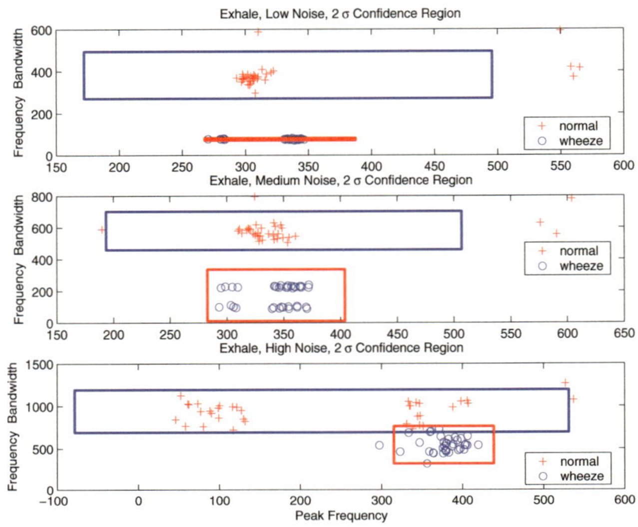

Fig. 8. Noise impact on normal lung sound and wheeze

3.2.2 Impact of noise on sound characteristics

To find the lung sound diagnosis pattern after passing the wireless telemedicine system we transmitted both normal and wheeze lung sound through the system. As we illustrated before noise will impact on lung sound patterns. Figure 9(a) shows a typical normal breathing sound and figure 9(b) shows an expirational wheeze (these are from the Human Patient Simulator, i.e. HPS, which was set as a 50 year old truck driver with normal condition and with wheeze disease respectively) (33–35). When collecting the data, we used a ventilation machine to control the breath and the environment noise was set as low as possible. The top figures are the raw data measured directly from the HPS. Since the existence of some low-frequency noise such as skin-scraping noises, chest movement noises, etc., the breathing patterns are not obvious. We used a high-pass filter to eliminate the noise under 200 Hz. After filtering, the difference between normal and wheeze lung sound can be clearly seen from their time domain waveforms. In the frequency domain analysis, the wheeze can be further characterized by a substantial narrowing of spectrum, shifting of center frequency (towards low pitch in this example), etc.. For this example, sounds are obviously very clean with minimum noise corruption. Lung Sound patterns are significantly altered when noise artifacts are present. Figure 9(c) shows the corrupted wheeze signal, both in its time-domain waveform and frequency-domain spectrum. It is clear that in a noisy environment, the characteristics of a wheeze are distorted to the point that it is no longer possible to recognize sound patterns.

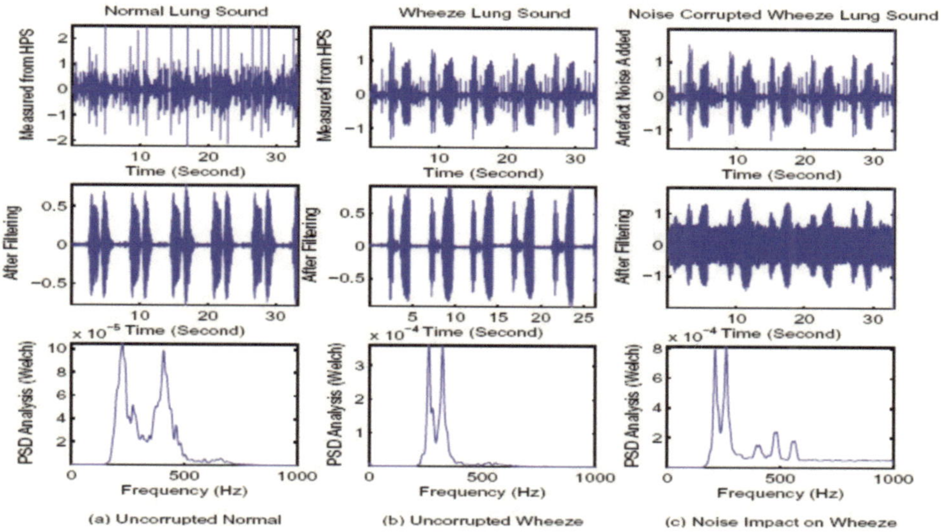

Fig. 9. A normal sound, a wheeze, and noise impact on sound patterns

3.2.3 Lung sound diagnosis after passing the wireless telemedicine systems

We shall reduce the noise by adaptive noise cancelation (ANC) method, see (33–35) for the details of ANC method, and use frequency domain characteristics of exhale signal to show the pattern of lung sound signals. Previous section told us that there is an optimized compression ratio or quantization level (in bits) for a particular signal-to-noise ratio of communication channel. Here we select same simulation module in section 5, and to simplified the analysis we do not compress the signal. Simulation result shows the optimal quantization level is 2^8.
After we received the lung sound signal, we plotted the lung sound frequency domain parameter points in a x(peak frequency)-y(frequency bandwidth) plane. Figure 10 illustrates the lung sound diagnosis pattern. The top figure shows the points of original lung sound signal, the meddle figure show the points of lung sound signal passing the WLAN-based telemedicine system when the quantization level is 2^8 and the signal to noise ratio is 10dB, and bottom one shows points of received lung sound signal after ANC process. To make clear we drew a 2σ confidence region both for normal and wheeze lung sound extracted parameters. From the figures we can see that after signals are transmitted through the system, the wheeze pattern data points are no longer in the wheeze region due to the quantization errors and transmission errors, and they mix with normal region, which makes the diagnosis incorrect. Fortunately, after ANC process the wheeze pattern data points are separated from normal region again, which correct the diagnosis.
ANC method separates the wheeze pattern region from normal pattern region. And the bottom one of figure 10 shows that there is distance between the normal 2σ confidence region and the wheeze 2σ confidence region. This comes out a problem: is it possible to reduce original lung sound signal data further while still make correct diagnosis ? The answer is: Yes. Figure 11 shows the result. Here quantization level is not 2^8 but 2^4 (The length of original lung sound data becomes half), and the other parameters of the system are kept same. We can see from bottom one of figure 11 that after noise cancellation the wheeze pattern region can still be separate from normal pattern region, however the distance of the two lung sound pattern region becomes shorter. So we can transmit less lung sound data than optimal one

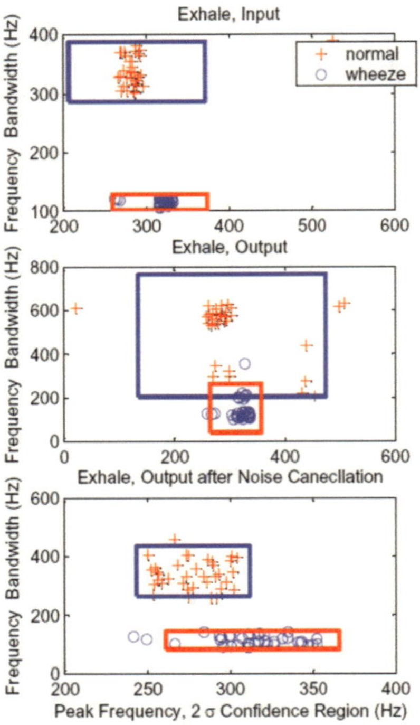

Fig. 10. Lung sound pattern when quantization level is 2^8

while can still distinguish wheeze lung sound to normal lung sound at receiver side, but the probability of error diagnosis will increase. There is a trade-off between them.

4. Security impacts of wireless channels

4.1 Weakness in wireless-based telemedicine systems

As wireless systems use an open medium, all the data transmitted or received over a wireless system like WLAN is susceptible to attacks from both passive eavesdropping and active interfering. There are several main common security threats in WLAN networks such as eavesdropping, deny of service, theft of service, etc. For example, an attacker can use some utilities like NetStumbler (47) to monitor all active access points in the area, and start Ethereal (48) to look for additional information. The attacker can then capture the packets with Airsnort (49), and crack the WEP key. With WEP key, an attacker can further sniff layer 3-7 packets. Portable medical equipment and sensors based on SCADA technology, increasingly utilize WiFi networks and thus are vulnerable to a combined wireless / SCADA attack. Such SCADA attacks would include Unauthorized Command Execution, SCADA Denial of Service, SCADA Man-in-the-Middle, Replay, and Malicious Service Commands. A focus on protection of the WiFi network is an essential step in reducing these vulnerabilities (14). As such security becomes one of the most pressing and challenging problems faced by WLAN networks (28). When a telemedicine system uses WLAN to transmit or receive medical signal, security becomes extremely important. Security features such as authentication and encryption are always considered, and the goal is to make WLAN traffic as secure as wired traffic (37).

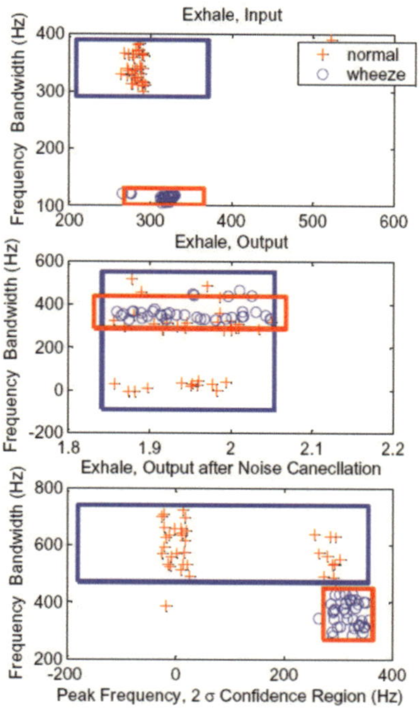

Fig. 11. Lung sound pattern when quantization level is 2^4

Bluetooth is another widely used wireless network standard. Though the security of Bluetooth is enhanced, malicious nodes can still use Denial of Service (DoS) attacks to prevent victims going through Bluetooth LAN access points.

4.2 Enhancement of WiFi security using 802.11i standard

WiFi alliance (52) defined two authentication standards i.e., WPA (Wi-Fi Protected Access) and WPA2. WPA was based on IEEE 802.11i standard (40), and used to replace WEP (Wired Equivalent Privacy). One major improvement in WPA is the TKIP (Temporal Key Integrity Protocol) which dynamically changes encryption keys when the WiFi is used. TKIP is combined with the much larger initialization vector to provide greatly improved protection from attacks against WEP. Moreover, WPA also provides MIC (Message Integrity Code) to greatly improve payload integrity. WPA2 is the advanced version of WPA which implemented the full mandatory parts of 802.11i. In addition to the TKIP and MIC, it also implements a new AES (Advanced Encryption Standard) based algorithm and CCMP (Counter Mode with Cipher Block Chaining Message Authentication Code Protocol) to enhance the security.
There are two modes for both WPA and WPA2: enterprise and personal. Enterprise WPA and WPA2 use IEEE 802.1X protocol (41), which is based on EAP (Extensible Authentication Protocol), and distributes different keys to each user through RADIUS authentication server. Figure 12 shows the authentication procedures (50). When an 802.11 mobile node (supplicant) tries to connect to the WLAN network, the access point will sent out EAP-Request identity packet, and the mobile node will response with the EAP-response packet that will be forwarded to the RADIUS server. The authentication server then begins the authentication procedures including sending out challenge and verifying challenge response. If mobile

node passes the authentication, RADIUS will accept the request, and allow normal traffic. Otherwise, RADIUS will reject the request and block all non-EAP traffic.

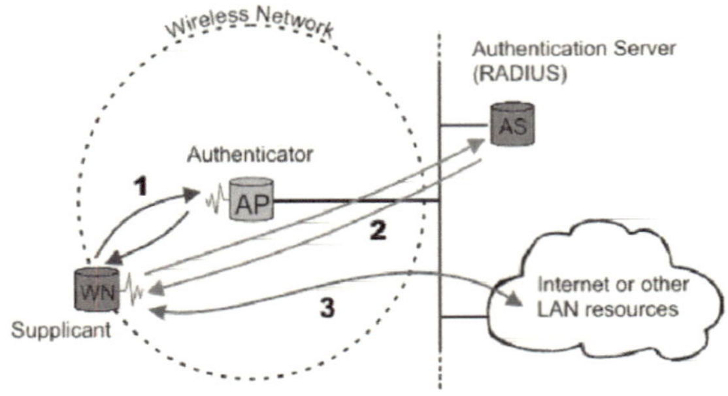

Fig. 12. EAP authentication

Personal WPA and WPA2 do not use RADIUS server to authenticate but utilize less scalable Pre-shared Key (PSK). In PSK mode, each mobile node is given the same passphrase.

4.3 Enhancement of security at home or residential areas

In most personal and residential areas where RADIUS is not available, the WLAN medical sensor nodes will use the PSK mode for both WPA and WPA2. Instead of using a complex and expensive authentication server, each user must enter a passphrase (up to 63 ASCII characters or 64 hexadecimal digits) to access the network. When using the ASCII characters, a hash function reduces it from 504 bits (63 characters $\times$ 8 bits/character) to 256 bits. For the PSK mode, the security level depends on the strength and secrecy of the passphrase, and is vulnerable to some attacks such as password cracking attacks, brute force attack, etc. Aircrack is one tool used to retrieve WPA and WPA2 PSK keys (44).
There are several ways to strengthen the PSK mode:

- Generate passphrases at their discretion, and pre-store on the medical sensor node to avoid re-entry;
- Employ a PBKDF2 (Password-Based Key Derivation Function) key derivation function;
- Bypass weak passphrase, and only allow passphrase using 40 characters or more.

Alternatively, mobile sensor nodes and access points can choose some privately defined security protocols to enhance the security level in residential areas. There are several such protocols, such as WAPI (WLAN Authentication and Privacy Infrastructure) (51). People may also implement high complexity authentication protocols based on their research and preference. However, as those methods are not standardized, people need to have the access to change the firmware of access points. Moreover, while private protocols are a good step, they do not ensure security. A prime example is the Lightweight Extensible Authentication Protocol (LEAP) developed by Cisco Systems which blocks all access until the client provides authentication credentials before a session key and access to the network is granted. ASLEAP is a tool to exploit LEAP. "Within months, some helpful person invested their time into generating a cracker tool. Publicizing the threat was a service to everyone, but I leave it as an exercise for readers to determine what satisfaction is obtained by the authors of tools that turn threat into reality and lay waste to millions of dollars of investments (45)."

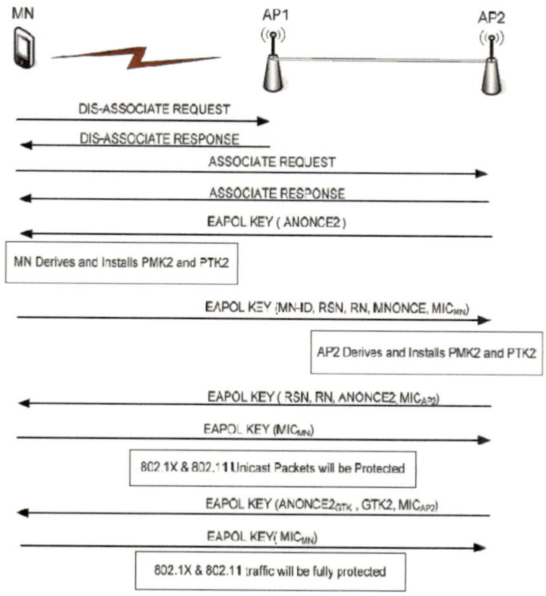

Fig. 13. Secure Fast Roaming Packet Streams

4.4 Secure session based fast roaming

WiFi-based telemedicine networks will normally comprise multiple access points in healthcare centers or at home to have full coverage. WiFi medical sensor nodes can roam freely between access points once they have been authenticated and associated to the telemedicine network, which means a sensor node can move in and out of coverage of different access points, and always associates with the strongest RF signal as it moves across the WiFi network. When a sensor node starts a roaming procedure, it will disassociate from the current access point and subsequently associate with the desired access point without losing connection and current communication session. And no new authentication is needed when a sensor node swap the access points. To do this, the WiFi sensor node will still keep catching neighbor access points' information from their beacon packets and/or probe response packets when it associates an access point. A roaming process will be triggered when one or more of following conditions meets (30):

1. RSSI (receive signal strength indication) from current access point is too low;
2. RSSI difference between neighbor access point and current access point is larger then threshold;
3. Excessive interface or noise for current access point;
4. Excessive retries when re-associates to access point;
5. Current access point has insufficient capacity;
6. Other transmission error exceed threshold; etc.

Medical sensor nodes must complete roaming and be able to pass data within 100-200 milliseconds when it decides to roam to a new access point (36). Figure 13 shows detailed roaming procedures when a WiFi mobile node moves from the coverage of one access point to another.

4.5 Problems with standard wireless security tactics

While it is essential to implement standard security methods, one needs to realize that individually each method is not enough. For example, disabling SSID broadcasting has no impact on network traffic. This is one layer of defense for a wireless network. A determined hacker tools like Kismet will probe wireless networks and by default the WAP responds with a message that contains its SSID. MAC filtering attempts to restrict access to known devices; but tools like Macshift (windows) and Macchanger (Linux) allow spoofing of MAC addresses to work around this defense.

Multiple layers of defense and complex defenses are the best methods of promoting security.

4.6 Wireless SCADA system concerns

In addition to the computers, laptops, and handheld devices, medical environments are increasingly integrating medical equipment and sensors into their wireless networks. Wireless smart beds automate patient charting, wireless robots bring pills to patients, wireless smart intravenous (I.V.) pumps deliver medication into patients (16), wireless heart monitoring tracks patients' heart health and adjusts medication accordingly (1), and various other wireless medical technologies are becoming common place (2; 8; 25; 39). Such medical equipment and sensors are supervisory control and data acquisition (SCADA) systems.

In July 2010, vulnerabilities of SCADA systems hit the mainstream news with the discovery of the Stuxnet trojan. The Stuxnet trojan attacked Siemens PLCs, using a default password hard-coded in the Siemens Simatric WinCC software to access the SCADA MS SQL database. Stuxnet readily infiltrated systems that were NOT directly connected to the internet. Even before Stuxnet the President's Critical Infrastructure Protection Board and the Department of Energy realized the serious nature of SCADA vulnerabilities and developed 21 steps to improve the security of SCADA systems (42). DoD initiated a series of SCADA Security Workshops, which include a plugfest for live vulnerability testing of SCADA systems (43). There have been a number of examples of "war driving" to attack SCADA systems. The Maroochy Shire Sewage Spill in 2000, where a disgruntled employee accessed wireless sewage pumping stations, released millions of liters of raw sewage into nearby rivers and parks. SCADA attacks can take the form of unauthorized command execution, SCADA denial of service, SCADA man-in-the-middle, replay attacks, and malicious service commands.

With these examples in mind, one can easily envision wireless attacks aimed at wireless medical equipment and sensors. Patient charting could be manipulated. Medication dosage could be changed. Medical "war driving" would be localized, but trojans aimed at specific wireless medical equipment could impact large numbers of patients across the nation or even across the globe. The idea of deploying these wireless tools is to reduce errors by enabling doctors and nurses to input critical data on the spot and offer immediate and "reliable" access to patient information and records. Yet pursuit of this worthy goal via wireless and SCADA technologies introduces new and frightening vulnerabilities. There are some basic steps that can be applied to wireless medical equipment and sensors:

- Identify all wireless connections.
- Perform risk assessments and audits.
- Establish red teams.
- Limit access by MAC address.
- Disable SSID broadcasting.

- Lock down backdoors and change default passwords
- Disconnect unnecessary wireless connections
- Appropriately configure firewall
- Implement manufactures security features.

Some more in-depth security tactics would be:

- Install a wireless IDS (46)
- Encrypt bluetooth channels (a method which could be revised for any WiFi traffic)
- Utilize anomaly-based behavior analysis of wireless network traffic (4)

4.7 Advanced wireless security protection methods

This section will discuss a scheme to successfully trace attacking paths from malicious nodes as well as segregate and protect systems from these malicious nodes (3). It can be implemented in both WLAN (WiFi) and WPAN (Bluetooth, Zigbee). Another method mentioned in this section are Wireless Self Protection Systems. In combination with standard security methods, these methods build a multilayer defense for wireless security.

4.7.1 Wireless covert channel signaling

Denial of service (DoS) attacks is one of active interfering attacks using which an attacker can cause congestion in WLAN or WPAN network either by generating an excessive amount of traffic itself, or by making other nodes generate excessive amounts of traffic. Besides common DoS attacks incurred in wired networks which transmit falsified route updates or reduces the TTL (time-to-live) field in the IP header, etc., WLAN or WPAN networks have their own unique DoS attacks. For example, an attacker can cause a particular node to continuously relay dump data to use up the battery of that node. DoS attack is a serious problem for WLAN or WPAN networks for medical applications, especially when the they networks are connected to a scatternet or a local area network. In this case, because malicious nodes from anywhere in the scatternet or anywhere in the LAN can launch the DoS attacks, they can block time-essential or even life-threatening information from being sent through the networks or disable the WLAN or WPAN networks. Covert channel signalling can be used to trace DoS attack paths back to the malicious nodes:

Establish Cover Channels

An end-to-end authentication may prevent DoS attacks from being launched, however if two nodes collude, DoS attacks are still quite feasible (10). To detect malicious nodes in a WLAN or WPAN network, schemes of covert channels have been designed (3; 21), which are implemented in baseband layer, logical link control layer, and service discovery layer. Those covert channels may inject probabilistically device information through the access points, and based on the injected information the DoS victims may reconstruct the complete path from the packets.

Trace Back with Covert Channels

When tracking back function is enabled, the WLAN or WPAN access points write their MAC addresses (each has 48 bits) or IP addresses (each has 32 bits for IPv4 or 48 bits for IPv6) into the designed covert channel of packet headers probabilistically (3; 20). When the victim receives the packets, necessary information can be extracted from the covert channels of those packets. To make the tracing back more accurate and robust, access points need to insert the checksum into the packets header fragments. Checksum function should be random and unpredictable to the attacker. A random hash function, for example, can be used (9).

Reconstruct Attack Paths

When the victim node receives a set of packets which were marked by access points with a certain probability, it extracts the embedded bits from the covert channel. After removes the duplicates, it then sorts the blocks that have the same checksum. By combining all the fragments, the victim will recover the original address chain information (3; 9). The attacking path from the malicious node to the victim is reconstructed.

4.7.2 Wireless self protection systems

Wireless Self Protection Systems (WSPS) are an advance security method capable of detecting complex attacks and responding to these attacks. WSPS uses abnormality metrics collected from multi-channel packet monitors and signal analyzers. These metrics form a foundation to recognize potential attacks, which allows appropriate responses. The collected signal, channel and frame metric attributes are unique for each wireless network device (5). Figure 14 shows the flowchart of WSPS.

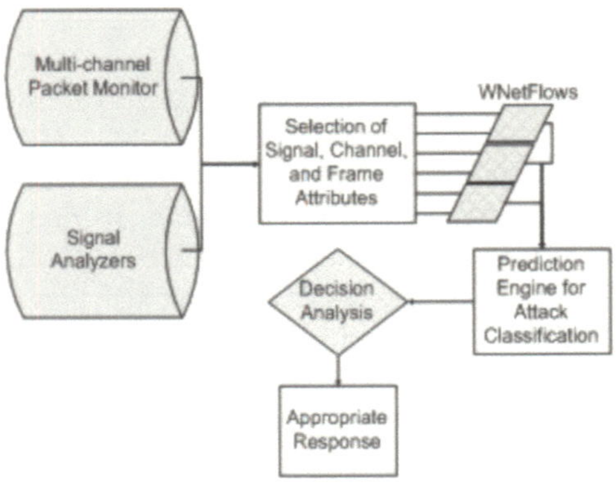

Fig. 14. WSPS Flowchart

Signal attributes can include device name, encryption type, signal strength, and source type (client station, WAP, etc.). These are good for detecting man-in-the-middle attacks and MAC attacks. Channel attributes can include channel number, frequency used, IEEE standard used, AP and master device names, and channel reuse. Frame attributes can include sequence ID, date and time, source and destination (MAC and IP), packet size, frame type, application name, source rate, and frame sequence number. Good for detecting replay and address spoofing (12).

Wireless network flows (WNetFlows) are developed and explored by anomaly based behavior analysis to identify relevant attributes of normal traffic (6). Metric attributes combine to form a WNetFlow-key for each WNetFlow. Common attributes of the WNetFlow keys are utilized to determine specific traffic types. Based on the WNetFlows, a prediction engine classifies the attack. When an attack is identified, then a decision analysis function dynamically determines an appropriate response in order to minimize vulnerabilities from that attack. Some actions that can be taken include deauthentication of the attacker, utilizing the attack signal power to identify the attacker location and physically stopping the attack, and shutting down WAPs in order to stop the attacker (5). Experimental results show that the WSPS approach can protect from wireless network attacks with an average detection rate of 99.13% for experimented attacks (4).

5. Conclusions

In this chapter, medical signal accuracy in a WLAN-based telemedicine system was studied. Relationships of medical information processing and wireless communication channels were discussed in an integrated medical information system containing the key function blocks: DCT transform, data compression, quantization, wireless channels, and IDCT transform. Explicit interactions between complexity and errors of each block were derived. Transmission errors are directly proportional to transmission rates and channel noise level, while data compression and quantization errors are inversely proportional to their respective compression ratios and quantization levels. There is a fundamental trade-off between overall information errors in these blocks. For example, the less the compression ratio is, the less the data size becomes. Consequently, the data can be transmitted at a slower transmission speed. For a given resource such as bandwidth and signal-to-noise ratio, there exists an optimal allocation that maximizes overall information accuracy after passing information processing and communication channels. Relationships between information resource allocation and medical lung sound diagnosis pattern were examined in detail. When applied to medical information processing, it becomes clear that in an integrated medical information processing and wireless communication system, a small deviation from the optimization point of resource allocation can result in a significant change in overall errors, leading to less accurate and unreliable diagnosis. Lung sound signals were used to show the trade-off between signal pattern accuracy and resource allocation. Lung sound pattern was correctly recognized after proper resource optimization and noise cancelation.
Security challenges and methods were also examined in a wireless-based telemedicine system. Enhanced security technologies both in enterprise areas and personal areas were reviewed. Secure fast roaming and wireless SCADA systems were introduced. Finally, two advance security methods for wireless telemedicine systems, i.e., wireless covert channel signalling and wireless self protection systems were discussed.

6. References

[1] W. T Abraham, et al., Wireless pulmonary artery haemodynamic monitoring in chronic heart failure: a randomised controlled trial, *The Lancet, Vol. 377, Iss. 9766, Pgs. 658 - 666,* 19 Feb., 2011.

[2] L. Burnes Bolton, DrPH, RN, FAAN, et al., Smart Technology, Enduring Solutions: Technology Solutions Can Make Nursing Care Safer and More Efficient, *JHIM, FALL 2008, vol. 22 / No. 4*

[3] Q. Cheng, H. Qu, Enhancing Bluetooth Security with Covert Channel Signaling, *IEEE and IFIP Int. Conf. on Wireless Communications Networks,* June 2004.

[4] S. Fayssal, S. Y. Al-Nashif, Anomaly-Based Behavior Analysis of Wireless Network Security, *Fourth Annual International Conference on In Mobile and Ubiquitous Systems: Networking & Services, 2007. MobiQuitous 2007. pp. 1-8.* doi:10.1109/MOBIQ.2007.4451054

[5] S. Fayssal, Y. Al-Nashif, B. uk Kim, S. Hariri A Proactive Wireless Self-Protection System, *ACM International Conference on Pervasive Services (ACM ICPS 2008).*
[6] S. Fayssal, Wireless self-protection system, *Dissertation for The University of Arizona*, 2008, 155 pages.
[7] B. Firoozbakhsh, N. Jayant, S. Park, and S. Jayaraman, Wireless communication of vital signs using the Georgia Tech Wearable Motherboard, *2000 IEEE International Conference on Multimedia and Expo, ICME, Volume 3, 2000 Page(s):1253 - 1256 vol.3*, 30 July-2 Aug.
[8] T. Gao, et al., Wireless Medical Sensor Networks in Emergency Response: Implementation and Pilot Results, Technologies for Homeland Security, *2008 IEEE Conference on In Technologies for Homeland Security, 2008 IEEE Conference on (2008)*, pp. 187-192. doi:10.1109/THS.2008.4534447 Key: citeulike:4460555
[9] M. T. Goodrich, Efficient Parket Marking for Large-Scale IP Trace back. *CCS'02, November 18-22, 2002, Washington, DC, USA*
[10] V. Gupta, S. Krishnamurthy, and M. Faloutsos, Denial of Service Attacks at the MAC Layer in Wireless Ad Hoc Networks, *Report, Dept of EECS, UC Riverside.*
[11] S. Haykin, *Communication systems*, ISBN 0471178691, New York: Wiley, c2001.
[12] K. Hulin, C. Locke, P. Mealey, and A., Analysis of Wireless Security Vulnerabilities, Attacks, and Methods of Protection, *Information Security Semester Project*, Fall 2010
[13] T. B. Johnson, Thermal Agitation of Electricity in conductors, *Phys. Rev., Vol. 32*, July 1928.
[14] D. Kelley, Why SCADA Security Matters–And What You Should Know About It. /emph http://www.esecurityplanet.com/views/article.php/3901856/Why-SCADA-Security -Matters–And-What-You-Should-Know-About-It.htm
[15] I. Korn, *Digital Communications*, Van Nostrand Reinhold Company Inc., New York, 1985.
[16] L. Siv-Lee, L. Morgan, Implementation of Wireless Intelligent Pump IV Infusion Technology in a Not-for-Profit Academic Hospital Setting, *Hospital Pharmacy, Thomas Land Publishers Inc., Vol. 42, No. 9, Sept. 2007. http://thomasland.metapress.com/content/x280t2318u35l716/*
[17] S. Lehrer (2002). *Understanding Lung Sounds*, 3rd ed., W.B. Sounders, 2002.
[18] S. McGarrity, 802.11b PHY Simulink Model, *802.11b baseband physical layer, wireless communication*, Aug, 26th, 2002.
[19] H. Pasterkamp, S. Kraman and G. Wodicka, Respiratory sounds, *Am. J. Respir Crit Care Med. Vol. 156, pp.974-987*, 1997.
[20] T. Peng, C. Leckie, R. Kotagiri, Adjusted Probabilistic Packet Marking for IP Traceback, Department of Electrical and Electronic Engineering, The University of Melbourne, Victoria 3010, Australia, 2001
[21] S. Savage, D. Wetherall, A. Karlin, and T. Anderson. Practical Network Support for IP Traceback. *In Proceedings of the 2000 Acm Sigcomm Conference*, August 2000.
[22] A. M. Sayeed, A signal modeling framework for integrated design of sensor networks, *IEEE Workshop Statistical Signal Processing*, 28 Sept.-1 Oct. 2003 Page(s):7.
[23] B. Sklar, Digital Communications: Fundamntal and Applications. *ISBN 0-13-084788-7, Prentice Hall PTR Publishers, second edition*, 2001.
[24] A. Sovijarvi, P. Helisto et al., A new versatile PC-based lung sound analyzer with automatic crackle analysis (HeLSA); *repeatability of spectral parameters and sound amplitude in healthy subjects, Technology & Health Care.* 6(1), 1998 Jun, pp. 11-22.
[25] R. S. Tolentino, S. Park, Hospital RFID-Based Patient u-Healthcare Design over Wireless Medical Sensor Network, *Database Theory and Application, Bio-Science and Bio-Technology*

Communications in Computer and Information Science, 2010, Vol. 118, 299-308, DOI: 10.1007/978-3-642-17622-7_31
[26] H. Qu, L. Y. Wang, Y. Zhao, Integrated Information Processing and Wireless Communication: Complexity Analysis, *The International Conference on Communication Systems and Applications (CSA'06)*, July 3-5, 2006, Alberta, Canada.
[27] H. Qu, L. Y. Wang, Q. Cheng, E. Yaprak, H. Zheng, Wireless-Based Medical Information Processing: Integrated System Analysis and Simulation, *Proceedings of the International Conference on Telehealth (Telehealth'06)*, July 3-5, 2006, Alberta, Canada.
[28] H. Qu, Q. Cheng, E. Yaprak, Using Covert Channel to Resist DoS attacks in WLAN, *Proceedings of the International Conference on Wireless Networks (ICWN'05)*, Page.38-44, June 27-30, 2005, Las Vegas, USA..
[29] H. Qu, Q. Cheng, and E. Yaprak, Unconfined E-health care system using UMTS-WLAN, *International Journal of Modelling and Simulation, Issue 4*, 2006, ACTA Press.
[30] H. Qu, J. Cheng, Q. Cheng, L. Y. Wang, WiFi-Based Telemedicine System: Signal Accuracy and Security, *2009 International Conference on Computational Science and Engineering*, Vancouver, Canada August 29-August 31.
[31] H. Wang, L. Y. Wang, and H. Qu, Wireless-Based Identification of Patient Dynamics: Analysis and Quantization Design, *Volume 2 of the proceddings of the 11th WSEAS International Conferences on SYSTEMS*, Agios Nikolaos, Crete Island, Greece, July, 2007.
[32] L. Xiao, M. Johansson, H. Hindi, S. Boyd and A. Goldsmith, Joint optimization of communication rates and linear systems, *IEEE trans. on automatic control, vol. 48, no. 1*, Jan. 2003.
[33] H. Zheng, H. Wang, L. Y. Wang, and G. Yin, Time-Shared Channel Identification for Adaptive Noise Cancellation in Breath Sound Extraction, *Journal of Control Theory and Applications, Number 3, Volume 2*, August 2004, ISSN: 1672-6340, pages 209-221.
[34] H. Zheng, H. Wang, L.Y. Wang, and G. Yin, Lung Sound Pattern Analysis for Anesthesia Monitoring, *Proceedings of 24th American Control Conference*, June 8-10, 2005.
[35] H. Zheng, H. Wang, L.Y. Wang, G. Yin, Cyclic System Reconfiguration and Time-Split Signal Separation with Applications to Lung Sound Pattern Analysis, *IEEE Transactions on Signal Processing*, Vol. 55 Issue 6 Part 2, pp. 2897-2913, June 2007
[36] Cisco Compatible Extensions for WLAN Devices (CCXv1-v4).
[37] S. Weatherspoon, Overview of IEEE 802.11b security, *Network Communications Group, Intel Corporation. Intel Technology Journal*, 2000.
[38] LAN MAN Standards Committee of the IEEE Computer Society, Part 11: Wireless LAN Medium Access Control (MAC) and Physical Layer (PHY) Specifications ANSI/IEEE Std 802.11b, 2000.
[39] Shoreline Research, Wireless Solutions in Healthcare: Expanding Point of Care Practices and Services in Hospitals, *A Bluesocket BluePaper*.
[40] IEEE Standard for Information technology telecommunications and information exchange between systems local and metropolitan area networks specific requirements Part 11: Wireless LAN Medium Access Control (MAC) and Physical Layer (PHY) specifications Amendment 6: Medium Access Control (MAC) Security Enhancements, 2004.
[41] IEEE standard for local and metropolitan area networks Port-based network access control, 2001.
[42] U.S. Department of Energy: 21 Steps to Improve Cyber Security of SCADA Networks. *http://www.oe.netl.doe.gov/docs/prepare/21stepsbooklet.pdf*

[43] SCADA Security Workshop, *http://www.drighten.com/Events/index.html*
[44] *http//www.aircrack-ng.org*
[45] William Arbaugh and Jon Edney at Real 802.11 Security.
[46] http://www.ijcaonline.org/archives/volume5/number8/934-1312
[47] http://www.netstumbler.com/
[48] http://www.ethereal.com/
[49] http://en.wikipedia.org/wiki/AirSnort
[50] http://en.wikipedia.org/wiki/802.1x
[51] http://www.suntzureport.com/wapi/wapi.pdf
[52] http://www.wi-fi.org/

4

Design Criteria for Large eHealth Infrastructure Systems

Thomas Grechenig, Barbara Avana, René Baranyi,
Wolfgang Schramm and Anna Wujciow
Vienna University of Technology – Research Group for Industrial Software (INSO)
Research Industrial Systems Engineering (RISE)
Austria

1. Introduction

We live in a time where ubiquitous access to information is part of our daily lives. Most of us use the Internet for sending or receiving information every day. We store data about our daily lives and thanks to social networks, we are able to stay in contact with other people even easier than before. Interestingly one of the most important aspects in our private lives has not yet made the jump into the digital world: our health. While every doctor's office, hospital and insurer keeps a specific set of information about the progress of their patients' health, the patient itself rarely has the possibility to either read or contribute this set of information. In addition these piles of health information are completely disjoint. This means, that whenever a patient visits a physician, this patient him- or herself has to update the doctor about all the medical events that have happened since the last visit. For the patient, this is not necessarily an easy task. Not only is it very difficult for the average the patient to remember what happened when, but it is also very difficult for a layman to articulate these facts correctly.

This is where eHealth comes into play. EHealth infrastructures, when done properly, can help to aggregate data, provide the right information to the right people and most importantly give control about health related information back to the patient. EHealth itself is not a technology per se, but a collection of tools and technologies, which combine healthcare topics with computer technologies. These tools include telemedicine, electronic health records, electronic medical records, computer aided diagnosis, hospital information systems and many more. When talking about large health infrastructures, usually regional, national or international eHealth networks and systems are meant (Eysenbach, 2001).

The most common goals of large eHealth projects include a personal health record (PHR), confirmation of a patient's insurance status and electronic medication. Electronic medication in particular has the potential to positively affect daily health care. Not only does eMedication reduce paper work for health care providers (HCP), pharmacies and insurers, but also allows a streamlined process for preventing accidental prescription of medications with a negative cross interaction.

Planning eHealth strategies for healthcare providers or a nationwide healthcare system is one of the most critical aspects when starting programs or initiatives for eHealth and telemedicine implementation. The planning aspect involves building a strategic vision to align the goals of politic representatives or senior management with the needs of the e-Health marketplace. Technology management and system implementation relate to managing the diffusion of eHealth innovations, redesigning work practices so that both workers and users can work virtually (e-work), and addressing issues of user acceptance or failure arising from the implementation and evaluation of an eHealth system (Tan et.al, 2005).

Before approaching such a project, the vision on the strategic or political level must be carried to the institutions, which would be responsible for the eHealth or telemedicine project development. On the operational level of the institutions concrete measures are analyzed and planned. The technicians on the technical level are responsible for the implementation of the strategic infrastructure programs or application design.

Any sufficiently large IT infrastructure project on a regional, national or international level can be cognitively described along four major abstraction levels:

1. Political/Public Level - Political/Public Criteria (PC)
2. Institutional Level - Institutional Criteria (IC)
3. Operative Level - Operational Criteria (OC)
4. Technical Level - Technical Criteria (TC)

Engineering practices target only the technical level, while making quaint references to the existence of an operational level that might influence purely technical issues and decisions. The existence and the importance of the institutional level and the political level are usual ignored, if not outright denied in technical textbooks and university curricula. This is in strong contrast to the fact, that projects hardly ever fail on the technical level, and if so, only as a result of failures on the other levels.

This chapter presents an insight into the most important design criteria with their associated requirements and pitfalls on the four levels.

2. Political level

Every large-scale eHealth project begins on a political level. Politics in this context denotes not only a governmental body, but can also be a collection of persons inside a company or organisation. A functioning political level is essential for a successful eHealth project. Issues on the political level always have direct impact on the underlying levels, most critical on the technical.

First and foremost the ultimate goals of the project have to be defined. A system with aim to reduce healthcare costs will have other requirements than a project which is simply used to check the insurance status of a patient or a project with the aim to create a nation-wide personal health record. The important questions to ask are:

- What do we want to achieve with the new eHealth infrastructure?
- Who are the end-users?
- Will this project involve the creation of the specification and the implementation, or only the specification?
- How will the industry be included?
- Depending on the project goal: Who will be the stakeholder groups?

Only when these questions are answered discussions on a broader level can happen. Every decision that is made on this level determines the possible implementation, rollout and risk mitigation strategies, which are needed for a successful completion.

Most infrastructure projects are riddled with multiple conflicting goals, less than perfect responsibility delineations, infighting amongst participants and stakeholders and unclear budgetary and timing constraints. There will usually be an overwhelming number of documents claiming the contrary and brand name consulting companies involved to maintain the facade of orderly project management. This big mess during every project stage is not necessary. With clear communications, removal of typical "ego" personas, the early inclusion of patient and physician representatives and a complete project transparency, many of the problems arising from this pile of stakeholder can be prevented or at least diminished.

The level of the political criteria (PC) is sometimes under-estimated and sometimes over-estimated. Overestimation often occurs at that group of people whose daily business is in the public sphere, media and political space. Just as useful it is for a large eHealth infrastructure system that the locally political representatives engage themselves in the relevant ministries or trade spokesmen try to deal seriously with the topic, as inappropriate is often a direct public debate between different political representatives on the subject area of the eHealth system.

A general large eHealth system therefore needs across a common will of all parties to build such an infrastructure. If it is not possible to establish such consensus, the establishment as such must be called into question.

Underestimation of the criteria on political aspects is done regularly by technical specialists in the medical field or information technicians who are involved with building the infrastructure. As positive the value of the overall system of the level of medical or information technology may be, no system can be implemented against the public, the policy or against established cultural practices. In smaller IT environments it may be possible to set up systems against the established processes and users may adapt to the systems - this is a tradition in the 40 years of information technology. But in a system that affects nearly every citizen of a country and a very large protected practitioners group, the use case against the known tasks in everyday life results to a failure of the system.

In the triangle Nation / Health Sector / Citizen or Patient the right relationship of all parties has to be identified for each question or problem, then the potential of the use of eHealth, electronic health record or nationwide health telematic systems can be discussed (see fig. 1).

Promotion and ownership of the system are necessary for the public political discourse and a professional decision-making process.

The following criteria can be identified on the political level:

- **Consideration of cultural aspects and historical development in healthcare**
- **Appropriate and necessary innovation to implement the main systems for eHealth**
- **Healthy Growing: Creating a healthy eHealth Infrastructure Step-by-Step**
- **Appropriate design of the media presentation, dealing with fears and enhance Acceptance**
- **Appropriate allocation at the general governmental level**
- **Representation in parliament and other representative organisations for citizens**
- **Appropriate legislative measures to accompany the implementation process and operation of the system**

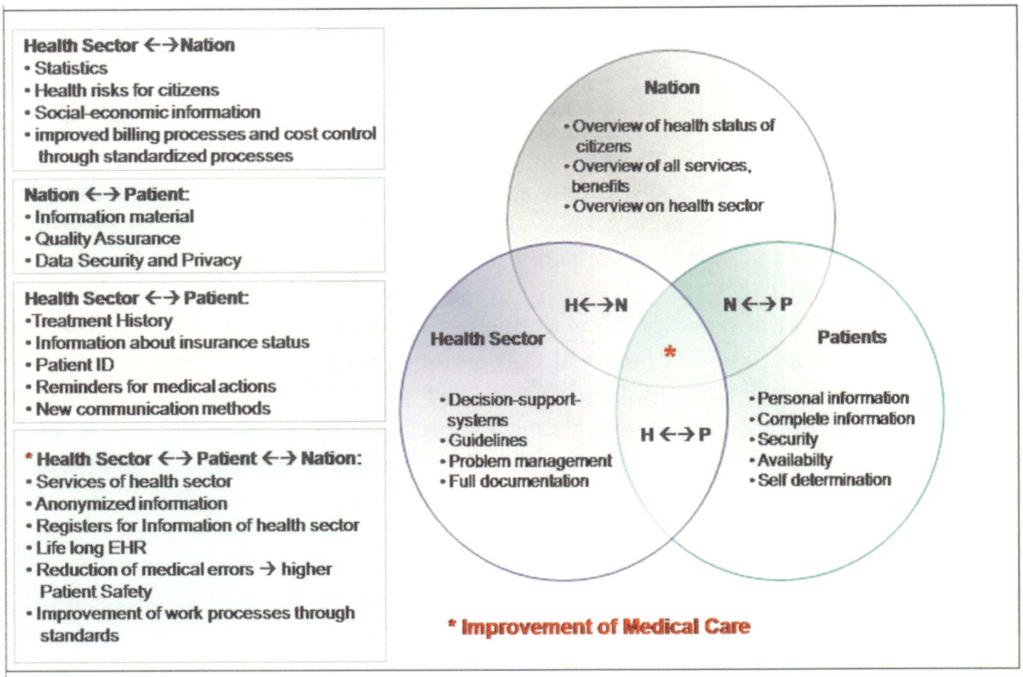

Fig. 1. Triangle of potentials of eHealth and health telematic systems (Larsen E., 2003)

2.1 Consideration of cultural aspects and historical development in healthcare

Of course there are always exciting innovations and of course innovative work flows can be introduced as part of new technology, but the basis of trust is gained with the possibility to use that which has been always used or to handle situation how they were previously feasible to handle.

Mapping the history means that the understanding, translation and analysis of it is a necessary prerequisite for a valid construction of the new system. It will not be made obsolete entirely, but re-implemented.

On the opposite the "electronification" of healthcare brings options and opportunities that appear for the patient as a pleasant relief. If a process previously was extremely difficult, such as the collection of a lesion, and which can be done in future by electronic delivery and saves a long way, certainly from the point of acceptance of the system is a hit.

2.2 Appropriate and necessary innovation to implement the main systems for eHealth

Until now different application modules for systems in eHealth have been identified by previous research and development as important to be implemented in a future-proof eHealth infrastructure. The most important of them are Electronic Health Records (EHR), eMedication systems and emergency data sets.

2.2.1 Electronic health records

One of many problems for a physician when diagnosing and treating a patient is to perform an accurate anamnesis. Many patients are not able to properly communicate a medical or medication history. This of course can lead to treatment mistakes, which in the worst case may end with the death of the patient. Therefore many large-scale eHealth projects also include an electronic health record platform. An electronic health record is the systematic collection of electronic health information about individual patients or populations (Gunter & Terry, 2005). This means, that every citizen is associated with a data set consisting of her or his medical history. Depending on the reason behind the electronic health record implementation, this may include diagnoses, hospital stays, medication history, etc. Ultimately a thoroughly implemented electronic health record can provide a safer and more effective healthcare for the patient by providing the physicians with the necessary information in every step of the treatment process. For this to work the support of the physicians is absolutely necessary.

When implementing an electronic health record, the project has to deal with two main user groups: patients and health care professionals. Both groups usually have strong opinions about this topic, which in turn will cause heated debates during the project phase. In sections 2.4 and 3 the fears and agendas of patients and health care professional are discussed in greater detail.

2.2.2 Emergency information

If a significant political resistance against a large scale electronic health record system is foreseeable, it is often advisable to start with an electronic health record with limited functionality. Such a minimal electronic health record could for example only include a patient's emergency information (e.g. allergies, contact person). The advantage with this approach is the possibility to start the rollout with a relatively low risk application, and then add additional functionality when the running system has a high stable performance (technical and political wise). In many cases this approach helps to avoid costly discussions and public debates.

2.2.3 Medication interaction

One of the most useful applications an eHealth system can include is the interaction check between multiple prescribed medications. Since a patient's complete treatment process usually involves multiple doctors, prescription with medications with adverse effects, can form. This can easily be avoided with an electronic medication system, which checks every prescription for potential hazards. Since a potential off-label use of medication lies at the discretion of the physician, such checks should ideally also be performed at the time of prescription in the doctor's office, not only at the time of dispensation at the pharmacy.

2.3 Healthy growing: Creating a healthy eHealth infrastructure step-by-step

In theory there are two main possibilities for creating a large eHealth infrastructure.

First: Include all conceivable state-of-the-art features into the project. This will create, at least on paper, a fully featured system that can be used to do everything even remotely eHealth related.

Second: After defining the immediate goals of the project, the next step is to evaluate possible implementation approaches and to test the waters for eventual resistance from potential stakeholder groups. The art when using this approach is to align the project goals with technical and political possibilities while maintaining the essential functionality required for a meaningful system.

While in theory the first approach could yield a fairly complete system, in reality it will be almost impossible to fully implement it. Every health topic causes debates on a political level, the more people involved or affected, the more intense these debates will be. The political and public resistance in such a project can easily reach critical levels up to the point where the project would be required to stop, or to be heavily reengineered. In practice, the second approach has a greater chance of actual finishing close to the planned duration. An early alignment between project goals and the opinion of involved stakeholders helps to alleviate public and political resistance. When taking this step, people should still be educated about the future possibilities while assuring that these future steps will only be performed if feasible and meaningful.

2.4 Appropriate design of the media presentation, dealing with fears and enhance acceptance

Health topics invoke strong emotions in everybody affected. There will be heated public debates from the first project presentation until after the project launch. There can be no general rule on how to prevent these discussions, since the political and public environment is different for each project. Typical attack points include project costs, technical safety of the final solution, changes in clinical workflows, and the general usefulness of the project. Certain parties will not hesitate to play with end-users' fears to motivate a movement against the project. Public disputes do not necessarily need to have a negative impact, in the contrary: Public disputes also provide the possibility for the project team to present their views and therefore the possibility to turn the public opinion into a favourable one. For this strategy to work the project needs to provide complete transparency about the intended project goals, the architecture, the implemented security measures and the level of involvement of political and industrial parties. Appropriate media presentation, the right information at the right time is needed.

Health in general and eHealth in particular are topics, which invoke emotional debates on the political and on the public level. Therefore it is essential that from early project stages on, the project goals, purpose and technologies are open and transparent. The end-user needs to know what individual information is stored in which way, who will be able to access it, and how the individual can control his or her information.

A typical fear of physicians includes the fear of increased control from payer organisations. A complete digitalisation of the treatment process and the traceable association between a treatment task introduces a transparency into a doctor's daily work, which is completely new to this field. Currently doctors are also required to meticulously document every step of a patient's treatment, but there are very few possibilities for outside institutions to actual verify that these steps really have been performed as stated. The only way to deal with this fear is to turn it into an advantage for the doctor. An accurate documentation provides assurance about previous treatments and illnesses and therefore increases the physician's treatment confidence.

Patients' fears are fundamental similar to the fears of the physicians. The fear to be a complete transparent patient for everyone to see is more than justified and must be taken seriously. The newspapers are full of reports about compromised IT systems. While these incidents are isolated events, they create an atmosphere of uncertainty. There are few technological possibilities to absolutely secure an IT system on a physical and application level, but these measures have to be open for discussion from early project stages on. Only a complete transparent and open specification of these security measures, where experts are allowed to freely comment can the project reassure concerned users. If does not take these security concerns seriously, it will have to deal with fearful patients and an increasingly worse public opinion.

2.5 Appropriate allocation at the general governmental level

A large eHealth Infrastructure system is as far as possible recognized as an "all-party" system because it makes little sense for investment with more than 10 or 15 years effect, is again and again re-questioned if a government or management changes. It is the duty of engineers to take precautions to ensure that certain political streams can be completely changed in the course of establishing and to anticipate that these streams can be integrated either easily or have no effect on the system at all.

2.6 Representation in parliament and other representative organisations for citizens

Main principles of the new system are established in a time period in which the parliamentary political discourse doesn't care much about it. But since a negative reaction of the competent parliamentarians, regardless of their fraction, at a time, where the technology can only be slightly changed, the involvement of specialists in the respective groups in the parliament at a reasonably early stage is certainly important.

Depending on the type of construction and the procurement of technology in the process of tendering and contract awards there are extensive public debates over task and award decision. In many countries this is controlled and steered of the respective industrial players, therefore the parliamentary needs to be informed properly.

Therefore it is necessary to have a general political statement, owner or writer of it. This must be done with professional modesty and neutrality. Political processes and large eHealth infrastructure systems are long-term projects, and therefore a only short-term successful fractionation is not advised for receiving overall success.

2.7 Appropriate legislative measures to accompany the implementation process and operation of the system

Appropriate legislation must be provided to grant a stable basis for the large scale/nationwide implementation and to minimize risks in the setup through policy enforcement. The best condition for the functioning of such an eHealth system and also the most important initial planning action is and remains the provision of a proper legal basis for the system establishment. Without such a legal basis any perfectly established system can be swept away after two or three years of construction by a political storm.

3. Institutional level

A large-scale eHealth project consists of several involved institutions. Every institution included in such a project has its own agenda and goal. This goal is not necessarily equivalent with the success of implementing a large-scale eHealth project in time and in budget. Long established institutions tend to fear that they risk losing influence and power if they are not able to increase and state their importance and needs in a large project. EHealth projects in particular contain a lot of institutions with longstanding traditions (e.g. general practitioners or hospitals) and every one of them wants their fair share of influence. So the final goal (from the political level) should be that every institution in the project feels an immediate benefit from such a system and suffers no visible loss in reputation or

influence. Even though this is hard to achieve – it might be advisable to give the institutions the impression, that their goals and requirements are the most important ones. The final system needs to combine requirements from all participating institutions (these requirements need to be discussed and adapted for the final system - see Fig. 2). To make that happen, the project initiators need to know which institutions are involved and what their respective agenda is. You should bring their goals to the table and start a solution finding when it is defined which institutions will participate. The results of this process should give the political level the opportunity to compare the benefits and costs of the various options resulting from the institutions' requirements/wishes/necessities. It is important to remember, that the duration of the solution finding process increases with the amount of involved institutions and the nature of their respective goals. It might be a good starting point to initially align goals between the institutions. Another issue might be the public perception on this process. Some institutions might misuse the general opinion of citizens for their agendas. e.g. a institution may spread fears among people by releasing only parts of the results of the discussion process. These may be avoided by providing transparency throughout every institution and the general population (see also chapter 2.4).
The above stated aspects can be summarized into the following important points of the institutional level:

- **Identify Institutions:** Which institutions are involved and what agenda or goal do they have?
- **Describing benefit:** What is the benefit for the system for the institutions?
- **Solution process:** The goals of every institution should be discussed with them. The requirements of the solution finding process should be taken into consideration by the political level.
- **System acceptance:** among the institutions there are different stages of acceptance. Some of them will like the system and some will not like it at all. You have to determine why acceptance among some groups is low and try to increase it.

Usually a large-scale eHealth project consists of many stakeholders/roles from various institutions with different sights. Because of the uniqueness of every large scale eHealth project the institutions and the involved roles will not always be the same but a few of these institutions will be part of nearly every large-scale eHealth project:

- **Primary and secondary healthcare centres:** These healthcare centres represent institutions, which are responsible for delivering the initial care in most countries. They might be users or promoters of a large-scale eHealth system. The centres are essential for promoting and increasing acceptance among citizens, because they are the first or even the single point of contact in terms of healthcare.
- **Health Insurances:** depending on the national healthcare funding, public or private health insurances play major roles in budgeting and funding of healthcare services.
- **Hospitals:** hospitals consist of multiple user groups which potentially will access the final system.
- **Pharmacies:** a pharmacy is a user of a eHealth system or a promoter for it.
- **Nursing and Nursing homes**: After-hospital-care is often offered by nursing services or nursing homes. Even if immediate patient referral is usual, data of patients are seldom taken from one institution to the other. Integrated care will have to be considered on supporting IT systems.
- **Patients:** the patient delivers data to an eHealth system or uses it. Patients are very heterogeneously distributed and therefore it is difficult to find the appropriate solution

to the requirements raised by them especially if there is no representative (which is normally the case) present.

See Fig.2 for the different roles and sights of a large-scale eHealth project.

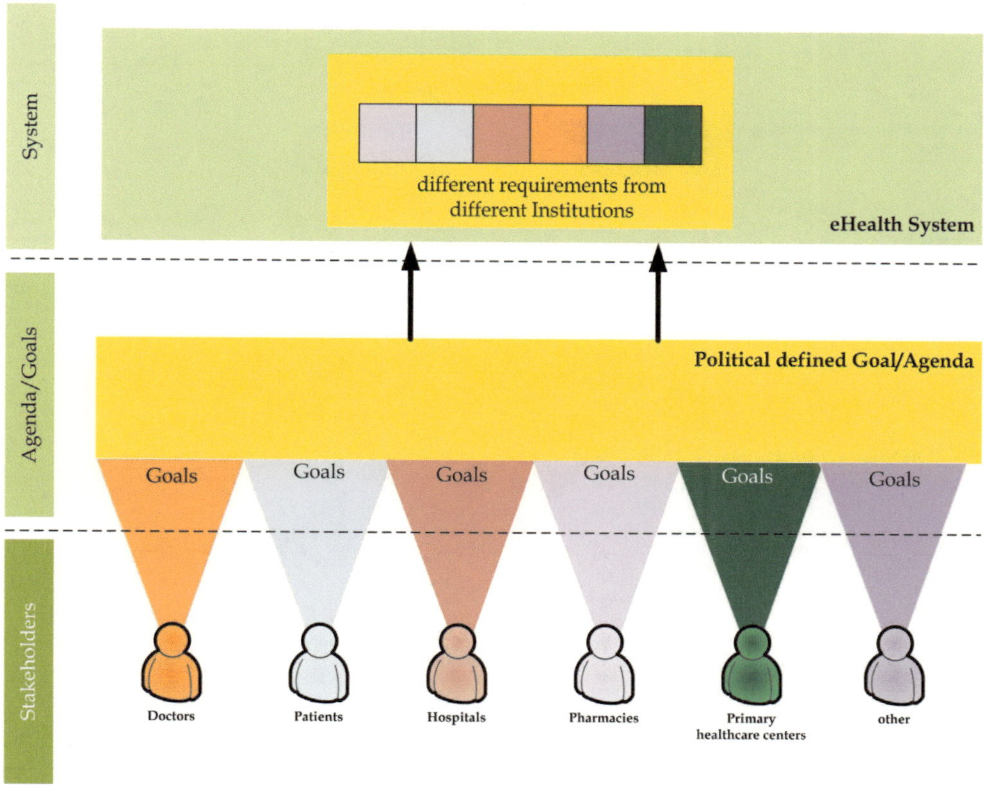

Fig. 2. Different roles and sights

Acceptance among institutions might be the most important part in the design of an eHealth system - what is the best (in terms of technical planned and designed) system worth if nobody is using it?

But the acceptance has to be widespread among every involved institution (or even further, to institutions who are not directly involved) and not focused on one group. Normally there are institutions, which have a high acceptance towards a new eHealth Systems and institutions which have lower acceptance. First it should be determined why the acceptance might be low (e.g. their goals might not be met) and then try to increase it by actively including them in further requirements engineering phases.

An approach to satisfy all stakeholders, is to integrate them in the design process very early and iteratively. Fig.. 3 shows this iterative process for the design of a large scale health IT network.

3.1 System acceptance for primary and secondary healthcare centers

As initial point of contact in most of the care cases, the primary and secondary healthcare centers play a major role in opinion formation. Doctors and their institutional representatives tend usually to have a rather critical role for larger eHealth-Systems connecting different institutions. They fear the worsening of their situation, more control over their working procedures and their charging/accounting.

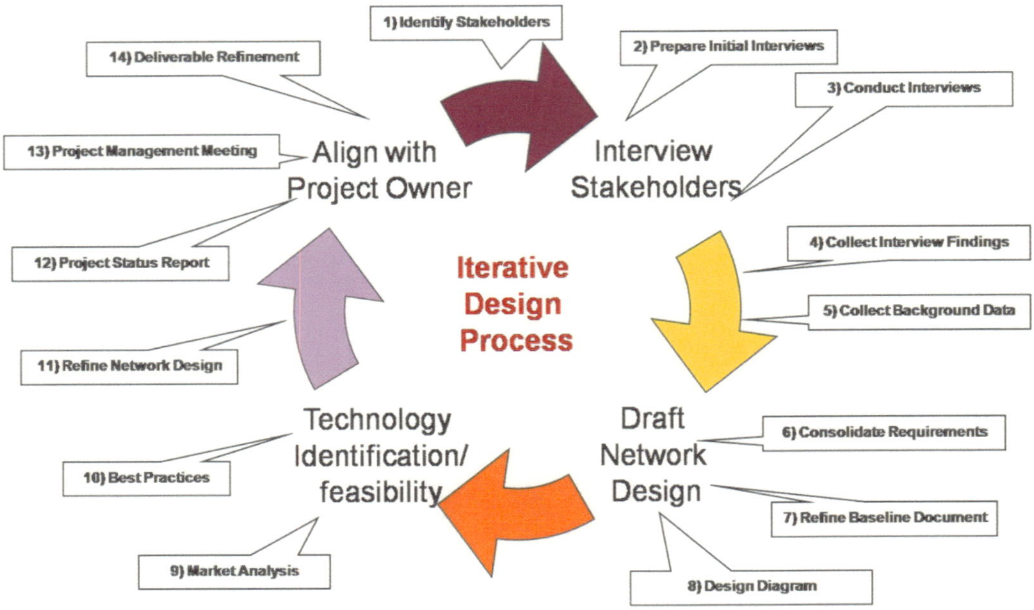

Fig. 3. Iterative design process for a large scale health network

But eHealth-Systems with telemedical use cases such as second-opinion-possibilities, specialisation and remote working can bring many advantages to primary healthcare providers. A new interaction room and a joint task force for care for patients can be created. Many healthcare professionals also are very innovative and interested in new technologies. It is in the hand of the system operators/owners to win these professions for the new eHealth systems, even if often the system owners as budget-holders are natural opponents to them.

3.2 System acceptance for health insurances

The system of mutual insurance against common risks of illness (modern social security) was built as a process of industrialization at the end of the nineteenth century, first at factory level, and has then developed into a general public system. In almost every nation with social security system, there exist the obligatory social and health insurances and beyond them the private insurances.

Health insurance companies can benefit from eHealth systems by making efforts to compete with other health insurers in offering faster, modern and appropriate services to the citizens. eHealth systems integrating insurances usually are planned for the billing process connecting directly to the healthcare providers. The requirement of neutral bodies, which provide individual citizens with reliable information on the quality of certain medical services would be a natural task for them. As budget holder and the payer they could be a trust worthy informant for the individual citizen.

3.3 System acceptance for hospitals

Hospitals belong to the so-called acute-care institutions that are required to provide 24x7 emergency operation. The funding and management of such institutions is subject to its own laws, interventions from outside without understanding these structures are generally not appropriate. Individual hospitals are often focused on the latest practices in specific disease areas (cancer clinic, heart clinic, cosmetic surgery, etc.). These two special features give some hospitals - either for geographical or medical reasons - a kind of unique position in the medical supply area and the position to be able to build and operate their own eHealth systems autonomously. The role of hospitals in a nationwide eHealth system therefore has to be clearly defined; interfaces and interoperability of the hospital legacy system to the new eHealth systems play a major role in the overall acceptance, as hospitals also are usually holding most of the patients' data.

3.4 System acceptance for pharmacies

Interestingly pharmacists are experienced and good traders and find usually common ways to pursue new tasks in interoperable and entity-connecting eHealth infrastructure systems. Easy to imagine, for example, it would be the pharmacist, who could serve as regional patient data lawyer, because he himself is not treating actively and still has a certain sound medical understanding and is trusted over any doctors for the patient as a neutral instance. Next to the normal business case of selling medicines new business cases such as the mentioned data lawyer or medical consultant can be supported by eHealth systems.

3.5 System acceptance for nursing and nursing homes

With the increased life expectancy in developed countries, the home care and nursing market will develop further and eHealth systems can offer a technological basis for this, supporting patients needs and rights. From the perspective of medical documentation is to be noted that a large-scale eHealth system in principle should offer the possibility to document the treatment and disease progression in non-clinical care area in a compact way to serve the spirit of integrated care and to achieve complete supplementary documentation for care during a full care process of a patient. Transparency of medication for different institutions, referral from hospital care to home care with all necessary patient data improve the treatment result of nursing professionals with decreasing the error rates due to lack of information.

3.6 System acceptance for patients

As already mentioned in chapter 2.4 the acceptance among patients is an important aspect for a successful launch of any eHealth project. The remarkable and paradoxical fact is, that the main and relevant "Institution Patient" for the development of a large-scale eHealth system has no clearly established interest group to defend their requirements and goals individually. Healthcare institutions have emerged from issues as financing, profession and qualification, access, community care and abuse prevention. The resulting institutions are now mandated to take over these roles for patients.

The topics here are patients' rights, protection of privacy, access to authentic medical information, data sovereignty of the patient, availability of information to qualified hospital staff in an emergency, etc. (Batami, 2001). All these are issues that require special and clear accentuation obtained from the patient's perspective.

A starting point for further studies can be found in (Hackl, 2009) where the acceptance and fears towards an EHR of patients is reviewed and in (Hoerbst, 2010) where this is discussed from the point of view from physicians.

4. Operational level

The operational level is where the actual administration and management of an eHealth system occurs. The eHealth system maintains sensitive data; therefore everything should be tracked, measured, analyzed and planned accordingly. The operational level has to fulfil the needs raised by the technical level and the political level - so the operational level may start with acquiring the requirements from the technical and political level.

In the operational level a few important aspects need to be answered and discussed:

- **Adaptability and framework quality:** can your system be adapted when new requirements arise?
- **Locality of medical or e-Health services:** from where and by whom can the service be accessed?
- **Accessibility and Ownership of patient or treatment data:** who is the owner of the data and how can it be accessed?
- **Maintainability of systems and networks:** The developed standards need to be maintainable with respect to future organizational changes and/or technological advancement within the given environment of human or infrastructural resources.
- **Integratability and interoperability of heterogeneous systems:** how can new systems or services be integrated into the eHealth infrastructure? The technical design and standards must ensure ongoing information flow between all nodes of the network and system, considering heterogeneous existing IT infrastructures.
- **Transparency of data transmission and audits:** data transmissions should be traceable by the users.

These aspects are described in more detail in the next sections.

4.1 Adaptability and framework quality

A large-scale eHealth project will not be static - it will continuously grow in size (in terms of users or user groups and requirements). So these requirements or users should be able to be easily integrated into the system. The choosing of a flexible and adaptable framework is necessary to allow the ease of adaptation. This is not reduced to only technical changes but also to organizational ones. If there is an organizational change, which might be happen throughout a long large scale eHealth project, the operational level has to continue the work. This might be achieved by a flexible and easy adaptable framework.

4.2 Locality of medical or e-health services

It should be determined what the purpose of a service or system is and who the users are. Where are access points for the end-users and should it be accessible from everywhere with no restrictions (e.g. a PHR which is accessible from every web browser) or should this be restricted (e.g. a HIS can only be accessed from within a hospital)? Depending on this purpose adequate security measures (e.g. VLAN or VPN on network level) should be taken into consideration. A system or service, which is available from everywhere, is potentially more susceptible to unauthorized access and fraud, e.g. when someone has stored his medical data in a PHR and his login and password is stolen by malicious software the thief can easily access the data from everywhere. As opposed to this it would be more difficult if the thief has to be in the same LAN or can only access a system or service from a specific terminal.

4.3 Accessibility and ownership of patient or treatment data

The ownership of patients' data is in most cases determined by juridical restrictions, which are different in every country (e.g. who is the owner of the data in a national EHR). If the eHealth project is set in more than one country, juridical advice might be necessary from all participating states. Even if this is not the case the chance for patients to have control over their own data might be a great benefit of the system/service.

To access the data it is necessary, that the system or service is available when the end-user needs to access it. See chapter 5.4 for further information about reliability and availability.

4.4 Maintainability of systems and networks

Highly available, fault-tolerant large-scale systems and networks tend to be hard to configure and maintain. Simplicity of maintenance has to be guaranteed on any level of network design to make integration processes for further components as easy as possible. Defining a update-cycle may positively influence the maintainability. When it comes to maintenance a definition of service level agreements or operational level agreements are necessary to deliver a highly available system - which is needed in an eHealth project with sensitive data involved. The end user also might want to know when maintenance is happening. When it comes to problems while using the system, a single point of contact for the end user is useful, where he can ask questions or address new problems.

4.5 Integratability and interoperability of heterogeneous systems

This design criteria is strongly related but not limited to future developments (i.e. applications, services or new infrastructure components). Often large eHealth projects need to include interfaces to clinical and billing systems - so the integratability and interoperability has to be available from the beginning and not exist only in some future implementation. This is important especially when integrating new services or connecting heterogeneous systems. To ensure this, without too much additional implementation effort, standards should be used where possible. There are multiple available standards to choose from e.g. IHE or HL7. An evaluation of available standards to fit the systems is required to find the right standard.

4.6 Transparency of data transmission and audits

EHealth systems contain sensitive data (e.g. health status of a patient). If this data is stolen there will be a huge reputation loss for the system, especially if this was not the fault of the patient himself (e.g. application bugs). There also might be scenarios, where a health care professional is looking at medical metadata without a reason and the patient wants to know about this. Everything, which is stored, changed or read, should be documented and logged - this includes who has taken an action and when it happened. Audits allow the complete tracking of who accessed what and when, without knowing the content of the accessed data. This can only be achieved by encrypting the sensitive data and therefore this has to be integrated into the design process on the operational level.

5. Technical level

The technical level is where the actual implementation occurs. Mistakes on this level, for example insufficient security measures may lead to catastrophic consequences in the future. A large eHealth project can only work if the other levels support and not hinder the technical progress of the project. Issues on a political level nearly always have a direct impact on the technical implementation and therefore on the whole project. These issues often lead to missed deadlines, increasing financial requirements and possibly to loss of support in the public.

The main design criteria on the technical level can be classified into the following categories:

- **Security**: Measures to guarantee a secure system on a physical level and on the application level.
- **Usability Engineering**: Criteria for a successful usability engineering process.
- **Scalability:** Aspects of extending the project on a technical level.
- **Infrastructure Reliability**: Aspects of maintaining sufficient system availability.

5.1 Security and privacy implementation

Security is by far the most important aspect in the implementation of any health related system. Insufficient security measures may lead to major problems on a personal and political level. Health care information about a person is not only important to the individual but may also be valuable to other parties (e.g. employer, insurer). Therefore it is essential, that the access to this information is sufficiently and future proof secured (Dantu, 2007). An official compromised system will also have major implication on a political level. In the worst case it will require a complete suspension of either the on-going project (e.g. if a pilot system has been compromised) or the running system. A suspension of such a system has not just negative image implications for all participating parties, but will also require a high amount of financial resources to fix it on a technical level. Many modern large-scale IT projects utilize the Common Criteria for Information Technology Security Evaluation (CC) standard (ISO/IEC 15408) for defining and assessing their security requirements. This approach has the advantage, that because of CC's generic nature, it can be customized to the project's individual needs.

There are three main categories of security concepts, which have to be observed when designing an eHealth infrastructure:

- **On-site security:** Securing the physical components of the eHealth infrastructure.
- **Communication security:** Securing the communication between the separate components.
- **Application security:** Securing the application components.

5.1.1 On-site security

On-site security deals with all aspects of securing the physical components, which are either used to store, or access confidential information. These components may include the server infrastructure of a centralized electronic health record storage, computer systems in a medical practice or smartcard readers that are used to control the health care professionals or patients access to the health infrastructure. Depending on the political environment, the requirements for on-site security may differ from the security requirements of the general population (e.g. allowing lawful inspection on one hand and technically eliminating unwanted inspections on the other hand). On-site security is usually implemented by organizational measures (e.g. limit physical access to core components).

5.1.2 Communication security

Communication security can be split into two parts:

- Securing the physical connection.
- Securing the transmission channel.

While establishing onsite-security is achieved by restricting access to network centres, this cannot be achieved organizationally for the actual physical link (i.e. fibre channels connecting the sites). As there is no practical defence against eavesdropping on network traffic on the wire The network traffic can be disclosed by touching (fast prism-splice devices generating a non disruptive Y-connection for the eavesdropper) or even non-touching methods (e.g. appraising Rayleigh-scattering) all inter-site connections have to be considered as insecure. While eavesdropping on the fibre links could be protected against by hardware encryption modules, this would not protect against eavesdropping at the core routers themselves or at the handover points to client locations or the central application servers.

Hence all confidential traffic within the network cannot be secured by the network itself but rather needs to be secured by point-to-point encryption (typically achieved by asymmetric or hybrid cryptosystems) between client and services endpoints. Therefore securing the actual transmission need to be handled on an application level.

5.1.3 Application security

Application security measures deal with all aspects of securing the actual application components. This not only includes the infrastructural backend components but also all interfaces that are used to connect to the system. As mentioned previous in the previous section, a secure transmission cannot be guaranteed on the physical level. Depending on various environmental factors (e.g. laws, regulations) various cryptographic methods may be utilized. An important aspect is that the cryptographic technology can be upgraded without losing previous data.

If external components are going to be allowed to access the system, security specification must be in place in time. Further, organisations have to be nominated or created to perform a security validation against the individual components. In addition the system as a whole has to undergo regular security audits.

5.2 Usability engineering and user tests

The general aim of large-scale eHealth projects is to give the target population access to medical information in a way that is not possible at the time of the project inception. Depending on the ultimate project goal, various usability aspects have to be taken into account. Especially in regional, national or international projects a diverse population is present. These projects deal with a young population, handicapped people, elderly people and people with a diverse educational background. If the end-user is required to participate in the resulting eHealth system (e.g. a nationwide health insurance card) the system has to be designed in a way that no one is excluded. The unique character also prohibits the unreflected exclusive use of usability engineering best practices. If an insufficient amount of effort is applied in this project phase, the project will provide additional points to attack the project by its opponents. The nature of such a large project also requires, that usability tests are continuously performed and that the end-user interfaces are engineered around these usability test results. The main challenge in usability engineering of health related IT projects, is aligning usability requirements with security requirements. If for example the access to the eHealth system requires a smartcard with a not individual selectable six digit PIN, it will result in a low acceptance with the potential security risk of everybody writing the PIN directly on the card.

5.3 Scalability for change process implications

Scalability in large IT systems refers to all aspects of extending the projects either vertical or horizontal. While the concrete project extensions are defined and decided on a political level, it is advisable, that the technical level includes potential scalability aspects already in the core architecture. A typical problem when extending a running system is a closed core architecture. If a system is designed and implemented only for the specification of the initial project, without including the possibilities to extend the system, any extension will require a significant higher amount of financial resources and will cause an increased project duration.

Typical extension scenarios include:

- Including additional regions.
- Including additional user groups.
- Adding electronic health record related topics.
- Adding electronic prescription.

Every additional functionality will also involve a certain degree of horizontal extension; therefore both aspects will have to be evaluated before approaching any extension project.

5.3.1 Horizontal extension

A horizontal extension of an eHealth system is the inclusion of a larger target audience. This usually means the inclusion of a new region, different health care professional (HCP) specialities or a patient population. There are various political and technical reasons behind such a horizontal extension. Many national eHealth infrastructure projects tend to start with only a few regions for the pilot testing and then include new regions after the successful pilot completion. Another possible scenario is that legal requirements prohibit a certain target population from participating in an eHealth infrastructure project in the implementation phase, but, since such a project usually takes several years, may be allowed to participate at a later stage.

On the technology level a horizontal extension requires measures to increase networking and backend infrastructure. When attaching new regions to the existing network, it is necessary to evaluate the current state of broadband availability. While urban and suburban regions usually have a good availability of current broadband technologies like DSL, Cable, UMTS, etc., this cannot necessarily be said for rural regions. When planning a large eHealth infrastructure project it is therefore essential to define strategies on a technological level on how to cope with differences in networking infrastructure. For example: If the new system requires an always-on connection from the HCP, it will create problems when attaching an HCP in a region without broadband Internet access.

5.3.2 Vertical extension

A vertical extension in comparison describes the addition of new features in the eHealth infrastructure. An example for this is the addition of a nationwide electronic health record to a system where only a limited emergency dataset exist. As described in section 2.2 there could be multiple reasons for adding functionality to an eHealth infrastructure. While a horizontal scalability mostly requires measures for increasing performance when adding more users to the system, a vertical extension requires sufficient extensibility on an application and backend level. In modern software development process, these extensibility mechanisms are not new, but they have to be careful planned. Extending a system, which was not built for extensibility, requires higher financial resources and a longer duration to finish.

5.4 Reliability to support eHealth systems availability

Availability is the probability that the system is operating properly when it is requested for use. A system, which is used 24/7 to access critical data, which is the case for most eHealth systems, requires an availability of almost 100%. A high and reliable system availability from a political point of view is especial important in the months following the project launch. Every significant offline time, even below an hour, will create negative press and will lower the acceptance rate. To avoid this unnecessary project risk, it is important to introduce modern redundancy and general availability technologies and methodologies in the infrastructure and application architecture. By now, there are more than sufficient technical possibilities to facilitate the necessary availability.

Several categories of events can lead to unavailability of the system:

- Failure of the underlying hardware (e.g. switches, servers, data storage components)
- Failure of the housing infrastructure (flooding, power, air condition etc.).
- Broken physical connections (e.g. cabling)
- Very high latency (i.e. longer than network timeouts) due to excessive arbitrary usage of the network by other users

To avoid unavailability due to component failures a concept of redundant everything is required. In theory "everything" means really everything: not only switches, cables, power supplies, buildings, air condition units, power lines, but also operating systems and maintenance staff. In extreme cases, redundant switches would have to be from different vendors utilizing different operating systems to protect against systemic failures in operating systems. This also means that the maintenance staff is required to have different training and different operating procedures to protect against systemic procedure errors that could lead to downtime. High latency can be avoided by implementing sufficient Quality of Service (QoS) methods. The concrete QoS settings will have to be established during the first pilot and test phases. Ensuring availability is one of the major functions of every infrastructure operations centre. Permanent monitoring and automatic alerting in case of system failures (or system fail-over) guarantees short response times and normal system operations.

6. Natural order of criteria levels

Institutional criteria (IC) map the needs of the different stakeholders within their historically grown environments of the health system: e.g. patients have to learn about the idea and the use of a large scale health IT system; doctors need to be taught about their role, pharmacies hold a special role with e-prescriptions and can e.g. become independent "personal health data lawyers" for patients; hospitals can and will provide professional EHR services and have to define their role within the health telematics system; insurances play a crucial role in building up the infrastructure and have to redefine their organizational role within the opportunities of the new infrastructure.

Political criteria (PC) manage the mindsets and common national notion of the health telematics. Such a project will fail if public trust in the system vanishes. Trust will vanish e.g. if growth is not done step by step on the basis of serious field tests. Public acceptance must not be lost in any phase of construction. Another important political criteria is a countries' own health system history: any reasonable system has to build on that history and migrate step by step. Cultural aspects will be highly important in actual use and acceptance. We will not highlight this issue here in further detail as these reflections lead beyond the scope of the focus at hand.

We need to emphasize though that according to our experiences in several projects any nation-wide public health IT project has to obey a hidden rule of criteria priority:

$$PC > IC > OC > TC.$$

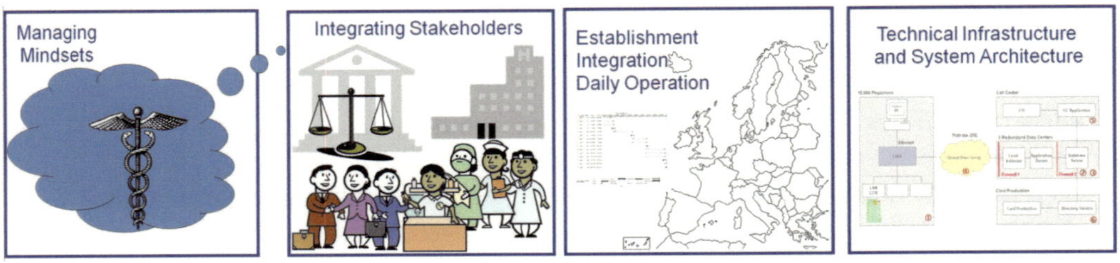

Fig. 4. Natural Order of Criteria Levels

The view of the public and the attitude of the people are most critical for the success of a nation wide health IT system. Some examples: even a perfect understanding and coordination between doctors, insurances and ministries will be a weak instrument against a publicly discussed case for e.g. patients' health data misuse by employers or by credit banks (PC > IC).

If one of the stakeholders (e.g. insurances) is hurt in its basic interests they will (openly or secretly) foul the process of construction large scale or national health telematics. No matter how complete your project organization is, you cannot build the system against a stakeholder (IC > OC).

Your technical components and architecture can be highly elaborated and sophisticated and all-problem-solving, but your system will be a fail, if e.g. your roll out scenarios and project integration concepts are not realistic, competitive or do not match with the given industrial and administrative facts (OC > TC).

Managing the whole process of establishing a state-wide health IT infrastructure affords a thorough reflection of the above priority levels as a constant attitude from the drivers of the project. If obstacles arrive in the process of establishment the team in charge has to identify the cause and its criteria level. Removing the obstacle and finding the solution will usually be done within the according level of the nuisance. Solving IC problems by e.g. TC means will always fail. Yet, to our experience this type of level mismatch phenomenon does appear frequently within such large public IT projects. This phenomenon then becomes the cause of unstructured decision making: e.g. institutional top-management (who is in charge of the global vision and general goals of the system) will discuss small technical details. - The operative team in charge of such a project needs to maintain a sane process of decision making respecting the cited levels of construction criteria.

7. Conclusion

The introduction of large eHealth systems cannot be done in a day. Before approaching such a project, the participating parties need to define common goals and draft an approach of how they are going to achieve these goals. When this is done the planning and implementation of the project can begin. During this phase many discussions with representatives from the affected population will happen. Each of these groups will have certain reasons either for or against this project and won't hesitate to mobilize a public movement to support their claim. Therefore it is essential that these discussions are handled correctly.

Every new large eHealth project has unique problems and goals which need to be included in the design process throughout the whole process from the project start to the project end.

Table 1 summarizes the aforementioned design criteria, which can be used to reduce risks, increase acceptance and give guidance from the political to the technical level of a large-scale eHealth project. Naturally the mentioned design criteria can be enhanced with project specific design criteria, e.g. on the operational level rollout mechanisms, program or project management, maintenance and operation aspects and can be seen as flexible starting point to categorize typical large scale eHealth infrastructure projects.

The authors have been in charge for consultancy and engineering tasks in many eHealth projects: from the technical implementation of ePrescription or modules for electronic health record systems (technical level), over the management, operations and maintenance of existing systems (operational level), to the consultancy of e.g. hospital IT managers (institutional level) and up to the consultancy of Health Ministries of different countries (political level). In the respective levels the identified criteria have been applied, though not in an explicit way, but in as analysis, precondition and alignment of the relevant tasks. This chapter therefore summarizes the experiences to a catalogue which can be applied, checked and amended in future tasks in the health systems area.

Building a modern large or nation-wide health infrastructure provides several promising options in administrative as well as medical progress. In its mature stage, nations will coordinate their health professionals and health budgets in a more effective way not only on the domestic level. They will cooperate and share resources in integrated environments on an international level. The technical-organizational way to arrive at this advanced stage is still very long to go. Brute-force top-down approaches will fail dramatically. The great objective "Unity in Diversity" in health IT connecting all people and institutions into one system needs an organic bottom-up approach. E.g. WHO top-down approaches can support and guard that but are unfit to be the main drivers of that process. Drivers and promoters are regional and national. Integration and connection in health IT must succeed on the national level first. - Overall the whole process requires a permanent attitude of unity from all stake-holders. May it last more than a decade: IT today provides the means of merging doctors, clinics, hospitals, nursing homes, pharmacies, ministries, and insurances into one coordinated health service provider for the benefit of all of us.

8. Acknowledgment

The authors want to thank all colleagues at INSO and RISE, who support the research in Medical Informatics and successfully work in the implementation of smaller and larger eHealth projects. Their vast experience has supported the content and categorization for this chapter.

Levels	Design criteria	Chapter
Political Level = Political Criteria (PC)	• Consideration of cultural aspects and historical development in healthcare • Appropriate and necessary innovation • Healthy Growing: Creating a healthy eHealth Infrastructure Step-by-Step • Appropriate design of media presentation, dealing with fears and enhancing Acceptance • Appropriate allocation at the general governmental level • Representation in parliament and other representative organisations for citizens • Appropriate legislative measures to accompany the implementation process and operation of the system	See Chapter 2
Institutional Level = Institutional Criteria (IC)	• System Acceptance for Primary and secondary healthcare centers • System Acceptance for Health Insurances • System Acceptance for Hospitals • System Acceptance for Pharmacies • System Acceptance for Nursing and Nursing homes • System Acceptance for Patients	See Chapter 3
Operational Level = Operational Criteria (OC)	• Adaptability and framework quality • Locality of medical or e-Health services • Accessibility and Ownership of patient or treatment data • Maintainability • Integratability and interoperability of heterogeneous systems: • Transparency of data transmission and audits	See Chapter 4
Technical Level = Technical Criteria (TC)	• Security • Usability Engineering • ScalabilityInfrastructure • Reliability	See Chapter 5

Table 1. Design criteria

9. References

Batami S., 2001, Patient data confidentiality and patient rights, in *International Journal of Medical Informatics*, vol. 62, issue 1, pp. 41-49.

Dantu R., Osterwijk H., Kolan P., Husna H., 2007, Securing medical networks, *in Network Security*, Volume June 2007, Issue 6, pp 13-16.

Eysenbach G, 2001, What is e-health? In *Journal of Medical Internet Research.* http://www.jmir.org/2001/2/e20/ (online journal)

Gunter T.D.and Terry N.P. 2005. The Emergence of National Electronic Health Record Architectures in the United States and Australia: Models, Costs, and Questions in *J Med Internet Res* 7(1.)

Hackl W., Hoerbst A. & Ammenwerth E. 2009. The Electronic Health Record in Austria: Physicians' Acceptance is Influenced by Negative Emotions, in *Studies in Health Technology and Informatics*, vol. 150, pp. 140-144.

Hoerbst A., Kohl, C., Knaup, P., and Ammenwerth, E. 2010. Attitudes and behaviors related to the introduction of electronic health records among Austrian and German citizens, in *International Journal of Medical Informatics*, vol. 79, pp. 81-89.

Larsen E., 2003, *Standards Insight: An Analysis of Health Information*, 2003 Annual HIMSS Conference

Tan J., et.al, 2005, *e-Health Care Information Systems*, Jossey-Bass.

5

QoS in Telemedicine

Phumzile Malindi
Walter Sisulu University
South Africa

1. Introduction

Telemedicine can be defined as the use of information and communication technology (ICT) to deliver medical services and information from one location to another. In other words, telemedicine can be seen as a way of distributing medical expertise and services to medically underserviced areas such as remote and rural areas using ICT as a communication platform. Though any communication system can be used in telemedicine, rapid development in computer technology and easiness to purchase has led to more amenability to computer-based telemedicine technologies which are IP-based.

Services offered by telemedicine are designed to help improve healthcare access and information service while reducing the isolation of healthcare providers and residents in rural areas. Telemedicine can also reduce the time and allay the costs of rural patient transportation significantly. Telemedicine includes applications in areas such as pathology and radiology, as well as consultations in specialties such as neurology, dermatology, cardiology, and general medicine. Telemedicine is also used for Continued Medical Education (CME), administration, research and development. Table 1 shows a summary of telemedicine application categories.

- Initial urgent evaluation of patients, triage decisions, and pre-transfer arrangements.
- Medical and surgical follow-up and medication checks.
- Supervision and consultation for primary care encounters in sites where a physician is not available.
- Routine consultation and second opinions based on history, physical exam findings, and available test data.
- Transmission of diagnostic images.
- Extended diagnostic work-ups or short-term management of self-limited conditions.
- Management of chronic diseases and conditions requiring a specialist not available locally.
- Transmission of medical data.
- Public health, preventive medicine, and patient education.

Table 1. A Summary of Telemedicine Application Categories (Source: Grigsby et al., "Analysis of Expansion of Access to Care Through Telemedicine, Report 4, Study Summary and Recommendations for Further Research," Center for Health Policy Research, Denver, CO, December 1994, p.43)

From the applications listed in Table 1, the services offered by telemedicine can be grouped as follows:

- Tele-education
- Tele-consultation
- Tele-monitoring
- Tele-management (or combination of tele-monitoring and tele-consultation)
- Tele-diagnosis
- Medical data exchange

The scope of this chapter is to present a holistic approach to the provision of quality of service in an IP-based telemedicine system. Methods of mitigating some of the problems that degrade the quality of real-time traffic when transmitted over packet networks are discussed, which include DiffServ/MPLS, error concealment and low-bit rate coding.

2. Need for QoS in telemedicine

Telemedicine makes it possible for rural patients in health clinics who need special medical care to have face-to-face consultations with specialists that are situated in a hospital or another medical institution that is far away. In other words, it enables the nurse in a primary health center to send the medical sounds, images and video, which are captured using medical peripherals such as medical video scopes (Octoscope; Colposcope; Dermascope; Rectoscope; Iriscope; Endscope, etc.), Stethoscope, cameras and other medical instruments, to a doctor in a secondary or tertiary medical center to be used to make a diagnosis for a patient.

For the telemedicine to be effective, it must be able to emulate the onsite face-to-face consultation experience. That is, the telemedicine system must provide quality video, image and audio or sound transmission in both real-time and store-and-forward modes. Quality audiovisual communication is also essential in order for the physician at the distant end to better approximate an on-site physical examination so as to make a correct diagnosis from the received medical sounds, images and/or video.

According to Nanda and Fernandes (2007), it is essential in a critical medical environment that the networking applications perform with a surgical precision; otherwise the outcome could be fatal, both for patients as well as the future of networking in telemedicine. For this to be possible, it is necessary that the information signals reach the end location with high degree of reliability and predictability. Such systems are said to have stringent real-time QoS constraints, of which if not met can lead to disaster; for example, the unbounded delay and jitter in the control system of telerobotic surgery can lead to control loop instability and mission failure (Szymanski and Gilbert, 2010). Lastly, the availability of resources is also imperative in health networks, because the generated traffic may be crucial for the patients' health and life (Zvikhachevskaya et al., 2009).

2.1 Quality of service

According to ITU-T recommendation E.800, QoS can be defined as the collective effect of the service performances, which determine the degree of satisfaction of the user of service (Afullo, 2004). Muhammed et al. (2006), describes QoS as the ability of the network to provide a service with an assured service level, and it is building block for reaching quality end-user experience (QoE); that is, QoS in the network ensures that the user gets quality usable services. These two definitions show clearly, that there is a relationship between the performance of the system and the satisfaction of the user of the services provided by the system.

In the technical context, QoS is a set of attributes that can be used to define the network's capability to meet the requirements of the user and application (Kilkki, 2008). QoS parameters include delay (or latency), jitter, bit rate (throughput) and packet loss rate (Aidarous & Plevyak, 2003; Malindi & Kahn, 2008; Tulu & Chatterjee, 2008), and according to Salatian et al. (2011), network resource availability also plays a role in QoS, where delay represents the maximum delay bound that is acceptable to the application; jitter reflects variations in delay; bit rate, also called throughput, refers to data rate that the system can transfer or the rate at which packets are transmitted in a network, packet loss rate refers to the percentage of packet lost among all the delivered packets in a given time interval, and network resource availability is the infrastructure associated with the transmission of data (Salatian et al., 2011).

2.2 Profile of the telemedicine traffic

Typical telemedicine application includes the transfers of basic patient information, transfers of high resolution images such as radiographs, computer tomography (CT) scans, magnetic resonance imaging (MRI) pictures, ultrasound, pathology images, video images of endoscopes or other procedures, patient interviews and examinations, consultations with medical specialists and health care educational activities; therefore, telemedicine traffic includes medical images, video, audio and data from different telemedicine applications or services. These applications may be classified as store-and-forward, near real-time and real-time, where store-and-forward is used for non-emergent situations where the consultation may be made within the next 24 - 48 hours, real time involves transmission of the information as it is acquired and is sometimes interactive like two-way telephone conversation, or two-way face-to-face video conferencing consultation, and near real-time is used for emergent situations where certain data is transmitted immediately to help during consultation that is in process or to be in process soon.

Each of these telemedicine applications has its own QoS requirements (Malindi and Kahn, 2008; Skorin-Kapov and Matijasevic, 2010), ranging from low to high bandwidth, delay tolerance to delay intolerance, and tolerance to packet losses to packet loss intolerance. These QoS requirements vary depending on the type of traffic, type of service, and the context in which the service is invoked. For example, in an emergency situation, a remote specialist diagnosis may require near real-time transmission of medical data, while in a different, non-emergency situation, the patient data is transferred (with tolerance for delay) to a remote location to be analyzed by a specialist (Skorin-Kapov and Matijasevic, 2010). Often the real time applications have stringent network requirements than other applications. According to Feng et al. (2010), the variety of telemedicine applications produces traffic with diverse network requirements and some telemedicine traffic, such as tele-diagnostic with interactive audio and video transmission, may require very high bandwidth, and strict delay and jitter requirements. For example, interactive video communication requires low delay of 200 to 300 ms round-trip and an average jitter that is not more than 30 ms, and for speech the latency is also 200-300 ms and jitter must be limited to 50ms (Cisco Systems, 2002; Sze et al., 2002; Hassan et al., 2005; Tobagi, 2005). According to Szymanski and Gilbert (2010), telerobotic surgery may tolerate maximum delays of up 250 ms and a relatively small jitter of the order of 10s of milliseconds. Some telemedicine applications such as remote surgery may also require guaranteed level of availability in addition to latency and jitter requirements mentioned above. Such applications are referred to as safety-critical or life-critical applications and the type of QoS they require from the network is sometimes referred to as hard QoS. According to Vergados et al. (2006), Vouyioukas et al. (2007), Zvikhachevskaya et al. (2009), Skorin-Kapov and Matijasevic, (2010), the basic requirements for the different types of telemedicine are presented in Table 2.

Application Type	Required throughput	Small delay	Small jitter	Context sensitive
Tele-consultation	High	Yes	Yes	Yes
Tele-diagnosis	High	Yes	No	Yes
Tele-monitoring	Low	No	No	Yes
Tele-education	High	No	No	No
Access to DB	Low/High	No	No	Yes

Table 2. QoS Requirements for telemedicine services

2.3 Factors affecting the quality of service

Quality transmission of video and sound depends on four variants: acquisition (or recording), coding, transmission and reproduction. For example, in video communication, the type and the resolution of camera used, the coding standard used, the communication network used, and the resolution of the display at the receiver will contribute to the overall quality of the video at the receiver, whereas in sound transmission it is the acoustic response of the microphone or the stethoscope used, the coding standard used, the communication network used, and the frequency response of the speakers at the receiver will contribute to the quality of the sound at the receiver. Each of these variants has some limitations, which make it impossible to achieve the ideal quality of the signal being transmitted as a result in most cases a compromise is reached between the ideal and the practical quality transmission.

As alluded to in the introduction, most of the telemedicine system are IP-based and the default and traditional datagram delivery service used in IP-based networks is called best-effort service. This type of service delivers the packets as fast as possible, using, in most cases, first-in-first-out (FIFO) scheduling mechanism, which delivers the datagram to the output port in the same order as they came from the input port without giving preference to any type of traffic. For slightly loaded network this service can be sufficient, but if the network is congested queuing losses and queuing delays can make the network not to be suitable for real-time and critical traffic. Another problem with IP network is the link-state routing protocols that are used to distribute IP routing information throughout a single autonomous system (AS) in an IP network; that is, Interior Gateway Protocols (IGPs). These IGPs like Intermediate System-Intermediate System (IS-IS) protocol, and Open Shortest Path First (OSPF) protocol create a shortest path matrix for each router and then forward traffic along this shortest path. Unlike ATM's PNNI, IP routing protocols do not have a Connection Admission Control (CAC) mechanism to balance network traffic along multiple paths. The result is under-utilization of certain links, creation of hot spots in the network and congestion along the shortest path route. These congestions can cause long queues, resulting in serious degradation for applications that are running due to packet loss, latency, and jitter thus compromising the quality of service. Additional to IP debilities, other factors, such as transmission errors and limited bandwidths, can also jeopardize the quality of service required by telemedicine applications.

3. Provision of quality of service

IP network is a packet-based network, which is an unpredictable system with parameters that are variable according to network usage. In order to overcome the challenges posed by such a system and still be able to provide quality transmissions the following are proposed:

i. Traffic differentiation and prioritizing
ii. Traffic engineering and protection
iii. Error control and concealment
iv. Using encoding schemes that will produce low bit rates without compromising much on quality in order to cater for low capacity systems.

3.1 Traffic differentiation and prioritizing

IETF has proposed some mechanisms to compensate for the best effort debilities of IP-based networks in order to make IP suitable for almost all the different multimedia applications. These mechanisms or technologies, which include IntServ, DiffServ, and MPLS, have been proposed to provide QoS in IP-based multiservice networks. All the three mechanisms are able to guarantee the appropriate QoS treatment to real-time traffic concerning its special delay, jitter, packet loss and bandwidth requirements. However, the drawback of IntServ is that it suffers from scalability problems (Aidarous & Plevyak, 2003; Leon-Garcia & Widjaja, 2004). Hence most of the literature on provision of QoS has been concentrating on the combination of DiffServ and MPLS as the enablers of QoS in IP networks. Where DiffServ is used to divide traffic into a small number of classes, and MPLS is used for traffic engineering and to offer IP QoS services efficiently over diverse layer-two backbone networks (Patrikakis et al., 2003).

One of the reasons for the adoption of a combination of DiffServ and MPLS, is that, though MPLS offers traffic engineering and great savings in terms of switching speed, it still lacks an effort to distinguish among the flows of different delay characteristics, and drop precedence in order to meet the two conditions that are necessary for true QoS as proposed by Fineberg (2003), which are guaranteed bandwidth, and class-related scheduling and packet discarding treatment. Secondly, using DiffServ alone cannot guarantee QoS since DiffServ does not influence a packet path, and therefore during a congestion or failure, even high-priority packets would not get guaranteed bandwidth. Pairing MPLS with DiffServ can compensate these downsides, so that DiffServ can be responsible for classifying the traffic according to different flow characteristics, while MPLS is responsible for providing a connection-oriented environment that enables traffic engineering. According to Ghazel and Saïdane (2008), the integration of DiffServ with MPLS guarantees the QoS for a broad range of multiservice traffic by offering traffic policy and classification in diverse QoS classes of the transport data plane.

3.1.1 Traffic differentiation

The diversity in network resources that are needed for different e-health application, as well as various levels of urgency in medical situations makes the DiffServ model an appropriate architecture for QoS provision (Vergados, 2006). DiffServ divides traffic into a small number of classes with each class being identified by a mark called DSCP, which is carried in the six-bit differentiated field of the IP header. DiffServ defines Classes of Service (CoS), called aggregates, and QoS resource management functions with node-based, or per-hop, operation. The CoS definitions include a behaviour aggregate (BA) which has a specific requirements for scheduling and packet discarding, and an ordered aggregate (OA) which performs classification based on scheduling requirements only, and may include several drop precedence values. Thus, OA is a coarser classification than a BA and may include several BAs. DiffServ offers per hop behaviour (PHB) to BA, which includes scheduling and packet discarding, and PHB scheduling class (PSC) to OA, which only concerns scheduling. The value of the DSCP field is used to specify a BA (or class), which is used by DiffServ-compliant nodes for choosing the appropriate PHB. Per-Hop Behaviors refers to specific forwarding treatments of traffic aggregates or packets in a DiffServ network, which includes packet scheduling, queuing, policing or shaping behavior of a node on any given packet belonging to a BA. There are four standard PHBs that have been defined: the assured forwarding (AF) PHB, expedited forwarding (EF) PHB, class-selector PHB, and default PHB. Where AF PHB is designed to give a reliable service even in times of congestion; EF PHB is designed for traffic that is required to be guaranteed enough resources to ensure that it receives its minimum guaranteed rate (Ibe, 2002, p.227); class-selector PHBs are designed to preserve backward compatibility with the IP-Precedence scheme defined in RFC1812 and default PHB is the standard best-effort treatment that nodes (routers) perform when forwarding traffic (Ibe, 2002, p.228; Aidarous and Plevyak, 2003, p.119; Leon-Garcia and Widjaja, 2004, p.719). AF PHB can be further subdivided into twelve PHBs to make the total of fourteen PHBs in all. The twelve AF PHBs are divided into four PSCs, and each of the PSCs consists of three sub-behaviours, which are related to different packet discarding treatment.

3.1.2 Traffic prioritization

Once the traffic has been classified, it needs to be ranked according to the order of priority it deserves and thereafter set the per-hop behavior (PHB) that closely suite its QoS requirements.

Usually, the traffic is classified according to the content and not the context, however, Skorin-Kapov and Matijasevic, (2010) have proposed that the service context in terms of emergency or patient critical versus non-emergency and non-critical is also crucial in traffic scheduling mechanisms. Vouyioukas et al. (2007) alluded to the importance to distinguish between the requirements for real-time and non-real time, medical for diagnosis and non-diagnosis. Emergency sections need to be prioritized over non-emergency sessions to ensure the best coordination (Gouveia et al. 2009). The following table can be used for prioritizing:

Traffic	Priority
Emergency services and Tele-surgery	Highest
Real-time Tele-consultation and Tele-management	High
Tele-diagnosis and Tele-monitoring	Medium high
Tele-education	Medium low
Medical data exchange	Low

Table 3. Prioritization of telemedicine traffic

3.2 Traffic engineering and protection

Once the traffic has been classified and arranged according to its priority levels, traffic engineering (TE) is needed, which is a process of controlling how the traffic flows through the network as to optimize resource utilization (Xiao et al., 2000). This is done in order to prevent uneven network traffic distribution which can cause high utilization or congestion in some part of a network, even when total capacity of the network is greater than total demand (Xaio et al., 2002). Uneven distribution may be due to the fact that packets tend to follow the shortest path of route, thus resulting in the shortest path being highly utilized and congested, while a longer path remains under-utilized. This uneven traffic distribution in the core network can result in QoS problems such as packet loss, latency, and jitter increase as the average load on a router rises, even when the network utilization is low. Additional to congestion, another problem that can be encountered is route failure, which can result in packet loss and quality of service degradation if not attended to quickly. The IntServ and DiffServ QoS schemes, mentioned above, do not eliminate traffic congestion or provide fast rerouting, but provides differentiated performance degradation for different traffic during network congestion. Therefore, additional to DiffServ, there is still a need for managing network resources such as bandwidth, and controlling routing and traffic in order to minimize congestion and provide fast re-route in the event of route failures so that traffic oriented performances, such as latency, jitter, and packet loss, can be improved.

3.2.1 Traffic engineering using MPLS

In order to facilitate efficient and reliable network operations while simultaneously optimizing network resource utilization and traffic performance, the IETF has introduced multi-protocol label switching (MPLS), constraint-based routing (CR) and an enhanced link state IGP.

MPLS is an IETF specified framework that provides for efficient designation, routing, forwarding, and switching of traffic flows through the network. It approaches the QoS by attempting to address the shortcomings of the IP routing, which include speed, scalability, QoS management and traffic engineering. In traditional IP networks each router makes an independent forwarding decision on each packet as it traverses the network. This decision usually involves a complex manipulation of a large routing table to determine the next hop of a packet. MPLS also uses IP addresses either Ipv4 or Ipv6, to identify end points and intermediate switches and routers. This makes MPLS networks IP-compatible and easily integrated with traditional IP networks. However, unlike traditional IP, MPLS flows are connection-oriented and packets are routed along pre-configured Label Switched Paths (LSPs). MPLS also slightly modifies the IP packet format to include a new Shim Label header, called the MPLS header, which contains a label field. MPLS works by tagging each packet with an identifier to distinguish the LSPs. This identifier is contained within the label field and it consists of fixed-length value, called label, which is used as index into table, which specify the next hop, and new label. When a packet is received, the MPLS router uses this label, instead of the traditional IP destination address, to deliver the packet along the selected path or LSP, and then looks up the LSP in its own forwarding table to determine the best link over which to forward the packet, and the label to use on this next hop. The 32-bit MPLS header sits between the layer 2 (data link layer) header and the layer 3 (network layer).

In a DiffServ/MPLS network MPLS edge nodes need to be DiffServ-enabled in order to engineer the network with traffic engineering that is applied on per class basis. This type of traffic engineering is referred to as DiffServ-aware MPLS traffic engineering (DS-TE) and its essential goal is to guarantee network resources separately for each traffic in order to improve and optimise its compliance with QoS requirements. The essential goal of DS-TE is to guarantee network resources separately for each type of traffic in order to improve and optimise its compliance with QoS requirements (Minei, 2004). This makes it possible to establish separate LSPs for different classes, taking into consideration resources available to each class. For example, a separate LSP can be established for each type of real-time or premium traffic, and these LSPs can be given higher priority than other LSPs (Goode, 2002). DS-TE enables the introduction of the concept of LSP priorities, where some LSPs are marked as more important than others, and it also allows the more important LSPs to be able to confiscate resources from the less important LSPs; that is, pre-empting the less important LSPs. This is done to ensure that important LSP always establishes along the optimal path regardless of the existing reservations, and when LSP needs to reroute in the event of node or link failure, important LSPs have a better chance of finding an alternative path. It is also done to ensure that when high-priority-bandwidth is not needed for real-time traffic, it can be used for lower priority class of traffic that is carried on less important LSPs (Goode, 2002; Minei, 2004). Each LSP has two priorities associated with it: a setup priority and a hold priority. The setup priority controls access to the resources for an LSP at the time of LSP establishment, and the hold priority control access to the resources for an LSP that is already established. The fundamental requirement for DS-TE is to be able to enforce different limits on the percentage of a link's bandwidth for different sets of aggregation of traffic flows of the same class, which are placed inside an LSP; that is, DS-TE must enforce different bandwidth constraints (BCs) to different sets of traffic trunks (TT). This implies keeping track of how much bandwidth is available for each type of traffic at a given time on all the routers throughout the MPLS network. To address this, Le Faucheur and Lai introduced the concept of a class type (CT), which is the set of traffic trunks crossing a link, that are governed by a specific set of bandwidth constraints. This CT is used for the purpose of link bandwidth allocation, constraint based routing and admission control. Once a traffic trunk has been assigned to a CT it will remain an element of that same CT on all links. Each CT may carry traffic from more than one class of service (RFC 3564, 2003). According to RFC 3564 (2003), the DS-TE solution must support up to 8 CTs. Those 8 CTs are referred to as CTc, $0 \leq c \leq MaxCT\text{-}1 = 7$; that is, CT0 through CT7. The DS-TE solution must enforce a different set of bandwidth constraint for each CT, and a DS-TE implementation must support at least 2 CTs. LSPs that are traffic engineered to guarantee bandwidth from a particular CT are referred to as DS-TE LSPs, and in current IETF model, a DS-TE LSP can only carry traffic from on CT. By convention the best effort traffic is mapped to CT0.

3.2.2 Traffic protection

Once the high-priority traffic has been classified and the important LSPs have been established, the high-priority or premium traffic can be mapped on these important LSP to allow it to utilize the resources available for the premium class. To make sure that this premium traffic is less affected by route failures, the important LSP will have Fast Reroute enabled so that when there is a route failure the premium traffic can be switched to the protection LSP, which is established around the 'working' or operational LSP as an alternative route in the event of any link/s or router/s along the working LSP fail. This traffic protection and fast rerouting is essential for applications that cannot tolerate packet loss in order to make sure that premium traffic is less affected by route failures.

3.3 Error control and concealment

One of the inherent problems with any communication channel is the introduction of errors to the data being transmitted through it. According to Wang and Zhu (1998), transmission errors can be roughly classified into two categories: random bit errors and erasure errors. Random bit errors are caused by the imperfections of physical channels, which result in bit inversion, bit insertion, and bit deletion. Erasure errors, on the other hand, can be caused by packet losses, or system failures for a short time (Wang and Zhu, 1998). These errors of transmission channel can be effectively corrected by channel coding methods such as forward error correction (FEC) and automatic repeat request (ARQ) or a mixture of them (Sullivan and Wiegand, 2005). Both FEC and ARQ channel coding methods improves the reliability of the information being transferred by adding additional bits to the transmitted data stream, which of course increases the amount of data being sent. However, these two traditional methods do not provide the bounded delay that is required for real-time traffic as a result other types of error-control mechanisms such as error resilience and error concealment have been proposed in addition to ARQ and FEC schemes (Wu et al., 2000; Stanković et al., 2003).

3.3.1 Error resilience

Error resilient schemes deal with packet loss on the compression layer by considering the semantic meaning of the compression layer and attempt to limit the scope of damage caused by the packet loss on the compression layer. The standard error resilient schemes are resynchronization, data partitioning, and data recovery (Arankalle, 2003; Wu et al., 2000).

In resynchronization the encoder must introduce resynchronization markers in the video bitstream at various locations (e.g. beginning of the frame in MPEG -1/2, H.261/263, or periodically in MPEG 4) so that when the decoder detects an error, it can hunt for this resynchronization marker to regain synchronization with the encoder, thereby preventing error propagation across different segments of the video bitstream, which are separated by the markers. These markers are designed such that they can be easily distinguished from all other codewords and a small perturbation of these codewords (Villasenor et al., 1999; Wang et al., 2000; Du et al., 2003).

Data partitioning is a technique, which involves segmenting the bit stream into segments. This is based on the fact that some bits in the encoded video bitstream are more important than others within the same bitstream. For example, DCT coefficients are less important than GOB headers, motion vectors, and Macroblock information bits. Hence an error occurred in the received DCT information has less impact on the decoded quality than bit errors received in group of block (GOB) headers, motion vectors, and Macroblock information bits. Because of this unequal data importance within the encoded video bitstream, it is possible to separate the bitstream into two layers of importance to allow each to be protected according to its level of importance; that is, unequal error protection (UEP). This helps during the decoding to prevent the errors occurring in one segment from affecting other segment (Katsaggelos, Ishtiaq, Kondi, Hong, Banham and Brailean, 1998).

One of the shortcomings of using resynchronization markers alone is that, after detecting an error in a video bit stream and resynchronizing to the next resynchronization marker, the video decoder discards all the data between the two resysnchronization markers. This is due to the fact that the decoder cannot be certain of the exact location, between the two resynchronization markers, where the error has occurred. Reversible variable-length codes (RVLCs) alleviates this problem and enable the decoder to better isolate the error location by enabling data recovery in the presence of errors. RVLCs are VLCs that are wrapped in an error correcting code; that is, they are having the prefix property when decoding them in both the forward and reverse directions. This enables RVLCs to be uniquely decoded in both forward and reverse direction. So when a decoder detects an error while decoding a bit stream in a forward direction, it jumps to the next resynchronization marker and decodes the bit stream in the backward direction until it encounters an error, and based on the locations of these two errors, the decoder can recover some of the data between the two consecutive resynchronization markers that would otherwise have been discarded (Talluri, 1998). According to Li et al. (2000), RVLC can be used in conjunction with data partitioning, where data partitioning is used to separate the less important information bits from the most important information bits and RVLC is used in coding the most important information bits so that the decoder is able to recover data within the erroneous segments (Villasenor et al., 1999; Li et al., 2000). RVLC has been adopted in both MPEG-4 and H.263, in conjunction with insertion of synchronized markers (Wang et al., 2000).

3.3.2 Error concealment

Error concealment is implemented at the receiver by the decoder, usually after data recovery, in order to hide the effects of errors once they have occurred. It improves the quality of the decoded sequence in the presence of errors when the error rate is not that high. There are three types of concealment: temporal concealment, spatial concealment, and motion-compensated concealment. Temporal concealment replaces a corrupted area with a pixel values in the same location in the previous decoded frame, and it is only effective if there is a little change from the previous frame. Spatial concealment replaces the distorted block by a spatial interpolation between adjacent error-free blocks. It is used for those situations where temporal concealment is not effective, for example, where there is high motion or scene change. Motion-compensated concealment estimates the motion vectors for the lost block rather than simple assuming no motion. (Riley and Richardson, 1997, p.124).

3.4 Coding for low-bit rates

Rural and cellular-based telemedicine systems have limited bandwidths (Zvikhachevskaya et al., 2009; Salatian et al., 2011), which can affect the QoS. One approach to deal with low bandwidth and service contention in a rural setup is to use data compression to shrink larger files to smaller files so that they can occupy less space and become faster to transfer over the network. This decreases the delay, and jitter, while increasing the throughput (Salatian et al., 2011). This enables the transmission of bandwidth-hungry traffic like video using a system with a limited capacity.

The Digital Imaging and Communication in Medicine (DICOM) committee has adopted various JPEG variants, such as lossy and lossless JPEG, JPEG-LS, and JPEG 2000. For medical images, which are having a diagnostic use, medical image compression techniques have primarily focused on lossless methods, where the signal can be reconstructed exactly from its uncompressed format (Pattichis et al., 2002). For digital video, the DICOM committee has adopted MPEG 2 for diagnosis video. However, due to its high bandwidth requirements and frame synchronization problem, MPEG 4 standard can be used for real-time diagnosis video and for non-diagnosis video applications such as video conferencing, H.263 may be acceptable (Pattichis et al., 2002). The advancement in video coding has led to the development of H.264 by Joint Video Team (JVT), which is a joint venture between ISO's MPEG and ITU-T's VCEG. The official title of the H.264 standard is Advanced Video Coding (AVC); however, it is widely known as by its old working title, H.26L, and by its ITU document number, H.264 or as ISO MPEG 4 Part 10, or just MPEG AVC. The main objective of H.264 standard is to provide means to achieve substantially higher video quality as compared to what could be achieved using any of the existing video coding standard. It has a number of advantages that distinguish it from existing standards, while at the same time, sharing common features with other existing standards. These advantages include up to 50% in bit rate saving compared to H.263 or MPEG 4, high quality video that is consistent at high and low bit rates, error resilience, and network friendliness that makes it possible to transport H.264 bit streams over different networks. These advantages make H.264 an ideal standard for several video applications such as video conferencing, storage and broadcast video. According to Panayides et al. (2010), H.264/AVC provides for efficient (size wise) and timely (real time) encoding.

4. Performance evaluation of the proposed QoS

In the preceding section techniques for providing a holistic QoS in IP-based telemedicine system were discussed and here the performance of the proposed solutions are evaluated. First will be the network functions (DiffServ and MPLS), second will be the coding standard, and thirdly will be the error control and concealment.

4.1 DiffServ/MPLS evaluation

First is the evaluation of the performance of DiffServ with MPLS in a multiservice IP-based network. The simulation is performed with only DiffServ first and thereafter with a combination of both DiffServ and MPLS, and as part of this performance evaluation different schedulers were evaluated to determine the most appropriate one for real-time traffic, which is delay and delay variation sensitive, in a differentiated services environment. Topology used is as shown in Figure 1.

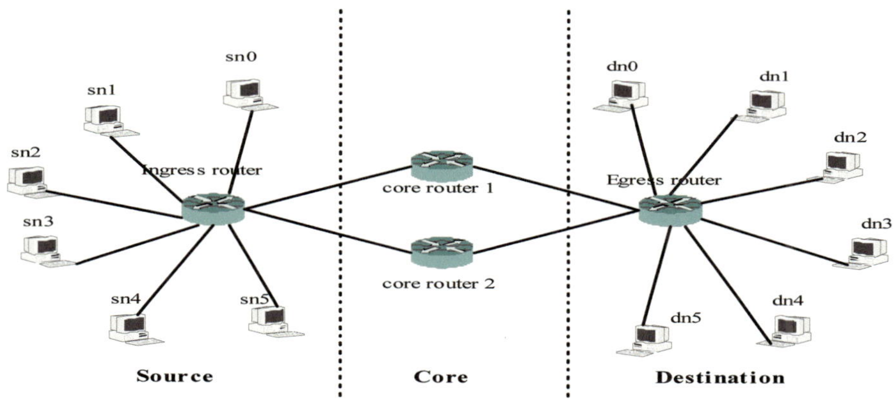

Fig. 1. Simulation setup

Each site in the network is capable of communicating using video, voice or data and these applications can either run one at a time or simultaneously. Since most of rural systems have a limited bandwidth, the core links are represented by bidirectional E1 links (2.048 Mbps).

4.1.1 Traffic source definition

Multi-service traffic involves data, voice and video traffic. Data traffic is usually transmitted using Transport Control Protocol (TCP) while real-time traffic such as voice and interactive video are transmitted using User Datagram Protocol (UDP). To simulate data applications,

Telnet and FTP traffic sources are going to be considered. To simulate speech traffic, which is characterized by alternating spurts and periods of silence, an ON/OFF process is going to be used. Since the ON (or OFF) periods do not have a heavy-tailed distribution, a non fractal version of the ON/OFF model with an exponential distribution of on and off times is suitable. So voice traffic is simulated by the G.711 audio codec, which transmit data over RTP. The G.711 codec outputs data at a constant rate of 64 kbps with a frame size of 240 bytes, and in the case of IP-based networks, these frames are encapsulated by the IP/UDP/RTP protocols that augment the basic frame size with their headers resulting in packet sizes of 280 bytes for IPv4 and 300 bytes for IPv6, and transmission rates of 74.667 kbps for IPv4 and 80 kbps for IPv6. The parameters for speech traffic ON/OFF source are given in Table 4.

Traffic type	Mean ON duration (seconds)	Mean OFF duration (seconds)	Peak rate (Packets/second)
Voice	0.35	0.65	80k

Table 4. Simulation parameters for the voice

These ON/OFF parameters for VoIP are widely used in literature (Rakocevic, 2003) and are taken from measurements by Deng (1995). For data sources, the packet size is 1500 bytes for each type.
The real-time video is simulated using a trace driven source. These traces are generated from 'Mr Bones' (a movie by a South African comedian, Leon Schuster), which is encoded using H.264 at 600 kbps.

4.1.2 Service definition

To support service differentiation, the simulated model specifies the following class:

- Premium for real time traffic that requires low latency, low jitter and low loss, which is classified as EF.
- Silver for data services like telnet and FTP, which is classified as AF11 for Telnet and AF 12 for FTP
- Best effort for non-emergent traffic such as e-mail

4.1.3 Simulation results

Nine schedulers: PQ, SCFQ, SFQ, WFQ, WF2Q+, LLQ, WIRR, RR, and WRR, were compared using the three QoS parameters: packet loss, [one way] delay, and jitter. Two traffic types were used for simulation: video trace and constant bit rate (CBR) traffic for other traffic source. Two queues were configured to support both EF and BE aggregates. Video was transmitted as premium traffic using EF services, while CBR was transmitted using BE services. To avoid synchronization problems, background traffic was generated with several CBR sources whose rate was chosen from a uniform random distribution in the range [10 kbps, 100 kbps], while the starting time was chosen from a uniform random distribution in the range [0 s, 5 s]. The simulation was done using packet sizes ranging from 64 to 1600 bytes.
The simulation results revealed that WFQ has the lowest average jitter values which are less than 1.55 ms, followed by LLQ with average values which are less than 1.65 ms, PQ and RR with average values that are less than 1.7 ms, and then others. The simulation results also

revealed that when it comes to one way delay (OWD) PQ and LLQ have the lowest average one-way latency values which are less than 17.5 ms, followed by RR with average values of less than 19 ms, and then others.

The second scenario simulated was to check the ability of DiffServ to provide QoS of service when the network is heavy loaded and also its ability to do fast rerouting in the event of node or link failure when it is used alone.

The results revealed that as the number of video traffic is increased the one way delay and delay variations also increase as shown in Figure 2. However, when MPLS was incorporated in the simulation it was found that both the one way delay and jitter were reduced as shown in Figure 3. The simulation results also revealed that in the event of link or node failure, MPLS has an ability to do fast rerouting.

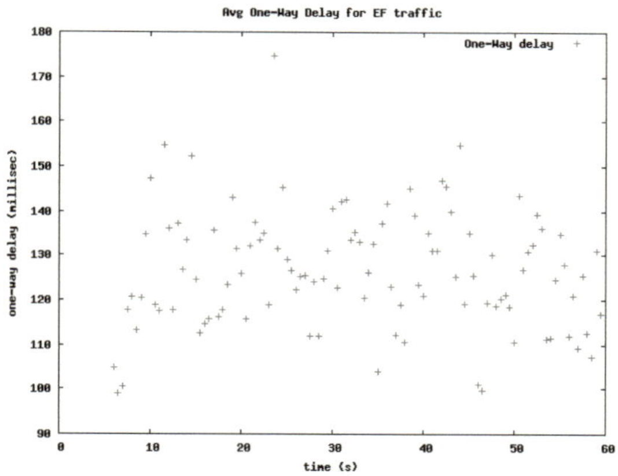

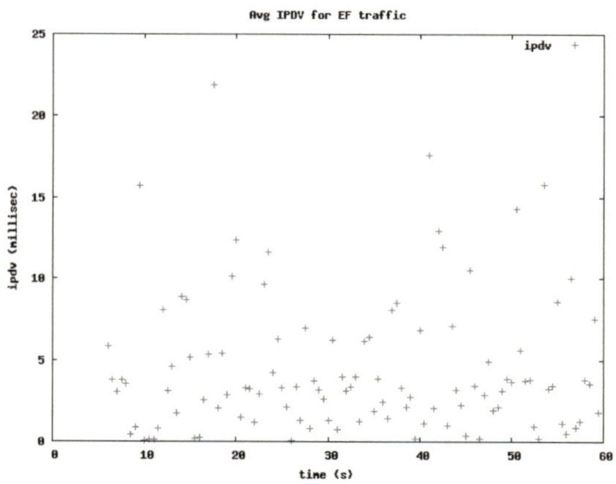

Fig. 2. One Way Delay (OWD) and Jitter (IPDV) for DiffServ only

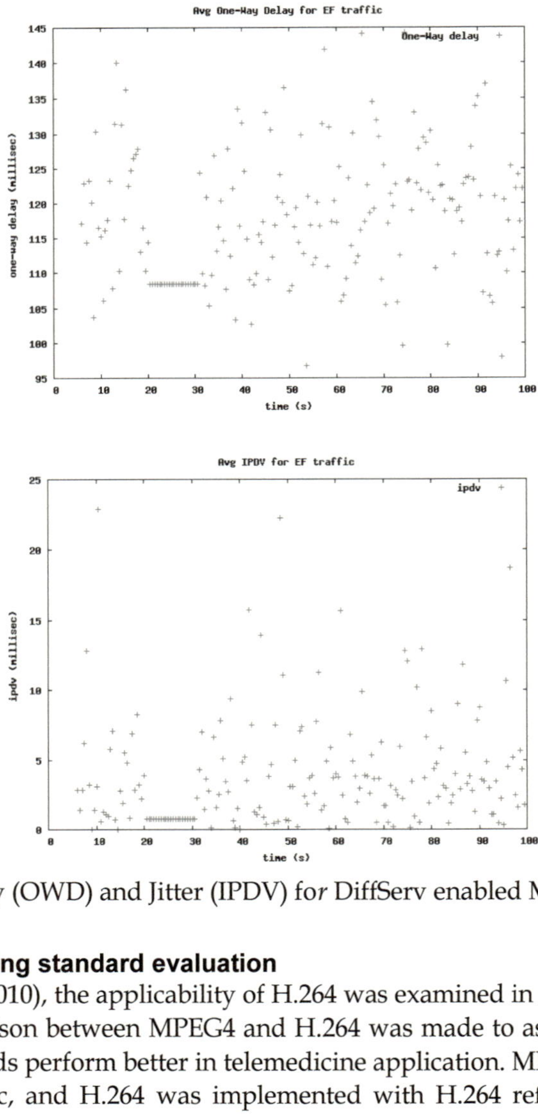

Fig. 3. One Way Delay (OWD) and Jitter (IPDV) for DiffServ enabled MPLS

4.2 Low bit-rate coding standard evaluation

In a study by Zoha (2010), the applicability of H.264 was examined in telemedicine reference model and a comparison between MPEG4 and H.264 was made to assess which of the two video coding standards perform better in telemedicine application. MPEG was implemented with MoMuSys codec, and H.264 was implemented with H.264 reference model version JM6.1e.

With the test conditions for MPEG 4 set to match those of H.264, the results achieved showed that H.264 performs much better than MPEG 4 (Zoha, 2010).

4.3 Error control and concealment evaluation

Tests of the performance of the H.264 in an erroneous environment were also performed by the author to check the error resiliency of the H.264 using evaluation process steps as depicted in Figure 4.

A raw YUV digital video sequence, called "Mother & Daughter", was downloaded in CIF format from the site http://www.tkn.tu-berlin.de/research/evalvid/cif.html, and processed by JM1.7 codec to generate a H.264 bitstream at 213.95 kbps. After encoding the trace files were generated, then followed by all the perceptual video evaluation process steps depicted in Figure 4. Errors were introduced in the communication process in order to simulate link-level errors and losses. Then the quality of video was evaluated before and after transmission using peak signal-to-noise ratio (PSNR), Video quality measurement (VQM), and Double stimulus impairment scale (DSIS) measurements. Common compression artifacts such as blockiness (or block distortion), and blur (loss in the detail that occurs around edges, typically due to the quantization of transform coefficients representing higher frequencies) were also evaluated.

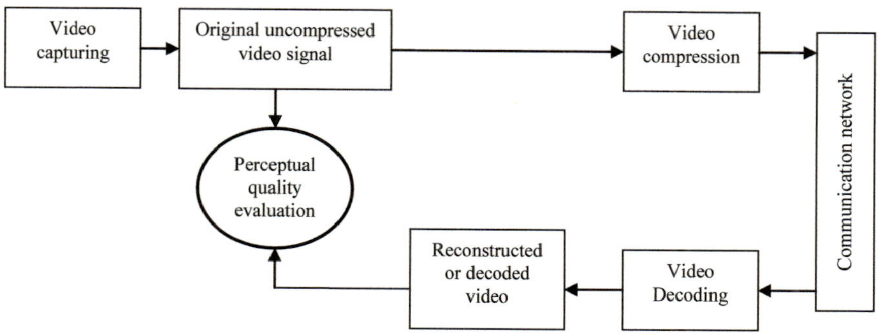

Fig. 4. Perceptual video evaluation process

The first test was done without any Intra-coded macro-blocks (MBs), and the second test was done with Intra-coded MBs, which are used in H.264 encoding to prevent error propagation (Shi et al., 2008). The results of the tests are presented in Figures 5, through 8, and Table 5.

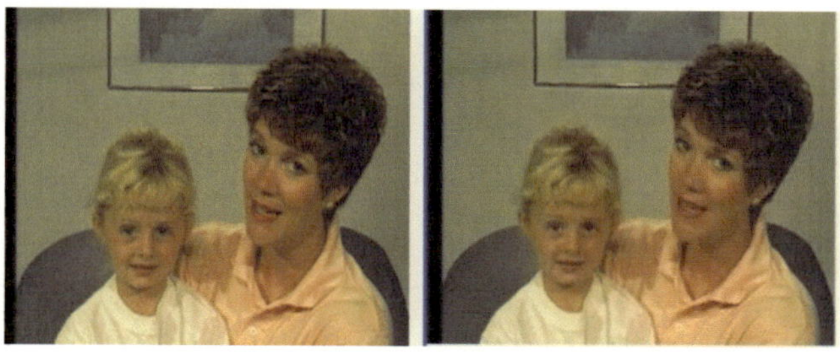

Fig. 5. Original and encoded video before transmission

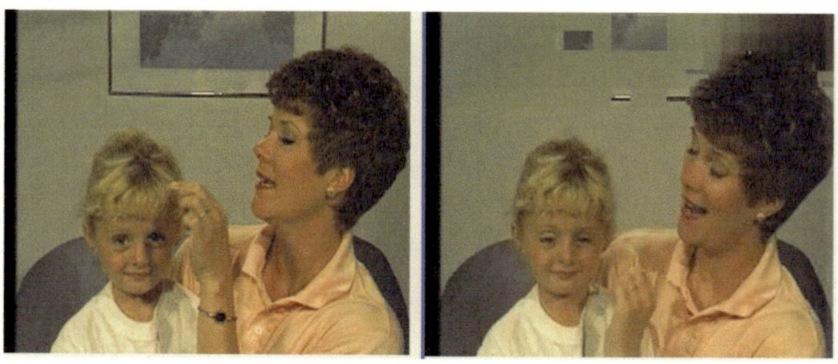

Fig. 6. Original and received video (without Intra-coded MBs) after transmission

Where Figure 5 shows the original (raw) and processed (encoded and decoded) video before transmission, Figure 6 shows the Original and received video (without Intra-coded MBs) after transmission, Figure 7 shows the original video and the received video (with Intra-coded MBs) after transmission, and Figure 8 shows the PSNR plots of the three conditions: before transmission, after transmission (without Intra-coded MBs), and after transmission (with Intra-coded MBs).

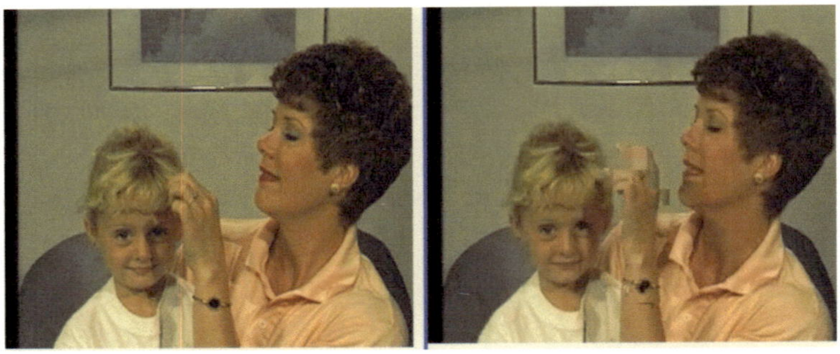

Fig. 7. Original video and the received video (with Intra- coded MBs) after transmission

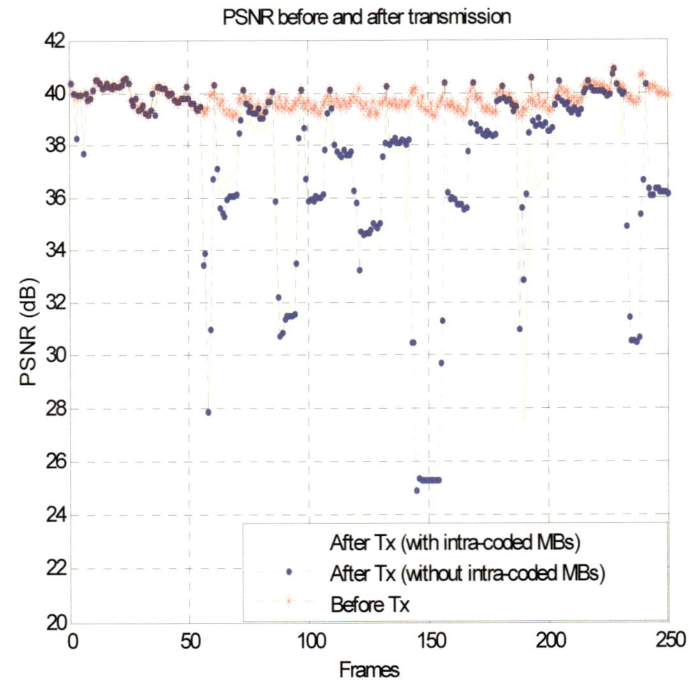

Fig. 8. PSNR quality plots before and after transmission

Table 5 gives a summary of the values of the mean PSNR, VQM and DSIS scores, and impairments such as blurring, blockiness and jerkiness of the encoded video before and after transmission..

Processed video under measurement	Mean PSNR (dB)	VQM score	DSIS score	Blurring %	Jerkiness %	Blockiness %
Before transmission	39.77			21	28	26
After transmission (without intra- MBs)	37.28	0.50	3.0	25	28	51
After transmission (with Intra-MBs)	38.35	0.38	3.5	22	28	37

Table 5. Summary of mean PSNR, VQM score, DSIS Score, and perceptual effects

From the PSNR plots, the received decoded pictures, and the results in Table 5 it can be seen that the errors introduced by the channel can have a profound effect on the quality of the transmitted video. However, using Intra-coded MBs, during coding can help minimize the effects of the errors. This is can be observed in the images of the received videos in Figures 6(right)-7(right). For example, in Figure 6(right) the fingers of the left hand, picture on the wall and the tip of the head of the mother is distorted due to the errors introduce by the channel, whereas in Figure 7(right), which is the video that is encoded with Intra-MBs, that only the hand of the mother has been affected by errors. This means then that the erasure effect that is caused by the packet loss and errors in the channel can be minimized by using resynchronization (or Intra-coded MBs), which prevents error propagation. This is also evident from the summary of the evaluation results in Table 5.

5. Conclusion

This chapter presents a holistic approach to the provision of quality of service in IP-based telemedicine system. Methods of mitigating some of the problems that degrade the quality of real-time video when transmitted over packet networks are be discussed. These include mechanisms to compensate for packet networks idiosyncrasy, especially IP best-effort debilities, in order to meet the latency and jitter requirements of real-time traffic. Secondly, to cater for erroneous channel and limited bandwidth, the solution includes adopting coding techniques that will provide coding efficiency, high quality video that is consistent at high and low bit rates, resilience to transmission errors, scalability, and network friendliness, which will result in perceived quality improvement, high-compression efficiency to suite the limited bandwidth, and possibility of transportation over different types of networks.

To facilitate quality of service within IP networks, DiffServ has been adopted in this study so as to provide differentiated services for different classes by using mechanisms that include packet classification, policing, class-based queuing and scheduling, and random early detection. To complement the DiffServ and provide a holistic approach to the provision of QoS, traffic engineering using MPLS was incorporated. MPLS provides connection-oriented paths in a connectionless IP environment. It also provides fast reroute during link or route failure, thus minimizing packet loss that can cause quality degradation and unavailability. The two technologies: DiffServ and MPLS compliments each other to minimize delay, jitter and packet loss.

Since almost every telemedicine system includes real-time video, which is bandwidth hungry, reduction of video transmission rate is required in order to transmit it in real-time over the band-limited channel that is available in most of the rural and mobile communication systems used in telemedicine. Tests have shown that H.264 is the best candidate for low bit rate video compression. Tests have also shown that H.264 has a superior built-in error resiliency to guarantee better quality even under erroneous transmission conditions.

6. References

Afullo, T.J.O. (2004). Quality of Service in Telecommunications - The Custormer's Perspective, *Proceedings of IEEE AFRICON 2004, 7th AFRICON Conference in Africa*, Vol. 1, pp. 101-106, ISBN: 0-7803-8605-1 Gaborone, Botswana, September 15-17, 2004.

Aidarous, S. & Plevyak T. (Eds) (2003). *Managing IP Networks: challenges and Opportunities - IEEE Press Series on Network Management*, John Wiley & Sons, New Jersey, ISBN 978-0471392996.

Cisco Systems, (2002). *Cisco AVVID Network Infrastructure Enterprise Quality of Service Design: Solutions Reference Network Design*, August 2002, Available from: http://docstore.mik.ua/cisco/pdf/Cisco AVVID Network Infrastructure.pdf

Du, B.; Maeder, A. & Moody M. (2003). ECC Video: An Active Approach for Error Resilience. *Proceedings of VIIth Digital Image Computing: Techniques and Applications*, 10-12 December, Sydney, pp.1027-1036, ISBN 0-643-09041-X.

Feng, S.; Liang, Z. & Zhao, D. (2010). Providing Telemedicine Services in an Infrastructure-Based Cognitive Radio Network. *IEEE Wireless Communications*, February 2010, pp. 96-103, ISSN 1536-1284.

Fineberg, V. (2003). QoS Support in MPLS Networks. MPLS/Frame Relay Alliance *White Paper*, [March 2004] Available from: www.mfaforum.org/tech/MPLSQOSWPMay2003.pdf

Ghazel, C. & Saïdane, L. (2008). Migration from Traditional Networks to Converged Next Generation Networks Architecture with Guaranteed Quality of Service, *Proceedings of the International Conference on Convergence and Hybrid Information Technology 2008*, pp. 417-424 ISBN, 978-0-7695-3328-5, Daejeon, Korea, August 28-29, 2008..

Goode, B. (2002). Voice Over Internet Protocol (VoIP). *Proceedings of the IEEE*, Vol. 90, No. 9, pp. 1495-1517, September 2002, ISSN 0018-9219.

Gouveia, F.C.; Rebahi, Y.; Planella, P.R. & Magedanz, T. (2009). *Network Protocols and Algorithms*, Vol. 1, No. 2, ISSN 1943-3581, pp.99-112.

Hassan, H.; Garcia, J.-M. & Brun, O. (2005). Generic modeling of multimedia traffic sources, Report No05350, *Proceedings of the 3rd International Working Conference on Performance Modeling and Evaluation of Heterogeneous Networks (HET-NETs'05)*, pp. 14/1-14/10, Ilkley, West Yorkshire, U.K., July 18-20, 2005.

Ibe, O.C. (2002). *Converged Network Architectures: Delivering voice and Data over IP, ATM, and Frame Relay*, John Wiley & Sons, New York, ISBN 0471202509.

Kilkki, K. (2008). Quality of Experience in Communication Ecosystem. *Journal of Universal Computer Science*, Vol. 14, No. 5, pp. 615-654.

Leon-Garcia A. & Widjaja I. (2004).Communication Networks: Fundamental Concepts and key Architectures, 2nd edition. McGraw Hill, Boston, ISBN 0-07-246352-X.

Li, A.H.; Kittitornkun, S.; Hu, Y.-H.; Park, D.-S. & Villasenor, J. (2000). Data Partitioning and Reversible Variable Length Codes for Robust Video Communications, *Proceedings of*

2000 IEEE Data Compression Conference (DCC'00), (March 2000), pp. 460-469, ISBN: 0-7695-0592-9 Snowbird, Utah, March 28-30, 2000..

Malindi, P. & Kahn, M.T. (2008). Providing QoS for IP-Based Rural Telemedicine Systems". *Proceedings of the Third International Conference on Broadband Communications, Information Technology & Biomedical Applications,* pp. 499-504, ISBN 978-1-4244-3281-3, Pretoria (Gauteng, South Africa), November 23-26, 2008.

Minei, I. (2004). MPLS DiffServ-aware Traffic Engineering, *White Paper,* Juniper Networks Inc., Sunnyvale, CA, USA

Muhammed, N.; Chiavelli, D.; Soldani, D. & Li, M. (2006). Introduction, In: *QoS and QoE Management in UMTS Cellular Systems,* Soldani, D.; Li, M. & Cuny, R. (eds.), p. 1-8, Wiley & Sons, [January 2011], Available from: http://onlinelibrary.wiley.com/doi/10.1002/9780470034057.ch1/summary

Nanda, P. & Fernandes, R.C. (2007). Quality of Service in Telemedicine, *Proceedings of the First International Conference on the Digital Society, ICDS 2007, Telemedicine workshop,* ISBN 0-7695-2760-4, Guadeloupe (French Caribbean), January 2-6, 2007.

Panayides, A.; Pattichis, M.S.; Pattichis, C.S.; Schizas, C.N.; Spanias, A. & Kyriacou, E. (2010). An overview of recent end-to-end wireless medical video telemedicine systems using 3G, *Engineering in Medicine and Biology Society (EMBC), 2010 Annual International Conference of the IEEE* , pp.1045-1048, Buenos Aires, Argentina, August 31-September 4 2010

Patrikakis, C.H.; Despotopoulos, Y.; Rompotis, A.; Boukouvalas, C.; Pediaditis, G. & Lambiris A. (2003). OLYMPIC: Using the Internet for real time coverage of major athletic events. *International Conference on Cross Media Service Delivery,* May 30-31, 2003, Santorini, Greece.

Pattichis, C.S.; Kyriacou, E.; Voskarides, S.; Pattichis, M.S.; Istepanian, R. & Schizas, C.N., (2002). Wireless Telemedicine Systems: *An Overview. IEEE Antenna's and Propagation Magazine,* Vol. 44, No. 2, April 2002.

Rakocevic V., (2003). Impact of End-to-end QoS Connectivity on the Performance of Remote Wireless Local Networks. *Proceedings of the IASTED Communication Systems and Networks Conference (CSN 2003),* ISBN 0-88986-388-1, Benalmadena, Spain, September 8-10, 2003.

[RFC3564]: Le Faucheur, F. & Lai, W., (2003). Requirements for Support of Differentiated Service-aware MPLS Traffic Engineering, July 2003, [March 2004] Available from: http://www.ietf.org/rfc/rfc3564.txt

Riley, M.J. & Richardson I. E.G. (1997). *Digital Video* Communication. Artech House, Boston, ISBN 978-0890068908.

Salatian, A.; Adepoju, F. & Oborkhale, L. (2011). Using Wavelets to Improve Quality of Service for Telemedicine. *International Journal of Advanced Science and Technology,* pp. 27-34, ISSN 2005-4238, Vol. 27, February 2011

Shi, Y.; Zhu, X.; Xia, J. & Yin, H. (2008). A Fast and Efficient Spatial Error Concealment for Intra-coded Frames, *Proceedings of the Congress on Image and Signal Processing, 2008 (CISP '08),* pp. 264-267, ISBN 978-0-7695-3119-9, 27-30 May 2008

Sikora, T. (2005). Trends and Perspective in Image and Video Coding". *Proceedings of the IEEE,* Vol. 93, No. 1, January 2005, pp. 6-17.

Skorin-Kapov, L. & Matijasevic, M. (2010). Analysis of QoS Requirements for e-Health Services and Mapping to Evolved packet System QoS Classes. *International Journal of Telemedicine Applications,* Vol. 2010, Hindawi Publishing Corporation.

Stanković, V.; Hamzaoui, R. & Xiong Z. (2003). Live video streaming over packet networks and wireless channels, *Proceedings of PV2003 13th Packet Video Workshop*, Nantes, April 2003.

Sullivan, G.J. & Wiegand, T. (2005). Video Compression - From Concepts to H.264/AVC Standard, *Proceedings of the IEEE*, Vol. 93, No. 1, January, pp.18-31.

Sze, H.P.; Liew, S.C.; Lee, J.Y.B. & Yip, D.C.S. (2002). A Multiplexing Scheme for H.323 Voice-Over-IP Applications, *IEEE Journal on Selected Areas in Communications*, Vol. 20, No. 7, September 2002.

Szymanski, T.H. & Gilbert, D. (2010). Provisioning mission-critical telerobotic control systems over internet backbone networks with essentially-perfect QoS, *IEEE Journal on Selected Areas in Communications*, Vol.28, No.5, pp.630-643, June 2010.

Talluri, R. (1998). Error-Resilient Video Coding in ISO MPEG-4 Standard". *IEEE Communication Magazine*, June 1998, pp.112-119.

Tobagi, F.A. (2005). A Top Down View of Quality of Service", *ST Journal of Research*, Vol. 2, No. 1, Networked Multimedia, pp.6-30.

Tulu, B. & Chatterjee, S. (2008). Internet-based telemedicine: An empirical investigation of objective and subjective video quality. *Dicision Support Systems*, Vol. 45, Issue 4, ISSN 0167-9236, pp. 681-696, November 2008.

Vergados, D.J.; Vergados, D.D. & Maglogianis, I. (2006). Applying Wireless DiffServ for QoS Provissioning in Mobile Emergency Telemedicine. *Proceedings of the Global Telecommunications Conference, 2006. GLOBECOM '06*, San Francisco, CA, USA, 27 November - 1 December 2006.

Villasenor, J. D.; Zhang, Y. -Q. & Wen, J. (1999). Robust Video Coding Algorithms and Systems, *Proceedings of the IEEE*, Vol. 87, No. 10, October 1999, pp. 1724-1733.

Vouyioukas, D.; Maglogiannis, I. & Komnakos, D. (2007). Emergency M-Health services through high-speed 3G systems: simulation and performance evaluation, *Simulation*, Vol. 83, No. 2, pp. 329 - 345.

Wang, Y. & Zhu, Q.-F. (1998). Error Control and Concealment for Video Communication: A Review", *Proceedings of the IEEE*, Vol. 86, No. 5, May 1998, pp. 974-997.

Wang, Y.; Wenger, S.; Wen J. & Katsaggelos A.K. (2000). Error Resilient Video Coding Techniques, *IEEE Signal Processing Magazine*, Vol. 17, No. 4, July 2000, pp.61-89.

Wu, D.; Hou, Y.T. & Zhang, Y.-Q. (2000). Transporting Real-Time Video over the Internet: Challenges and Approaches, *Proceedings of the IEEE*, Vol. 88, No. 12, December 2000, pp.1855-1876.

Xiao, X.; Hannan, A.; Bailey, B. & Ni, L.M. (2000). Traffic Engineering with MPLS in the Internet, *IEEE Network Magazine*, Vol. 14, No. 2, March/April 2000, pp. 28-33.

Xiao, X.; Telkamp, T.; Fineberg, V.; Chen, C. & Ni, L.M. (2002). A practical approach for providing QoS in the Internet backbone, *IEEE Communications Magazine*, Vol. 40, No. 12, December 2002, pp. 56-62.

Zoha, M.U. (2010). Applicability of H.264 in Telemedicine Reference Model, *International Journal of Advanced Science and Technology, (IJAST)*, Vol. 27, (February 2010), pp. 7-11, ISSN 2005-4238.

Zvikhachevskaya, A.; Markarian, G. & Mihaylova, L., (2009). Quality of Service consideration for the wireless telemedicine and e-health services. *Proceedings of the 2009 IEEE conference on Wireless Communications & Networking Conference (WCNC'09)*, ISBN: 978-1-4244-2947-9 5-8 April, 2009, Budapest, Hungary.

6

On Redefining Telemedicine Paradigm: An Innovative Integrated Model for Efficient Implementation of Healthcare Delivery in Developing Countries

K.V.Sridhar and K.S.R.Krishna Prasad
National institute Of Technology Warangal (AP)
India

1. Introduction

There is varied accounts of the history of telemedicine in the published literature as well as in popular discourse. A careful review of these accounts reveals a common characteristic, despite significant variability between them. None of the reports has seriously considered the full story of telemedicine, including its continuity in medical practice in one form or another from ancient times to the present, the enduring necessity of connectivity in the delivery of medical care, the various transformations of telemedicine over the ages, or most importantly the contexts that sustained interest in this modality of practice. These accounts do not pay adequate attention to the rich context that prompted the early experimentation in the use of telecommunication technology in the delivery of healthcare and that continues to guide its development and transformation into the future. Delving into the detailed history of telecommunications as well as accounts and analysis of various national and regional initiatives aimed only at addressing the issues of healthcare access, quality, and cost . Nonetheless, the unintended detour gives a valuable insight and a genuine appreciation of the complexity and difficulty of designing optimal health systems that serve all segments of the population and that assure equity of access to standardized care at affordable prices. Indeed, gaining a better understanding of the broader context for the initiation, development, and persistence and the unique role a telemedicine can play in redressing intransigent problems in healthcare delivery as we go forward into an increasingly complex healthcare environment.

Tracing the history of long-distance communication from its humble origins in semaphore, and much later the telegraph, and radio to advanced digital communication and computer processing systems and even the recent trends in the transformation of telemedicine from simple "connectivity" tools to "versatility' tools in the mainstream of medical care, such as the use of telemedicine for clinical decision support, prescription ordering, disease management, patient empowerment, and disaster preparedness / response. These new application areas appropriate in various clinical settings and environments. However, they are not limited to connecting distant participants. Hence, it raises a question whether the term "telemedicine" still applies to these applications under our broader discussion of the nomenclature in this field. This chapter makes a special effort to place telemedicine development in its proper context, not simply as a technological innovation but as an effective solution to persistent problems in healthcare delivery including inequitable access to care in the population at large, uneven distribution of quality, and unabated cost inflation. Indeed, the persistence of these problems has provided the strongest rationale for the development and growth of telemedicine. The search for telemedicine's roots revealed the enduring need for connectivity in medical care in ancient times and the failure of repeated initiatives and national programs to address problems of inequity of access to healthcare in the population, discrepancies in quality of care between areas and regions, and unabated cost inflation in modern times. There is a great difference between the developing and the developed world on issues of health and healthcare services. The emphasis of the developing world is on basic survival (such as providing better access to healthcare and increasing the quality of health) whilst in the developed world, the emphasis is on reducing public funding for healthcare. Indeed, the rapid increases in healthcare costs and finding ways to control them have become the most important health policy issues for the developed world in the past few decades (Industry Canada, 2006).

The case for telemedicine rests on its promise to address some aspects of all of these problems in one form or another. Whereas the importance of these problems is universally acknowledged, for many observers, the efficacy of telemedicine remains a promise. For others, it has already been demonstrated at a reasonable level of confidence. In response to this discrepancy in perspective regarding the true merit of telemedicine, we have tried to highlight the scientific evidence available to date, in order to achieve as much closure on the question as possible. Also, since evaluative research will continue to occupy centre stage, we have attempted to identify the methodological requirements for this research as we pursue the search for more conclusive evidence regarding the true merit of telemedicine.

2. Health scenario in India

India is a second most highly populated ancient country with rich history, culture, and traditions coupled with geography and environment that encompasses the entire spectrum of conditions and bio-diversity. A large segment of population resides in rural and suburban areas, which lack adequate health infrastruction. To ensure that all sections of the society is able to fully participate in its development and progression has been, continues to be, and will do so in future, a challenge to one and all. With its more than a billion population, there exists a finite limit of elasticity in providing healthcare in terms of infrastructure, facility, manpower and funds. Wide disparities continue to persist between the various income groups, communities, states and even the districts within a state. With a predominantly rural population that are distributed over wide geographical locations, apart from the densely populated urban areas, providing even the basic and minimally acceptable healthcare has been and continues to be the priority of Indian health administrators. Further this is compounded by the following factors like:

- Low paying capacity of the rural population
- Lack of investment in health care in rural areas
- Inadequate medical facilities in rural & inaccessible areas
- Problem of retaining doctors in rural areas where they are required to serve & propagate widespread health awareness.
- Specialist doctors cannot be retained at rural areas as they will be professionally isolated and become obsolete and even monetary incentives also cannot prevent it.

2.1 The facts on India's health care situation are as follows

- 620 million live in rural India (National Council for Applied Economic Research (NCAER))
- Bed-Population ratio 1.85 per thousand (2005) Vs. ideal of 1:500 Central bereau of health intelligence CBHI)
- Doctor-patient ratio in the country is one doctor for nearly 2,000 persons (in the US it is 1:400),
- 2 million beds are required as against 0.7 million available.
- 700 hospitals of 250 beds each are required every year.
- only 9% of 1 billion people are covered health schemes.
- only 0.9% of GDP for health (WHO recommends 5%)
- 5% of annual family income spent towards curative health care.

The distribution of specialists in India is indeed lopsided. There are more neurologists and neurosurgeons in Chennai, than in all the states of North eastern India put together. Similarly tertiary care hospitals are also concentrated in pockets with large segments of the population having no access.

India is short of 600,000 doctors, 1 million nurses, and 200,000 dental surgeons to achieve 1:10,000 doctor-patient ratio. A recent survey by the Indian Medical society has found 75% of qualified consulting doctors practice in urban centers and 23% in semi urban areas and only 2% from rural areas whereas majority of the patients come from rural areas. . Contagious, infectious and waterborne diseases such as diarrhoea, amoebiasis, typhoid, infectious hepatitis, worm infestations, measles, malaria, tuberculosis, whooping cough, respiratory infections, pneumonia and reproductive tract infections dominate the morbidity pattern, especially in rural areas. However, non-communicable diseases such as cancer, blindness, mental illness, hypertension, diabetes, HIV / AIDS, etc. are also on the rise. Health being a State of subject in every human life, the data in regard to **Doctor-patient ratio** (D:P)in various State Government Hospitals is not maintained centrally. The doctor-patient ratio, varies from case to case depending upon various factors like the type of disease, nature of specialization, type of patient-care required i.e. indoor/outdoor. According to the Medical Council of india, the present allopathic doctor-population ratio at present works out to 1:1722.

The health of a nation is the product of many factors and forces that combine and interact. Economic growth, per capita income, literacy, education, age at marriage, birth rates, information on health care and nutrition, access to safe drinking water, public and private health care infrastructure, access to preventive health and medical care and the health insurance are among the contributing factors. Given that many conditions are preventable, every health care interaction should include prevention support. When patients are systematically provided with information and skills to reduce health risks, substance use, stop using tobacco products, practice safe sex, eat healthy foods, and engage in physical activity can dramatically reduce the long-term burden and health care demands of chronic conditions. To promote prevention in health care: awareness rising, change in thinking, stimulate the commitment of patients and families, health care teams, communities and policy-makers is crucial. A collaborative management approach at the primary health care level with patients, their families and other health care actors is a must to effectively prevent many major contributors to the burden of disease. Given that many conditions are preventable, every health care interaction should be recorded.

The advances in medical science and biomedical engineering on one side and Information and Communication Technology (ICT) on the other are offering wide opportunities for improved health care. Despite making great strides in overall development and uplifting of largely rural-based, thickly populated urban areas and essentially economically challenged sections of the society, providing proper and desirable levels of health care to them still remains an unfulfilled dream.

Telemedicine is supposed to contribute quality health care to those in need irrespective of socio economic ,density, geographical disparities and should be available for the benefit of all people located in dense urban, rural, remote and inaccessible places, and to further enhance its end-to-end capability. An efficient telemedicine network would mean that a large amounts of data (like medical records) is generated and maintained. These databases would be accessible on a national/ international telemedicine grid. Software and hardware is needed to manage all this, and organizations to take care of the operations.

Most decision-makers, managers, health care professionals and citizens lack basic information on telemedicine services and potential. This has resulted in misconceptions, resistance to telemedicine and relative lack of progress in project initiation. Telemedicine is still not recognized as a technical programme within the ministries of health and is not a unit at the ministries of telecommunications. The idea of being treated from one's home is very comforting and is proving to be cost-effective. Driven by the aging population, the increased medical requirements in remote locations, and the recent advancements in technology, the world market for telemedicine is forecast to reach $18 billion by 2015 (Source: Global Industry Analysts Inc.). Hence, telemedicine will soon play a very important role inhuman life. This has resulted in dealing with telemedicine projects as pilot or demonstration projects despite the fact that they are fully functional and operational in most cases. Developing Countries does not have the necessary legal and administrative framework to incorporate telemedicine service in the national health care systems. There is a need to develop plans or to create frameworks to introduce telemedicine services at the national level. Full understanding and commitment by top management to telemedicine should be secured and seen as essential for the success of telemedicine projects. Introduction of telemedicine as part of the national health care system requires thorough study and consideration at all levels. There is an acute need for telemedicine services with special emphasis on tele-consultation, tele-education and tele-radiology. Continuous medical education has become an integral element of patient care in an ever-expanding field of medicine. Tele-education can help as many health care professionals in remote areas deprived from any means of continuing education, the heterogeneous background of health care professionals with different medical and health backgrounds, the lack of organized health education.

Various organizations & researchers defined Telemedicine as :

Definition 1

The delivery of health care services, where distance is a critical factor, by health care professionals using info & Communication Technologies for exchange of valid information for diagnosis, treatment & prevention of diseases & injuries, research & evaluation and for the continuing of health care providers all in the interest of advancing the health and their communities.

---World Health Organisation

Definition 2

TM N/ W is to provide quality, cost effective patient care to underserved rural communities &Providing access to specialty care with in rural community needs of patient is met by decreasing travel time, cost & lost wages and impact of time & distance on morbidity.

--- University of Tennesse Med center

Definition 3

Rapid access to shared and remote medical expertise by means of Telecommunications & Informatio Technology. No matter where the patient or relevant information is located.

--European Commissions Health care Telematics program

Definition 4

The use of electronic medical info. & Comm. To provide and support health care when distance separates the participants

---www.Hospitalmgt.net

Definition 5

T.M is the use of medical info. Exchange from onsite to another via electronic Communication to improve patients health or status of health care provider.

---American Telemedicine Association

Def6

T.M. is the investigation , monitoring and management of patients and education of patients & staff using systems which allow ready access to expert advice & patients info. No matter where the patient or relevant info is located.

----European Health Telematics research programme

Other Definitions

T.M services provide means to improve accessibility to high quality health care in case of shortage of appropriate health professionals or the necessary medical expertise or skills at the site of the patient.

T.M thus covers a broad spectrum of services such as tele-consultation, second opinion, homecare and training and builds on technologies such as video-conferencing supported by the exchange of medical images and medical records as well as remote Monitoring. Communication infrastructures include ordinary telephone landlines, internet connections of various speeds and in many instances also satellite links to enable health care in remote and isolated areas.

T.M is a generic term covering the application of a variety of proven electronic and communication techniques in providing healthcare. Telemedicine offers the potential to alleviate the severe shortage of medical specialists in developing countries.

However the traditional approach to telemedicine relies on real-time video interaction between the specialist and the referring physician or patient). Digital imaging and the availability of ISDN lines have extended the reach of this technology in developed countries, but it remains impractical and uneconomic in remote and resource poor areas. However, medical diagnosis and management can often be achieved with the use of textual descriptions and still images. This "store-and-forward" approach to telemedicine simulates the working patterns of radiologists, pathologists, and those of certain clinical specialties such as dermatology, infectious diseases.

After critical investigations in all the above definitions stated revealed that the root cause or locus for origination of TM is POOR DOCTOR TO PATIENT RATIO (D:P). In all the definitions stated it is true only in geographically isolated or less densely populated developed countries . While in high densely populated developing countries like india , china and many other countries all over the world the situation is different where there is an acute shortage of physicians and medical specialties. Due to high cost and poor living conditions, people below the poverty line are not ready to afford their earnings and time towards health care.

In view of various definitions stated without looking into the fact of D:P, it is now essential to **Redefine** TM in such a way so as to include the phrase **To improve Doctor to Patient Ratio**.

While many visionaries believe that increasing Doctors is solely the solution to the above problem of poor D: P. Investigations & surveys in many health care modalities have revealed that early detection of any abnormality can reduce the risk of health. Preventive Health care reduces the number of patients and hence the need for more doctors, thereby increasing virtually D: P.

2.2 Preventive healthcare

Preventive healthcare involves measures taken to identify and minimize risk factors for disease, improve the course of an existing disease and screening for early detection of diseases in people who do not yet have any signs or symptoms. Early recognition and prevention of disease is an important part of healthcare because it detects disease at the initial and curable stages thereby preventing complications and co-morbidities. It is also cheaper and effective than treating a full-blown disease at a later stage. It also involves health promotion, which is aimed at modifying the individual's social circumstance and lifestyles so that their health is improved (or maintained) and disease is prevented. Another aspect of Preventive Healthcare is the early identification of high-risk individuals prone to major life-threatening illnesses like heart disease and cancers. This helps in taking timely, precautionary lifestyle modification measures or treatment. The ultimate goal of screening is to help people live longer, healthier lives.

2.3 Why is preventive healthcare so crucial?

Some diseases like cancers cannot be cured if they are diagnosed at an advanced state while some disorders like heart disease may result in sudden death without any previous warning signs. Prevention, in such cases, is not only better than cure but is often the only option for a healthy life. Modern lifestyles don't leave people with quality time for healthy routines. It then becomes necessary that periodic health checkups be done for early detection of risk factors and diseases. Diabetes, Obesity, Hypertension, Stress, High Cholesterol, Heart Diseases. Most of the diseases are "silent", We often do not have any early symptoms. Hence regular screening tests are the only way for early detection. All these diseases are quite debilitating. They seriously impair normal life and if left untreated, lead to complications and may even cause death. Fortunately, these diseases can be easily prevented and even fully cured if detected early. Some of these diseases can be 'managed' so that one can lead a near normal life. All that one need to do is to make slight modifications in your lifestyle, eat regularly and responsibly, exercise, avoid stress, and sleep well. Regular health check - ups coupled with these lifestyle changes, can go a long way in the prevention, early detection and cure of these diseases.

2.4 Integrating prevention into health care

Due to public health successes, people are ageing and are increasingly living with one or more chronic conditions for decades. This places new, long-term demands on health care systems. Not only are chronic conditions projected to be the leading cause of disability throughout the world by the year 2020; if not successfully prevented and managed, they will become the most expensive problems faced by our health care systems. People with diabetes, for example, generate health care costs that are two to three times those without the condition, and in Latin America the costs of lost production due to diabetes are estimated to be five times the direct health care costs. In this respect, chronic conditions pose a threat to all countries from a health and economic standpoint.

Many costly and disabling conditions - cardiovascular diseases, cancer, diabetes and chronic respiratory diseases - are linked by common preventable risk factors. Tobacco use, prolonged, unhealthy nutrition, physical inactivity, and excessive alcohol use are major causes and risk factors for these conditions. Trends in tobacco use will increase in the foreseeable future especially in developing countries. The ongoing nutritional transition expressed through increased consumption of high fat and high salt food products will contribute to the rising burden of heart disease, stroke, obesity and diabetes. Changes in activity patterns as a consequence of the rise of motorized transport, sedentary leisure time activities such as television watching will lead to physical inactivity in all but the poorest populations. Many diseases can be prevented, yet health care systems do not make the best use of their available resources to support this process. All too often, health care workers fail to seize patient interactions as opportunities to inform patients about health promotion and disease prevention strategies.

2.5 Current systems of health care

Many diseases can be prevented, yet health care systems do not make the best use of their available resources to support this process. All too often, health care workers fail to seize patient interactions as opportunities to inform patients about health promotion and disease prevention strategies.

Most current health care systems are based on responding to acute problems, urgent needs of patients, and pressing concerns. Testing, diagnosing, relieving symptoms, and expecting a cure are hallmarks of contemporary health care. While these functions are appropriate for acute and episodic health problems, a notable disparity occurs when applying this model of care to the prevention and management of chronic conditions. Preventive health care is inherently different from health care for acute problems, and in this regard, current health care systems worldwide fall remarkably short.

2.6 How can health systems respond to this challenge?

Given that many conditions are preventable, every health care interaction should include prevention support. When patients are systematically provided with information and skills to reduce health risks, they are more likely to reduce substance use, to stop using tobacco products, to practice safe sex, to eat healthy foods, and to engage in physical activity. These risk reducing behaviors can dramatically reduce the long-term burden and health care demands of chronic conditions. To promote prevention in health care, awareness rising is crucial to promote a change in thinking and to stimulate the commitment and action of patients and families, health care teams, communities, and policy-makers.

A collaborative medical data management approach at the primary health care level with patients, their families and other health care actors is a must to effectively prevent many major contributors to the burden of disease.

Many health care institutions have been investing in computerized systems for years, but only to automate the administrative or back-office work within the institution. New information systems are being designed to enable health information exchange across systems and institutions. Evidence suggests the use of secure, standards-based Health Information Technology and the timely, electronic exchange of health information could improve patient care, increase efficiency, and result in:

- Higher quality care through adherence to treatment protocols and guidelines;
- Reduction in adverse drug events and detection of pending patient error;
- Fewer duplicative treatments and tests;
- Administrative efficiencies through decreased paperwork;
- Improved population health and coordination of clinical care as a result of timely and appropriate access to individual and community health information;
- Early detection of infectious disease outbreaks around the country;
- Disease management tracking; and More complete data sources for use in research and policy.
- Comprehensive data on patients' conditions, treatments and outcomes.

Therefore Electronic Medical Records(EMR) A model emerged to be a dominant frame work for TM evaluation & research. Rapid technological development in IT which has lead to the emergence of new ways of managing information. Specifically for health care, the need for portability & instant communication has transformed use of EMR to create a more complete source of health care data management.

The Electronic Health Record (EHR) is a longitudinal electronic record of patient health information, shown as Appendix, generated by one or more encounters in any care delivery setting. Included in this information are patient demographics, progress notes, problems, observations, laboratory tests, diagnostic, treatments, therapies, drugs administered medications, vital signs, past medical history, immunizations and radiology reports etc. The EHR automates and streamlines the clinician's workflow. The EHR has the ability to generate a complete record of a clinical patient encounter, as well as supporting other care-related activities directly or indirectly via interface—including evidence-based decision support, quality management, and outcomes reporting.

EHR systems support physicians and other healthcare professionals in the delivery of care management services. Although published literature on the use of EHR systems in care management in solo and small group practices is very limited, there is a growing recognition of the role of EHR systems to support individual and population-based care management in medical practices. Independent of practice size, EHR systems support physicians and care teams in multiple care management areas, including patient self-management, individual and population management, delivery system design, and clinical decision support system.

2.7 Integrated health care

The Electronic Health Record (EHR) has been a key research field in medical informatics for many years. It refers to the complete set of information that resides in electronic form and is related to the past, present, and future health status or health care provided to a subject of care. Currently, many medical information systems are used in healthcare organizations: Hospital Information System (HIS), Radiology Information System (RIS), Picture Archiving and Communication System (PACS), Laboratory Information System (LIS) and so on. These EHR data is stored in many different formats in a multitude of medical information systems. Typical formats include relational database tables, structured document-based storage in various formats, and unstructured document storage such as digitized hardcopies maintained in a classic document management system. Clinicians must rely on the comparison and inter-confirmation among those data to make more accurate clinical diagnoses, treatment plans and preventive measures in their daily work. But with the rapid development of modern medical information technology, the modality and amount of EHR data can be incredibly large in a digital hospital environment. It is a very tedious and inefficient work for clinicians to extract valuable information directly from the raw form of those complex multi-modal EHR data. As a consequence, effective visualization methods are needed to reveal the hidden information carried by them.

Since 1990s, much work has been done to visualize different kinds of EHR data. Most of those work only focused on the visualization of one or several kinds of EHR data partially. But actually, these data should not be isolated from each other for diagnosis purpose. It is far from enough to visualize them separately. We must treat them as a whole during visualization, i.e., make an integrated visualization. As the complexity and multiplicity of EHR data grows, this work becomes a big challenge.

Nowadays, there is almost no single working EHR system due to the research level of medical informatics. Most EHR data of an individual is generated and recorded during his visits in various hospitals. An unified structure to represent the multi-modal EHR data as various clinical acts is needed. If a method is formulated to organize those data according to the two dimensional act-time relationships, thus we can achieve the integrated visualization based on this method. After analysing the characteristics of each kind of EHR data, some appropriate visualization forms are designed and implemented as an integrated viewer. By this means, we provide the clinicians an overall scene of the patient's personal history, present health status, and future care plans to be held. The integrated viewer figure .1 can, not only help the clinicians in their daily work, but also is useful for telemedicine consultation

2.8 Integrated Lifetime Health Record (LHR)

A repository of information regarding the health of a subject of care, in a form able to be processed by a computer that is stored and transmitted securely and accessible by multiple authorized users using different applications. It has a standardized information model which is independent of an EHR system. Its primary purpose is the support of continuing, efficient and quality integrated health care and it contains information that is retrospective, concurrent and prospective.

An integrated Lifetime Health Record (LHR) is fundamental for achieving seamless and continuous access to patient medical information and for the continuum of care. These can be achieved through the convergence of Information and Communication Technology (ICT), medical content and health knowledge. Through this convergence, the patient LHR can be shared among healthcare professionals and across healthcare facilities regardless of where the previous visit was. In contrast, the fragmented and paper-based medical records have significant limitations such as illegibility, unavailability, sheer physical volume (over time), difficult transferability and integration between providers and institutions, and the necessity to record the same data many times (duplication) on different documents (Roman *et al.*, 2006; Coiera, 2003; Pories, 1990). These problems become worse in situations where patients are able to freely visit any healthcare facilities for the same medical problem, and where the patients can be referred to an appropriate hospital anywhere in the country.

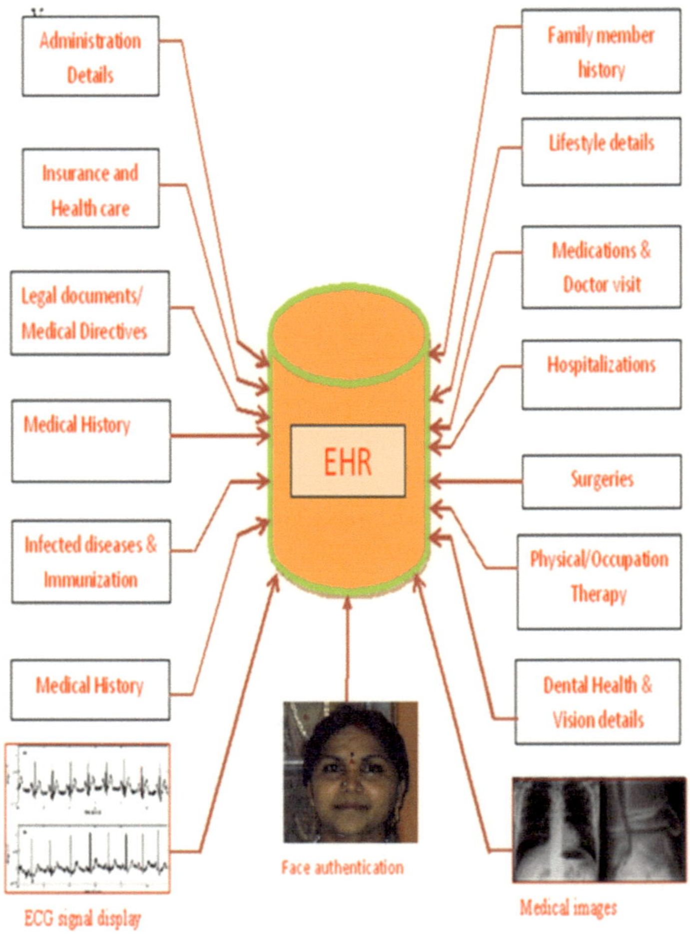

Fig. 1.

All countries in the globe, had taken initiatives to implement an integrated Electronic Health Record (EHR) system in their public health system either locally or nationwide. However, the aim has not yet been fully realised. The efforts are actively progressing towards finding the best approach in implementing integrated LHR on all levels of public healthcare facilities. Every stage of the development of the LHR initiatives had presented peculiar challenges. The best lessons are those of someone else's experiences. This chapter presents an overview of the development approaches to be undertaken in developing countries in implementing a national LHR in the public health system. The major challenges elicited from the review, including integration efforts, process reengineering, funding, people and law regulation are to be considered. If suitable, this chapter will provide guidance for best practices to implement the LHR for developing nations.

This LHR is expected to aid rehabilitation by maintaining health record of the human subjects, predicting various abnormality well in ahead and suggest health tips which are easily adaptable, hence avoid any sudden /unexpected degradation of health.

Widespread adoption of LHR has the potential to help consumers and patients manage their own health, help doctors and hospitals to immediately gather relevant information to best treat an individual patient, improve tracking of chronic disease management, and provide for early detection of infectious disease outbreaks around the country. LHR also provide:

- Cognitive support for healthcare professionals and patients to help integrate patient specific data where possible and account for any uncertainties that remain. Help healthcare professionals to help integrate evidence-based practice guidelines and research results into daily practice.
- Instruments that allow providers to manage a portfolio of patients and highlight problems as they arise within both individual patients and populations.
- Rapid integration of new instrumentation, biological knowledge, treatment modalities, etc., into a "learning" healthcare system that encourages early adoption of promising methods but also analyzes all patient experience as experimental data.
- Accommodation of growing heterogeneity of locales for provision of care, including home instrumentation for monitoring and treatment, lifestyle integration, and remote assistance.
- Empowerment of patients and their families in effective management of healthcare decisions and execution, including personal health records (as contrasted to medical records held by care providers), education about the individual's conditions and options, and support of timely and focused communication with professional

Some telemedicine systems set up at high cost are lying unused due to lack of technical skill in handling. Today most PHCs have the basic infrastructure, including a personal computer, and a little additional investment on Web camera, speaker and Internet connection is all that is required. Using simple computer system based health portal, doctors at a remote location can view the specialist and share medical data. The patient can also interact with the specialist. It operates on any available connectivity. The twin option of store and forward, and real time consultation, gives the physician at one end the opportunity to raise his doubts, and the specialist at the other end, the flexibility to answer queries later, if both are not free at the same time. The platform also offers a multi-specialty telemedicine software solution, and is designed to enable quick and easy creation of telemedicine referrals.

The data in Electronic Medical Records prepared in this way is archived in a structured fashion. Further, the progressive medical history of the patient can be maintained. ECGs (electro cardiogram), X rays and other scanned diagnostic images can also be stored and viewed both by patient/remote hospital/ primary health centre as well as the super speciality hospital to facilitate better diagnosis. The audio-video exchange helps specialists talk to patients in remote locations. The specialist at a tertiary care hospital can make a better assessment of a patient's condition. The audio-video interface happens in real time and saves time on patient care despite distances. All the data sits on a central server.

3. Conventional approach to electronic health records

Today's predominant approach to implementing electronic health records involves purchasing an information system to automate, or script care processes. The vendor may provide a "starter set" but commonly the healthcare provider has to build its pick lists to support data capture, its decision or communication support logic, etc. As the provider uses the system, the electronic health record is created "for free" as a byproduct of using the automated care process (Stead & Hammond, 1988). When care takes place in an area of the practice that is not yet automated, the record catches up through "after-the-fact" data entry. The vendors often seek to increase the coverage of the record by providing a suite of applications that work together supported by a common database. Data elements are mapped into standard formats, such as Health Level 7 (HL7), for exchange with parts of the vendor's suite that are not well integrated into the database or products from other vendors. Much of that mapping is repeated practice by practice because exchange standards clarify what the data element is, such as a drug orderable, but not what it means, such as its chemical ingredients, dose-form and strength. This automation approach is workable if the patient population and the healthcare provider are largely self-contained and if the provider can afford IT staff to handle the setup and data mapping, and the clinical process expertise to adapt practice and systems to avoid unintended consequences. Even when all of those conditions fall into place, the provider does not obtain the quality and safety benefits of electronic records until the automation of each part of the practice is complete enough to fill out the record. Once the automation is complete, the information system makes the process rigid, providing a barrier to change over time as new business demands are experienced, as advances in biomedical science alter in substantive ways approaches to defining and confirming specific diagnoses and as communities of patients and providers alter their approach toward managing health problems., Automation and transaction processing have their place supporting well defined, small scale work processes that can be done over and over again with little variation – when specific treatment of disorders is clearly defined for some period, e.g. hernia repair, cardiac angiography, adjuvant chemotherapy for some malignancies. However, healthcare often attempts to extend the use of automation to more complex situations that require general problem-solving and both inter-dependencies and variations in work processes to manage combinations of disorders. Examples include: connectivity – linking people to each other and systems; decision support – making choices clear; and data mining – discovering relationships among data. Even when healthcare uses domains other than automation, they are often bolted onto a pre-existing core of automation. This core limits the range of scale of the data, knowledge, processes and roles that can be accommodated.

3.1 Features of the proposed model

1. To provide security to the medical data so that only authorized persons can view the details.
2. The data needed for the health record should be collected with a higher degree of flexibility.
3. The health record data collected should be organized and stored in a single file so as to reduce storage space needed.
4. Real time modification/updating of the data collected as it changes from episode to episode.

5. Compressing the medical data to reduce the memory required to store and to reduce the time of transmission.
6. Dynamic transmission and reception of the medical data between various terminals in the network of expert doctors and patient attendant at rural places.

3.2 Modular implementation of the model

Module 1

Module 1 of the Model implements an authentication algorithm that provides security to access the database of LHR. If a new record is to be created then a facial image of the person is captured from the integrated webcam and an authentication code runs using PCA based Eigen face recognition technique. To open an existing record, the facial image of the individual is again captured and is compared with the existing image templates that are already trained in the present database. Security to the database is provided in such a way that the contents of the record is accessible or viewed only when the individual facial features matches with the one that is already exist in the database. Here the individual health records that include wide range of health information regarding a human subject is created in a highly flexible and structured manner. This module includes the real time patient image capture process as soon as his record is created. The features of the facial image are stored as a set of coefficients along with other data.

Module 2

In this module the images present in the database are subjected to the advanced compression techniques to reduce the memory needed to store them in the Electronic Health Record of a person. Because of its excellent performance in medical image compression and various advantages such as reduction in computational efficiency, no boundary extensions, memory savings, parallel processing. Lifting wavelet Transform along with the SPIHT is applied to the images. The compression can be performed to various levels using the threshold that can be adjusted using the SPIHT. Corresponding decompression is applied at the receiver end to perform reconstruction of the images from the coefficients present in the file.

Module 3

Module 3 presents the application representation part for the authorized person to create, retrieve and modify the patient's database. Here the electronic health record of the person can be created which includes his medical history details, medical images, pathological reports, signal reports such as ECG, EEG etc. While opening the database of a person the authentication process is included so as to provide security to the subject's medical data. Flexibility is provided so that a person can enter any details and can view any details at a time so that he can provide the rest of the details at a later time if needed. The application is created in an innovative way so that it identifies the images of a particular patient from a set of images in the database converts them to intensity coefficients ,compresses them and stores them in the EHR.

Module 4

Module4 consists of the data representation part which includes representing various details of the subject as needed .This part also consists of the modification module which facilitates the dynamic updation/modification of any data in the medical record as it changes from the patient's visit at every episode Various numbered options are provided to the application so that the person can view different details, images and signal reports by just entering the option provided beside the choice. The option for viewing the images in the subject's database is designed / written in a way that the coefficients from the specified positions will be collected and image is constructed from them. The data will be extracted from the file and arranged at corresponding position for the accurate representation of the dynamic data on the static form.

Module 5

This module consists of real time transmission and reception algorithms implemented in an innovative way so as to reduce the time of medical data transfer. The transmission algorithm is developed in such a way that only the dynamically changing data or the vital data which is to be diagnosed is sent to the Expert Center for immediate referral from the individual LHR. The reception algorithm then dynamically updates the LHR from the data received and rebuild the entire form for further inspection by the Expert physician.

Snapshots of the Lhr model developed

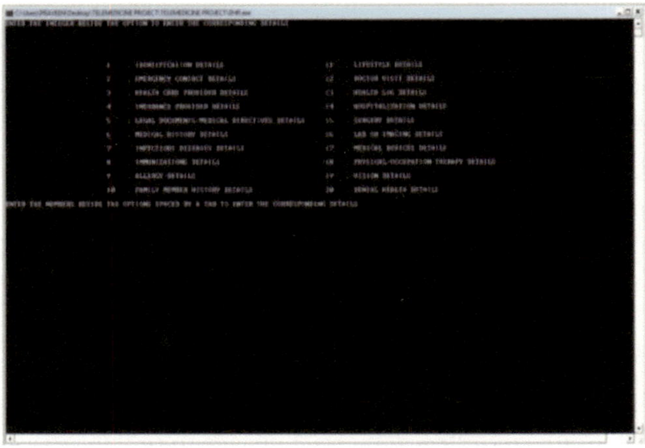

Fig. 2.

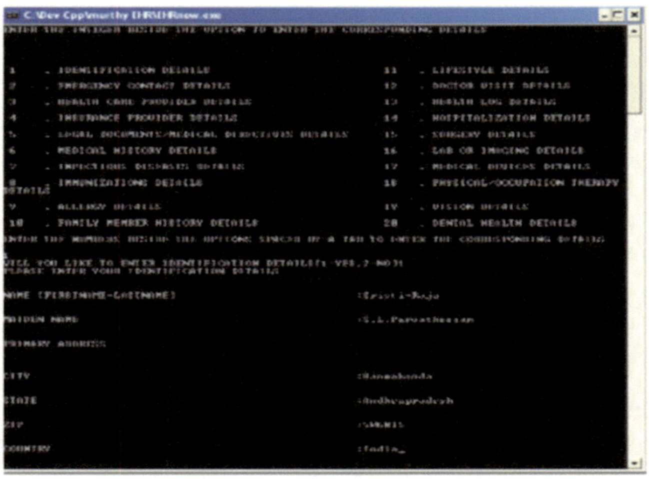

Fig. 3.

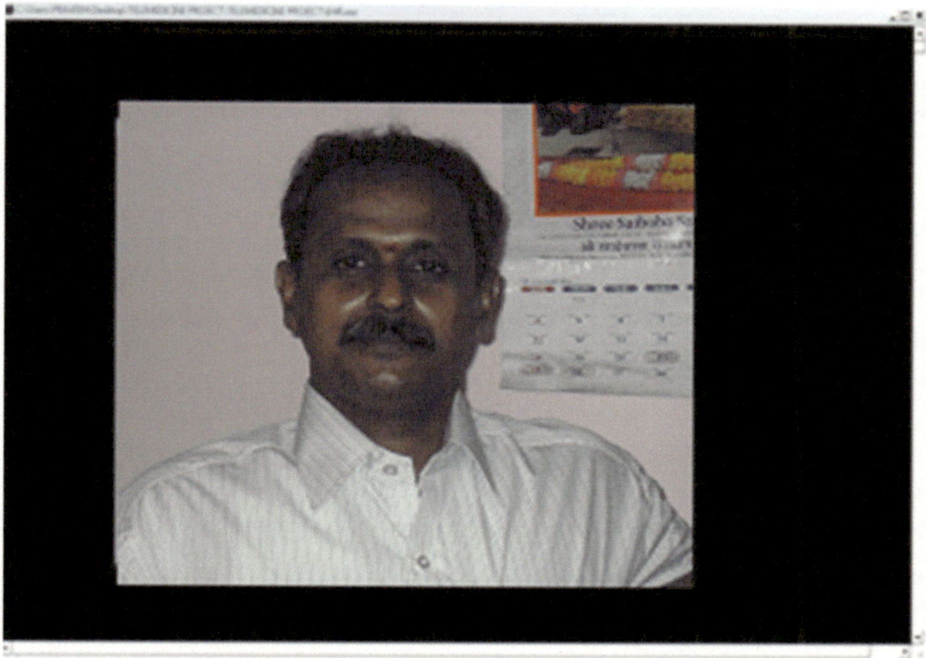

Fig. 4.

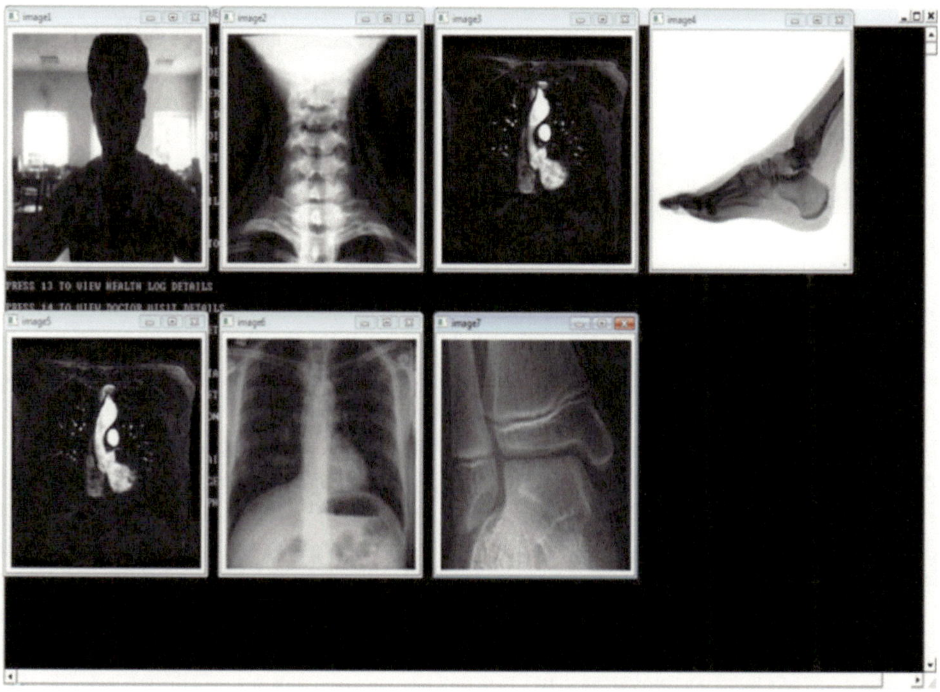

Fig. 5.

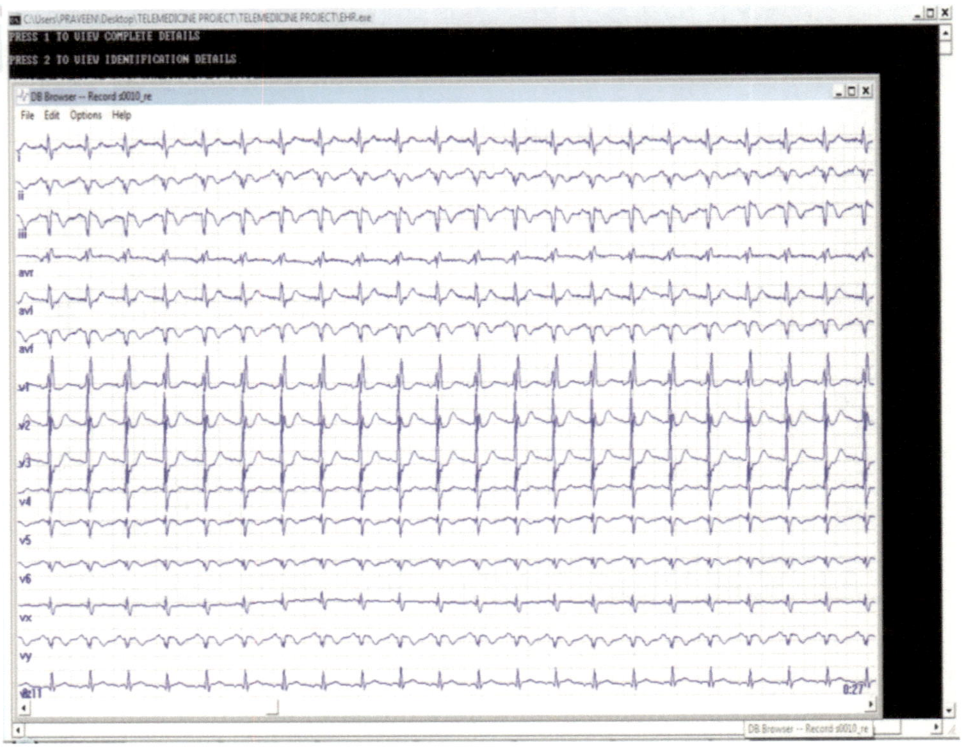

Fig. 6.

4. Conclusion and future scope

As this model developed and brought out as executable file form it easy for any level of user to create ,update, store and transmit using menu driven selection of various features in LHR. This model has been tested as an integrated module with all the features discussed above and is currently being adapted in a small scale at two of the local hospitals successfully. The presented model can further be made more secure by adding different security based algorithms along with encryption of the medical data to ensure higher degree of authentication to the EHR. Lossless compression models on heterogeneous medical data can be replaced in place of the existing algorithms. The model can be augmented with various transmission protocols such as wireless transmission which includes Bluetooth, infrared so as to increase the availability and flexibility for the users. It calls for a shift in the paradigm from thinking of the electronic health record as a by-product of automating practice, to thinking of it as a visualization of signals accumulated across scales of biology, time and geography.A paradigm shift from the current 'biomedical model' to a 'socio-cultural model', which should bridge the gaps and improve quality of rural life, is the current need. A revised National Health Policy addressing the prevailing inequalities, and working towards promoting a long-term perspective plan, mainly for rural health, is imperative.

5. Appendix

Lhr telemedicine form

A. Identification B. Emergency Contacts

Name (Last) (First) (Middle)			
Maiden Name			
Primary Address			
City	State	Zip	Country
Alternate Address			
City	State	Zip Code	Country
Home Phone	Work Phone		
Cell Phone	Email Address		
Date of Birth	Sex: ☐ Male ☐ Female		
Height	Weight	Eye Color	Hair Color
Race	Birthmark/Scars		
Blood/RH Type	Special Conditions	Marital Status	
Occupation			
Company Name			
City	State	Zip Code	Country

In Case of Emergency, Notify: Primary Contact Name (last) (First) (Middle)			
Relationship			
Address			
City	State	Zip Code	Country
Home Phone	Work Phone		
Cell Phone	Email Address		
In Case of Emergency, Notify: Secondary Contact			
Name (last)	Name (middle)	Name (first)	
Relationship			
Address			
City	State	Zip Code	Country
Home Phone	Work Phone		
Cell Phone	Email Address		

Phone Number	Languages Spoken
Primary Health Insurance Carrier	Policy Number
Secondary Health Insurance Carrier	Policy Number

In Case of Emergency, Notify: Medical Contact	
Doctor *(Indicate Specialty)*	
Phone Number	
Dentist	Telephone Number
Pharmacy	Telephone Number

C. Healthcare Provider

Healthcare Provider Specialty		Primary Care Physician ☐ Yes ☐ No		Phone	Emergency Phone No.(after hours)
Name				Email Address	
Group or Association				Fax	
Address				Web Address/URL	
City	State	Zip Code	Country		

D. Insurance Providers

Insurance Provider Type				E-mail Address		Fax	
Company Name				Web Address/ URL			
Address				Primary Insured Person-Name		Social Security No.	
City	State	Zip Code	Country	Name of Employer			
Contact – Name		Phone		Address			
Identification-Group Number		Member(ID) Number		City	State	Zip Code	Country
Contact Information-Phone		Emergency Phone No.(after hours)		Phone Number			

E. Legal Documents/Medical Directives

☐ Living Will ☐ Durable Power of Attorney for Healthcare ☐ Power of Attorney				Fax			
Document Location (Physical Location)				Contact (Name of person who has access to the document)			
Location Name (for example Bank of America)				Address			
Address				City	State	Zip Code	Country
City	State	Zip Code	Country	Contact Information			
Legal Representative (Name of person who you have assigned legal authority)				Home Phone		Cellular Phone	
Address				Pager		E-mail Address	
City	State	Zip Code	Country	Work Phone		Work E-mail Address	
Contact Information				Fax			
Home Phone		Cellular Phone		Date Filed			
Pager		E-mail Address		Organ Donation:			
Work E-mail Address		Work Phone		Organ Donor ☐ Yes ☐ No		State Where Registered	

☐ Living Will ☐Durable Power of Attorney for Healthcare ☐ Power of Attorney				Fax			
Document Location(Physical Location)				Contact (Name of person who has access to the document)			
Location Name (for example Bank of America)				Address			
Address				City	State	Zip Code	Country
City	State	Zip Code	Country	Contact Information			
Legal Representative (Name of person who you have assigned legal authority)				Home Phone		Cellular Phone	
Address				Pager		E-mail Address	
City	State	Zip Code	Country	Work Phone		Work E-mail Address	
Contact Information				Fax			
Home Phone		Cellular Phone		Date Filed			
Pager		E-mail Address		Organ Donation:			
Work E-mail Address		Work Phone		Organ Donor ☐ Yes ☐ No		State Where Registered	

F. Medical History(Check appropriate)

☐ Acquired Immunodeficiency Síndrome(AIDS) or HIV Positive:	Date of Onset	☐High Blood Pressure	Date of Onset
☐ Arthritis		☐ Hypoglycemia	
☐ Asthma		☐ Jaundice	
☐ Bronchitis		☐ Kidney Disease	
☐ Cancer		☐ Low Blood Pressure	
☐ Chlamydia		☐ Mental Retardation	
☐ Diabetes		☐ Pain or Pressure in Chest	
☐ Dizziness		☐ Palpitations	
☐ Emphysema		☐ Periods of unconsciousness	
☐ Epilepsy		☐ Rheumatic Fever	

☐	Eye Problem		☐	Rheumatism	
☐	Fainting		☐	Seizures	
☐	Frequent or Severe Headaches		☐	Shortness of Breath	
☐	Glaucoma		☐	Stomach Liver or Intestinal Problems	
☐	Gonorrhea		☐	Syphilis	
☐	Hearing Impairment		☐	Tuberculosis	
☐	Herat Condition		☐	Tumor	
☐	Hemodialysis		☐	Thyroid Problems	
☐	Herpes		☐	Urinary Tract Infection	
☐	High Blood Cholesterol		☐	Other	

G. Infectious Diseases

Disease	Age	Date	Remarks
Chicken Pox			
Hepatitis			
Measles			
Mumps			
Pertussis /Whooping Cough			
Pneumonía			
Polio			
Rubella			
Scarlet Fever			
Other			

H. Immunizations:

	Booster 1	Booster 2	Booster 3

Immunization for	Age	Date	Age	Date	Age	Date
Diptheria						
Hepatitis B						
Measles						
Mumps						
Pertussis/Whooping Cough						
Polio						
Rubella						
Smallpox						
Tetanus						
Tuberculosis						
Typhoid						
Other						

Allergy/Sensitivity Type *(include medications foods environmental or other)*	Reaction	Date last Occurred	Treatment

Display for ECG/XRAY/NMR/CT

J. Family Member History

	Mother	Father	Sibling(s)	Grandparent	Children
Enter ages of relatives					
If deceased, indicate age and cause of death					
Check all items that apply for their present state of health or any illnesses they have had					
Alcoholism					
Arthritis					
Asthma					
Cancer					
Diabetes					
Emphysema					
Glaucoma					
Herat Condition					
Hemodialysis					
Hepatitis					
High Blood Cholestrol					
High Blood Pressure					
Kidney Disease					
Mental Retardation					
Rheumatic Fever					
Seizures					
Smoking					
Stomach Liver or Intestinal Problems					

Stroke					
Thyroid Disorders					
Tuberculosis					
Tumor					
Other					

K. Lifestyle

☐ Alcohol	Drink(s) Per Week	Number of Years
☐ Smoking	Pack(s) Per Day	Number of Years
☐ Exercise	Type(s) of Exercise	Days Per Week

L. Health Log (Noninfectious major illnesses. Include pregnancies and childbirth)

Date Diagnosed	Doctor	Nature of Health Problems	Age at Onset	Condition Status	Remarks *(Such as, medications, special tests, x-rays, length of hospital stay, surgery and so on)*

M. Medications

Note: Include all prescription medications, (such as nitroglycerin) over-the-counter medications (taken on a regular basis), vitamin supplements, and herbal remedies

N. Doctor Visits

Date	Doctor	Reason	Diagnosis

O. Hospitalizations

Hospitalization Type (includes emergency room visits)		Diagnosis
Admission Date	Discharge Date	
Doctor		
Hospital		
Reason		Complications

Hospitalization Type (includes emergency room visits)		Diagnosis
Admission Date	Discharge Date	Admission Date
Doctor		
Hospital		
Reason		Complications

P. Surgeries

Date	Doctor	Results

Hospital	
Surgical Procedure	
Description	Comments

Date	Doctor	Results
Hospital		
Surgical Procedure		
Description		Comments

Q. Lab or Imaging (Examples: X-ray, MRI, Mammogram)

Test Type	Date	Test Type	Date
Requesting Doctor	Administered by	Requesting Doctor	Administered by
Reason		Reason	
Result		Result	

Test Type	Date	Test Type	Date
Requesting Doctor	Administered by	Requesting Doctor	Administered by
Reason		Reason	

Result	Result

R. Medical Devices (Examples: pacemaker, insulin pumas, breathing devices)

Device Type	Doctor	Device Type	Doctor
Hospital	Date	Hospital	Date
Reason		Reason	

S.Physical/Occupation Therapy

Therapy Type	Start Date	Stop Date	Frequency	Therapist

T. VISION

Date of Visit	Physician	Date of Visit	Physician
Vision RX		Vision RX	

Date of Visit	Physician	Date of Visit	Physician
Vision RX		Vision RX	

U. Dental Health

Date of Visit	Dentist	Problems	Resolution

6. References

[1] I. Iakovidis, "Towards Personal Health Record: Current situation, obstacles and trends in implementation of Electronic Healthcare Records in Europe", International Journal of Medical Informatics vol. 52 no. 128 (1998), pp. 105 -117.

[2] Knut Bernstein. :"Modeling and implementing Electronic Health Records in Denmark, Electronic Health Record Definition, Scope, and Context by ISO/TC". Report on HIT in USA, Chpt.7,2008.

[3] WHO-Strategy 2004-2007 Ehealth for Health care delivery ,Marketing and Dissemination, CH-1211 ,p 44, Geneva Switzerland,2004

[4] M. Eichelberg :"Electronic Health Record Standards - a brief overview", at ITI 4th International Conference on Information Communications Technology(2006) Publisher: Ieee, Pages: 1-1,ISBN: 0780397703.

[5] *Blobel, Bernd* : "Authorization and access control for electronic health record systems" International Journal of Medical Informatics,73(3),pp.251-257, (2004-03-31).

[6] Future of Health Information Exchange and Electronic Health Records by Richard.

[7] Knut Bernstein,M B-Rasmussen, S Vingtoft, S K Andersen, Christian N: "Modelling and implementing Electronic Health Records in Denmark. "

[8] Ali Nasser Al-Solbi "Towards the development of e-health implementations in developing countries", IADIS International Conference WWW/Internet 2007.

[9] HSF Fraser ,Paul B, Deshen M ,Sharon C, Burke Weter" Implementing electronic medical record systems in developing countries" Informatics in Primary Care ;13:83–95 # 2005 PHCSG, British Computer Society.

[10] Electronic Health Records: A Global Perspective

[11] A Work Product of the HIMSS Enterprise Systems Steering Committee and the Global Enterprise Task Force ,August 2008 .
[12] Sanjay P. S,Stacie N,Victor W.A. M,N Prakash,Samir C,Pradeep Ray,Saroj Mishra "Electronic Medical Records: A Review Comparing the Challenges in Developed and Developing Countries", Proceedings of the 41st Hawaii International Conference on System Sciences - 2008.
[13] Esther S. Hing, Catharine W. B, David A. Woodwell, Electronic Medical Record Use by Office-Based Physicians and Their Practices: United States, 2006, Advance Data No. 393 , October 26, 2007.
[14] Prrior.F, "Communication technology for Telemedicine" proceeding of national forum IEEE, 1996.
[15] Luciano Beolchi "Telemedicine glossary" 5th edition 2003.
[16] "Electronic health record overview", National Institutes of Health National Center for Research Resources, April 2006.
[17] "SVD-Based Projection for Face Recognition", Chou-Hao Hsu and Chaur-Chin Chen IEEE EIT 2007 Proceedings, pp 600-603.
[18] "Three-Dimensional SPIHT Coding of Volume Images with Random Access and Resolution Scalability" Emmanuel Christophe, and William A. Pearlman EURASIP Journal on Image and Video Processing Volume 2008.
[19] "Nonlinear Wavelet Transforms for Image Coding via Lifting", Roger L. Claypoole, Jr., Senior Member, IEEE, Geoffrey M. Davis, Wim Sweldens, Member, IEEE, and Richard G. Baraniuk, Fellow, IEEE IEEE TRANSACTIONS ON IMAGE PROCESSING, VOL. 12, NO. 12, DECEMBER 2003.
[20] "A new fast and efficient image codec based on SPIHT", Amir Said, William A. Pearlman, IEEE circuits and system for video technology Vol 6, June 1996.
[21] "An Internet based telemedicine system", Zhenyu Guo and John C. Moulder, IEEE2000.
[22] "A Biometric Method to Secure Telemedicine Systems", G. H. Zhang, Carmen C. Y. Poon, Member, IEEE, Ye. Li, and Y. T. Zhang, Fellow, IEEE.
[23] Baturalp R. Arslan', Metin Tulgar, Peder C. Pedersen, Kaveh Pahlavan, Beyhan Cengiz', and Ahmet Arslan':"ADVANCES IN WIRELESS TELEMEDICINE: IMPROVEMENTS AND CHALLENGES FACING WIRELESS ULTRASOUND",
[24] Absar Kazmi', "Bluetooth Telemedicine Processor for MultichannelBiomedical Signal Transmission via Mobile Cellular Networks", Mohd Fadlee A. Rasid and Bryan Woodward ieee transactions on information technology in biomedicine, vol. 9, no. 1, march 2005.
[25] W. P. Santamore, C. Homko, J. Marble, J Wald, and A. A. Bove "Improving Heart Failure Care by Using a Telemedicine System",. Proceedings of the 26th Annual International Conference of the IEEE EMBS
[26] San Francisco, CA, USA • September 1-5, 2004
[27] "Telemedicine in HealthCare System", Amin Moghadas, University of Texas at San Antonio, USA, Mo Jamshidi, University of Texas at San Antonio, USA, Mehdi Shaderam, University ofTexas at San Antonio, USA.
[28] "Face Verification Based on Singular Value Decomposition and Radial Basis", Function Neural Network", Yunhong Wang, Tieniu Tan and Yong Zhu.

[29] "Face Recognition Using Improved Fast PCA Algorithm", Neerja and Ekta Walia, 2008 Congress on Image and Signal Processing.

[30] "FACE IMAGE RETRIEVAL BY PROJECTION-BASED FEATURES", Chaur-Chin Chen, Yu-Shu Shieh, Hsueh-Ting Chu, The Third International Workshop on Image Media Quality and its Applications, IMQA2008. I. Daubechies and W. Sweldens, "Factoring wavelet transforms into lifting schemes," J. Fourier Anal. Appl., vol. 4, pp. 247-269, 1998.

[31] W. Sweldens, "The lifting scheme: A new philosophy in biorthogonal wavelet constructions," in Proc. SPIE, vol. 2569, 1995, pp. 68–79

[32] A VLSI Architecture for Lifting-Based Forward and Inverse Wavelet Transform by Kishore Andra, Chaitali Chakrabarti, Member, IEEE, and Tinku Acharya, Senior Member, IEEE.

[33] A. R. Calderbank, I. Daubechies,W. Sweldens, and B.-L. Yeo, "Wavelet transforms that map integers to integers," Appl. Comput. Harmon. Anal., vol. 5, pp. 332–369, July 1998.

[34] H. Chao, P. Fisher, and Z. Hua, "An approach to integer wavelet transforms for lossless for image compression," in Proc. Int. Symp. Computational Mathematics, Guangzhou, China, Aug. 1997, pp. 19–38.

[35] J. Shapiro, "Embedded image coding using zerotrees of wavelet coefficients,"IEEE Trans. Signal processing, vol. 41, pp. 3445–3463, Dec.1993.

[36] A. Said and W. A. Pearlman, "A new, fast, and efficient image codec based on set partitioning in hierarchical trees," IEEE Trans. Circuits Syst. Video Technol., vol. 6, pp. 243–250, June 1996..

[37] Michael D. Adams and Faouzi Kossentini: Reversible Integer-to-Integer Wavelet Transforms for Image Compression: Performance Evaluation And Analysis

[38] Li-bao zhang and Ming-quan zhou, :" Embedded Reversible Medical Image Compression Using Integer Wavelet Transform." Proceeding ICIC'06 Proceedings of the 2006 international conference on Intelligent computing: Part II Springer-Verlag Berlin, Heidelberg ©2006 ISBN:3-540-37274-1 978-3-540-37274-5

Novel Prediction Based Technique for Efficient Compression of Medical Imaging Data

Josip Knezović, Mario Kovač, Martin Žagar,
Hrvoje Mlinarić and Daniel Hofman
University of Zagreb
Croatia

1. Introduction

The annual volume of imaging data in modern paperless hospitals can approach up to 10 terabytes, heavily pressing the storage and transmission requirements (Choong et al., 2007). Utilizing efficient compression techniques for those data in order to reduce associated costs is very attractive from both viewpoints: financial and organizational (Sanchez, Abugharbieh & Nasiopoulos, 2009; Sanchez et al., 2008). Although lossy techniques can yield better compression results, due to possible compression artifacts in the compressed image, they are less favored compared to lossless compression techniques in certain medical applications such as image-based diagnosis, archival etc. Compression itself helps in alleviating storage requirements for medical imaging system. Additionally, it also helps in accommodating the on-line transmission and availability of patient diagnostic imaging data which is essential for future electronic health frameworks.

Moreover, new approaches in medical imaging such as 3D and 4D imaging and bio–modeling produce even greater amounts of image data. For efficient storage and transmission of those data and utilization of systems that exploit 3D and 4D imaging technologies, compression is inevitable. In this field, at least certain parts of images are required to be stored and transmitted without any loss of information. The lossless compression algorithm that we propose can also be efficiently employed for at least those vital parts of interest in this kind of applications (Zagar et al., 2007).

Important property of image data is high degree of correlation among neighboring pixels which is crucial for any compression technique since it makes it possible to decorrelate the samples using some sort of prediction–based modeling. If employed modeling technique effectively models the spatial correlation among neighboring pixels, remaining data will be mostly decorrelated and easily coded with an entropy coder. On the other hand, it is well known that image data are nonstationary, i.e. properties of image regions vary all over the image (Memon & Wu, 1999). Accordingly, it is necessary to adapt the model to the changing image characteristics. Another assumption of local stationariness is very well applicable to the image data. This means that for arbitrarily small image regions, the model adapted to the dominant local property will be effective inside the region. Predictive image coding in which the prediction error of the current pixel is coded has shown to be the most effective technique in lossless image compression. Using prediction, image data are decorrelated prior

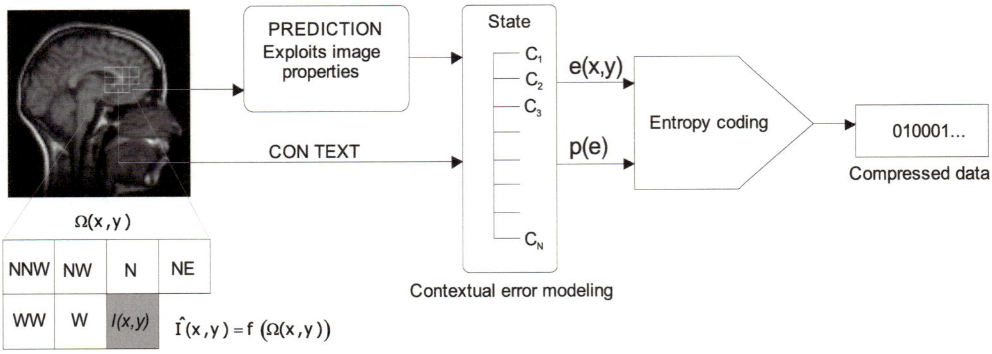

Fig. 1. Block scheme of predictive image coding

to the entropy coding so that better compression is achieved. In the framework of sequential, backward adaptive lossless image compression, predictive image coding can be formulated as composed of the following steps as shown in Figure 1:

1. Prediction of the current pixel based on the casual set of surrounding pixels - pixel prediction.
2. Contextual error modeling: Determination of the conditional probabilistic context in which the current prediction error occurs (Memon & Wu, 1999).
3. Entropy coding of the prediction error in the detected probabilistic context - entropy coding.

In this work a new predictive model for lossless image compression is proposed. The model is based on classification and blending of static predictors which is followed by heuristic contextual error modeling. The classification is performed in order to capture and model higher order redundancies inside the local image region. Then, on the causal set of classified neighboring pixels, the set of selected static predictors is dynamically blended to produce the prediction. The idea behind the blending of predictors is to find a dominant property inside the current image region while taking other properties into account. The dominant property will have the biggest impact on the final, blended predictor. Based on our proposed predictor, we developed two lossless image compression codecs characterized with high compression efficiency. First codec neglects computational complexity while the second proposal employs an effective technique which reduces the computational requirements of the first proposal while maintaining compression efficiency.

2. Proposed Predictive Coding Method

We treat image as a two-dimensional array $I(x,y)$ of pixel grey intensity values of width W and height H, where $0 \leq x < W$ and $0 \leq y < H$. Pixels are observed sample by sample in raster scan order, from top to bottom, left to right. In the assumed backward adaptive approach, the encoder is allowed to use only past information that is also available to decoder. This means that for forming the prediction only previously observed pixels are used, as shown in Figure 1. In fact, only a small subset of previously encoded pixels is used to form the causal template. Predictor from Figure 1 uses causal context of surrounding pixels for the prediction of the current pixel :

$$\hat{I}(x,y) = f(\Omega(x,y)) \tag{1}$$

In simple prediction schemes that use small causal context the compass point notation for surrounding pixels is used which is also illustrated in Figure 1. For example *N* denotes North pixel, *W* denotes the West pixel from the current pixel, *NE* North–East, *NW* North–West etc. After the prediction is performed, the model outputs the prediction error. This means that instead of coding the real pixel value, the pixel prediction $\hat{I}(x,y) = f(\Omega(x,y))$ is performed and the prediction error $e(x,y) = I(x,y) - \hat{I}(x,y)$ is further encoded by the statistical encoder. As previously observed, a typical image can be treated as composed of regions with varying dominant properties such as edges, textures, smooth regions, noisy regions etc. Those properties pose different and conflicting constraints on the prediction function if it is required to adapt to the region properties. The main properties of image regions and their requirements on the predictor are given in (Seemann & Tischer, 1997). If we consider a linear predictor:

$$\hat{I}(x,y) = f(\Omega(x,y)) = \sum_{I(i,j)\in\Omega} a_{i,j} \cdot I(i,j), \tag{2}$$

then we can formulate the following constraints on the predictor coefficients $\{a_{i,j}\}$ depending on the dominant property of the current region:

- **Smooth regions** in which the intensity of pixel doesn't change require that $\sum a_{i,j} = 1$. For planar region it is required for at least one of $a_{i,j}$ to be negative so that the gradient can be estimated.
- **Noisy regions** require the minimum magnitude of noise is introduced into prediction which implies that $\sum |a_{i,j}|$ should be as small as possible. Therefore, the best approach for noisy regions is the use of averaging prediction function.
- **Edges and textured regions** constitute the most important visual part of images (Seemann & Tischer, 1997). Edges require some kind of adaptation mechanism in the predictor to provide the detection and orientation of the edge. Textures are the most difficult to model and they can be considered as combination of noise and edges.

In general, image regions can be viewed as composed of structures mentioned before with one or two dominant properties; therefore the choice for predictor to satisfy given constraints is very often in conflict. The best choice for the most cases is to assume the noisy property and corresponding constraint as suggested in (Seemann & Tischer, 1997) where the blending of static predictors is proposed which practically gives the final predictor to be an averaging predictor.

The effectiveness of any prediction scheme depends on its ability to adapt to different image regions. This precludes the use of static predictors if efficient prediction is required. Typical, heuristically tuned switching predictors use a set of static prediction functions and heuristics to determine which function will be used for the prediction of the current pixel. Such predictors include GAP from the CALIC algorithm (X. Wu and N. Memon and K. Sayood, 1995), MED predictor from the LOCO-I and JPEG–LS standard (M.J. Weinberger and G. Seroussi and G. Sapiro, 1998), etc. The main drawback of switching predictors is the lack of robustness in the presence of nontrivial image structures. Another approach is to use adaptive predictor which we also propose. There is a large spectrum of adaptive predictors with various mechanisms of adaptation and complexities such as LS–based predictors (G. Motta and J.A. Storer and B. Carpentieri, 2000; X. Li and M.T. Orchard, 2001) and blending predictors (Seemann & Tischer, 1997;

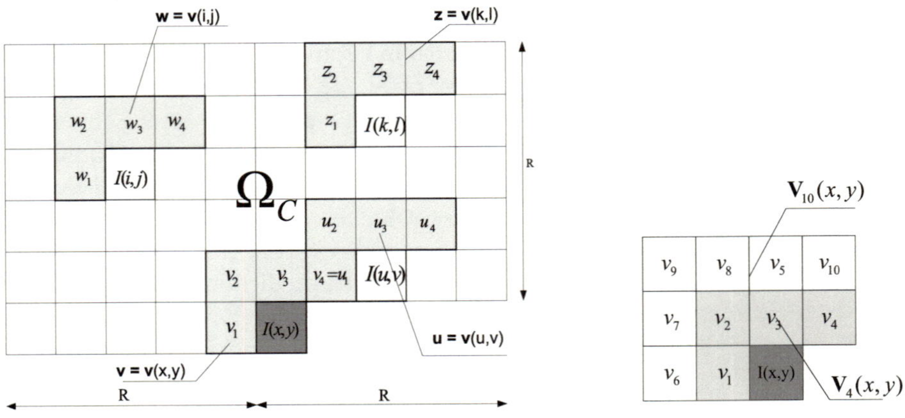

(a) Causal context (b) Vector template

Fig. 2. Contextual elements of proposed predictor

Seemann et al., 1997). The aim of the prediction scheme proposed in this paper is to predict well in all various image regions with moderate computational complexity.

2.1 Proposed predictor

In order to efficiently model different image structures we propose adaptive predictor based on the idea of predictor blends (Seemann & Tischer, 1997). The blending predictor is extended with dynamic determination of blending context on a pixel–by–pixel basis. The set of predictors

$$\mathcal{F} = \{f_1, f_2, \cdots, f_N\}$$

is composed of N static prediction functions adjusted to predict well in the presence of specific property. For example simple predictor $f_W = I(x-1,y)$ is known to predict well in the presence of sharp horizontal edge. The classification process determines the set of neighboring pixels on which the blending of $\mathcal{F}$ is performed. It is similar to initial step of vector quantization design substantially simplified in order to be usable in symmetric, backward adaptive algorithm (M.J. Slyz and D.L. Neuhoff, 1994). The process of blending of selected predictors will finally produce an averaging predictor which is known to predict well in the noisy regions. This way, the final predictor will try to adapt to the most relevant image properties while detecting and adjusting to the dominant property in the current local region, whether it is an edge, a planar region or even a texture with nontrivial coarseness and period. Figure 2 depicts basic elements of proposed prediction scheme. Ω_C denotes the causal context used by the predictor. It is a rectangular window of radius R composed of previously encoded pixels on which the search procedure for classification is performed. Each pixel from the Ω_C and currently unknown pixel $I(x,y)$ is associated with its vector template $\mathbf{v}(x,y)$ that is composed of d closest causal neighboring pixels as shown in Figure 2(b). As an example, the vectors of size $d = 4$ ($\mathbf{v}_4(x,y)$) and $d = 10$ ($\mathbf{v}_{10}(x,y)$) are shown. In Figure 2(a) the vectors of size four are used. The Euclidean distance between associated vectors will be used for classifications of pixels into the *current* cell of pixels *similar* to the current pixel $I(x,y)$, just like in VQ design (A. Gersho, 1993; A. Gersho and V.M. Gray, n.d.). In order to reduce the complexity of proposed scheme some basic simplifications are introduced. First, as shown by

Slyz and Neuhoff, we do not perform full vector quantization. Rather, only the *current* cell in which the current pixel lies needs to be calculated (M.J. Slyz and D.L. Neuhoff, 1994). Next, the cell population, i.e. number of pixels that go into the cell together with the current pixel's vector, is set as constant M at the beginning of the coding process.
Proposed prediction scheme operates as follows:

Classification and Blending Predictor CBP

1. *Iteration:* Iterate for every pixel $I(x,y)$ in the image.
2. *Classification:* For each pixel $I(i,j) \in \Omega_C$ compute the Euclidean distance $D(i,j)$ between its corresponding vector $\mathbf{v}(i,j)$=$\mathbf{w}$ and the current pixel's vector $\mathbf{v}(x,y)$=$\mathbf{v}$:

$$\begin{aligned} D(i,j) &= ||\mathbf{v}(i,j) - \mathbf{v}(x,y)|| \\ &= ||\mathbf{w} - \mathbf{v}|| \\ &= \textstyle\sum_{k=1}^{d} |w_k - v_k|^2 . \end{aligned} \tag{3}$$

   Based on the computed distances, determine M pixels from Ω_C that belong to the current cell, i.e. with the smallest vector distances from the current pixel's vector. The current cell will be used as blending context Ω_B for $\mathcal{F}$. This step is similar to nearest neighbor selection in VQ design.

3. *Predictor penalties:* For every predictor f_k the penalty G_k is calculated by the following equation:

$$G_k = \sum_{I(i,j)\in\Omega_B} (\hat{I}_k(i,j) - I(i,j))^2, \tag{4}$$

   where $\hat{I}_k = f_k(i,j)$ is the prediction of $f_k \in \mathcal{F}$ for the pixel $I(i,j) \in \Omega_B$.

4. *Final predictor blending:* Based on the penalties we form the prediction for the current pixel $\hat{I}(x,y)$ as:

$$\hat{I}(x,y) = F(x,y) = \left[\frac{\left(\sum_{k=1}^{N} \frac{1}{G_k} \cdot \hat{I}_k(x,y)\right)}{\sum_{k=1}^{N} 1/G_k} \right]. \tag{5}$$

   The prediction for the current pixel is the weighted sum of predictions of all the predictors from $\mathcal{F}$ with weights inversely proportional to corresponding penalties. The penalty of predictor reflects its prediction accuracy on the blending context. If the predictor predicts well, its contribution, i.e. its weight in the final prediction will be higher. The predictors that do not predict well on the current blending context will eventually be blended out by associated large penalties. The denominator in (5) normalizes the final prediction so that the sum of weights equals to 1.

5. *Error correction:* On the blending context Ω_B calculate *typical* error of the final predictor as:

$$\bar{e}(\Omega_B) = \frac{1}{M} \sum_{I(i,j)\in\Omega_B} (F(i,j) - I(i,j)). \tag{6}$$

   Based on the typical error of blending predictor F the final prediction for the current pixel is further refined as:

$$\dot{I}(x,y) = F(x,y) + \bar{e} = \hat{I}(x,y) + \bar{e}. \tag{7}$$

   This final step of proposed predictor captures typical bias of the blending predictor F on the classified set of pixels Ω_B that are the part of similar structure as current pixel.

Through the classification and blending process, proposed predictor adjusts itself to the dominant local property. The blending allows other non–dominant properties to be included in the final predictor, although with less contribution. This is crucial difference compared with switching predictors that don't have the capability to model nontrivial image structures with mixture of properties. Note that pixels from the search window that do not belong to the region with the same dominant property as the region in which current pixel resides will not be included in the current cell and thus they will not be part of the blending context.

2.2 Contextual error modeling

Although the prediction step removes statistical redundancies within image data, there are remaining structures in the error image which cannot be completely removed using only previously applied prediction step (Memon & Wu, 1999). Those structures are removed using contextual modeling of prediction error, where the context or the state is the function of previously observed pixels, errors or any other relevant variables. As reported by Wu, the heuristic method that uses both, previous pixels template and causal error energy estimate is best suited for this purpose (Wu, 1997). Wu's contextual model is composed of two different submodels: (1) Model with large number of states that is used for prediction error feedback; and (2) Model with low number of states used for error probability estimation. On the other hand, Wu's predictor is a heuristic predictor with low degree of adaptation and our proposal is highly adaptive predictor with already built in error feedback mechanism (error correction step in the prediction). This implies that our mechanism needs smaller and less complex contextual model for estimation of symbol probabilities. Therefore it is built as follows: Besides of the high correlation with texture pattern, current prediction error is also highly correlated with the errors on neighboring pixels. This is modeled with the error discriminant

$$\Delta = d_h + d_v + 2|e_w|, \tag{8}$$

where

$$d_h = |W - WW| + |N - NN| + |N - NE|, \tag{9}$$

and

$$d_v = |W - NW| + |N - NN| + |NE - NNE|, \tag{10}$$

are horizontal and vertical gradients around the current pixel, and e_w is the prediction error on the west pixel W from the current pixel. Δ is uniformly quantized into eight levels to produce the state of the model (Wu, 1997). Every state contains the histogram table which is used for probability estimation of the prediction error in the current state. Because of the context dilution effect, this contextual model is required to have small number of states.

2.3 Entropy coding of prediction error

The final step of proposed image compression algorithm is entropy coding of the resulting prediction error. For the given error symbol and given probability estimate obtained from the contextual state, the codeword is computed by the entropy coder. This codeword is output as the final result of predictive image coding algorithm. Our proposal uses highly efficient implementation of adaptive arithmetic coding (P.G. Howard and J.S. Vitter, 1994).

3. Selective computation of Predictor Blends

In this section we extend our Classification and Blending Predictor CBP with the goal to reduce the computational requirements of the method while maintaining its compression efficiency. We achieve this by implementing an effective heuristic approach in the predictive part of the compression method.

Our optimization is based on the observation that the changes in the predictor, i.e. the changing of predictor weights, i.e. coefficients, mainly happens on the boundaries of image regions. For example, once computed prediction parameters in the CBP predictor remain mostly unchanged while the coder is in the local region with dominant property such as smooth or planar region. Noticeable change in the CBP predictor parameters happens when the coder reaches out of the one local region and enters into another with a new dominant property. Shortly, this change happens on the edge areas. Based on this fact, we propose a novel way of reducing the number of required computations in the predictor by preserving the predictor coefficients as long as we are inside a local region. This idea is implemented in the CBP predictor in a way that when the magnitude of the prediction error on the current pixel is beyond a predefined threshold, we trigger the compute-intensive calculation of the predictor weights in the CBP. As long as the prediction error magnitude is below the threshold, previously calculated predictor weights are used for the prediction of the current pixel. This way, we evict the pixel-by-pixel computation of predictor weights, and perform it only on pixels on which the current predictor fails beyond a predefined threshold. This technique is motivated by the Edge Directed Property of LS–based predictor reported in (X. Li and M.T. Orchard, 2001).

Modified prediction scheme operates as follows:

Selective Classification and Blending Predictor SCBP

1. *Initialization:* Set the previous prediction error to zero.
2. *Iteration:* Iterate for every pixel $I(x,y)$ in the image.
3. *Selective computation:* Check the previous prediction error. If it is less than the predefined prediction error threshold T_e, skip the computation and go to step 6; otherwise go to step 4.
4. *Classification:* For each pixel $I(i,j) \in \Omega_C$ compute the Euclidean distance $D(i,j)$ between its corresponding vector $\mathbf{v}(i,j)$=$\mathbf{w}$ and the current pixel's vector $\mathbf{v}(x,y)$=$\mathbf{v}$:

$$\begin{aligned} D(i,j) &= ||\mathbf{v}(i,j) - \mathbf{v}(x,y)|| \\ &= ||\mathbf{w} - \mathbf{v}|| \\ &= \textstyle\sum_{k=1}^{d} |w_k - v_k|^2 . \end{aligned} \tag{11}$$

   Based on the computed distances, determine M pixels from Ω_C that belong to the current cell, i.e. with the smallest vector distances from the current pixel's vector. The current cell will be used as blending context Ω_B for $\mathcal{F}$. This step is similar to nearest neighbor selection in VQ design.

5. *Predictor penalties:* For every predictor f_k the penalty G_k is calculated by the following equation:

$$G_k = \sum_{I(i,j)\in\Omega_B} (\hat{I}_k(i,j) - I(i,j))^2, \tag{12}$$

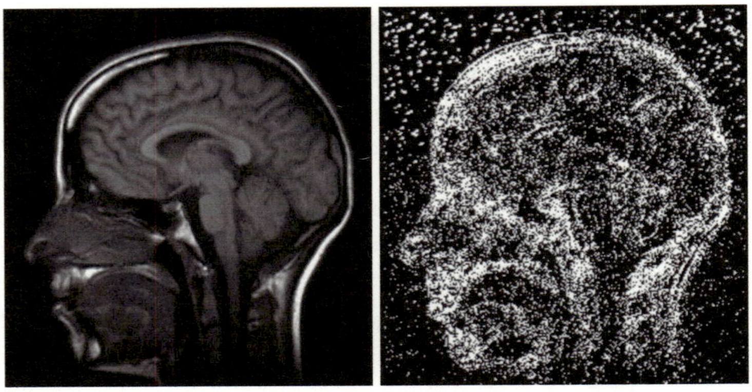

Fig. 3. Effects of selective computations of predictor weights

where $\hat{I}_k = f_k(i,j)$ is the prediction of $f_k \in \mathcal{F}$ for the pixel $I(i,j) \in \Omega_B$.

6. *Final predictor blending:* Based on the blend penalties we form the prediction for the current pixel $\hat{I}(x,y)$ as:

$$\hat{I}(x,y) = F(x,y) = \left[\frac{\left(\sum_{k=1}^{N} \frac{1}{G_k} \cdot \hat{I}_k(x,y) \right)}{\sum_{k=1}^{N} 1/G_k} \right]. \quad (13)$$

The prediction for the current pixel is the weighted sum of predictions of all the predictors from $\mathcal{F}$ with weights inversely proportional to corresponding penalties.

7. *Error correction:* On the blending context Ω_B calculate *typical* error of the final predictor as:

$$\bar{e}(\Omega_B) = \frac{1}{M} \sum_{I(i,j) \in \Omega_B} (F(i,j) - I(i,j)). \quad (14)$$

Based on the typical error of blending predictor F the final prediction for the current pixel is further refined as:

$$\dot{I}(x,y) = F(x,y) + \bar{e} = \hat{I}(x,y) + \bar{e}. \quad (15)$$

This final step of proposed predictor captures typical bias of the blending predictor F on the classified set of pixels Ω_B that are the part of similar structure as current pixel.

Based on the step of selective computation in which the algorithm checks whether the current predictor penalties form the prediction which is reasonably accurate, we omit a number of computations of predictor weights which do not contribute substantially to the overall prediction efficiency and therefore the compression. On the other side, this simple, yet effective technique reduces the computational complexity of our first proposal, a CBP predictor.

As an illustration, Figure 3 shows the effects of applying Selective Classification and Blending Predictor SCBP on a sample medical image. Left image is the original while on the right side, white pixels denote the positions for which the recomputation of the predictor penalties was performed. More specifically, we set the recomputation threshold T_e to zero, meaning that only the perfect prediction on the previous pixel will not trigger the predictor recomputation. For this particular case, this resulted in reduction of predictor blend calculations by a factor of 2.05 and reduced the computation time by 39% of the original CBP predictor. At the

Predictor	Prediction function	Description
f_1	N	North pixel to the current pixel
f_2	W	West pixel to the current pixel
f_3	NW	Northwest pixel to the current pixel
f_4	NE	Northeast pixel to the current pixel
f_5	$N+W-NE$	Planar region predictor
f_6	$2N-NN$	Planar region predictor horizontal
f_7	$2W-WW$	Planar region predictor vertical

Table 1. Set of static predictors

same time the compression efficiency measured by zero–order entropy of prediction error was unnoticeably increased by approximately 2%. More details are given in the Section 4 where we demonstrate our experimental results.

4. Experimental results

In this section we show the experimental results obtained with our proposed predictors. We also show the results obtained while implementing our predictors in complete lossless image codecs. Proposed predictors have several parameters that can be varied in order to balance between the compression ratio and the computational complexity. These are, as illustrated in Figure 2:

1. Radius R of the classification context which defines the size of the classification template Ω_C on which the current cell is estimated. Increasing R, the algorithm has more chance to capture the structure of the current region, but at the cost of requiring more computations.
2. Population size M of the current cell. Captures the similar pixels to the current pixel for blending of predictors. If this parameter is too small the resulting predictor is overspecialized and having too few samples to effectively model the local region. On the other hand, higher value of would result in pixels in the current cell that are not similar enough to the current pixel. This will also jeopardize the final predictor efficiency to predict well in the current region.
3. The size of the vector template d. Vector template is composed of d closest already observed pixels. In proposed predictor we experimented with the vector size 1 to 10 as shown in Figure 2(b). The higher vector size, the higher capability to capture more complex structures. Also higher vector size demands more computations.
4. Set of predictors $\mathcal{F}$. Exhaustive tests on a large number of medical test images had shown that the set $\mathcal{F}$ should contain simple static predictors that are suited to various regions, such as oriented edges, planar regions, smooth regions etc. Our experiments resulted in best choice for set $\mathcal{F}$ to be:

$$\mathcal{F} = \{N, W, NW, NE, N+W-NW, G_W, G_N\}, \quad (16)$$

where $G_W = 2N - NN$ and $G_N = 2W - WW$. Table 1 gives the details of the static predictors used in our experiments. We use compass point notation for surrounding pixels,

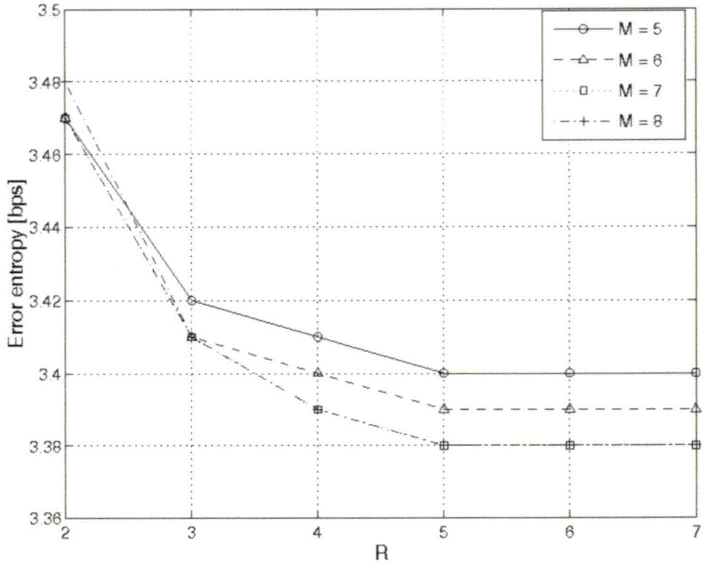

Fig. 4. Average zero order entropy of prediction error

i.e. W denotes west pixel, N denotes a pixel placed on the North side of the current pixel, NN denotes pixel placed two pixels to the North of the current pixels and so on. We selected a set of seven predictors that include horizontal and vertical edge predictors and planar predictors. The process of blending of selected predictors will finally produce an averaging predictor which is known to predict well in the noisy regions. This way, final predictor will try to adapt to most relevant image properties while detecting and adjusting to the dominant property in the current local region, whether it is an edge, a planar region or even a texture with nontrivial coarseness and period The set includes simple predictors suited for edges, planar predictor and predictors with gradient modeling for planar regions. Through the blending process the final predictor has the form of averaging predictor which is suited for noisy regions and for modeling higher structures such as textures.

Figure 4 shows the average zero-order entropy of the Classification and Blending Predictor CBP obtained on a test set of images shown in Figure 5. The zero-order entropy is shown in bits per symbol (bps) versus radius of the classification template and with the cell population M as a parameter. The vector size was fixed to four. As can be seen, the entropy saturates for $R > 6$ and $M > 7$. That clearly shows that increasing the radius and cell size beyond these limits will result in diminishing returns in terms of compression while increasing computational time. Consequently, in Table 2 we show experimentally chosen working parameters of the CBP and SCBP predictors that we will further use in the comparison with other popular predictors for lossless image compression. We used these settings in experiments in which we employ our predictors as parts of the complete image compression algorithms. Notice that due to the decreased computational requirements, SCBP predictor can afford larger classification template Ω_C with higher radius $R = 6$ as opposed to CBP with the $R = 5$.

Predictor	Radius R	Cell size M	Vector size d	Threshold T_e
CBP	5	7	4	–
SCBP	6	7	4	0

Table 2. Working parameters for CBP and SCBP

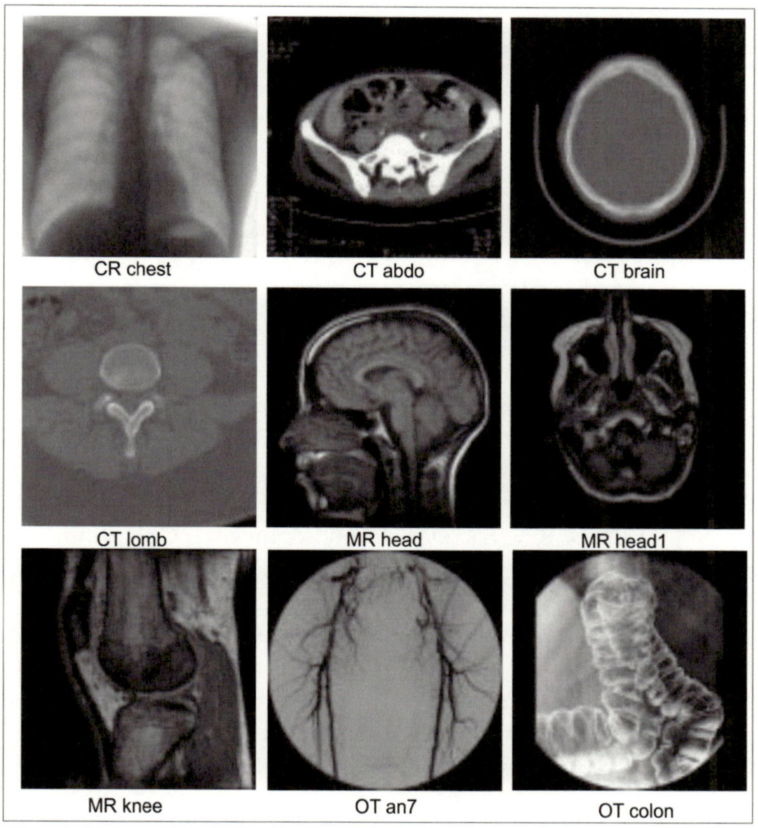

Fig. 5. Test set of medical images

In order to demonstrate the performance of proposed predictors we will show their results on the set of nine medical images obtained with varying modalities (Meyer, 2005; S. Barré Medical Image Samples, 2004). Those images are grey level images with 8 bits per pixel precision and their thumbnails are shown in Figure 5.
We compared our predictors CBP and SCBP with several popular predictors used in predictive lossless image compression algorithms in Table 3. The results show the zero-order entropy of the prediction error in bits per symbol for the same test set of medical images. GAP predictors is static heuristically tuned predictor used in the CALIC algorithm (Wu, 1997), and MED is the predictors from LOCO-I algorithm which is used as JPEG-LS standard (M.J. Weinberger and G. Seroussi and G. Sapiro, 1998). Our predictors outperform other predictors for all images in the set except for *CT abdo* where MED predictor performed best. CBP was slightly better than SCBP for all test images.

Image	GAP(CALIC)	MED(JPEG–LS)	CBP	SCBP
CR Chest	2.49	2.52	**2.28**	2.29
CT Abdo	2.73	2.67	**2.72**	2.75
CT Brain	1.93	1.79	**1.17**	1.19
CT Lomb	2.59	2.46	**2.19**	2.19
MR Head	4.75	4.80	**4.55**	4.65
MR Head1	4.82	4.85	**4.51**	4.55
MR Knee	5.20	5.24	**5.12**	5.16
OT An7	4.28	4.20	**4.17**	4.19
OT Colon	3.91	3.84	**3.75**	3.77
Average	3.63	3.60	**3.38**	3.42

Table 3. Zero–order entropy of prediction error (bps)

We built two complete lossless image codecs that incorporate CBP and SCBP predictors, contextual error modeling described section 2.2, and arithmetic coding. We call them Classification and Blending Predictive Coder CBPC and Selective Classification and Blending Predictive Coder SCBPC, respectively. To compare both coders we show their compression efficiency in the Figure 6. We show the compression ratios obtained on the test set. From the figure, we can see that the SCBPC encoder closely follows the CBP although with reduced computational complexity. Geometric mean of compression ratios is within 2% of the CBP results. Additionally, Figure 7 illustrates the time savings of SCBPC encoder compared to CBPC encoder on the test set. On average, SCBPC encoder has reduced the execution time by more than 35% compared to CBPC method.

Finally, Table 4 shows the results of our CBPC and SCBPC coders compared with the results of popular lossless coders for our test set of medical images. The first column shows the compression ratios of the CALIC algorithm (Memon & Wu, 1999), the second column the JPEG-LS results (M.J. Weinberger and G. Seroussi and G. Sapiro, 1998) and the third column shows the results of JPEG 2000 lossless compression that uses reversible wavelet transform (Santa-Cruz & Ebrahimi, 1997). Last two columns show the results of CBPC and SCBPC encoders respectively. Our both coders outperform other coders. CBPC obtained the best compression ratios on all test images except for *CT abdo* where it was slightly outperformed by JPEG–LS. SCBPC closely followed CBPC encoder beating other encoders on all images except on *CT abdo*.

5. Conclusions

The results obtained with our proposed compression algorithms are encouraging. Proposed approach of modeling the image as composed of regions with the mixture of dominant and non–dominant properties has shown to be useful for lossless image compression. On the other hand, it should be noted that the increase in compression performances comes with the increase in computational complexity. This was extensively studied and resulted in the heuristic approach described in this work. Our predictors are moderately more complex than predictors used in contemporary lossless compression algorithms such as CALIC and

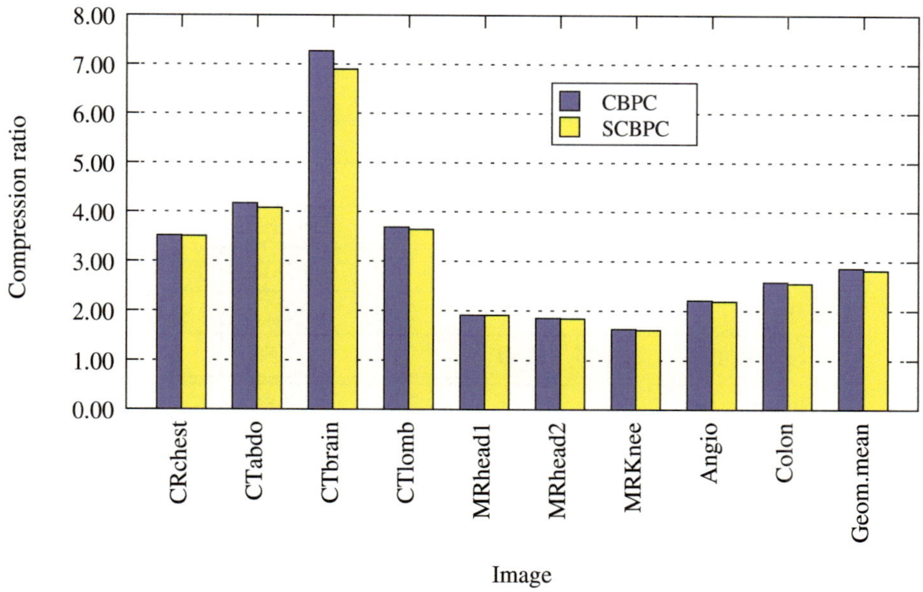

Fig. 6. Compression efficiency of SCBPC and CBPC

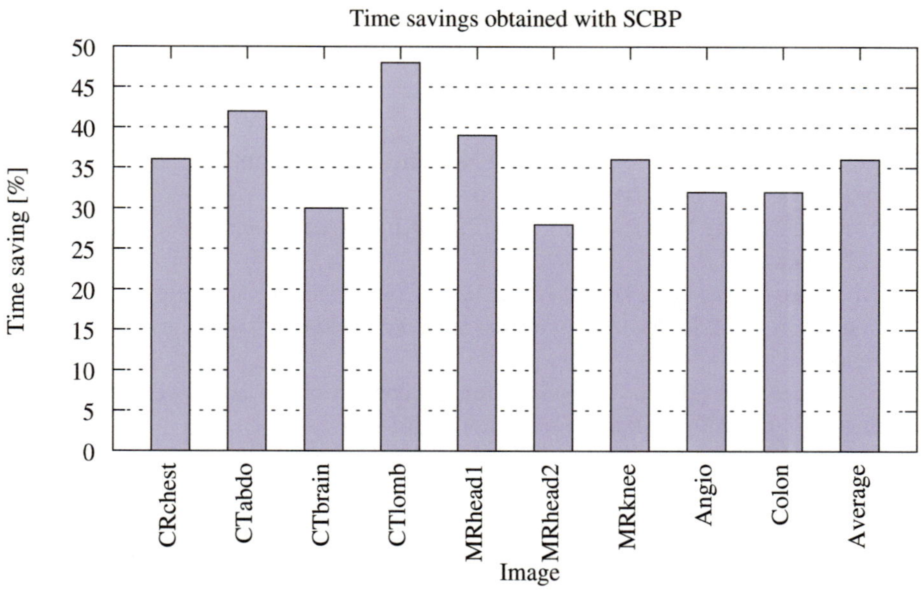

Fig. 7. SCBP and CBP: Time savings

Image	CALIC	JPEG–LS	JPEG2000$_R$	CBPC	SCBPC
CR Chest	3.40	3.35	3.17	3.52	3.51
CT Abdo	3.52	4.23	3.09	4.17	4.08
CT Brain	6.45	6.20	5.67	7.27	6.90
CT Lomb	3.62	3.42	3.36	3.69	3.64
MR Head	1.87	1.80	1.79	1.91	1.91
MR Head1	1.80	1.73	1.70	1.85	1.84
MR Knee	1.61	1.57	1.57	1.63	1.61
OT An7	2.16	2.18	2.02	2.21	2.19
OT Colon	2.49	2.50	2.32	2.58	2.55
Geom.mean	2.72	2.71	2.52	2.86	2.82

Table 4. Obtained compression ratios

JPEG–LS, but less complex than highly–adaptive predictors that can be found in proposals based on least squares approach (X. Li and M.T. Orchard, 2001). Also, the complexity of proposed predictors can be tuned for both goals: better compression and faster time by changing its parameters which can be set on a image basis.
As part of the future work, we plan to investigate possible extension of our image compression techniques to 3D and volumetric medical data. In this framework, we would propose to have regions of data that will be stored using lossless compression, while other, less relevant parts could be compressed with lossy algorithms. Additionally, prediction template can be extended by incorporating three dimensions rather than using two dimensions as is currently the case.

6. References

A. Gersho (1993). Optimal Vector Quantized Nonlinear Estimation, *Proc. 1993 IEEE Int. Symp. on Information Theory*, San Antonio, p. 170.

A. Gersho and V.M. Gray (n.d.). *Vector Quantization and Signal Compression*, Kluwer Academic Publishers.

Choong, M., Rajasvaran, L. & Bister, M. (2007). Cost–effective handling of digital medical images in the telemedicine environment, *International Journal of Medical Informatics* 76: 646–654.

Dikbas, S. & Zhai, F. (2010). Lossless image compression using adjustable fractional line-buffer, *Sig. Proc.: Image Comm.* 25(5): 345–351.

G. Motta and J.A. Storer and B. Carpentieri (2000). Lossless Image Coding via Adaptive Linear Prediction and Classification, *Proceedings of The IEEE* 88(11): 1790–1796.

Knezović, J. & Kovač, M. (2003). Gradient Based Selective Weighting of Neighboring Pixels for Predictive Lossless Image Coding, *Proc. 25th Int. Conf. Information Technology Interfaces ITI 2003*, Cavtat, Croatia, pp. 483–488.

M. Boliek and A. Zandi (1995). CREW: Lossless/lossy Image Compression – Contribution to ISO/IEC JTC 1.29.12, *ISO Working Document ISO/IEC JTC1/SC29/WG1 N196* .

Memon, N. & Wu, X. (1999). Recent developments in context-based predictive techniques for lossless image compression, *IEEE Computer* 10: 127–136.

Meyer, B. (2005). Tmw page, http://www.csse.monash.edu.au/ bmeyer/tmw/index.html.

Miaou, S.-G., Ke, F.-S. & Chen, S.-C. (2009). A lossless compression method for medical image sequences using jpeg-ls and interframe coding, *Information Technology in Biomedicine, IEEE Transactions on* 13(5): 818 –821.

M.J. Slyz and D.L. Neuhoff (1994). A Nonlinear VQ–based Lossless Image Coder, *Proc. 1994 Data Compression Conference*, IEEE, Snowbird, UT, pp. 491–500.

M.J. Weinberger and G. Seroussi and G. Sapiro (1998). The LOCO–I Lossless Image Compression Algorithm: Principles and Standardization into JPEG–LS, *HP Laboratories Technical Report HPL-98-198* .

Neves, A. J. R. & Pinho, A. J. (2009). Lossless compression of microarray images using image-dependent finite-context models, *IEEE Trans. Med. Imaging* 28(2): 194–201.

P.G. Howard and J.S. Vitter (1994). Fast and Efficient Lossless Image Compression, *Proc. 1994 Data Compression Conference*, IEEE, Snowbird, UT, pp. 351–360.

S. Barré Medical Image Samples (2004). http://www.barre.nom.fr/medical/samples/, WWW.

S. Forchhammer and X. Wu and J.D. Andersen (2004). Optimal Context Quantization in Lossless Compression of Image Data Sequence, *IEEE Transactions on Image Processing* 13(4): 509–517.

Sanchez, V., Abugharbieh, R. & Nasiopoulos, P. (2009). Symmetry-based scalable lossless compression of 3d medical image data, *IEEE Trans. Med. Imaging* 28(7): 1062–1072.

Sanchez, V., Nasiopoulos, P. & Abugharbieh, R. (2008). Efficient lossless compression of 4-d medical images based on the advanced video coding scheme, *IEEE Transactions on Information Technology in Biomedicine* 12(4): 442–446.

Sanchez, V., Nasiopoulos, P. & Abugharbieh, R. (2009). Novel lossless fmri image compression based on motion compensation and customized entropy coding, *Trans. Info. Tech. Biomed.* 13: 645–655.

Santa-Cruz, D. & Ebrahimi, T. (1997). An analytical study of jpeg 2000 functionalities, *Proceeding of IEEE Data Compression Conference*, IEEE, pp. 49–52.

Seemann, T. & Tischer, P. (1997). Genralized Locally Adaptive DPCM, *Proc. 1997 Data Compression Conference*, IEEE, Snowbird, UT, pp. 473–488.

Seemann, T., Tischer, P. & Meyer, B. (1997). History–Based Blending of Image Sub-Predictors, *Proceedings of PCS'97 Picture Coding Symposium*, VDE–Verlag, Berlin, Germany, pp. 147–151.

Sriraam, N. & Eswaran, C. (2008). An adaptive error modeling scheme for the lossless compression of eeg signals, *IEEE Transactions on Information Technology in Biomedicine* 12(5): 587–594.

Wu, X. (1997). Lossless Compression of Continuous-tone Images via Context Selection, Quantization, and Modeling, *IEEE Transactions On Image Processing* 6(5): 656–664.

X. Li and M.T. Orchard (2001). Edge–Directed Prediction for Lossless Compression of Natural Images, *IEEE Transactions on Image Processing* 10(6): 813–817.

X. Wu and N. Memon and K. Sayood (1995). A Context–Based, Adaptive, Lossless/nearly–lossless Coding Scheme for Continuous–Tone Images, ISO Working Document ISO/IEC/ SC29/WG1/N256.

Zagar, M., Kovac, M. & Bosnic, I. (2007). Lossless and lossy compression in 4d bio-modeling, *Proceeding of the First International Conference in Information and Communication Technology & Accessibility*, pp. 271–276.

Zhang, Y. & Adjeroh, D. A. (2008). Prediction by partial approximate matching for lossless image compression, *IEEE Transactions on Image Processing* 17(6): 924–935.

8

Clinical Decision Support Systems

Dejan Dinevski, Uroš Bele, Tomislav Šarenac,
Uroš Rajkovič and Olga Šušteršič
Faculty of Medicine, University of Maribor, University Clinical Center Maribor
Faculty of Organizational Sciences, University of Maribor and
Faculty of Health Sciences, University of Ljubljana
Slovenia

1. Introduction

In the chapter we are presenting the theoretical background, state of the art and modern research trends of Clinical decision support systems (CDSS). The challenges for success are derived and our experience is described with the presentation of a good practice example of employing CDSS in telemedicine.

CDSS systems are increasingly often integrated into telemedicine clinical practice. In addition to using the same resources, namely digitally coded clinical data, CDSS systems are able to enhance the quality of telemedicine services in many cases.

CDSS are computer applications that are designed to help health-care professionals with making clinical decisions about individual patients (Shortliffe and Cimino 2006; Berner 2007). In other words, CDSS are active knowledge systems, which use two or more items of patient data to generate case-specific advice (Wyatt and Spiegelhalter 1991).

These kinds of software use relevant knowledge, rules within a knowledge base and relevant patient and clinical data to improve clinical decision making on topics like preventive, acute and chronic care, diagnostics, specific test ordering, prescribing practices (National Electronic Decision Support 2003; Pearson, Moxey et al. 2009). A CDSS correlates data about patient traits with a trustworthy knowledge base to guide a clinician with patient-specific advice, assessments or recommendations. Clinicians, health-care staff or patients can manually enter patient characteristics into the computer systems; alternatively, electronic medical records (EMR) can be queried for retrieval of patient characteristics. These kinds of decision-support systems allow the clinicians to spot and choose the most appropriate treatment. Provided decision-support is based on processes of sophisticated outcomes assessment and algorithms that use knowledge bases to inquire after the newest developments about best practice (Remmlinger 2002; Garg, Adhikari et al. 2005).

Regardless of how we choose to define CDSS, we have to accept that the field of CDSS is rapidly advancing and unregulated. It has a potential for harm, if systems are poorly designed and inadequately evaluated, as well as a huge potential to benefit, especially in health care provider performance, quality of care and patient outcomes (Delaney, Fitzmaurice et al. 1999; Pearson, Moxey et al. 2009).

2. Clinical decision-making

There are some principal categories to take into account while striving for excellent decision-making: a) accurate data, b) applicable knowledge, c) appropriate problem-solving skills (Shortliffe and Cimino 2006).

Patient data must be adequate to make a valid decision. The problem arises, when the clinician is met with an overwhelming amount of specific and unspecific data, which he/she cannot satisfactorily process. Therefore it is important to assess when additional facts will confuse rather than clarify the patient's case. For example, usual setting for such a problem are intensive-care units, where practitioners must absorb large amounts of data from various monitors, be aware of the clinical status, patient history, accompanying chronic illnesses, patient's medication and adverse drug interactions, etc. - and on top of that make an appropriate decision about the course of action. The quality of available data is of equal importance. Measuring instruments and monitors should be as accurate as technologically possible, since erroneous data could have serious adverse effect on patient-care decisions.

Knowledge used in decision-making process must be accurate and current. It is of major importance that the deciding clinician has a broad spectrum of medical knowledge and access to information resources, where it is possible to constantly revise and validate that knowledge. For a patient to receive appropriate care, the clinician must be aware of the latest evidence-based guidelines and developments in the area of the case in question. It is in clinician's hands to bring proven therapies from research papers to the bedside. CDSS analogously needs an extensive, well-structured and current source of knowledge to appropriately serve the clinician.

Above all, good problem-solving skills are needed to utilize available data and knowledge. Deciding clinicians must set appropriate goals for each task, know how to reason about each goal and take in to account the trade-offs between costs and benefits of therapy and diagnostics. In further reflection, we should not neglect, that skilled clinicians draw extensively from their personal experience.

By incorporating patient-specific data and evidence-based guidelines or applicable knowledge base, the CDSS can improve quality of care with enhancing the clinical decision-making process (General Practice Electronic Decision Support 2000).

In order to be able to construct applicable CDSS, it is imperative to have a broader-based understanding of medical decision-making as it occurs in the natural setting. Designing CDSSs without understanding the cognitive processes underlying medical reasoning and decision analysis is pliable for ineffectiveness and failure for implementation into everyday clinical workflow (Patel, Kaufman et al. 2002).

2.1 Clinical decision analysis (problem solving)

Decision analysis is a quantitative evaluation of the outcomes that result from a set of choices in a specific clinical situation and is the methodology usually chosen for clinical problem solving. This process is often implicit and occurs within internal algorithms and heuristics (mental shortcuts) that the clinician has developed and acquired over time. Decision analysis, by requiring a specific model structure and assessment of various likelihoods and values of the outcomes, makes the decision process explicit and more inclined to examination, discussion, and re-validation. Decision models are often used as analytic tools to conduct cost-effectiveness analyses, since this methodology can be used to find the expected value of predicted outcomes.

The range of clinical problems appropriate for decision analysis is vast. Such problems focus upon a specific decision, where there is a tradeoff involved, which means that one of the choices considered is not necessarily unambiguously superior. As an example, a diagnostic test carries some risk, but it trades off with more appropriate therapy and better patient outcome when treatment is directed by the results of that test. Decision-making is rarely a clear-cut process - it therefore inevitably involves compromises.

In general, decision analyses have been developed to:

- Assist in clinical decision-making for a specific individual patient;
- Estimate optimal strategies for classes of patients with specific clinical characteristics in given situations;
- Link estimates of both clinical and economic outcomes (cost-effectiveness analysis) to help in forming issues regarding health policy;
- Provide estimates of expected outcomes in situations where classical methods such as randomized trials are either impossible or impractical.

There are several advantages of using decision analysis to investigate options involving a single patient. Placing the problem in an explicit, analytic context forces clinicians to make their assumptions clear. Decision analyses can directly incorporate issues regarding quality of life and how the particular patient values various outcomes. An example of such a decision analysis is weighing the risks and benefits of prophylactic mastectomy (breast removal) and oophorectomy (removal of ovaries) for patients with BRCA1 or BRCA2 mutations. One has to combine several kinds of data - estimates of the increased risks of ovarian and breast cancer for women with the mutations, general cancer incidence and last but not least, the risks that the surgical procedures impose. The analysis in a certain point of time demonstrates, using the best currently available data, that life expectancy for women who carry such mutations was increased by as much as 5.3 years with prophylactic mastectomy and by as much as 1.7 years with prophylactic oophorectomy.

Developing and constructing a decision analysis follows a logical series of steps (problem-solving). Problems or errors in any step can alter the eventual results; thus, proper adherence to each of these steps is important both from the view of a researcher conducting an analysis and a clinician interpreting the results. The steps are (Roberts 2011):

- **Frame the question** - The process of defining the scope and boundaries of the particular clinical situation to be analyzed. In other words at this stage one is to analyze the new data which suggest a problem and identify the problem as it appears.
- **Structure the clinical problem** - Structuring the problem simply means constructing a decision model that represents the relevant components of the problem. We need to think through what the alternative solutions might be and create a list of alternatives - hypotheses. In the clinical setting these might be potential therapeutic options for a set diagnosis. The mathematical representation of a decision model is called a decision tree and is composed of several different elements. Elements combined into trees contain an amount of detail arbitrarily designated. There is a permanent tension between increasing the level of detail to be as clinically realistic as possible versus the feasibility of model construction, validation, and presentation. The more detail desired, the more difficult the model is to construct, validate, and present. However, the less detailed the analysis and the greater the number of simplifying assumptions, the more vulnerable is the analysis to attack for lacking clinically meaningful elements.
- **Estimate the relevant probabilities** - Once a decision tree has been structured, the numeric values of various probabilities need to be determined. There are many sources

of data that can be used to make these determinations. Although there is a generally accepted hierarchy of study quality (randomized controlled trial > cohort study > administrative databases > systematic reviews), such ratings are not always useful for decision analysis since the particular study type may not be conducive in estimating a given parameter. As an example, a randomized controlled trial is an excellent source for comparing one therapy versus another, but it is a poor source of data regarding the incidence of a particular disease. Thus, it is important to tailor the data source to the type of data required.

However there might not be enough evidence to assign relevant probabilities to candidate solutions or even to structure the clinical problem and find suitable alternative solutions in the first place (see previous step). Thus the process is bound to reform with a new search to fill the present "knowledge gap". Potentially many iterations of this cycle of data gathering and hypotheses generation may occur until the decision-making clinician has enough clarity to move on through the process. Clinical decision-analysis is hence a fundamental fuel for further research, evidence collection and problem re-evaluation - all for the purpose of finding suitable solutions that will help resolving the clinical situation. CDSS can be programmed in a way that they rearrange themselves for a specific problem, search for relevant evidence and even create new knowledge (Coiera 2003).

- **Estimate the values of the outcomes** - Different solutions to a problem have different outcomes. The structure of the problem defines the specific outcome measure to be used. For example, if death was a possible outcome of one or more strategies, life expectancy would be an appropriate outcome measure. The most important aspect in assigning outcomes is that they are measured in the same units across all branches. A useful feature of decision analysis is that a given model can be evaluated using different outcome measures. As an example, in addition to survival, the clinician may want to track the effect of different therapies upon the rate of stroke, myocardial infarction, pulmonary embolization, etc., across various treatment options. The decision model can be analyzed using any of those outcomes.
- **Analyze the tree** - The preferred type of analysis of a problem utilizes the strategy that maximizes the expected value of the outcome. As an example, if the outcome of interest was life expectancy, the result of a decision analysis would be of the form: "the average life expectancy with strategy A is 11.3 years versus 8.6 years with strategy B; therefore strategy A is the optimal strategy." Such a tree might represent the choice between two therapies, where one is preferred in terms of life expectancy.
- **Test the model's assumptions** - The results obtained from a decision analysis depend upon the accuracy of the data used to estimate the probabilities and outcomes. It is rarely the case that estimates are known with complete certainty. One of the major advantages of decision analysis models is their ability to rapidly test their assumptions and input data - to validate the decision model by performing a sensitivity analysis. The model's answer can be compared with the "true" answer to validate the model structure by evaluating a tree using parameters for which the result is known *a priori*. As an example, in a choice between a more effective (but riskier) surgical therapy and a less effective (but safer) medical therapy, a sensitivity analysis that postulated a zero mortality rate for the surgical intervention should advocate the surgical arm since there would be no downside risk.

- **Interpret the results** - Interpreting the results of a decision analysis is often the most complicated task. The ability of a decision analysis to explore how the optimal strategy in a particular clinical situation changes with variation in assumptions (and therefore to identify areas for further data needs) is often one of the most powerful attributes of this type of analysis. Several details of an analysis should be examined prior to using the results to change practice: a) The patient population should closely match the patients seen by the clinician. b) The reader needs to assess the strength of the result (sensitivity analysis). If sensitivity analyses indicate that the optimal choice is strongly dependent upon a given parameter, one should try to develop accurate measures of the parameter estimate.

Reasoning in a medical context involves uncertainty to a high extent, combined with constrained resources it therefore leads to increased use of heuristic strategies. Greatest advantage of heuristics is in limiting the extent of purposeful search through data sets and knowledge bases. By reducing redundancy, heuristics have substantial practical value. A significant part of a clinician's cognitive effort is based on heuristic thinking, the reasoning is inductive with assigned probability for each possible choice. However, the use of heuristics introduces considerable bias in medical reasoning, often resulting in a number of conceptual and procedural errors. These include misconceptions about laws that govern probability, false understanding of manifestation of general rules to a specific patient at the point of care, neglect and false validation of prior probabilities and therapeutic actions. Above all, the cognitive biases that unavoidably affect a human-decision maker are often the hallmark of decision uncertainty (Holyoak 2005).

If the designers of CDSSs are to create effective systems which would be successfully implemented into the workflow, providing the clinician with the necessary support of their decision-making abilities, they must be ready to accept the general paths of clinical decision-making process, described above. Efficiently designed and correctly implemented CDSS can elicit extensive positive externalities to the health-workers' performance and improve patient outcome thus affect the gross quality of healthcare.

3. Structure of clinical decision support systems

CDSSs vary very much in their design. The basic principles of structure and design had also changed substantially in the last decade. Various traits of CDSSs are related to or have a direct effect on clinical effectiveness, functionality, error prevention, potential for acceptance in the clinical world, system portability, cost-effectiveness etc. It is thus important to characterize CDSSs in a way to best understand the diversity of CDSS. The knowing of classification, conjunct with an idea of general clinical decision-making processes described above, present a powerful set of basic facts that are useful for CDSSs designers and evaluators.

In this chapter, we will try to characterize CDSS, combining several resources to create a comprehensive classification that capture key elements of CDSS design and function (Coiera 2003; Sim and Berlin 2003; Shortliffe and Cimino 2006; Berner 2007; Greenes 2007). According to Sim and Berlin 2003, the CDSS can be categorized along 5 axes.

3.1 Context axes

1. **Clinical setting.**
    - Inpatient setting
    - Outpatient setting

2. **Clinical Task.**
   - Diagnostic assistance.
     Based on the patient's data and the system's knowledge base, the CDSS provides likely diagnoses. Diagnostic assistance can be coupled with complex data-retrieval systems, like ECG. It seeks to identify "what is true" for a specific patient.
   - Therapy critiquing and consulting.
     This function can for example be incorporated into clinician's order-entry. It assesses the therapy, looks for inconsistencies, errors, cross-references for drug interactions and prevents prescribing of allergenic drugs. It has been shown that the necessity of a clinician to provide a statement of an appropriate reason, if he is or she is not to follow the recommendations, significantly increases the clinical importance of CDSSs. The CDSS can use protocols and evidence-based guidelines, combined with patient's facts, acquired from EMR, to provide an optimal treatment plan and help following it. These kinds of CDSSs address the question "what to do" with a patient and are often combined with recommendations about further diagnostic processing (i.e. which tests to order, X-ray, CT etc.). Such software can generate additional questions as to provide even more specific advice about further therapy (and diagnosis).
   - Drug dosing or prescribing.
     CDSS have the power to reduce toxic drug levels, reduce medical errors, change prescribing in accordance to guideline recommendations and reduce time to achieving therapeutic control. If connected to EMR, the system can prevent prescription of drugs that cause allergic reactions. Such systems have been widely accepted, since they are well integrated into a routine part of the clinician's workflow and they provide automated order-entry forms and electronic transmission to pharmacies. Overall prescription of medication is one of the commonest tasks of a physician and also one of the commonest clinical tasks where CDSSs arebeing applied.
   - Test selection.
   - Alerts and reminders.
     An expert system that is integrated into a monitoring device or health-care information system (e.g. laboratory information system, EMR) can provide real-time sound, visual or tactile alerts thru various communication tools (e.g. e-mail, SMS, pager). Reminder systems are designed to remind the clinician of crucial tasks that need to be done before a certain event (e.g. fasting before endoscopy, no anticoagulants before abdominal surgery).
   - Information retrieval.
     Relevant information retrieval through world wide web or comprehensive knowledge bases.
   - Image recognition and interpretation.
     Clinical images from CT, MRI, angiograms etc. can nowadays be partially automatically interpreted. More importantly CDSS can function as a mass screening tool, where software flags critical images, which require clinician's special attention.
   - Prevention.
   - Screening.

- Expert laboratory system.
- Chronic disease management.

3.2 Knowledge axes

This axes deals with the sources, quality and customization of the CDSS's knowledge and data.

1. **Clinical knowledge source.**
   It can be derived from high-quality sources (e.g. randomized-controlled trials, systematic reviews, national or professional society guidelines) and/or from participation of clinicians that will eventually use the system.
2. **Data source.**
   The patient-specific data can be retrieved from computerized order entry, medical instrument (e.g. blood pressure measuring device), EMR or other data repository. The data may also be gathered from a paper chart or a person. In that case data must be entered in the system using a data input intermediary (see bellow). This characteristic affects the likelihood of CDSS adoption in practice to a high extent. It has been shown, that automatic computerized provision of data to the system (e.g. from EMR) is preferred.
3. **Data source intermediary** is a clinician who inputs data into data source (see above). Intermediaries could also be patients themselves.
4. **Data coding.**
   For various reasons (e.g. funding, epidemiology) it is desirable to use a widely use coding schema, i.e. ICD-10, SNOMED. Obviously the data could also be in plain text.
5. **Data customization.**
   The more CDSS produces patient-specific targeted recommendations, customized to age, gender, concomitant diagnoses etc., more it has a probability of clinical relevance and effectiveness.
6. **Update mechanism.**
   As stated above, knowledge base ought to be current and constantly up-to-date.

We can divide CDSS to knowledge based and non-knowledge based systems.

The knowledge-based systems (a.k.a. expert systems) mostly consist of three parts - the knowledge base, inference engine and the mechanism to communicate. They contain expert clinical knowledge about very specific facts and tasks and are able to reason with the input of data from all the various sources stated above. These systems usually use knowledge in form of IF-THEN rules and probabilistic associations between compiled data. The inference engine lies at the core of the artificial intelligence part of knowledge-based systems - it combines and correlates knowledge base rules with the patient's data. Basically the inference engine reasons with the given information to form new conclusions (Wikipedia 2011).

The non-knowledge-based systems rather use principle of machine learning in the form of i.e. neural networks or genetic algorithms, where computers learn from past experience and/or find patterns in clinical data of an individual.

3.3 Decision support axes

Addressing a suitable decision-making process is probably the most important dimension of CDSS.

1. **Reasoning method.** Some of CDSS reasoning engines are:

- Rule-based systems. A rule-based system uses different expert knowledge bases in form of expressions that can be evaluated as IF-THEN rules (production rules). Such a system is an example of heuristic approach in which individual logical statements in the form of production rules are obtained by observing human experts, or interviewing and debriefing them, and then combined in an attempt to emulate the reasoning processes of experts. This approach was first used in the MYCIN (Shortliffe 1976), with the goal of choosing appropriate antimicrobial therapy for a patient.
- Neural networks. Artificial neural network is a non-knowledge-based adaptive CDSS that uses machine learning to learn from experiences and recognize patterns in clinical information.
- Bayesian network. A typical knowledge-based decision-making system is the Bayesian network (a.k.a belief network or causal probabilistic network) that shows probabilistic relationships between sets of variables - diseases and symptoms, based on conditional probability according to Bayes theorem. It is a network with a explicit requirement, that the relationships be causal. Such a network helps to model the progression of a disease over time and the interaction between diseases; a big road-block however is that medical knowledge sometimes finds it difficult to directly specify what is the effect and what the cause.
- Model based systems. The latest achievement is patient specific modeling (see section 5.2.).
- Logical condition. Logical reasoning makes decisions according to the value of a given variable. The results of a decision-making process are different if the value is within or outside of the set boundaries.
- Data mining and machine learning. These methods are based on probabilistic decision-making according to the system's database. The ideal databases should be large and well constructed, so that they allow precise retrieval of patients similar to a current patient. Analysis of responses of those patients to various treatments is used to decide upon the best treatment for the current patient.
- Genetic algorhytm. As a non-knowledge-based method it uses iterative processes to rearrange itself and provide an optimal solution based on the patient data.

2. **Clinical urgency.**
   Provision of decision support to decisions that have to be made urgently. CDSS should first provide its function to issues with clear clinical priority, according to the principle "treat first what kills first". This characteristic leads to better patient outcomes and physicians performance.
3. **Recommendation explicitness.**
   Users are more likely to follow explicit recommendations, providing concrete course of action.
4. **Response requirement.**
   The using clinician may be required to provide justification for the way he/she responded to the recommendation provided by the CDSS. This could be done in a form of acknowledgement of recommendation, with a statement of what alternative action was taken and with an explanation for non-compliance.

3.4 Information delivery axes

This axes deals with the delivery of newly produced information to the user.

1. **Delivery format.**
   Paper-based, online (via internet or integrated into EMR), via other technology - phone, pager, e-mail etc.
2. **Delivery mode.**
   The recommendations can be delivered after the decision-maker has requested so or on the other hand it could be delivered without the consent in form of an alert, reminder or optimization request. In the first case the clinician has to make an additional effort, recognize when the advice would be useful, "go to the program" and enter data to request diagnostic or therapeutic assessment, thus the program is passive.The so-called "push systems" that automatically provide recommendations may be more effective and substantially more used. They play an active role with providing decision support as a byproduct of data-managing activities (e.g. monitoring, EMR supervision). System decision logic is in a way integrated within a patient's database that is already being gathered from various sources and provides results of its decision analysis without an additional effort of the clinician. A valid point to consider here is how to avoid so-called "alarm fatigue", where the clinician is over-warned to minor discrepancies which are otherwise noted and commonly understood.
3. **Action integration.**
   It is imperative, that the CDSS provides the ability to the decision-maker to exert the recommended actions with ease. For example, the software can, while providing prompts on therapy-critique, also provide direct links to order-entry forms and therapy planning section of EMR. The action of therapy change should be completed within a range of few clicks, for example with checking a mark. Action integration unambiguously adds to wider acceptance and usability of CDSS.
4. **Explanation availability.**
   It is a function, where the system provides an explanation of its recommendations, through e.g. links to evidence-based articles, books or directly from the knowledge base.

3.5 Workflow axes

CDSS can be seen as a process, however at the point of care it is virtually an intervention of technology, that could also act as an interruption. Systems that are synergistic with the institution's workflow are likely to experience higher usage and prove to be more effective in optimizing practitioner's performance.

4. Success factors of CDSS

Despite the fact, that the computerized CDSSs were continuously in development since the 1970s, their impact on routine clinical practice has not been as strong as expected. The potential benefits of using electronic decision support systems in clinical practice fall into three broad categories (Coiera 2003):

1. Improved patient safety (reduced medication errors and unwanted adverse events, refined ordering of medication and tests);
2. Improved quality of care (increasing clinicians' time allocated directly to patient care, increased application of clinical pathways and guidelines, accelerate and encourage the use of latest clinical findings, improved clinical documentation and patient satisfaction);

3. Improved efficiency of health-care (reducing costs through faster order processing, reductions in test duplication, decreased adverse events, and changed patterns of drug prescribing, favoring cheaper but equally effective generic brands).

Developing CDSSs is a challenging process, which may lead to a failure despite our theoretical knowledge about the topic. Understanding the underlying causes, which lead either to success or either to failure, may help to improve the efficiency of CDSS development and deployment in day-to-day practice. Failures can originate from various developmental and implementation phases: failure to technically complete an appropriate system, failure to get the system accepted by the users and failure to integrate the system in the organizational or user environment (Brender, Ammenwerth et al. 2006).

There is an estimation that 45% of computerized medical information systems fail because of user resistance, even though these systems are technologically coherent. Some reasons for such a high percentage of failure may derive from insufficient computer ability, diminished professional autonomy, lack of awareness of long-term benefits of CDSS-use and lack of desire to change the daily workflow (Zheng, Padman et al. 2005). There is also clear evidence that CDSS services are not always used when available, since too numerous systems' alerts are being overridden or ignored by physicians (Moxey, Robertson et al. 2010).

Despite the problems and failures that might accompany CDSSs, these systems have still been proven to improve drug selection and dosing suggestions, reduce serious medication errors by flagging potential drug reactions, drug allergies and identifying duplication of therapy, they enhance the delivery of preventive care services and improve adherence to recommended care standards.

Recent studies suggest that there are some CDSS features crucial to success of these systems (Kawamoto, Houlihan et al. 2005; Shortliffe and Cimino 2006; Pearson, Moxey et al. 2009; Moxey, Robertson et al. 2010):

- CDSS should provide decision support automatically as part of clinicians' workflow, since systems where clinicians were required to seek out advice manually have not been proven as successful.
- Decision support should be delivered at the time and location of decision-making. If the clinician has to interrupt the normal pattern of patient care to move to a separate workstation or to follow complex, time-consuming startup procedures it is not likely that such system will be good accepted.
- Systems that were provided as an integrated component of charting or ordering systems were significantly more likely to succeed than alone standing systems. Generally speaking, the decision-support element should be incorporated into a larger computer system that is already part of the users' professional routine, thus making decision support a byproduct of practitioners' ordinary work practices.
- Computerized systems have been reported to be advantageous over paper-based systems.
- Systems should provide recommendation rather than just state a patient assessment. For instance, system recommends that the clinician prescribes diuretics for a patient rather just identifying patient being cardiologically decompensated.
- CDSS should request the clinician to record a reason for not following the systems' advice (the clinician is asked to justify the decision with a reason, e.g. "The patient refused").
- It should promote clinicians' action rather than inaction.

- No need for additional clinical data entry. Due to clinicians' effort required for entering new patient data, they tend to avoid this process, which is essential for new decision support. Systems should rather acquire new data automatically (e.g. data retrieval from EMR).
- The system should be easy to navigate and use, e.g. with quick access and minimal mouse clicks for desired information.
- Timing and frequency of prompts are of great importance. For instance if there are too many messages, this might only lead to ignoring all of them and consequently to missing important information. The timing is as well of great importance - the alerts shouldn't appear at inappropriate times and interrupt the workflow.
- The presentation of data or information on CDSSs shouldn't be too dense or the text to small. Researchers also suggest the use of blinking icons for important tasks or the arrangement of interactions according to their urgency.
- Decision support results should be provided to both clinicians and patients. Studies have shown beneficial effect of such actions, because they stimulate the clinicians to discuss treatment options with patients, and consequently make the latter feel more involved in their medical treatment.
- Periodic feedback about clinician's compliance with system decision-making.

What these features have in common is that they all make it easier for clinicians to implement the CDSS into their workflow, thus making it easier to use. An effective CDSS must minimize the effort to receive and act on system recommendations. Clinicians found it also very practical if the CDSS would back up its decision-making with linking it to other knowledge resources across the intranet or Internet. In their opinion the safety and drug interaction alerts were the most helpful feature. Above all the organizational factors, such as computer availability at the point of care and technical perfection of CDSS hardware and software are crucial to implementation (Moxey, Robertson et al. 2010).

Kawamoto 2005 suggests that the effectiveness of CDSS remains mainly unchanged when system recommendations are stated more strongly and when the evidence supporting these prompts is expanded and includes institution-specific data. Similarly, the effectiveness and functionality remains unaltered when recommendations are made more specific. Interestingly the CDSSs didn't achieve wanted results when local clinicians were recruited into the system development process nor when bibliographic citations were provided to support the system made recommendations (Kawamoto, Houlihan et al. 2005).

To sum up, when developing CDSSs, there are factors beyond software and content that must be taken into consideration. Fundamental issues include availability and accessibility of hardware, sufficient technical support and training in use of the system, the level of system integration into clinical workflow and the relevance and timeliness of the clinical messages provided.

5. Examples of CDSS in practice

5.1 Historical examples: Leeds abdominal pain, MYCIN, HELP, Internist-1

There have been multiple attempts through history to construct a computer or program, which would assist clinicians with their decisions concerning diagnosis and therapy. Ledley and Lusted published the first article evolving around this idea in 1959. The first really functional CDSS didn't appear until the 1970s. We will review the following historical systems: Leeds abdominal pain, MYCIN, HELP and Internist-1.

F. T. de Dombal and his co-workers at University of Leeds developed Leeds abdominal pain. It used Bayesian reasoning on basis of surgical and pathological diagnoses. These pieces of information were gathered from thousands of patients and put into systems' database. The Leeds abdominal pain system used sensitivity, specificity and disease-prevalence data for various signs, symptoms and test results. With help of Bayes' theorem it calculated the probability of seven possible diagnoses resulting in acute abdominal pain: appendicitis, diverticulitis, perforated ulcer, cholecystitis, small-bowel obstruction, pancreatitis, and nonspecific abdominal pain. The system assumed that each patient with abdominal pain had one of these seven conditions, thus selected the most likely diagnose on the basis of recorded observations. Evaluation of the system was done by de Dombal et al. in 1972. It showed that the clinicians' diagnoses were correct in only 65 to 80 percent of the 304 cases, whereas the program's diagnoses were correct in 91.8 percent of cases. Surprisingly, the system has never achieved similar results of diagnostic accuracy in practice outside the Leeds University. The most likely reason for that is the variation of data that clinicians entered into the system for acquiring correct diagnoses (de Dombal, Leaper et al. 1972).

MYCIN was a consultation system that emphasized appropriate management of patients who had infections rather than just finding their diagnosis. The developers of this system formed production rules (IF-THEN rules), on basis of current knowledge about infectious diseases. The MYCIN program determined which rules to use and how to chain them together in order to make decisions about a specific case. System developers could update the system's knowledge structure rapidly by removing, altering, or adding rules, without reprogramming or restructuring other parts of the system (Shortliffe 1976).

The HELP system is actually an integrated hospital information system with the ability to generate alerts when data abnormalities in the patient record are noted. It can output data either automatically, in form of printed reports, or it can display specific information, if so requested. Furthermore, the system has an event-driven mechanism for generation of specialized warnings, alerts and reports (Burke, Classen et al. 1991).

Internist-I was an experimental CDSS designed by Pople and Myers at the University of Pittsburg in 1974. It was a rule-based expert system capable of making multiple, complex diagnoses in internal medicine based on patient observations. The Internist-I was using a tree-structured database that linked symptoms with diseases. The evaluation of the system revealed that it was not sufficiently reliable for clinical application. Nevertheless, the most valuable product of the system was its medical knowledge base. This was used as a basis for successor systems including CADUCEUS and Quick Medical Reference (QMR), a commercialized diagnostic CDSS for internists (Miller, Pople et al. 1982).

5.2 Selected contemporary examples of CDSS

ATHENA

The Athena decision support system was deployed in 2002 as a tool to implement guidelines for hypertension. It encourages blood pressure control and issues recommendations about a suitable choice of therapy, concordant with latest guidelines. It also considers co-morbidities of the specific patient in question. ATHENA DSS has an easily changeable knowledge base that specifies criteria for eligibility, risk stratification, set blood pressure margins, it includes relevant co-morbid states and guideline-recommendation, specific for patients with present co-morbidities. The knowledge base also comprises of preferences for certain drugs within antihypertensive drug groups according to the latest evidence. New pieces of evidence are constantly changing protocols of best hypertension management; ATHENA is thus designed to be accessible to clinicians for knowledge base-customization and to custom local interpretations of guidelines according to the local population structure and other factors. The system was designed to be independently integrated into a variety of EMR-systems, and is thus interchangeable and adaptable for various health information-systems. The effectiveness, accuracy and success of implementation has been researched and reviewed on many occasions (Goldstein, Coleman et al. 2004; Lai, Goldstein et al. 2004). Such systems as ATHENA can help with supporting general efforts of national and worldwide health care organizations in effective implementation and stricter following of issued guidelines in various fields of medicine.

In 2006 ATHENA DSS for opioid therapy was developed according to specific guidelines for the management of opioid therapy for chronic pain (Trafton, Martins et al. 2010).

This system uses EON architecture from the Stanford University. EON is a knowledge-based system that aids physicians with care of patients treated according to protocols and guidelines. It is constructed from set of software components that are embedded into a wider health information system, which uses patient-specific data. These software components are designed in such a way to be compiled together in various ways, mixed to create different decision-support functionalities. There are several components that are interrelated:

- Knowledge base encodes descriptions of clinical protocols; it is a source of evidence-based data for all other software components of EON.
- Problem solvers: They determine the right protocol for the patient, i.e. solve a task of placing the patient within the right therapy protocol, by addressing the knowledge base and incorporating patient's attributes (e.g. blood pressure measures and co-morbidities).
- Eligibility-determination component addresses the same knowledge base to match the factors in a patient with a certain protocol in order to ascertain if he/she is eligible for such a treatment,
- Database mediator is a conductor between all the components in EON and the database that stores patients' information. More sophisticated mediators already extract the relevant data and make relevant connections before presenting it to an EON problem-solver (Nguyen, Shahar et al. 1997).

ISABEL

Isabel is a web-based diagnosis decision support system that was created in 2001 by physicians. It offers diagnosis decision support at the point of care. The system is eligible for all aged patients, from neonates to geriatrics. Its database covers major specialties like Internal Medicine, Surgery, Gynecology & Obstetrics, Pediatrics, Geriatrics, Oncology, Toxicology and Bioterrorism. Isabel produces an instant list of likely diagnoses for a given set of clinical features (symptoms, signs, results of tests and investigations etc), followed by suggesting the administration of suitable drugs. This is executed by reconciling (i.e. pattern-matching technology) patient data sets with data sets as described in established medical literature. The system allows clinicians to follow their assumptions about differential diagnoses; it hence restricts searches to specific body systems, relatively to diagnoses in question. The system is interfaced with EMR, which allows it to extract existing diagnoses and other patient-specific data. Furthermore it contains a feature to help clinicians answer their questions with up to date knowledge from textbooks and journals.

Isabel uses Autonomy's natural language processing software as a search tool. The pattern of the clinical features entered is concept-matched with kernels of knowledge; then the best-matched kernels of knowledge (diagnoses) are returned for consideration. Autonomy's technology is based on advanced pattern-matching techniques (non-linear adaptive digital signal processing) rooted in the theories of Bayesian Inference and Claude Shannon's Principles of Information (Autonomy 2009). These enable identification of patterns that naturally occur in text, based on the usage and frequency of words or terms that correspond to specific concepts. Based on the predominance of one pattern over another within a piece of information, this technology enables computers to recognize when a particular document in question is about the searched subject. In this way, it extracts a document's digital essence and enables various operations to be automatically performed on that text.

Isabel has been extensively validated and been shown to enhance clinician's cognitive skills and thereby improves patient safety and the quality of patient care (Ramnarayan, Tomlinson et al. 2004; OpenClinical 2006).

LISA

LISA is a CDSS that consists of two main components. The first is a centralized Oracle database, holding all patient information about drug schedules, blood and toxicity results, doses prescribed etc. The database is accessible by health professionals from different sectors and locations. The second component represents a web-based decision support module, which is using the PROforma guideline development technology to provide advice about dose adjustments in treatment of acute childhood lymphoblastic leukemia. LISA is primarily concerned with providing support in the maintenance illness-period during which drug dose decisions have to be continually monitored and adjusted, as responses to these drugs vary significantly from patient to patient. Decision support is considered useful in this period, since many dose-errors have occurred in practice (Hurt, Fox et al. 2003). In order to give the patient an appropriate dosage of chemotherapeutics, the system uses PRO*forma* decision-making capabilities. It also contains an option, which allows a clinician to prescribe an alternative, not defined in the protocol. PRO*forma* bases its dose adjustment recommendations on five main data inputs defined in the protocol: current state, current platelet and absolute neutrophil count of the blood result on which the decision is being based, number of weeks that the patient has been at the current state and number of weeks that the patient has tolerated treatment.

Evaluational studies of LISA have concluded that the system is likely to be accepted by clinicians. Furthermore, the authors are predicting that the usage of LISA could lead to a decrease in non-compliance with the treatment protocol (Bury, Hurt et al. 2004).

Patient specific modeling

One of the promising novel concepts useful in CDSSs is Patient-Specific Modeling (PSM), which uses individualized computational models of human pathophysiology to model the dynamics of a wide variety of tissues and organs. It is not a CDSS per-se, we could rather think of it as functionality that adds-on and re-invents the process of clinical decision-making. Integrated into CDSSs it has a potential to even further improve diagnosis and optimize clinical treatment by predicting outcomes of therapies and surgical interventions. PSM is being pursued in well-funded projects, like the Virtual Physiological Human initiative (Viceconti, Clapworthy et al. 2007) and the International Physiome Project (Bassingthwaighte 2000).

Major advantage of PSM is that in contrast to regular diagnostic practices, which are based on averaged clinical trials, it provides tailored treatment and optimizes the individual therapy. While the training and experience of the physician prove to be the most valuable when deciding for the best treatment from an available range, this decision-making process often does not take into account all the data potentially available. Decision-making that bases on the results of simulations, which use models derived from patient-specific data, however, sometimes deal with basically immeasurable physical properties of tissues, e.g. tissue stress in the vessel-wall of a distending abdominal aneurysm (Doyle, Callanan et al. 2009). The results of such simulations enable judgment on effectiveness of a range of potential treatments before they are actually administered, preventing the patient from experiencing unneeded or ineffective treatments. We can think of such theoretical predictive data as descriptors that are used to very accurately asses values of outcome measures in a process of clinical decision-making

PSM has been studied and reviewed in modeling of blood vessels, bones, brain, skeletal muscle, heart and in modeling of the behavior of various tumors (Neal and Kerckhoffs 2010).

There are several basic elements, which are common to all fields of PSM in support of clinical decision-making. Data are obtained from the patient's medical record (EMR), e.g. from a virology genotypic assay or an angiography scan. The data is then used to construct a computational model, which is used to perform a complex workflow of simulations of a proposed protocol of treatment. Molecular dynamics simulations of drugs interacting with a range of viral proteins for example, provide results that are then interpreted to assess the efficacy of the treatment in question. This gives the physician an afore unimaginable ability to choose a treatment based on prior knowledge of how will that specific patient respond to it on a molecular-physiologic basis (Sadiq, Mazzeo et al. 2008).

Such patient-specific simulations require access to comprehensive patient data and an appropriate infrastructure for performing very large numbers of complex and demanding simulations. For this manner heterogeneous supercomputing grid technologies are used, which address, in real time, the outcome of many diverse emergency situations, such as the development and impact of hurricanes and earthquakes (Manos, S. et al. 2008). In the biomedical technology, high-performance computation has been used as a research capacity to investigate the interactions in many tissues with regard to biomolecular function and its interference due to disease, and all that in real time. Such real-time large-scale computation, meet the needs of the clinical environment, thus making "ultra patient-specific" clinical decision-support with PSM increasingly achievable.

Despite the attention that PSM has gotten in recent time, the evaluation of its predictive capability has not yet been tested on a large scale and is thus yet to become a standard in clinical care (Neal and Kerckhoffs 2010).

6. Good practice example - evaluating patient's health using a hierarchical multi-attribute decision model

With the possibility of employing CDSS in telemedicine, we take a closer look at a computerized model for the evaluation of a patient's health status in nursing care (Šušteršič et al., 2009). Holistic evaluation of a patient's health status is essential for solid decision making regarding the proper patient treatment. Our solution is based on a hierarchical multi-attribute decision model (HMADM) (Turban et al., 2004; Triantaphyllou, 2010). With this approach the practical efficiency of the Henderson's theoretical model of basic living activities (BLA) increases (Henderson & Nite, 1997).

Let us first present our solution from the structural point of view as described in chapter 2. With regard to the context axes, it deals with not only inpatients and outpatients but also with community nursing. It assists a nurse in practically all phases of the nursing process, including setting nursing diagnoses and nursing interventions. Its role also includes prevention, screening and chronic disease management. Special emphasis is on alerts and reminders.

The knowledge and data source axes are based on the theoretical BLA model. Data are collected directly from the patients or patients' records. The described CDSS is built upon widely used coding schemas such as ICNP and NANDA.

Decision making process is based on a combination of HMADM and expert systems. The knowledge base consists of a tree of criteria and rule based utility functions for every aggregated node in the tree. This way individual patient data are aggregated in an overall assessment of a patient's health status.

Concerning information delivery, the system is request-based with a special emphasis on the explanation of the evaluation results. Thus, the transparency of the nursing process as a workflow is enhanced.

The proposed HMADM can be applied both when analysing patient's health status and when explaining the results of the evaluation. Despite the holistic nature of the BLA approach, these models are not being sufficiently used in clinical practice (Šušteršič et al., 2002; Ozbolt & Bakken, 2006). A possible reason for limited use is the fact that a large number of parameters are used to describe a patient's health status. This means that it is difficult to gather information on all the parameters. Furthermore, the process of drawing a conclusion becomes very complex. However, the HMADM methodology helps to address these problems. (Potter & Perry, 2002; Gordon, 2009)

Increasing the operability of the BLA model can be achieved by understanding the model as a HMADM for evaluating patient's health. The model, which has been based on BLA (Šušteršič et al., 1999; Bohanec et al., 2000), is a comprehensive evaluation tool for the nursing care support process. This part of the patient's record becomes hierarchically structured and gains additional transparency, which facilitates the identification of nursing problems, setting of nursing diagnoses and planning of the appropriate nursing care.

Patient's changes in health status on the basis of the defined indicators are monitored at chosen time intervals. In terms of community nursing, where the model was tested, such intervals coincided with health visits or successive sessions using the tele-nursing approach. The model offers a helping hand to nurses as it reduces the possibility of overlooking problems that could otherwise lead to unwanted healthcare events.

Hierarchical multi-attribute decision models are primarily developed for option evaluation: each option, in this case a patient, is described by values of basic attributes and is evaluated according to the model. The final outcome is an overall evaluation for each option (patient). Furthermore, an evaluation result of the option makes it possible to investigate how the result was obtained. It also provides an insight into what specific attributes can be managed to improve the outcome. (Pöyhönen & Hämäläinen, 2001; Tsoukias, 2008)

The majority of current multi-attribute decision methods are aimed at the development of quantitative decision models (Triantaphyllou, 2010). In such models, all the attributes are continuous and utility functions are typically defined in terms of the attributes' weight, e.g. as a weighted-sum of lower-level attributes. In practice, however, the difficulty of understanding the underlying data behind the numerical results proves to be a common problem. The relationships between the attributes are linear, although the nature of the attributes often requires non-linear interdependence. In other words, different weights can be assigned to a single attribute depending on its relative importance. In contrast, Decision Expert (DEX) methodology (Bohanec & Rajkovič 1990), which is used in our approach, deals with discrete attributes, usually represented by words rather than numbers. The corresponding utility functions are represented by decision rules. Each rule represents one point or several equi-utility points of function values. The utility (aggregation) functions used in the DEX model are therefore not represented by formulae, such as weighted-sum, but are presented as tables of function values, i.e. decision rules (Rajkovič et al., 1988). This way, a HMADM can be built on non-linear discrete utility functions. It can be compared with the relative weights approach, where the weights depend on parameter values. If a parameter value changes, its relative importance (weight) can also be changed if required. By using the DEX interface, expressing and understanding such utility functions as sets of decision rules becomes suitable for being used in practice.

6.2 Model for patient's health status evaluation

A HMADM model, based on the BLA model, was developed by an expert team of nurses for the evaluation of patient's health and was tested in two health centres in Slovenia. This model uses indicators, which are measurable BLA criteria for describing a patient's health condition, as basic attributes. In the criteria tree, the BLA are hierarchically organized and, therefore, interconnected. Utility functions are presented as tables of decision rules. In accordance with those rules, the values and definitions of the higher level criteria are defined by the combination of the values and definitions of the lower level criteria, which enter the model as their predecessors. As a result, a comprehensive evaluation of a patient's health is obtained at the top of the criteria tree. The hierarchical structure of a comprehensive evaluation of the BLA is shown in Table 1, which represents a DEX output in tree form, including criteria descriptions. Each attribute is measured on a five-point scale: "problem to a very high degree" (vhd), "problem to a high degree" (hd), "problem to some degree" (sd), "problem to a lesser degree" (ld) and "no problem" (no).

```
COMPREHENSIVE EVALUATION        Evaluation of all basic living activities
├─PHYSICAL BLA                  BLA concerning physical patient's condition
│ ├─OEBt                        Oxygenation, Elimination, Body temp.
│ │ ├─Oxygenation               Mechanical inhalation and
│ │ │                              exhalation of air, circulation
│ │ ├─ELIMINATION               Movement & elimination of waste
│ │ └─BODY TEMPERATURE          The temperature of the body
│ ├─NPaS                        Nutrition and hydration,
│ │ │                              Physical activity, Sleep, Rest
│ │ ├─NUTRITION                 Nutrition and hydration
│ │ ├─PHYSICAL ACTIV.           Ability of body movement
│ │ └─SLEEP                     Sleep, restoration and rest
│ └─AdHD                        Avoidance of danger, hygiene and tidiness,dressing
│   ├─AVOIDANCE of DANG.        Physical, psychology and social security
│   ├─HYGIENE                   Tidiness and hygiene of body
│   └─DRESSING                  Dressing and undressing
└─PSYCHOSOCIAL BLA              BLA concerning psycho-social patient's condition
  ├─RRb                         Relationship with people,
  │                                communication, religious beliefs
  └─PltE                        Purposeful activit., Leisure time and Health educ.
    ├─PURPOSEFUL ACTIV.         Harmonisation of work and recreation
    ├─LEISURE TIME              Useful use of time
    └─EDUCATION                 Health education
```

Table 1. DEX printout of hierarchical structure of a comprehensive evaluation of BLA

The comprehensive evaluation model has 20 attributes comprising of 13 basic and 7 aggregate attributes. These correspond to the main attributes of the BLA criteria, covering items relating both to the patient's physical and psychosocial condition. They include: oxygenation, elimination, body temperature (OEBt); nutrition and hydration, physical activity, sleep and rest (NPaS); avoidance of danger from the environment, hygiene and tidiness, dressing (AdHD); relationships with people, communication, psychological and social needs, including religious beliefs (RRb); and purposeful activity, leisure time, health education (PLtE). The model also includes seven utility functions, one for each aggregate criterion, including the root of the tree which represents the final evaluation result. Each utility function is defined by a table of decision rules that determine the value of each aggregate attribute on the basis of the mutual dependence on lower-level attributes (immediate predecessor).

Here is an example of a decision rule on how the value of aggregate attribute is defined: if OEBt is assessed as a problem 'to some degree', NPaS as a problem 'to some degree' or worse and AdHD as being on the boundary between 'to a high degree' and 'to some degree', the overall patient's evaluation of physical BLA is evaluated as 'to a high degree'.

The utility functions (sets of decision rules) must be semantically appropriate, i.e. they must express correct nursing knowledge, so verification and validation play important roles. Two steps were included in the present model to achieve this: in the first, a group of chosen experts agreed on utility functions, taking into account existing knowledge from the literature and their experiences and, in the second, nurses validated the knowledge by using decision rules during their practical work.

6.3 Results of testing in practice

Testing of the HMADM took place in the community health care environment. The model was used during the entire treatment with a special emphasis on home visits. There were two main objectives of the testing: (i) to validate the nursing knowledge embedded in the model, especially with regard to the decision rules; and (ii) to test the actual operability of the model in practice, i.e. by testing during home visits.

During practical use of the model, transparent decision rules encouraged nurses to critically assess and to validate the nursing knowledge expressed by the rules. Nurses provided comments regarding the appropriateness of the proposed decision rules and the results of the evaluation of the BLA model. The extent to which the HMADM encouraged assessment of the interdependencies between various criteria was also observed.

Testing of the model was monitored during successive home visits. Each nurse used the model to evaluate their patients' health status on regular daily visits. Each nurse carried out between five and seven home visits daily, which were of a preventive and curative nature. At each visit, special emphasis was placed on analysing the patient's health with the set of BLA indicators.

Different patient groups were included, ranging from newborns to the elderly, either due to health promotion, prevention or recovery. Observed were different health problems such as nutrition problems, chronic diseases, wound management etc. An example of a 'comprehensive evaluation of BLA' of a newborn baby (NB) is presented in Table 2, where evaluations from three successive visits (NB1, NB2 and NB3) are listed. The root of the tree, which represents the final overall evaluation, shows how the baby's health condition or their need for nursing care changed from one visit to another. Considerable improvement of the baby's health can be observed. On the first visit the 'Comprehensive evaluation' was regarded as a problem to a 'very high degree', on the second visit as a problem to a 'high degree' and, on the third visit, just as a problem to 'some degree'. Table 2 breaks down the comprehensive evaluation result and shows that, at the first visit (NB1), there was a problem to a 'very high degree' for hygiene and education, and a problem to 'some degree' with elimination, sleep, avoidance of danger, RRb and leisure time. A nurse can easily see all of the existing problems and their actual values (degrees of problem) together with their propagation through the tree of attributes, including interrelationships, up to their influence on the overall evaluation. Such transparency improves understanding of the reasons for changes in the patient's health status and encourages nurses' critical thinking in terms of further actions that they need to take.

Option:	NB1		NB2		NB3
COMPREHENSIVE EVALUATION	**vhd**	⊕→	**hd**	⊕→	**sd**
├─**PHYSICAL BLA**	**vhd**	⊕→	**hd**	⊕→	**sd**
│ ├─**OEBt**	**sd**		**sd**	⊕→	**ld**
│ │ ├─OXYGENATION	no		no		no
│ │ ├─ELIMINATION	sd		sd	⊕→	ld
│ │ └─BODY TEMPERATURE	no		no		no
│ ├─**NPaS**	**ld**		**ld**		**ld**
│ │ ├─NUTRITION	no		no		no
│ │ ├─PHYSICAL ACTIV.	ld	⊕→	no		no
│ │ └─SLEEP	sd		sd		sd
│ └─**AdHD**	**vhd**	⊕→	**hd**	⊕→	**ld**
│ ├─AVOIDANCE of DANG.	sd		sd	⊕→	ld
│ ├─HYGIENE	vhd	⊕→	sd	⊕→	no
│ └─DRESSING	no		no		no
└─**PSYCHOSOCIAL BLA**	**vhd**	⊕→	**sd**	⊕→	**no**
├─RRb	sd	⊕→	ld	⊕→	no
└─**PLtE**	**vhd**	⊕→	**sd**	⊕→	**no**
├─PURPOSEFUL ACTIV.	ld	⊕→	no		no
├─LEISURE TIME	sd	⊕→	ld	⊕→	no
└─EDUCATION	vhd	⊕→	sd	⊕→	no

Table 2. Evaluation of a newborn from three successive evaluations

Changes in health indicators can also be followed graphically and Fig. 1 presents the changes during the three visits in the evaluation of physical BLA overall and its four improved sub-attributes: elimination, physical activity, avoidance of danger and hygiene; the condition remained unchanged for sleep. The nurses themselves could choose the indicators, which were then presented as a time series and this customization of the data eliminated the need for further data analysis. Changes in the values of the indicators from one visit to another can also be viewed as a helpful tool in the quality assurance processes.

Nurses who took part in the testing prepared their reports and structured interviews were carried out with each nurse. The reports and interviews served as the basis for a strengths, weaknesses, opportunities and threats (SWOT) analysis. The nurses indentified three main strengths: (i) the model supports holistic understanding necessary for identification of the nature and level of nursing problems; (ii) the computerized hierarchical structure enriches nursing documentation; and (iii) the possibilities of overlooking something important are reduced. Among the weaknesses, they emphasized the increased amount of work that was involved in using the model because of the need for consistently following a methodical work process. Opportunities suggested by the nurses were the development of electronic documentation and the consistent holistic evaluation of a patient's health status in the framework of the nurse's competencies. It could contribute to improved patient safety and also to the safety of members of the health team. On the basis of indicators and their values some adverse events can be predicted. If an adverse event occurs, we can explain the reasons and help determine personal responsibility. As the main threat, they listed their apprehension about computer-supported models being perceived as replacing nurses' creative thinking and work.

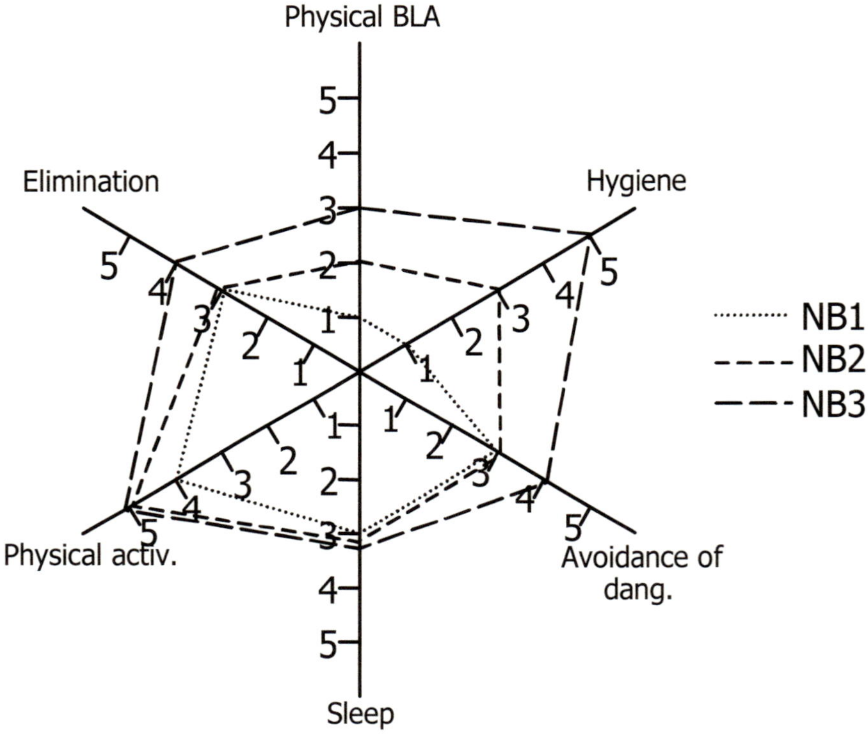

Fig. 1. Transcript of changes of the selected criteria of a newborn's Physical BLA during three visits

6.4 Towards higher quality of nursing and increased patient safety

The proposed CDSS uses the BLA model for assessing patients' health. It is built on multi-attribute decision-making theory in order to assess a patient's observed condition. The outcome is a a computer-calculated comprehensive evaluation based on the model. During clinical testing of the model in practice, transparency appeared to increase along the whole process and not only, as it was initially expected, during the phase of assessing patient health. This implies that patient data can be followed upward through the tree of criteria to the final estimate and an explanation can be provided of how the estimate was obtained and from where it originated. This way a contribution is made to an efficient evaluation that provides a holistic and transparent overview of the patient's condition. The structured approach based on the BLA tree assists nurses in keeping up with a large data set and their inter-relationships. This is especially vital when relatively small changes in some indicators may in combination with other indicators result in serious problems for the patient. A better understanding of the outcomes reduces the possibility of overlooking clinically important information. Together with appropriate nursing documentation, this computerized model can contribute to a higher quality of nursing and increased patient safety, as well as increased safety for health team members.

7. Conclusions, opportunities and roadblocks

It is clear that systems supporting clinical decision-making of doctors, nurses and other health-workers have an immense potential to benefit in their performance, provision of quality care and, what we strive for - better patient outcomes. In common sense, one can take better care of patients if one has superb knowledge about the clinical matters in question. For example, it could be said that with more information and knowledge a clinician has a better chance of solving a clinical problem in favor of the patient, the hospital and himself. The problem is that nowadays global knowledge about a topic is often overwhelming for a clinician to process at the point of care or in urgent situations. CDSSs incorporate patient-specific data and an applicable, well-structured and current knowledge base or evidence-based guidelines, thus serving the clinician with enhancing his/her clinical decision-making process. Such support of basic cognitive processes involved in medical thinking to some extent relieves the clinician and provides him with new, better-formed and possibly superior methods to take best care of the ill.

Many characteristics of CDSSs are related to clinical effectiveness, functionality, error prevention, potential for acceptance in the clinical world, system portability, cost-effectiveness etc., it is therefore important to fully understand the construction and different modalities of CDSS.

The most successful CDSSs deal with therapy critiquing and consulting and/or drug dosing or prescribing. Latest CDSSs use EMR to provide data for analysis, and they provide the ability to the decision-maker to exert the recommended actions with ease, being completely integrated into the information system. Developers of CDSSs should thus be aware that there are factors beyond software and content that must be taken into consideration. Fundamental issues include the level of system integration into clinical workflow and the relevance and timeliness of the clinical messages provided, availability and accessibility of hardware and sufficient technical support and training in use of the system. Reasons for difficulties in implementing CDSS into everyday clinical practice come mainly from programmers' insufficient understanding of medical reasoning and decision analyses. Such systems to some extent pose a threat to diminished clinicians' professional autonomy. Above all there is generally still a lack of awareness of long-term benefits of CDSS-use and lack of desire to change the daily workflow.

To encourage better health-processes, better individual patient care and better population health through CDSSs development, they need to be under constant improvement and their evolvement controlled from an appointed group of experts. To this end the American Medical Informatics Association developed a road map for action on CDSSs, regarding development, implementation and use. This road map comprises of three pillars, with their own subsets, which should bring sense into future evolvement and successful implementation of CDSSs (Lyman, Cohn et al. 2010).

1. Best knowledge available when needed;
   - Represent clinical knowledge and CDSS interventions in standardized formats.
     - There are multiple and most of the time very diverse types of formats used within CDSSs. The patient-specific data and thereafter computerized decision making is usually not exchangeable. This limits free interchange of patients between different institutions on national and international level. It thereby consequently limits the dispersion CDSSs and merits that global usage would bring.
   - Collect, organize and distribute clinical knowledge and CDSS interventions in a way that users easily find suitable material and incorporate it in their own information systems.
2. High adoption and effective use
   - Address policy, legal and financial barriers
     - The health care policy of e.g. European Union should support CDSSs implementation and development. One could expect that as EU directed the electronification of health care it should also direct further evolvement and implementation of CDSSs in everyday clinical practice. Review on research done in this field show multiple beneficial effects of using CDSS, resulting in better patient outcomes, enhanced health-care performance and consequently greater cost effectiveness of electronic health systems.
     - With implementing CDSSs in everyday practice, we are obliged to consider the legal consequences of its usage. The obvious conflict is if the decision of CDSS is in discordance with the clinician's opinion. For example, we should consider, what would mean if the clinician wouldn't agree with CDSSs recommendations, which would in common medical sense, be wrong, but the clinicians' actions would anyway result in medical error or even death. How much weight would bear a decision of CDSS? How could we prove that the outcome would be different or better by following CDSS's decision-making? On the other hand CDSSs can impose a regulatory role in following the current medical guidelines. In a way CDSS can prevent a clinician in making medical errors by alerting about e.g. EU-accepted guidelines. CDSS can be viewed as a tool to track clinician's actions. Such information, if comprehensive and detailed, could be of great importance in a court of law.
   - Improve the practice of deployment
   - Improve the ease of usage
3. Continuous improvement of knowledge and CDSS methods
   - Systematically capturing, organizing and examining existing CDSS deployments (e.g. http://www.openclinical.org)
   - Advance care-guiding knowledge by using the data readily available in EMR, thus improving clinical knowledge and health management.
   - Not only that EMR is time saving and basically essential for health information-system (and thus a CDSS) to function successfully and be integrated into a workflow, it is also a source of data for forming new knowledge. EMR can easily

provide data for clinical research, e.g. statistical analyses of patient outcomes, based on their illnesses and clinician's actions. The results of such analyses could be automatically invested into improving the power of CDSS's decision-making.

Despite all challenges in CDSS development and implementation, these systems have shown to be of great use. Further research and education in this area is therefore essential in order to utilize CDSSs to a higher extent in everyday clinical reality. The implications and positive externalities of CDSSs may well prove to be some of the strongest factors that will influence the health-care development in years to come.

8. References

Autonomy, I. (2009). Autonomy Technology Overview. I. Autonomy.

Bassingthwaighte, J. B. (2000). "Strategies for the physiome project." Ann Biomed Eng 28(8): 1043-1058.

Berner, E. S. (2007). Clinical decision support systems : theory and practice. New York, Springer.

Brender, J., E. Ammenwerth, et al. (2006). "Factors influencing success and failure of health informatics systems--a pilot Delphi study.
" Methods Inf Med 45(1): 125-136.

Bohanec, M., Rajkovič, V. (1990). DEX: an expert system shell for decision support. Sistemica, 1, (1990) 145 - 157.

Bohanec, M., Zupan, B., Rajkovič, V. (2000). Applications of qualitative multi-attribute decision models in health care. Int J Med Inform, 58-59, (2000) 191 - 205.

Burke, J. P., D. C. Classen, et al. (1991). "The HELP system and its application to infection control." J Hosp Infect 18 Suppl A: 424-431.

Bury, J., C. Hurt, et al. (2004). "A quantitative and qualitative evaluation of LISA, a decision support system for chemotherapy dosing in childhood acute lymphoblastic leukaemia." Stud Health Technol Inform 107(Pt 1): 197-201.

Coiera, E. (2003). Guide to health informatics. London : New York, NY :, Arnold ; Distributed in the USA by Oxford University Press.

de Dombal, F. T., D. J. Leaper, et al. (1972). "Computer-aided diagnosis of acute abdominal pain." Br Med J 2(5804): 9-13.

Delaney, B. C., D. A. Fitzmaurice, et al. (1999). "Can computerised decision support systems deliver improved quality in primary care?. Interview by Abi Berger." BMJ 319(7220): 1281.

Doyle, B. J., A. Callanan, et al. (2009). "Vessel asymmetry as an additional diagnostic tool in the assessment of abdominal aortic aneurysms." J Vasc Surg 49(2): 443-454.

Garg, A. X., N. K. Adhikari, et al. (2005). "Effects of computerized clinical decision support systems on practitioner performance and patient outcomes: a systematic review." JAMA 293(10): 1223-1238.

General Practice Electronic Decision Support, W. (2000). Strategic future directions / General Practice Electronic Decision Support Workshop. Canberra, A.C.T. :, Dept. of Health and Aged Care.

Goldstein, M. K., R. W. Coleman, et al. (2004). "Translating research into practice: organizational issues in implementing automated decision support for hypertension in three medical centers." J Am Med Inform Assoc 11(5): 368-376.

Gordon, M. (2009). Manual of Nursing Diagnosis, 12th ed, Jones and Bartlett, ISBN-13: 978-0763771850, Boston

Greenes, R. A. (2007). Clinical decision support : the road ahead. Amsterdam ; Boston, Elsevier Academic Press.

Henderson, V., Nite, G. (1997). Principles and Practice of Nursing, 6th ed, Collier Macmillan, ISBN-10: 0023535806, New York

Holyoak, K. (2005). The Cambridge Handbook of Thinking and Reasoning, Cambridge University Press.

Hurt, C., J. Fox, et al. (2003). Computerised advice on drug dosage decisions in childhood leukaemia: a method and a safety strategy. 9th Conference on Artificial Intelligence in Medicine in Europe, Protaras, Cyprus, Springer.

Kawamoto, K., C. A. Houlihan, et al. (2005). "Improving clinical practice using clinical decision support systems: a systematic review of trials to identify features critical to success." BMJ 330(7494): 765.

Lai, S., M. K. Goldstein, et al. (2004). "Insights from Testing the Accuracy of Recommendations from an Automated Decision Support System for Primary Hypertension: ATHENA DSS." MEDINFO CD: 1706.

Lyman, J. A., W. F. Cohn, et al. (2010). "Clinical decision support: progress and opportunities." J Am Med Inform Assoc 17(5): 487-492.

Manos, S., Z. S., et al. (2008). Life or Death Decision-making: The Medical Case for Large-scale, On-demand Grid Computing. CTWatch Quarterly. 4.

Miller, R. A., H. E. Pople, et al. (1982). "Internist-I, an Experimental Computer-Based Diagnostic Consultant for General Internal Medicine." New England Journal of Medicine 307(8): 468-476.

Moxey, A., J. Robertson, et al. (2010). "Computerized clinical decision support for prescribing: provision does not guarantee uptake." J Am Med Inform Assoc 17(1): 25-33.

National Electronic Decision Support, T. (2003). Electronic decision support for Australia's health sector : report to Health Ministers by the National Electronic Decision Support Taskforce. Canberra :, C'wealth Dept. of Health and Ageing.

Neal, M. L. and R. Kerckhoffs (2010). "Current progress in patient-specific modeling." Brief Bioinform 11(1): 111-126.

Nguyen, J. H., Y. Shahar, et al. (1997). "A temporal database mediator for protocol-based decision support." Proc AMIA Annu Fall Symp: 298-302.

OpenClinical, C. (2006). "Isabel - OpenClinical, AI Systems in Clinical Practice." from http://www.openclinical.org/aisp_isabel.html.

Ozbolt, JG., Bakken, S. (2006). Patient-care systems. In: Biomedical Informatics: Computer Applications in Health Care and Biomedicine, 3rd ed. Shortliffe, EH., Cimino, JJ. (Eds.), 564-584, Springer, ISBN-13: 978-0387289861, New York

Patel, V. L., D. R. Kaufman, et al. (2002). "Emerging paradigms of cognition in medical decision-making." J Biomed Inform 35(1): 52-75.

Pearson, S.-A., A. Moxey, et al. (2009). "Do computerised clinical decision support systems for prescribing change practice? A systematic review of the literature (1990-2007)." BMC Health Services Research 9(1): 154.

Potter, PA., Perry, AG. (2002). Basic Nursing: Essentials for Practice, 5th ed, Mosby, ISBN-13: 978-0323016629, St Louis

Pöyhönen, M., Hämäläinen, RP. (2001). On the convergence of multi-attribute weighting methods. Eur J Oper Res, 129, (2001) 569 - 585.
Rajkovič, V., Bohanec, M., Batagelj, V. (1988). Knowledge engineering techniques for utility identification. Acta Psychol (Amst), 68, (1988) 271 - 286.
Ramnarayan, P., A. Tomlinson, et al. (2004). "A novel diagnostic aid (ISABEL): development and preliminary evaluation of clinical performance." Stud Health Technol Inform 107(Pt 2): 1091-1095.
Remmlinger, E. (2002). Next generation clinical systems: is it time to jump? Annual Healthcare Information and Management Systems Society's Conference. Atlanta, USA. Session 49.
Roberts, M. S. (2011). Decision analysis. Up to date. M. D. Aronson. Waltham, MA, Up to date.
Sadiq, S. K., M. D. Mazzeo, et al. (2008). "Patient-specific simulation as a basis for clinical decision-making." Philos Transact A Math Phys Eng Sci 366(1878): 3199-3219.
Shortliffe, E. H. (1976). Computer-based medical consultations, MYCIN. New York, Elsevier.
Shortliffe, E. H. and J. J. Cimino (2006). Biomedical informatics : computer applications in health care and biomedicine. New York, Springer.
Sim, I. and A. Berlin (2003). "A framework for classifying decision support systems." AMIA Annu Symp Proc: 599-603.
Šušteršič, O., Rajkovič, U., Dinevski, D., Jereb, E., Rajkovič, V. (2009). Evaluating Patients' Health Using a Hierarchical Multi-attribute Decision Model. J Int Med Res, 37, 5, (2009) 1646-1654.
Šušteršič. O., Rajkovič, V., Kljajić, M. (1999). An evaluation of community nursing process in the frame of the international classification of nursing practice. In: ICNP and Telematic Applications for Nurses in Europe - the Telenurse Experience. Mortensen, RA. (Ed.), 243-249, IOS Press, ISBN-13: 978-9051994544,Amsterdam
Šušteršič, O., Rajkovič, V., Leskovar, R., et al (2002). An information system for community nursing. Public Health Nurs, 19, (2002), 184 - 190.
Trafton, J. A., S. B. Martins, et al. (2010). "Designing an automated clinical decision support system to match clinical practice guidelines for opioid therapy for chronic pain." Implement Sci 5: 26.
Triantaphyllou, E. (2010). Multi-criteria Decision Making Methods: a Comparative Study, Kluwer Academic Press, ISBN-13: 978-1441948380, Boston
Tsoukiàs, A. (2008). From decision theory to decision aiding methodology. Eur J Oper Res, 187, (2008) 138 - 161.
Turban, E., Aronson, J., Liang, TP. (2004). Decision Support Systems and Intelligent Systems, 7th ed, Prentice Hall, ISBN-13: 978-0130461063, New Jersey
Viceconti, M., G. Clapworthy, et al. (2007). Seeding the EuroPhysiome: a roadmap to the virtual physiological human. eHealth, STEP: A strategy for the EuroPhysiome.
Wikipedia, C. (2011). "Inference engine." Retrieved 2 February, 2011, from http://en.wikipedia.org/wiki/Inference_engine.
Wyatt, J. and D. Spiegelhalter (1991). "Field trials of medical decision-aids: potential problems and solutions." Proc Annu Symp Comput Appl Med Care: 3-7.

Zheng, K., R. Padman, et al. (2005). "Understanding technology adoption in clinical care: clinician adoption behavior of a point-of-care reminder system." Int J Med Inform 74(7-8): 535-543.

9

A 2.4GHz Non-Contact Biosensor System for Continuous Monitoring of Vital-Signs

Donald Y.C. Lie[1], Ravi Ichapurapu[1], Suyash Jain[1], Jerry Lopez[1],
Ronald E. Banister[2], Tam Nguyen[1,2] and John Griswold[2]
[1]*Department of Electrical & Computer Engineering, Texas Tech University, Lubbock*
[2]*Texas Tech University Health Sciences Center (TTUHSC),*
Texas Tech University (TTU)
USA

1. Introduction

In this chapter, we present a novel Doppler-based vital signs biosensor that can monitor the respiration and heartbeat rates of a person remotely without the need of any obstructions like patches, cords, etc. We will discuss the sensor operation principle and present three generations of systems that were designed to accurately extract the respiration rate and heartbeat of subjects using the Doppler radar principle. The systems have been realized using discrete custom off the shelf (COTS) parts. The first generation of the biosensor system consisted of discrete RF components system and a bulky SRS560 amplifier and filter box. Later generations of sensors consisted of custom designed printed circuits boards (PCBs) for the Doppler transceiver and for performing the analog signal processing. The data obtained using these non-contact biosensor systems was processed and logged in real-time using a LabVIEW© Graphic User Interface (GUI). Digital signal processing extracts the vital signs by filtering, auto correlating and calculating the Discrete Fourier Transform (DFT) of the waveforms. A comparison of performance among the three different generations of sensors shows that a quadrature transceiver system using autocorrelation can extract the respiration rates and heartbeat rates most accurately. Our single PCB version of the biosensor system was found to perform as well as the system using bulky components and SRS560 box. Good data accuracy has been observed on the quadrature radar sensor system with mean detection errors for respiration rate within ~1 beat/min and for heart rate within ~3 beat/min. The continuous vital signs data measured from these portable sensors can also be wirelessly transferred to healthcare professionals to make life saving decisions and diagnosis of symptoms. In the future, our vision is that a continuous log of these vital signs info can also be used to remotely monitor and gauge the recovery of patients, and even for the prevention or prediction of severe illnesses and complications.

1.1 Why non-contact vital signs monitoring?

Vital signs are measures of various physiological statistics often taken by the health professionals to assess the most basic body functions. Typical vital signs measured are: temperature, respiratory rate, heart-beat rate (i.e., pulse rate), blood pressure, and blood oxygen saturation. These numbers provide critical information about a patient's state and healthcare professionals (especially surgeons and anesthesiologists) value the vital-signs monitoring not only during the course of surgery, but also before and after a surgery is performed (Dorin, 2007). Tremendous progresses have been made recently in developing small and wearable sensors that can monitor the vital signs; however, their usage in either hospitals or homes is still rather uncommon. One reason is that many patients are not comfortable wearing the sensors, as they have leads and are attached to the patients using patches which cause discomforts. Unless implanted, the leads and the sensors can obstruct the free movement of the patient, causing irritations or distress. Also, in situations when patients have severe burns or injuries, it can be very difficult to attach these wearable sensors to the patients. Another major disadvantage of the wearable or implantable sensors is the battery lifetime. Most wearable devices cannot operate for more than 2-3 months on a single battery for continuous and intelligent monitoring, especially if sophisticated algorithms and wireless features are added on those sensors, draining significantly more power. Continuous vital signs monitoring on patients with pre-existing complications (e.g., seizure, stroke) can ensure timely treatment, and precious lives can be saved when early warnings are triggered. The focus of this chapter is to show our development of a novel *non-contact* biosensor technology for continuous vital signs monitoring.

The principle of non-invasive microwave measurement of respiration has been described in details since 1975, while the first non-contact microwave physiological motion sensor IC was not reported until 2001 (Lin, 1992; Droitcour A.D., et al., 2002). These non-contact sensors work on the principle of Doppler shift to sense heartbeat and respiration rate by monitoring the contraction and expansion of the chest wall. However, no such biosensor product has ever been successfully commercialized for heartbeat monitoring, probably due to the practical issues caused by background clutter, phase-nulling and DC offsets. We will demonstrate in this chapter that a quadrature transceiver sensor system with arc-tangent demodulation can be very promising for implementing this kind of biosensor with robustness and reliability (Park et al., 2007). In this work, we demonstrate the design, fabrication and testing of custom wireless sensors for non-contact monitoring of vital signs. These non-contact biosensors have a range of about 1 m and can be mounted on the ceiling or unto the patient's bed in either a hospital, nursing home or at the patient's residence for non-invasive, continuous monitoring of the heartbeat and respiration rate. In the future, an alert system and RFID can be also integrated to notify medical professionals should irregularities occur. The advantages of wireless non-contact sensors include that there is no need to attach the sensors to patients for acquiring vital signs data and they can draw power from the wall socket or battery (depending on where they are used) for long-term continuous monitoring. The sensor size limitations are relaxed as they are not worn or implanted. All factors above can help to make the sensors mass producible at low cost.

1.2 Overview of vital signs using a doppler radar

The principle of non-contact microwave measurement of respiration has been described since the work of Lin *et al.* (Lin, 1992). These sensors work on the principle of Doppler-shift to sense heartbeat and respiration rates by monitoring the motion of the chest wall. We are implementing a Doppler radar motion sensing system by transmitting a high frequency continuous wave (CW) electromagnetic signal that is reflected off the subject and then demodulated in the receiver of our biosensor system. Based on the Doppler effects, we know that if a target changes position with respect to time but has no net velocity, it gives us a reflected signal whose *phase* is in proportion to the time-varying position of the target. In our case as shown in Figure 1, a stationary person's chest has a periodic movement but no net velocity, and a CW radar system pointed to the chest as the target will receive a signal *Φ(t)* with its phase modulated by the time-varying chest position *x(t)*. On, multiplying the received signal with the original un-modulated signal from the same source, we can demodulate this phase information affected by the movement of the chest wall during heartbeat and respiration, and therefore heart and respiration rates can be determined. The peak-to-peak chest motion due to respiration in adults ranges from 4 mm to 12 mm (Droitcour, 2006), while the peak-to-peak motion due to the heartbeat is about 0.5 mm.

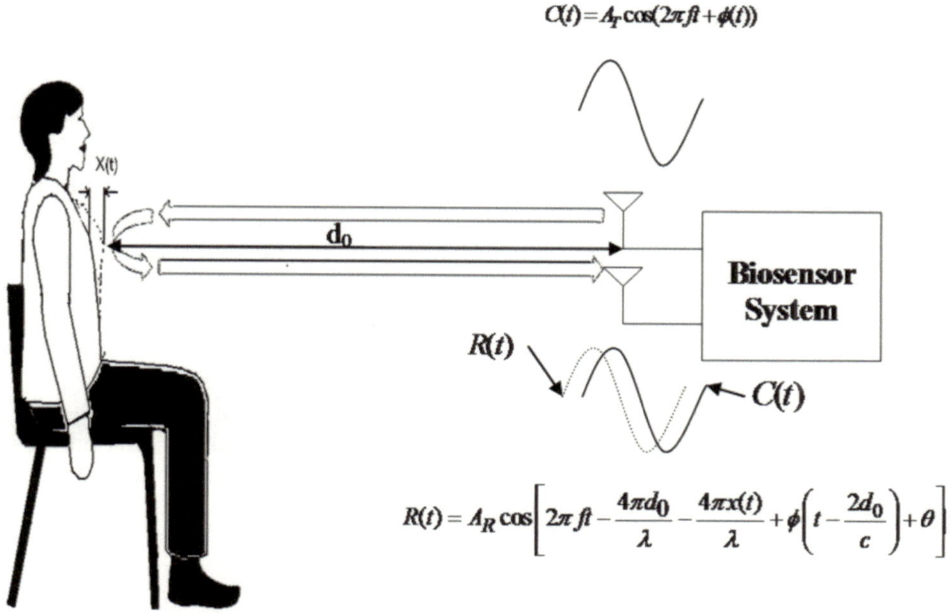

Fig. 1. Principle of operation of a Doppler-based noncontact vital-signs monitoring system

1.3 Applications of noncontact vital sign monitors

A good amount of research has been carried out recently and significant advancement has been made which have made it possible to use this Doppler technique to remotely monitor vital signs of a patient. The focus of this chapter is show how we have developed a portable non-contact biosensor technology for *continuous* vital signs monitoring. For severely burned patients and patients who suffer from serious Stevens–Johnson syndrome (SJS), it may be very difficult to attach the electrodes for vital signs monitoring; in these cases the Doppler-based non-contact vital signs monitor can be ideal to monitor the patient, reduce the risk of infection and can be safely monitored for longer duration of time. Another major advantage of our non-contact biosensor system is that it is very portable and can operate with low power, which makes it possible to monitor continuously for several weeks without having to replace batteries or power from a wall outlet. These Doppler radar based techniques can also detect *motion* and used to monitor patient movement. This can be a valuable asset to both surgeons and anesthesiologists as in some rare cases patients can start to move or have convulsions during the operating procedure which can be extremely dangerous. The Doppler radar can detect minute movements and can trigger an early warning to the

anesthesiologist/surgeon to make sure the patient is sedated. This motion sensing feature can also be used as a fall detection and prevention device (Wu et al., 2010).
Continuous monitoring of patients with preexisting conditions and complications (say, seizures, strokes, etc.) can ensure timely treatment to save precious lives as it can trigger early warnings to the caregivers and medical professionals (i.e., wireless-acute care). If continuous monitoring of vital signs is provided, a patient can be discharged early or sent to normal wards after surgical procedures, this will not only free up valuable space in the ER, but also save the patients considerable amount of money as ER care is very expensive. Other important applications for our biosensors include monitoring for sleep related disorders such as sleep apnea, sudden-infant-death (SID), etc. In additional, the vital sign sensors used in many hospitals throughout the world are not reliable as they generate a large number of *false positives*; the noncontact vital sensor will be useful and *complementary* to the traditional vital signs monitors as a perfect first-line-of-defense system to reduce the false positives of the vital signs monitoring system. This is especially true for the respiration rate monitoring.
To summarize, the advantages of wireless non-contact vital sign biosensors are many as they do not have to be attached to patients for monitoring vital signs and therefore are completely non-invasive. They are very portable and can operate for a long duration, drawing power from the wall outlet or battery depending on where they are used. These biosensors can even be realized on tiny integrated circuits (ICs) and be mass produced, making them very affordable. All these factors make the non-contact vital signs monitoring very attractive for the healthcare applications.
Currently, we have tested the prototype on a limited subject pool and have gotten some good results. We have to prove the accuracy of our system for vital signs monitoring for a lot more cases, though, to show its robustness. Therefore, we need to conduct extensive trials of our system on a diverse subject pool. We have to classify the system in terms of true and false positives and negatives in a clinical environment before qualifying and commercializing this sensor in the market place. Take one case for example to illustrate the serious needs for this kind of non-contact vital signs sensor, the Texas Tech Health Science Center and the nearby University Medical Center (UMC) system have more than 35 million patient admissions a year, while the magnitude of this problem of un-monitored patients (i.e., non-ICU and non-telemetry) is large and growing and has to be properly addressed, as they consist of approximately 10-20% of overall hospital codes! We believe that the portable non-contact vital signs and motion monitor has many advantages over the current monitoring systems and therefore are extremely attractive.

1.4 Current developments in noncontact vital sign monitoring

In the late 1990s, researchers in Bell Labs worked on integrating the Doppler radar sensing function in cell phones and other portable wireless communications devices to detect the user's heartbeat and respiration rates (Li et al., 2009). Using the BiCMOS chip set developed for cellular basestation RF transceiver front end specifications, an IC for the physiological motion sensing was developed and reported in 2001 (Droitcour et al., 2002). The chipset included a low noise amplifier (LNA), a double-balanced resistive mixer, a voltage-controlled oscillator (VCO), and an active balun buffer amplifier. The IC design was optimized for low noise and high linearity for the purpose of shrinking cellular network basestation's RF front ends, but it was demonstrated to also be suitable for building noncontact Doppler radar sensors (Li et al., 2009). To simplify the design, a direct-conversion based architecture was used. One of the critical challenges involved in integrating the microwave radar transceiver in a CMOS chip was the concern of high level of phase noise of CMOS VCO (Droitcour et al, 2004). Phase noise in the transmitted signals translates into amplitude noise on the baseband output signals in a radar system. It was shown that when measuring subjects at close distance, the range correlation effect reduces the adverse effect of phase noise significantly. Due to the range correlation effect the phase noise of the transmitted signal and the reference signal for the receiver from the same free-running VCO are correlated, making it possible to use an integrated free-running VCO. As a result, if we use the same VCO for the transmitted signal and as the LO (local oscillator) for the receive signal mixing, no phase-locked precision oscillator is needed for the non-contact sensor. This makes the fully integrated sensor chip easier. Another challenge is the detection null point. The null points occur at every quarter wavelength from the radar sensor to the subject. The detection accuracy drops significantly at these null points. To overcome this issue, quadrature receiver architecture was adopted to ensure that at least one of the two outputs is not at null (Park et al., 2007).

A. Arctangent demodulation:

It was recently demonstrated (Park et al., 2007) that arctangent demodulation in quadrature receivers achieves a high degree of accuracy in demodulation of small (heart signals) and large (walking) motion. By applying the arctangent operation to the ratio of I and Q output data, accurate phase demodulation can be achieved regardless of the target's position or motion amplitude. A particular challenge in this technique, however, is the presence of DC offset resulting from receiver imperfections and clutter reflections, in addition to DC information related to target position and associated phase. These DC components can be large compared to the ac motion-related signal, and thus cannot simply be included in digitization without adversely affecting the resolution. We have developed a method for calibrating the DC offset while preserving the DC information and capturing the motion-related signal with maximum resolution. Experimental results demonstrated that arctangent demodulation with DC offset compensation achieved a significant improvement in heart rate measurement accuracy over quadrature channel selection, with a standard deviation of less than 1 beat/min over a small number of "normal" people (i.e., 5 graduate students) for 40 to 60 sets of data is included in this chapter.

B. Double-sideband transmission/fetection and grequency tuning technique:

According to the Doppler radar theory, when the displacement of physiological motion is small compared to the wavelength and the received signal is in quadrature with the reference (φ=90°), the small angle approximation is valid and the received baseband signal is proportional to the displacement. Therefore, one would suggest that by decreasing the wavelength, the received baseband signal strength would increase, which means smaller wavelength would be more sensitive to the small physiological motions. To verify this, a radar sensor system operating at Ka-band was developed and reported (Xiao et al., 2005). It showed that the detection range can be extended without increasing the transmitted power or antenna gain. In fact, the transmitted power can be reduced. Detection distance of greater than 2m with less than 20-μW transmitted power as reported. That system used double-sideband transmission and detection method, which was found to achieve similar effect as the quadrature detection to avoid null-point problem when the difference in two sideband frequencies was properly adjusted. The frequency tuning technique (Xiao et al., 2006) was applied to adjust the separation of two sideband frequencies by tuning the IF LO. Although it is indirect conversion, the double-sideband architecture is also suitable for monolithic integration since no image reject filter is needed.

C. Complex signal demodulation and random body movement cancellation:

Complex signal Demodulation consists of expressing the received I and Q signals in the time domain in the form of Bessel functions using zero, first and second order Bessel functions (Li & Lin, 2008a) as shown below:

$$I(t) = \cos(\frac{4\pi x_h(t)}{\lambda} + \frac{4\pi x_r(t)}{\lambda} + \phi) = \sum_{k=-\infty}^{\infty} \sum_{l=-\infty}^{\infty} J_k\left(\frac{4\pi m_r}{\lambda}\right) J_l\left(\frac{4\pi m_h}{\lambda}\right)\cos(k\omega_r t + l\omega_h t + \phi)$$
$$= -2\left[C_{10}\sin(\omega_r t) + C_{01}\sin(\omega_h t) + ...\right]\cdot \sin\phi = -2\left[C_{20}\cos(2\omega_r t) + C_{02}\sin(2\omega_h t) + ...\right]\cdot \cos\phi$$

$$Q(t) = \sin(\frac{4\pi x_h(t)}{\lambda} + \frac{4\pi x_r(t)}{\lambda} + \phi) = \sum_{k=-\infty}^{\infty} \sum_{l=-\infty}^{\infty} J_k\left(\frac{4\pi m_r}{\lambda}\right) J_l\left(\frac{4\pi m_h}{\lambda}\right)\sin(k\omega_r t + l\omega_h t + \phi)$$
$$= -2\left[C_{10}\sin(\omega_r t) + C_{01}\sin(\omega_h t) + ...\right]\cdot \cos\phi = -2\left[C_{20}\cos(2\omega_r t) + C_{02}\sin(2\omega_h t) + ...\right]\cdot \sin\phi$$

Then a complex FFT is used to check the spectrum of the data (Li & Lin., 2008a):

$$S(t) = I(t) + j\cdot Q(t) = \exp\left\{ j\left[\frac{4\pi x_h(t)}{\lambda} + \frac{4\pi x_r(t)}{\lambda} + \phi\right]\right\}$$
$$= 2j\left[C_{10}\sin(\omega_r t) + C_{01}\sin(\omega_h t) + ...\right]\cdot e^{j\phi} + 2\left[C_{20}\cos(2\omega_r t) + C_{02}\sin(2\omega_h t) + ...\right]\cdot e^{j\phi}$$

Advantages:

1. The residual phase will not affect the relative strength between the odd order and the even order frequency components. The desired signal components (odd order tones) will always be present in the spectrum.
2. DC offsets exist in I/Q channels can lead to errors, but in complex demodulation they only affect the DC term. Therefore, the existence of dc offset does not affect obtaining the frequency of the desired signal components.
3. Some report that Complex FFT is computationally less intensive than regular FFT.

D. Comparison of arc tangent demodulation and complex demodulation for random Body movement cancellation:

Random Body movement is compensated by using a two sensor system placed in the front and back of the subject. The complex demodulation is not affected much by presence of baseband DC offset even with random body. Thus, the complex demodulation produces better results in the experiments carried out reported by (Li & Lin, 2008b). The critical issue of using arctangent demodulation for random body movement cancellation is how the presence of the baseband dc offset will affect the detection. This technique requires accurate calibration of the dc offset in order to properly reconstruct the angular information, which is troublesome and requires recalibration with motion of subject or changes in environment. However, the advantage of Arctangent Demodulation is the ability to eliminate the harmonics and inter-modulation interference (Li & Lin, 2008b).

E. Optimal carrier frequency:

The nonlinear property of sinusoidal transfer function not only causes the undesired effect of harmonics interference, but also causes inter-modulation between the respiration signal and the heartbeat signal. Therefore the detected strength of a desired signal (respiration or heartbeat) is determined by both the signal itself and the other signal (i.e., heartbeat affected by the much strong respiration). In contrast to a previous belief that the detection accuracy can always be increased by increasing the carrier frequency, some argues there is an optimum choice of carrier frequency (Li & Lin 2007a). At the so-called optimum carrier frequency, the heartbeat signal component can be maximized in the premise that the harmonics interference and the inter-modulation interference are not too large to affect the detection accuracy. According to simulation and experimental demonstration, the carrier frequency was found to be optimal up to the lower region of the Ka-band to improve the detection accuracy. Since each person has different signal amplitudes of physiological motions due to different body types, the carrier frequency may be tuned to optimize the detected heartbeat signal strength. Therefore, a transceiver with a broad tuning range can be desirable to optimize the performance for different subjects under test.

F. MIMO technology:

While Single Input Multiple Output (SIMO) systems in wireless communications can provide diversity gain, array gain, and interference canceling gain, they are still providing only one source signal. In the case of Doppler radar, even with a single TX (transmitter) antenna (Zhou et al., 2006), there can be many independent signals as scatterers such as objects in subject's vicinity will scatter radio waves (acting as secondary sources), resulting in independent phase shifts. When more than one target is in view, multiple TXs and RXs (receivers) providing multiple signal copies could be used to distinguish between the different sources of Doppler motion, and isolate the desired signals (Boric-Lubecke et al, 2005; Samardzija et al., 2005). Additionally a MIMO setup was utilized to cancel random body movement and was reported in (Li & Lin., 2008b). Two Doppler transceivers at the front and back of the subject were used to correlate the body movements. By exploring the multiple antenna systems and SIMO/MIMO signal processing, it has been experimentally demonstrated that it is possible to separate physiological signals from multiple subjects (Zhou et al., 2006; Boric-Lubecke et al, 2005; Samardzija et al., 2005).

G. UWB radar approach:

Ultra-wideband (UWB) radar can also be used for implementing a non-contact physiological motion sensing. Unlike the previously described continuous-wave (CW) approach, UWB radar transmits the signal in single pulses (Staderini, 2002). By analyzing the reflected waveforms, the small movement can be extracted. The potential advantage of the UWB approach is its high sensitivity to environmental changes, making it possible to effectively remove noises caused by environmental movements and motion artifacts, etc. (Immoreev, 2007; Pisa et al., 2008; Ossberger et al., 2004). However, UWB radar requires more complicated circuits to realize desired function such as pulse shaping and delay control.

2. Theoretical background and srchitectural selection

2.1 Continuous wave doppler radar

Radar is the acronym for Radio Detection and Ranging. Radar is an electromagnetic system that utilizes high frequency radio waves for the detection of objects. It operates by transmitting a wave or pulses and detecting the signal reflecting back from the object. Based on correlating the reflected signal and the transmitted signal various parameters like distance of the object, velocity of the object if it is in motion, area of cross section etc may be obtained. These radar systems have several advantages over optical line-of-sight based instruments, such as the ability to penetrate through some obstacles, operability with minimum performance degradation in rain, snow, and darkness, etc. Initially radar systems were mainly used in military applications but nowadays they find applications in areas of remote sensing for weather and exploration, air traffic control in airports, law enforcement for regulating speed on roads and highways, aircraft safety and navigation, nautical ranging and detection, space applications and recently for non-contact monitoring of vital signs (Skolnik, 1980). Radar systems can be generally divided into two types based on the signal being transmitted. They are pulsed radar systems and continuous-wave Radar systems. In a pulsed radar system, a short pulse is transmitted and there is a delay between consecutive pulses when the radar system tries to detect a reflection. In a continuous wave radar system, the radar emits a continuous wave and relative motion between the system and the object is detected either as a frequency shift or a phase shift. These radar systems cannot detect completely stationary objects as they will not cause any Doppler shifts in frequency, however they can still be very useful to detect the motion of the periodic chest wall of a stationary subject which causes a continuous phase shift depending on the position of the chest wall on which the continuous wave radar is incident. This is the main reason we find that most of the non-contact vital sign monitors employ a CW radar system to detect the respiration and heart rate of the subject. Another advantage of the CW system is that they are generally easier and cheaper to manufacture compared to pulsed radar based systems. However, the CW radar has some disadvantages too, and the major disadvantage being the coupling from the transmit chain into the receive chain either on the board itself or through the antennas which are generally closely spaced to minimize the size of the sensor system. This coupling of transmit power into the receiver can result in a time-varying or a constant DC offset, and this can limit the accuracy of detection significantly.

2.2 Principles of measurement of vital signs using a doppler radar

The Doppler shift in frequency in the general case is given as (Droitcour, 2006):

$$f_d(t) = \frac{2f}{c}v(t) = \frac{2v(t)}{\lambda} \tag{1}$$

Here $v(t)$ is the velocity of the target, λ the wavelength of the incident wave, and c is the velocity of the EM wave. However if the target is assumed to be stationary, this frequency shift can be viewed as nonlinear phase modulation as the phase signal $\Phi_r(t)$ is described as:

$$\Phi_r(t) = \frac{2f}{c}(2\pi x(t)) = \frac{4\pi x(t)}{\lambda} \tag{2}$$

Here $x(t)$ is the displacement of the chest wall. The transmitted signal from a continuous wave radar system is:

$$C(t) = A_T \cos(2\pi f t + \phi(t)) \tag{3}$$

Here f=frequency of operation and $\Phi(t)$ is the phase noise of the VCO and A_T is the amplitude of the transmitted signal. If we assume the distance from the subject to the biosensor system is d_0 and the time varying displacement of the chest is given as $x(t)$ then the distance travelled by the signal between the biosensor system and the target (chest wall of the subject under test) is given by:

$$d(t) = d_0 + x(t) \tag{4}$$

Now, the time delay between the transmitter and target is the distance travelled by the signal divided by the velocity of the wave *c*. However, as the chest has a time-varying displacement, the distance travelled by the signal at the time of reflection is given as:

$$d(t_{rf}) = d\left(t - \frac{d(t)}{c}\right) \tag{5}$$

Therefore the time delay by the time the signal is received is given as:

$$t_d = \frac{2d\left(t - \frac{d(t)}{c}\right)}{c} = \frac{2\left(d_o + x\left(t - \frac{d(t)}{c}\right)\right)}{c} \tag{6}$$

The signal at the receiver *R(t)* is a time-delayed version of the transmitted signal given by equation (3). We get the received signal to be:

$$R(t) = A_R \cos\left[2\pi f\left(t - t_d\right) + \phi\left(t - t_d\right) + \theta\right] \tag{7}$$

Here A_R is the amplitude of the received signal. Substituting for t_d from Eq.(6) in Eq. (7):

$$R(t) = A_R \cos\left[2\pi f\left(t - \frac{2\left(d_o + x\left(t - \frac{d(t)}{c}\right)\right)}{c}\right) + \phi\left(t - \frac{2\left(d_o + x\left(t - \frac{d(t)}{c}\right)\right)}{c}\right) + \theta\right] \tag{8}$$

$$R(t) = A_R \cos\left[2\pi ft - \frac{4\pi d_o}{\lambda} - \frac{4\pi x\left(t - \frac{d(t)}{c}\right)}{\lambda} + \phi\left(t - \frac{2d_o}{c} - \frac{2\,x\left(t - \frac{d(t)}{c}\right)}{c}\right) + \theta\right] \tag{9}$$

Here, the wavelength $\lambda = c/f$, and we know that the period of the chest movement for both heartbeat and respiration has a time period $T >> d_0 / c$, from this we can neglect the $4\pi x\left(\frac{d(t)}{c}\right)$ term in Eq. (9) and similarly in the phase noise term we can neglect $\phi\left(2\,x\left(t - \frac{d(t)}{c}\right)/c\right)$ as the displacement of the chest movement generally in the order of 1 cm is much smaller compared to the distance between the subject and the biosensor system which is generally 50 cm to 2m. On omitting these terms in Eq. (9) for reasons described above, the received signal becomes:

$$R(t) = A_R \cos\left[2\pi ft - \frac{4\pi d_o}{\lambda} - \frac{4\pi x(t)}{\lambda} + \phi\left(t - \frac{2d_o}{c}\right) + \theta\right] \tag{10}$$

From Eq. (10), we can see that the received signal *R(t)* resembles a time delayed version of the transmitted signal with *phase modulation*. The time delay is determined mainly by the distance d_0 between the biosensor system and the subject. The periodic motion of the target *x(t)* is superimposed as phase modulation. In order to determine the heart rate and respiration rate we need to demodulate this phase modulation to correlate the motion of the chest wall with actual heart rate and respiration rate.
From Eq. (10) we can see the wavelength has to be greater than at least twice the peak-to-peak motion *x*(t) of the chest wall. Otherwise we may get aliasing in the demodulated signal caused due to the under sampling of the phase modulated information by the sampling wave. So the lower limit on the possible choice of frequencies exists. The higher limit on the possible choices of operating frequency is given by the wavelength where the small signal approximation can no longer be applied which would complicate the analysis of the system.

2.3 Transceiver architectures and design

In the present section, we will discuss the choice of transceiver architectures and try to understand the advantages and disadvantages of each option in our attempt to determine which suits our application the best. As we have seen from the mathematical analysis above, the noncontact biosensor system needs to transmit CW at a fixed frequency. It needs to demodulate the phase modulated motion of the chest wall to determine the heart rate and the respiration rate. Transmitting CW at a fixed frequency can be easily accomplished by using a VCO tuned to the desired frequency. As Eq. (10) implies, the phase noise of the oscillator is an important parameter. If the VCO output is also used to drive the receive Local Oscillator (LO) inputs of the receive mixers, this will eliminate the need for a Phase-Locked-Loop (PLL) and also has an additional benefit of relaxing the phase noise requirements of the VCO by the phenomenon of range correlation. Depending on the range being targeted, a power amplifier can be added to boost output power. In order to obtain the vital sign information we need to down convert the received RF signals into baseband. This can be easily accomplished by mixing the received signal with a signal at the same carrier frequency, resulting in a conversion directly to baseband signals. This type of receiver is known either as a direct conversion or a homodyne receiver. A heterodyne receiver instead mixes the received signal with a LO signal at a different frequency, so the information is modulated on a non-zero intermediate frequency (IF) rather than being converted directly to baseband. This following section introduces the heterodyne and direct-conversion architectures, describes why the direct-conversion architecture is chosen for Doppler radar cardio-respiratory monitoring, and introduces the theory for Doppler radar monitoring with a CW system and a direct-conversion receiver.

2.3.1 Heterodyne transceiver architecture

In a heterodyne receiver, the input RF signal is mixed with a LO signal generated at a different frequency to the RF input signal, resulting in a signal at IF. This signal is filtered with a fixed bandpass filter and then amplified by a tuned IF stage amplifier and then demodulated directly or mixed down to baseband before demodulation. The receiver's basic architecture is shown in below. One major drawback with the heterodyne architecture is that it requires more circuits and passives as two-stage conversions are performed.

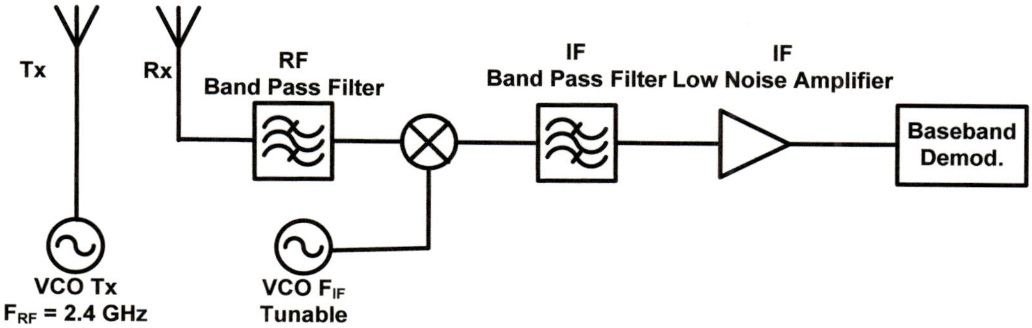

Fig. 2. Radar architecture using a heterodyne transceiver (single-channel)

2.3.2 Direct conversion or homodyne transceiver architecture

In a homodyne receiver, as shown in Figure 3, the received signal is mixed with a LO frequency at the same frequency as its carrier, converting the signal to baseband. The baseband signal is then filtered using a bandpass filter and then amplified by a baseband amplifier to the appropriate signal level for the digitizer (ADC) and demodulator. One major disadvantages of using a homodyne receiver for vital signs monitoring is the amount of DC offset introduced by the system; since the vital signs data is at very low frequency (0.3 to 3Hz), it can be difficult to demodulate the data in the presence of high DC offset so close to the desired frequency band. The DC offsets are caused by system imperfections like LO feed through, self mixing or by reflections from clutter or other nearby objects. The DC offsets can be as high as 200mV (Park et al., 2007) compared to the 1-10 mV respiration signals and the 10-100 μV heartbeat signals. Filtering this DC offset is essential to prevent saturation of ADC.

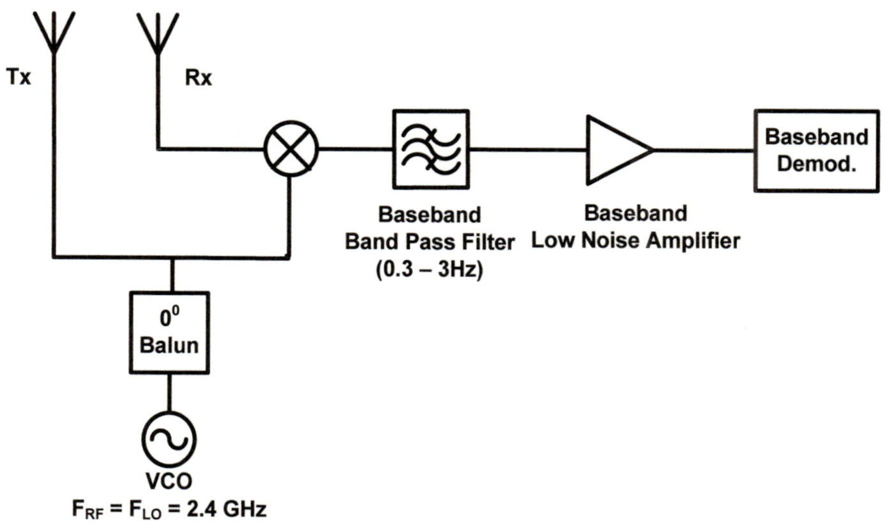

Fig. 3. Architecture of a Homodyne Transceiver

2.4 Transceiver architecture selection and design for vital signs monitoring

The direct conversion (homodyne) receiver for non-contact monitoring system has several advantages over a heterodyne receiver for applications that require continuous vital signs monitoring and therefore was chosen as the preferred architecture for our design. Some of the major advantages are:

a. *Range Correlation:* Range correlation is the process by which the phase noise of the transmitted VCO is correlated to the received signal cancelling out some of the phase noise of the received signal (Droitcour et al., 2003). This is an extremely valuable property of the direct conversion receivers as this can greatly relax the phase noise spec on the VCO. This is conceptually shown in the figure below.

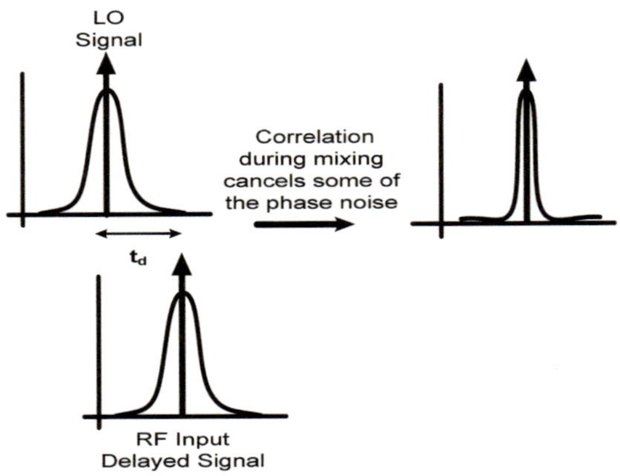

Fig. 4. Illustration of Range Correlation

b. *Simple Architecture and Design:* The direct conversion receiver is a simpler architecture to design as it is less susceptible to image and therefore does not require a RF bandpass image filter in the front end. It also uses the same VCO for both transmission and LO generation so it does not need a separate tuning stage for the baseband LO.

c. *Low Power Consumption:* The direct conversion receiver requires fewer components and therefore consumes lower power than a heterodyne receiver. During the operation as a portable non-contact vital sign sensor if we are operating these sensors from battery powered sources, we want to keep the power consumption to a minimum.

2.5 Single channel vs. quadrature (I-Q) radar systems

The Doppler radar transceivers can be built based on a single channel design or a quadrature design. In the system being reported in the current thesis, we built a single channel system initially and then switched to quadrature transceivers mainly to overcome the problem present in all Doppler radar transceivers: the phase-demodulation null points. These null points depend on the phase relationship between the LO and the received signal. This problem can be mitigated by using a quadrature receiver, which provides two receiver chains with a 90° difference in their LO phases.

We know from Eq 10 that the received signal which is the RF input to the mixer is:

$$R(t) = A_R \cos\left[2\pi ft - \frac{4\pi d_o}{\lambda} - \frac{4\pi x(t)}{\lambda} - \frac{4\pi y(t)}{\lambda} + \phi\left(t - \frac{2d_o}{c}\right) + \theta\right] \tag{11}$$

Here, *x(t)* is the signal due to respiration and *y(t)* is the signal due to the heart beat. Also the transmitted signal is used for driving the LO of the mixer, so the LO input to the mixer is:

$$C(t) = A_T \cos(2\pi f t + \phi(t))$$

On mixing these signals at the mixer and after filtering to obtain the desired low frequency components we get (Park et al., 2006):

$$D(t) = \cos\left[\theta + \frac{4\pi x(t)}{\lambda} + \Delta\phi(t)\right] \tag{12}$$

Here, $\Delta\phi(t)$ is the residual phase noise in the baseband demodulated signal (Park et al., 2006):

$$\Delta\phi(t) = \left[\phi(t) - \phi\left(t - \frac{2d_o}{c}\right)\right] \tag{13}$$

Also, θ is the constant phase shift dependant on the nominal distance to the target d_0 :

$$\theta = \left[\frac{4\pi d_o}{\lambda} + \theta_0\right] \tag{14}$$

The null and optimum demodulation points are the two extreme cases for the output signal given as a function of θ from Eq. (12). The optimum detection point occurs when θ is an odd multiple of $(\pi/2)$, In this case applying the small signal approximation as the cardiopulmonary signal information $x(t) << (\lambda/4)$ we get:

$$D(t) = \left[\frac{4\pi x(t)}{\lambda} + \frac{4\pi y(t)}{\lambda} + \Delta\phi(t)\right] \tag{15}$$

Now, assuming the displacements associated with respiration and heart rate can be modeled as sinusoids as a first order approximation, we have (Park et al., 2006):

$$D(t) \approx \left[R \sin 2\pi f_r(t) + H \sin 2\pi f_h(t) + \Delta\phi(t)\right] \tag{16}$$

Here, $R >> H$ *and* $f_h >> f_r$ and the demodulated output signal is linearly proportional to the cardio pulmonary information signals. For the optimum case of demodulation, we can easily demodulate the vital signs data after suitable amplification and filtering.
In the case of the null detection point, when θ is an odd multiple of π, we have

$$D(t) \approx 1 - \left[R \sin 2\pi f_r(t) + H \sin 2\pi f_h(t) + \Delta\phi(t)\right]^2 \tag{17}$$

If we assume the residual phase noise $\Delta\phi(t)$ *is* much smaller than the cardiopulmonary signals, we can neglect that term in Eq. 17. And expanding square terms we get:

$$D(t) \approx 1 - \left[R^2 \sin^2 2\pi f_r(t) + H^2 \sin^2 2\pi f_h(t) + 2HR \sin 2\pi f_r(t). \sin 2\pi f_h(t)\right] \tag{18}$$

Simplifying further we get:

$$D(t) \approx 1 - \frac{1}{2}\left[(R^2 + H^2) - R^2 \sin^2 4\pi f_r(t) - H^2 \sin^2 4\pi f_h(t) - 2HR(\cos 2\pi(f_h + f_r)t - \cos 2\pi(f_h - f_r)t)\right] \tag{19}$$

We can see that in the case of null demodulation point, we get a signal that has several distortion terms and the output signal is proportional to the square of the cardiopulmonary informational signals causing decreased sensitivity. Also, the only term that passes the low pass filter is the second order respiration term, along with the DC offsets associated with the output signal. It should be noted that the term being produced has twice the frequency of the true respiration signal. In addition, the respiration signals are much larger in magnitude than that of the heart rate signals, and at these null points there is a mutual coupling of the true heart and the respiration signals (which has a higher magnitude than the heart signal), making accurate demodulation of the heart rate signal very difficult at these null points.

In our current system with an operating frequency of 2.4GHz, we have a λ of 12.5 cm and we know from Eq. (14) this means we have a null point every 3.125cm. Since we cannot make such fine adjustments in the positioning of the vital signs monitoring sensor system, we need to implement a quadrature transceiver system that drives the in-phase and quadrature channels with a 90° phase shift such that when one channel is at a null point we have the other channel at an optimum point for demodulation. By either selecting the output closest to the optimal phase demodulation point or by intelligently combining the two outputs, phase-demodulation null points can be avoided and accurate results for both heart rate and respiration rate can be obtained. Another reason for implementing a quadrature receiver is that in direct conversion receivers, image rejection cannot be done with filtering, because the image signal and desired signal are in the same frequency space. So by using quadrature architecture we can convert each of the in-phase and quadrature frequency components individually to baseband so that the image signal can be rejected (depending on how good the I/Q matching is) to minimize its effect on the desired signal.

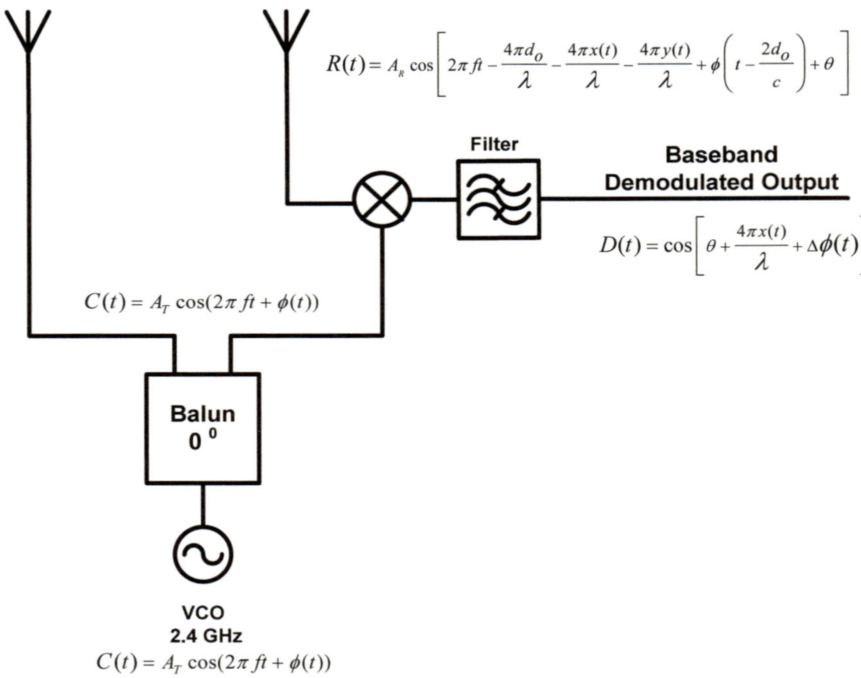

Fig. 5. System Diagram showing Demodulation with equations

2.6 Arctangent demodulation

As discussed above, the performance of single-channel Doppler Radar transceiver is known to be sensitive to the position of the target. For the worst case, the target can be at a "null" position that will produce virtually no signal due to its distance away from the radar at integer multiples of the quarter of wavelength (λ). Therefore, to avoid "optimum" and "null" extremities in the demodulated signal, we adopted a Quadrature Doppler Radar receiver system here. However, these in-phase and quadrature outputs need to be combined effectively to get accurate detection of the vital signs data. Arctangent combination of the I and Q signals has been shown to give highly accurate results (Park et al, 2007). We have also used this method to combine the quadrature data for demodulation in the present thesis work. In a quadrature system the two orthogonal baseband outputs are (Droitcour 2006):

$$I_B(t) = Cos\left[\theta + \frac{4\pi x(t)}{\lambda} + \frac{4\pi y(t)}{\lambda} + \Delta\phi(t)\right] \tag{20}$$

$$Q_B(t) = Sin\left[\theta + \frac{4\pi x(t)}{\lambda} + \frac{4\pi y(t)}{\lambda} + \Delta\phi(t)\right] \tag{21}$$

Here, θ is the constant phase shift dependent on the nominal distance to the target, $x(t)$ is the heart motion signal, $y(t)$ is the respiration motion signal, and

$$\Delta\phi(t) = \phi(t) - \phi\left(t - \frac{2d_O}{c}\right) \tag{22}$$

Here, $\phi(t)$ is the residual VCO phase noise translated in baseband, which depends on the nominal target distance. One can combine the I and Q channels in Eqs. (3) and (4) by using the arctangent function (Park et al., 2007). This gives us a resultant baseband signal:

$$\Phi_r(t) = \arctan\left(\frac{Q_B(t)}{I_B(t)}\right) \tag{23}$$

$$\Phi_r(t) = \arctan\left(\frac{Sin\left[\theta + \frac{4\pi x(t)}{\lambda} + \frac{4\pi y(t)}{\lambda} + \Delta\phi(t)\right]}{Cos\left[\theta + \frac{4\pi x(t)}{\lambda} + \frac{4\pi y(t)}{\lambda} + \Delta\phi(t)\right]}\right) \tag{24}$$

$$\Phi_r(t) = \left[\theta + \frac{4\pi x(t)}{\lambda} + \frac{4\pi y(t)}{\lambda} + \Delta\phi(t)\right] \tag{25}$$

A real system has several non-idealities like amplitude and phase mismatches and other hardware imperfections. There can be a significant DC offset term introduced by hardware imperfections and reflections from background clutter, etc. (Park et al, 2007) Due to these non-idealities, the demodulated signal using the arctangent function above changes to:

$$\Phi_r'(t) = \arctan\left(\frac{A_Q + A_E \, Sin\left[\theta + \frac{4\pi x(t)}{\lambda} + \frac{4\pi y(t)}{\lambda} + \Delta\phi(t) + \phi_E\right]}{A_I + Cos\left[\theta + \frac{4\pi x(t)}{\lambda} + \frac{4\pi y(t)}{\lambda} + \Delta\phi(t)\right]}\right) \tag{26}$$

Here, A_Q and A_I denote the dc offsets of Q and I channel, respectively, and A_E and ϕ_E are the amplitude error and phase error, respectively.

2.6.1 Comparison of arctangent demodulation and complex demodulation

We know from the above section that the arctangent combination gives us the resultant phase modulated vital signs information as shown in Eq. 26. Here, A_Q and A_I denote the dc offsets of I and Q channel respectively and are generally the most important parameters in determining the accuracy of the extracted heartbeat and respiration rate information. However, these DC offsets comprise of two components, one component is the "desirable DC offset" component that consists of some vital signs information and the other DC offset "undesirable DC offset" that consists of the DC offset caused by electronic components and caused by reflections from stationary or other objects in the vicinity of the subject. If this DC offset is improperly calibrated in the baseband, it leads to a shifted trajectory. When the trajectory is shifted the vital signs data is still present and can be extracted, but the difference is a changed harmonic level in the baseband spectrum. The arctangent method is reported to be more sensitive to these DC offsets especially in the presence of random body movements (Li & Lin., 2008b). Calibration of the DC offset can be a difficult problem because the DC offset is a dynamic variable and changes with environment, position of the subject, etc. To overcome the problems of DC offset calibration, we can also use a complex signal demodulation method to combine the I & Q channel data as described before.
The baseband signals can be expressed using Bessel's Functions as:

$$\begin{aligned} I(t) &= \cos(\frac{4\pi x_h(t)}{\lambda} + \frac{4\pi x_r(t)}{\lambda} + \phi) = \sum_{k=-\infty}^{\infty}\sum_{l=-\infty}^{\infty} J_k\left(\frac{4\pi m_r}{\lambda}\right) J_l\left(\frac{4\pi m_h}{\lambda}\right)\cos(k\omega_r t + l\omega_h t + \phi) \\ &= -2\left[C_{10}\sin(\omega_r t) + C_{01}\sin(\omega_h t) + ...\right]\cdot\sin\phi = -2\left[C_{20}\cos(2\omega_r t) + C_{02}\sin(2\omega_h t) + ...\right]\cdot\cos\phi \end{aligned} \tag{27}$$

$$\begin{aligned} Q(t) &= \sin(\frac{4\pi x_h(t)}{\lambda} + \frac{4\pi x_r(t)}{\lambda} + \phi) = \sum_{k=-\infty}^{\infty}\sum_{l=-\infty}^{\infty} J_k\left(\frac{4\pi m_r}{\lambda}\right) J_l\left(\frac{4\pi m_h}{\lambda}\right)\sin(k\omega_r t + l\omega_h t + \phi) \\ &= -2\left[C_{10}\sin(\omega_r t) + C_{01}\sin(\omega_h t) + ...\right]\cdot\cos\phi = -2\left[C_{20}\cos(2\omega_r t) + C_{02}\sin(2\omega_h t) + ...\right]\cdot\sin\phi \end{aligned} \tag{28}$$

, where $C_{ij} = J_i\left(\frac{4\pi m_r}{\lambda}\right)\cdot J_j\left(\frac{4\pi m_h}{\lambda}\right)$ determines the amplitude of each frequency component.

Hence, the DC components are given by:

$$DC_I = J_0\left(\frac{4\pi m_r}{\lambda}\right)\cdot J_0\left(\frac{4\pi m_h}{\lambda}\right)\cdot\cos\phi \tag{29}$$

$$DC_Q = J_0\left(\frac{4\pi m_r}{\lambda}\right)\cdot J_0\left(\frac{4\pi m_h}{\lambda}\right)\cdot\sin\phi \tag{30}$$

Then a complex FFT is used to combine the I & Q channels in the baseband (Li & Lin., 2008a):

$$\begin{aligned} S(t) &= I(t) + j\cdot Q(t) = \exp\left\{ j\left[\frac{4\pi x_h(t)}{\lambda} + \frac{4\pi x_r(t)}{\lambda} + \phi \right] \right\} \\ &= DC_{IQ} + 2j\left[C_{10}\sin(\omega_r t) + C_{01}\sin(\omega_h t) + ...\right]\cdot e^{j\phi} + 2\left[C_{20}\cos(2\omega_r t) + C_{02}\sin(2\omega_h t) + ...\right]\cdot e^{j\phi} \end{aligned} \tag{31}$$

Since $e^{j\phi}$ has a constant envelope of one, the effect of ϕ on signal amplitude can be eliminated. Applying the complex Fourier transform to the signal for spectral analysis, the residual phase will not affect the relative strength between the odd order and the even order frequency components. The desired signal components which are the odd order tones will always be present in the spectrum (Li & Lin., 2008b). DC offsets that exist in the I/Q channels and may lead to the error of measured vital signs, only affect the dc term of *S(t)* in Eq. (31). This DC offset can be extracted and safely removed by averaging the baseband signals and thus the existence of dc offset does not affect obtaining the frequency of the desired signal components making the complex signal demodulation more immune to DC offset mismatches. However, the complex signal demodulation method is affected by the even order harmonics that are still present in the baseband spectrum.

2.7 Summary on the architectural selection and theoretical background

A continuous-wave direct-conversion radar transceiver is the fundamental component of our non-contact vital signs monitoring system. Direct-conversion receiver architecture was chosen due to its simplicity, low power consumption, good performance, and lower fabrication cost compared to a heterodyne receiver. A quadrature receiver was used to avoid null points and it can provide us position-insensitive accurate results as null points can be difficult to avoid due to variations in the relative position of the subject (they occur every 3.125 cm at our operating frequency). Quadrature receivers consume more power and need more components making them more expensive than single channel systems.

3. Measured vital signs results and data analysis

3.1 Introduction

Our noncontact vital signs monitoring system consisted of a Doppler radar transceiver transmitting a continuous wave using a VCO, a single channel or quadrature receiver, custom analog baseband signal conditioning hardware and a custom GUI developed in Labview that performs digital signal processing, extraction of vital signs and logging of the data. For the purposes of calibration and comparison, a piezoelectric pulse transducer sensor was worn on a subject's hand and the signals from the transducer were used to compute the reference heartbeat signal. The in-phase (I), quadrature (Q) and reference channels were digitized simultaneously using a NI USB6000 ADC connected to a PC. The piezoelectric sensor was used to find the reference heartbeat rate which was compared with the rates computed by the Doppler sensor system using the Labview or Matlab software.

3.2 Experimental setup

Our experimental setup consisted of the Doppler noncontact radar transceiver, an analog signal processing system and a NI ADC connected to a PC running Labview. The subject was seated in a chair in an upright position and the piezoelectric pulse transducer sensor UFI 1010 was affixed to the subject's right hand index finger. The subject was then asked to sit straight and still in a chair for the measurements, and the antenna placement was adjusted to be approximately at the same level with the center of the subject's chest. The primary objective of this data collection was to determine whether the Doppler noncontact vital signs monitor can accurately extract the heartbeat and respiration rates of healthy, relaxed subjects in a well controlled environment with no background motion or presence of other humans in the vicinity of the Doppler radar system. During the course of the data collection, the subject was asked to remain still and to refrain from making any involuntary motions like scratching, talking or other movements for the complete duration of each measurement. The measurement setup is shown in the figure below.

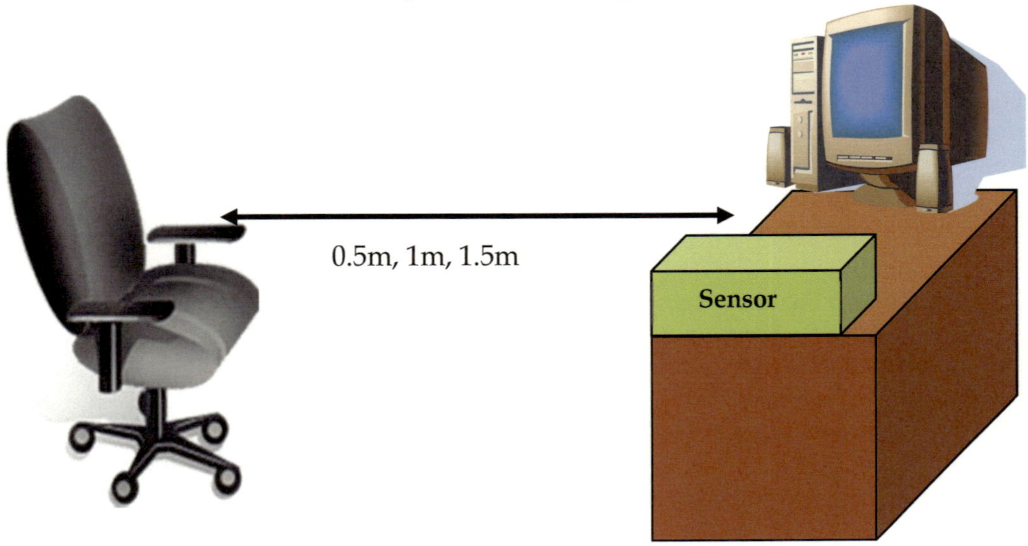

Fig. 6. Diagram showing the noncontact vital signs sensor measurement setup

3.3 Results and data analysis

In the present section we discuss the results of the data collected using our first, second and third generation systems and try to contrast and compare the differences in performance. For each reading that was collected, we compute the mean error, standard deviation and median. The mean error over several readings was computed and used to determine the accuracy of the system. As these Doppler radar based sensor systems are very sensitive to noise, background movement, stray reflections from clutters, etc., averaging the extracted respiration and heart rates becomes necessary. Momentary readings might be distorted due to sudden involuntary motion of the subject like sneezing, coughing etc. Also, another figure of merit for the sensor system is the standard deviation of the error. We can use the standard deviation as an estimate of the worst case accuracy range within which our system extracts the vital signs rates in this controlled environment.

3.3.1 First generation sensor system

This system was designed to initially show the proof of concept of the ability of extraction of vital signs using a Doppler transceiver. This system was a single channel system as shown in figure below. This system comprised of discrete SMA terminated Mini-circuits modules assembled together using SMA cables. The Analog Signal Processing (ASP) was done initially using a SRS 560 Preamplifier and Filter block. However, since the SRS560 block is bulky and expensive, we designed a custom ASP board. We compared the performance of both systems to verify that the ASP board performs as well as the SRS560, so we have replaced it with the custom ASP board. In this section we present the data collected by the SRS560 block and the ASP board, where the data was logged using the NI Data Logger that comes bundled with the NI USB ADC and logs the sampled voltage readings from each channel into a text file. The text file was analyzed using a MATLAB script and the respiration rate and heartbeat rate were extracted using only the autocorrelation function. The extracted heartbeat was compared to the piezoelectric reference from the finger pulse transducer sensor. From the data we can clearly see that the ASP board performs as well as or sometimes appears better than the SRS560 block. The mean and the standard deviation of the error of the extracted respiration rate of the ASP board are comparable to the mean and standard deviation of the error from the SRS560 block. We can conclude that the ASP board performs well and can be used as a replacement for the SRS560 block.

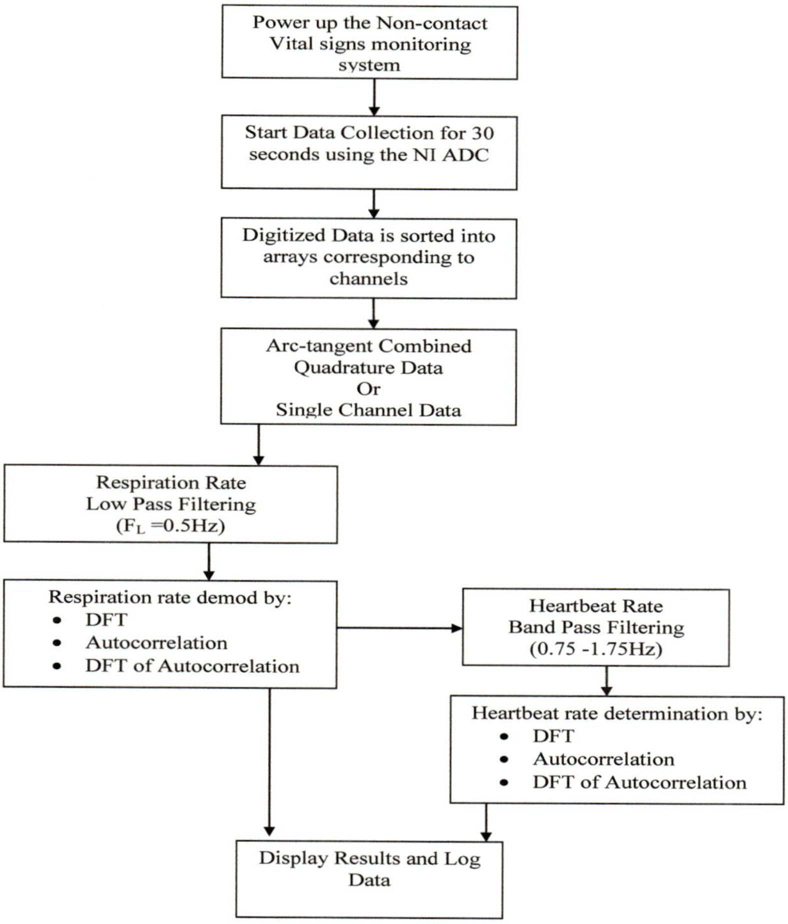

Fig. 7. Flowchart showing our sensor measurement sequence

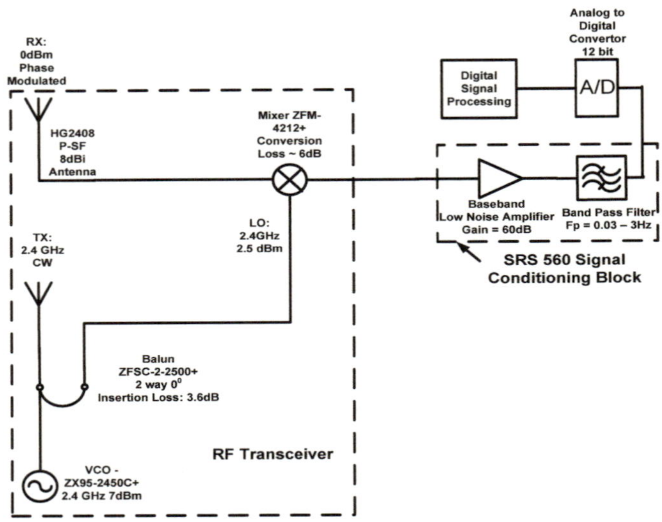

Fig. 8. First Generation noncontact vital signs system developed at Texas Tech U.

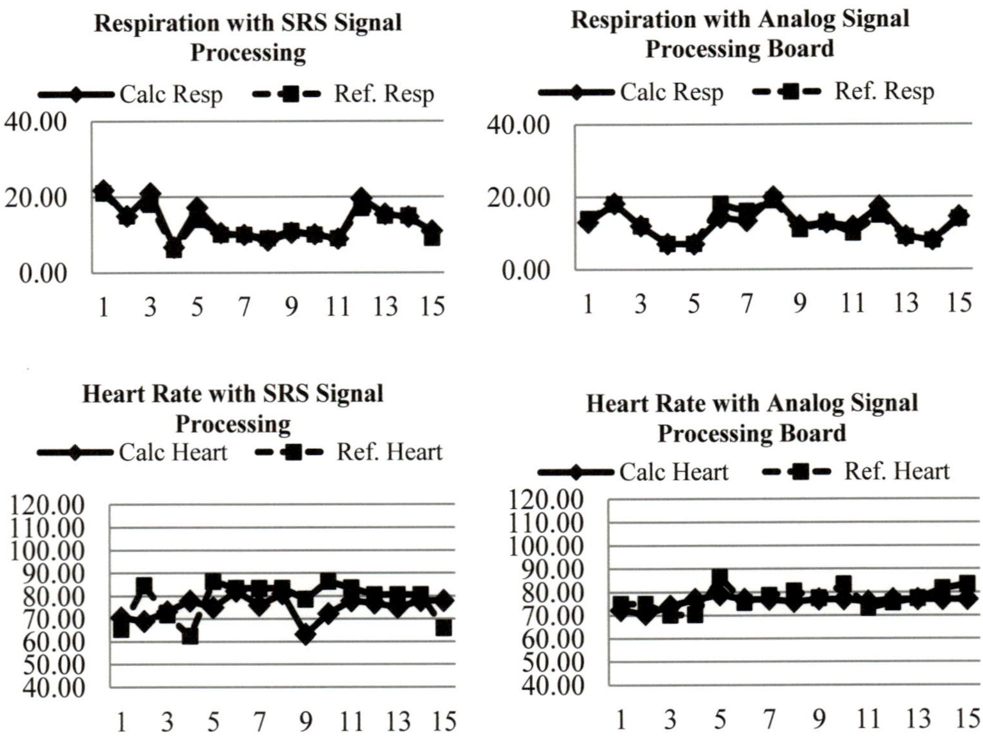

Fig. 9. (a). Respiration Data showing how well the system tracks the reference with the SRS560 Block (left); ASP board (right), (b). Heartbeat data showing how well the system tracks the reference with the SRS560 block (left); with our custom ASP board (right)

	SRS 560	ASP Board
Respiration (beat/min)		
Mean Error	0.76	-0.03
STDEV of Error	1.28	1.51
Heartbeat (beat/min)		
Mean Error	-3.38	-1.56
STDEV of Error	9.25	4.16

Table 1. Comparison of measured vital signs data using SRS560 vs. custom ASP board

3.3.2 Second generation sensor system

The second generation system is a Quadrature Doppler transceiver to get position-insensitive and accurate results compared to the first generation single channel system. It comprised of the first RF PCB that was designed to eliminate the bulkier SMA modules. We designed this system using our custom designed Analog PCB that comprises of Sallen-Key Active filters and an Op-amp based baseband Low Noise Amplifier. The system block diagram, the lab setup, the analog processing/filtering design, and pictures of two discrete RF and Analog PCBs are shown in the figures below.

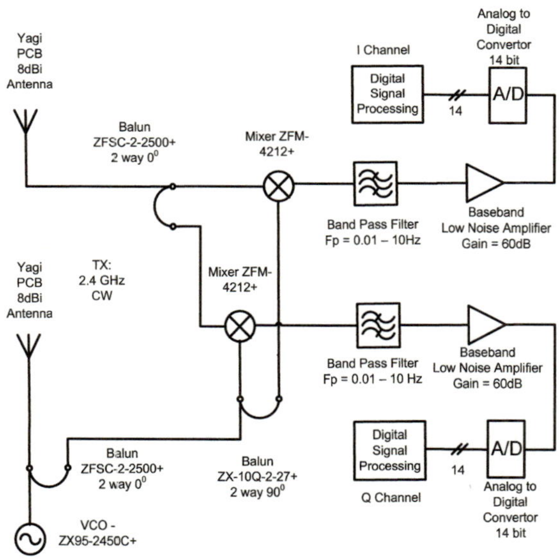

Fig. 10. Second generation sensor system with discrete components developed in Texas Tech

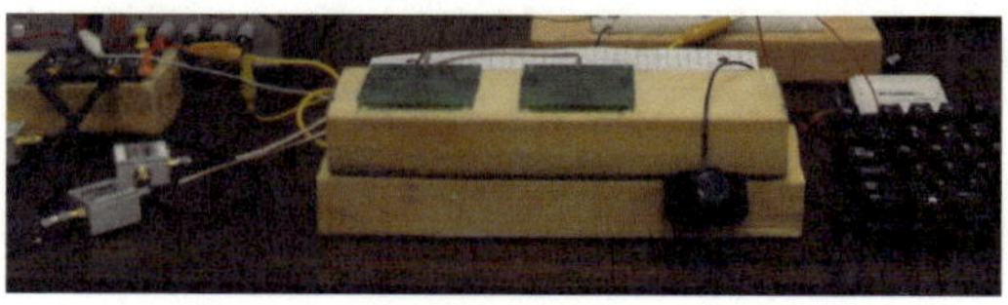

Fig. 11. A picture of the 2nd generation sensor with discrete components (PC not shown)

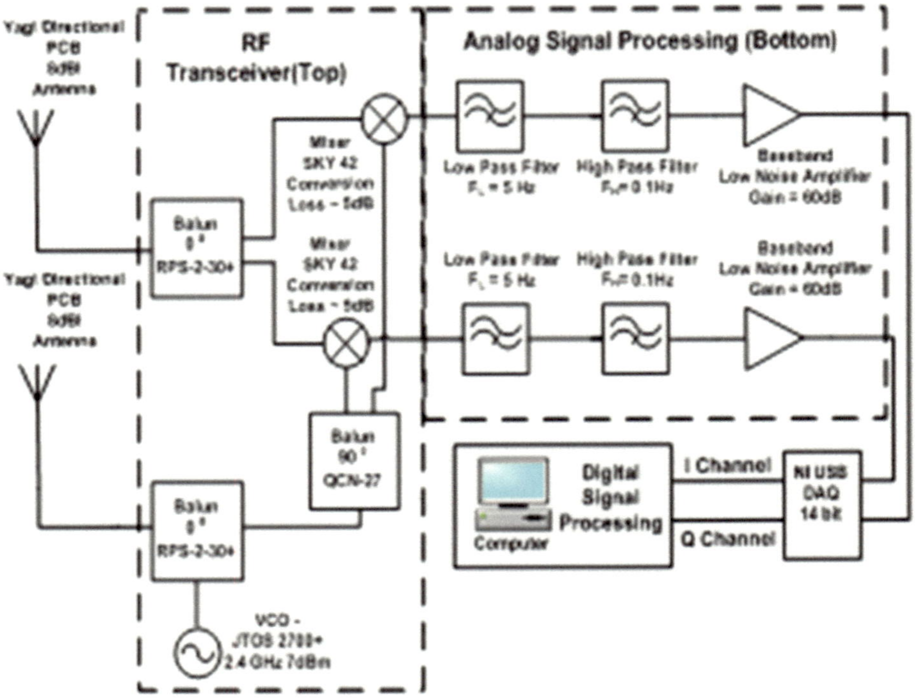

Fig. 12. Second generation sensor system with RF and Analog PCBs

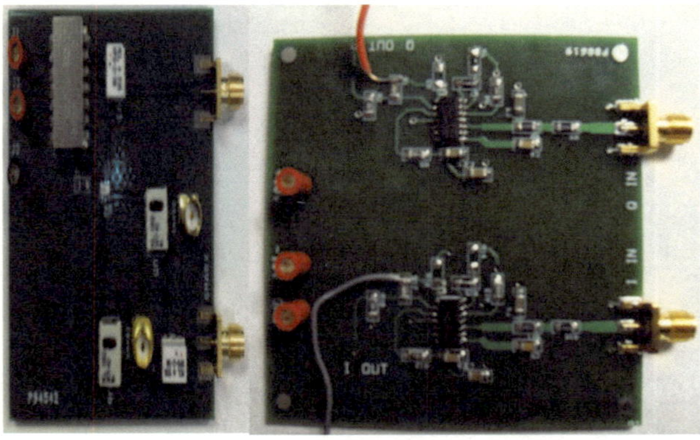

Fig. 13. Second Generation PCB system for our sensor: RF PCB (left); Analog PCB (right)

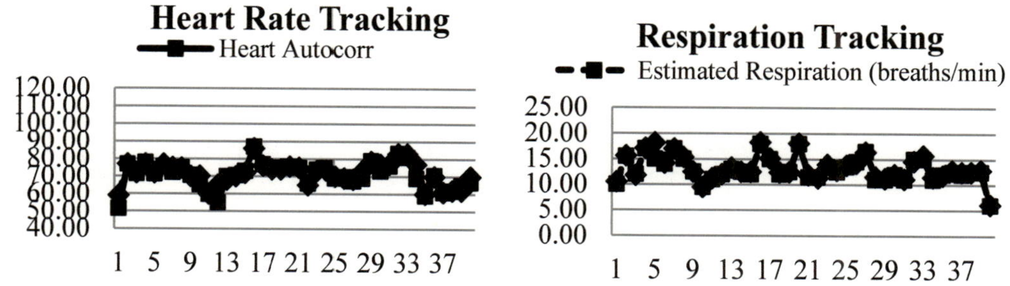

Fig. 14. 2nd Gen. sensor data tracks references for heartbeat (left) and respiration rate (right)

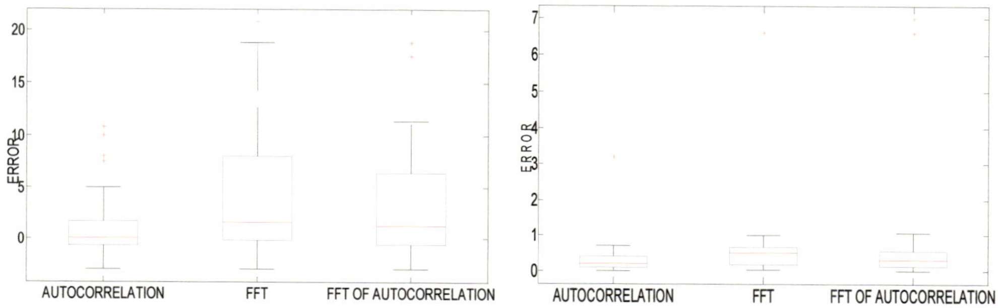

Fig. 15. Box plots of errors for 2nd Gen. sensor of heartbeat (left); respiration rate (right)

The duration of the data collection was 60 seconds for each dataset. The digitized data obtained from the ADC is processed in LabVIEW©. The sampled I and Q channels are initially combined using the arctangent function, then the combined data is filtered for respiration rate detection using a low-pass 500 order FIR filter with a cut-off of 0.75Hz and then filtered using a 1000 order band pass FIR filter for heart rate detection using pass-band of 1Hz to 1.5Hz. The Finite Impulse Response (FIR) filters have been designed using a Kaiser Window and Beta value of 6.5 for good main and side lobes characteristics. The extraction of vital signs is done by three different methods: Fast-Fourier-Transform (FFT) in the frequency domain, time-domain autocorrelation with peak detection, and FFT of the autocorrelation output. The filters and DSP to extract vital signs was done in NI's LabVIEW. The GUI displays the sampled data and results and logs all data (Ichapurapu et al., 2009a).

3.3.3 Third generation noncontact vital signs sensor system

In order to improve the portability of the system, we designed our third generation system to miniaturize the system further (Ichapurapu et al., 2009b). Compared to our earlier system, we made the following changes in this 3rd-gen. design: make the entire system into a single PCB as shown below; the duration of data collection is reduced to 30 sec (from 1 minute); implemented a pass band filter from 0.75 to 1.75 Hz (instead of 1-1.5 Hz) for the calculation of the heart rate. In both cases, the demodulated data was then analyzed and vital signs determined using all three methods mentioned above. For the third generation system the setup consisted of a single PCB based system as shown in Fig. 16 using YAGI antennas. The

Doppler measured vital signs data is shown in Figs. 17-18, which indicate very good data quality. A part of the GUI interface is shown in Fig. 19.

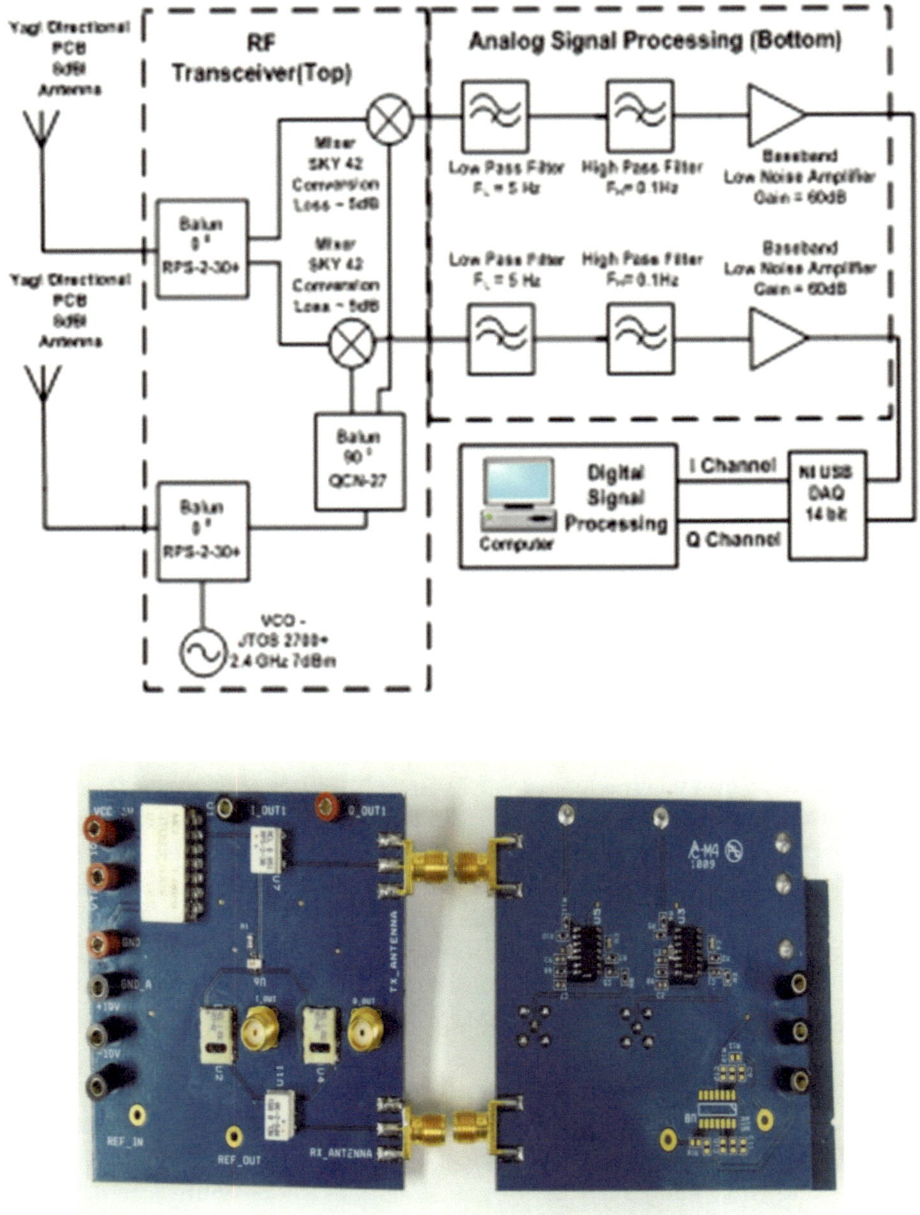

Fig. 16. Third Generation noncontact vital signs sensor system: system block diagram (TOP); single PCB sensor system (Bottom Left: RF PCB; Bottom Right: Analog PCB)

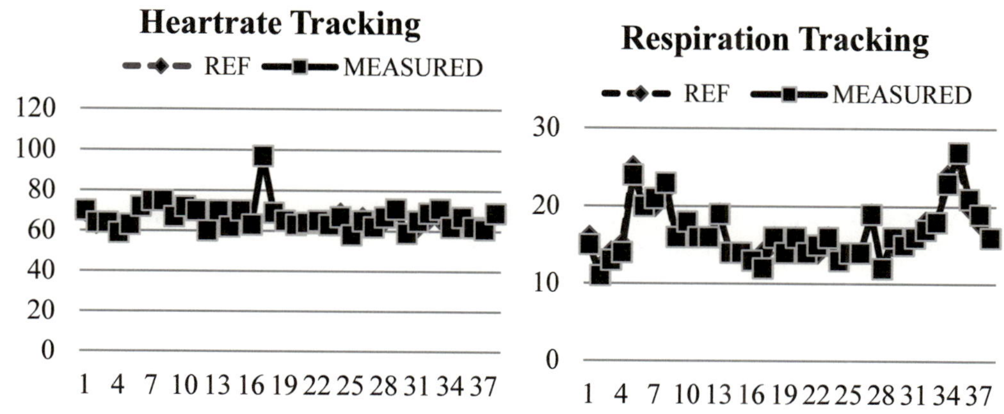

Fig. 17. Data showing how well our 3rd Generation non-contact vital signs sensor system tracks the reference for Heartbeat rate (left); Respiration rate (right)

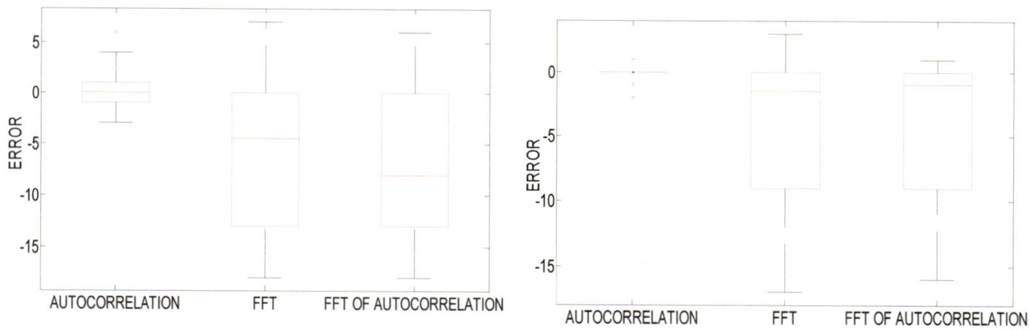

Fig. 18. Box plots showing the measured error distributions from our 3rd Generation non-contact vital signs sensor for the heartbeat rate (left) and respiration rate (right)

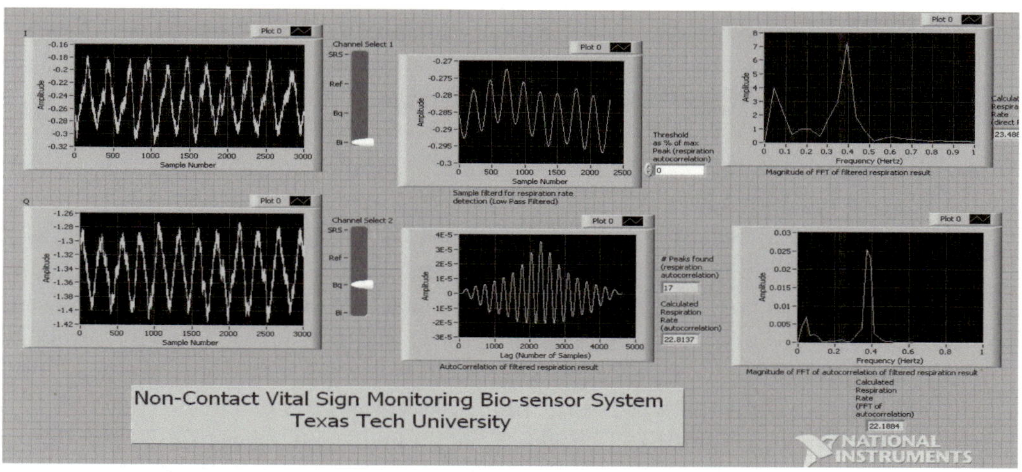

Fig. 19. A screenshot of our developed LabVIEW© GUI for the non-contact sensor system

4. Conclusions and future work

The Doppler radar non-contact system was used to measure the vital signs of a seated subject in a controlled environment. Data was collected using 4 different configurations including a single channel system with discrete RF components, and three different quadrature configurations. Good data accuracy was observed in the extracted vital signs. Quadrature transceiver with arctangent combination and autocorrelation showed the best accuracy for both respiration and heartbeat rate determination. Evaluating performance of the system using both the mean and standard deviation of these results gives us a good indication of the robustness of the system (using only the mean error can be misleading as the error in measurement can be positive and negative). As expected, the mean and standard deviation of the error increase as the distance of the subject from the sensor increases from 0.5m to 1.5m, due to the smaller SNR. Autocorrelation is a solid method with lowest extracted average error < 1 beat/min for respiration rate and average error < 3 beat/min for heart rate for 3rd generation sensor for most cases. Errors in extracted respiration rate are significantly smaller than those of the heart rates due to its larger signal strength. The continuous vital signs data measured from these portable sensors can be wirelessly transferred to healthcare professionals to make life saving decisions and diagnosis of symptoms. For future work, further miniaturization and performance improvement are needed on DC offset cancellation, and resolving the effects of the harmonics of respiration signal overpowering the heartbeat signal. We are working on making the algorithm more robust with some adaptive filtering techniques, where one might estimate the cutoffs for the heartbeat rate detection based on the respiration rate. Our vision is that a continuous log of these vital signs info can also be used to remotely monitor and gauge the recovery of patients, and even for the prevention or prediction of severe illnesses and complications. We also have to go through a couple of clinical trials to evaluate our non-contact vital signs sensor system in terms of false-positives and robustness in a clinical environment. Features such as RFID, motion-detection, etc. can also be integrated in the non-contact vital signs sensors.

5. References

Boric-Lubecke O., Lubecke V.M., Host-Madsen A., Samardzija D., Cheung K., "Doppler radar sensing of multiple subjects in single and multiple antenna systems", Proc. 7th Int'l Conf. on Telecomm. in Modern Satellite, Cable, Broadcasting Services, 1, 2005, pp. 7-11

Dorin A.F., "The Vitals of Vital Sign Monitoring", Supplement to Outpatient Surgery Magazine, August 2007

Droitcour A.D., Boric-Lubecke O., Lubecke V.M., and Lin J., "0.25 μm CMOS and BiCMOS single chip direct conversion Doppler radars for remote sensing of vital signs," IEEE Int. Solid State Circuits Conf. Dig., Feb. 2002, pp. 348-349.

Droitcour A.D., Boric-Lubecke O., Lubecke V., Lin J., and Kovacs G., "Range correlation effect on ISM band I/Q CMOS radar for non-contact vital signs sensing," IEEE MTT-S Int. Microwave Symp. Dig., June 2003, vol. 3, pp. 1945-1948

Droitcour A.D., Boric-Lubecke O., Lubecke V. M., Lin J., and Kovac G. T. A., "Range correlation and I/Q performance benefits in single chip silicon Doppler radars for noncontact cardiopulmonary monitoring," IEEE Trans. Microwave Theory and Techniques, vol. 52, pp. 838-848, March 2004

Droitcour A.D., "Non-contact measurement of heart and respiration rates with a single-chip microwave Doppler radar", Doctoral Thesis, Stanford University, CA (2006)

Hu W., Lie D.Y.C., Ichapurapu R., Kakade M.U., Mane S., Lopez J., Li Y., Li C., Banister R.E., Dentino A., Nguyen T., Zupancic S. and Griswold J., "An Intelligent Non-Contact Wireless Monitoring System for Vital Signs and Motion Detection", Proc. IEEE Int'l Conf. of System Science and Eng. (ICSSE), pp. 190-194, Taiwan, July 1-3, 2010

Ichapurapu R., Jain S., Monday T., Gregory J., Lie D.Y.C., Banister R.and Griswold J., "A 2.4GHz Non-Contact Biosensor System for Continuous Vital-Signs Monitoring", Proc. IEEE 10th Annual Wireless and Microwave Tech. Conf. (WAMICON), pp. 1-3, Clearwater, FL, USA, Apr. 20-21 (2009)

Ichapurapu R., Jain S., Kakade M.U., Lie D.Y.C., and Banister R.E., "A 2.4GHz Non-Contact Biosensor System for Continuous Vital-Signs Monitoring on a Single PCB", Proc. IEEE 8th Int'l Conf. on ASIC (ASICON), pp. 925-928, Changsha, China, Oct. 20-23 (2009)

Immoreev I.Y., "New practical application of ultra-wideband radars," Radar Conference EURAD 2007, 10-12 Oct. 2007.

Li C. and Lin J., "Optimal carrier frequency of non-contact vital sign detectors," Proc. IEEE Radio and Wireless Symp., Long Beach, CA, 2007, pp. 281–284.

Li C. and Lin J., "Complex signal demodulation and random body movement cancellation techniques for non-contact vital sign detection," Proc. IEEE MTT-S Int. Microwave Symp., Atlanta, GA, June 2008, pp. 567–570.

Li C. and Lin J., "Random body movement cancellation in Doppler radar vital sign detection," IEEE Trans. Microwave Theory Tech., vol. 56, 12, pp. 3143–3152, Dec. 2008.

Li C., Cummings J., Lam J., Graves E., and Wu W., "Radar remote monitoring of vital signs," IEEE Microwave Magazine, vol. 10, no. 1, pp. 47–56, 2009.

Lin J.C. , "Microwave sensing of physiological movement and volume change: A review," Bioelectromagnetics, 13, pp. 557–565, Dec. (1992)

Park B.-K., Yamada S., Lubecke V.M., and Boric-Lubecke O., "Single-channel receiver limitations in Doppler radar measurements of periodic motion", IEEE Radio and Wireless Symp., San Diego, CA, USA, pp. 99-102, 2006

Park B.K., Boric-Lubecke O., and Lubecke V. M., "Arctangent Demodulation with DC Offset Compensation in Quadrature Doppler radar Receiver Systems", IEEE Trans. Microw. Theory Tech., 55(5), pp. 1073-1079, May (2007)

Pisa S., Bernardi P., Cavagnaro M., Pittella E. and Piuzzi E., "Monitoring of cardio-pulmonary activity with UWB radar: a circuital model," Asia-Pacific Symp. on EMC, Singapore, May 2008.

Ossberger D., Buchegger T., Schimback E., Stelzer A. and Weigel R., "Non-invasive respiratory movement detection and monitoring of hidden humans using ultra wideband pulse radar," IEEE Int'll Workshop on Ultra Wideband Systems (IWUWBS), pp. 395-399, Piscataway, NJ, May 18-21, 2004

Samardzija D., Boric-Lubecke O., Host-Madsen A., Lubecke V.M., Sizer T. II, Droitcour A.D., Kovacs G.T.A., "Applications of MIMO techniques to sensing of cardiopulmonary activity", Proc. IEEE/ACES Int'l Conf. on Wireless Comm., Applied Computational Electromagnetics, 2005, pp. 618–621

Skolnik M. I., Introduction to Radar Systems, 2nd ed., New York: McGraw-Hill, 1980.

Staderini E.M., "UWB radars in medicine," IEEE Aerospace and Electronic Systems Magazine, Vol. 17, Issue 1, pp. 13-18, 2002

Xiao Y., Lin J., Boric-Lubecke O. and Lubecke V. M., "A Ka-band low power Doppler radar system for remote detection of cardiopulmonary motion," Proc. 27th IEEE Annu. Engineering in Medicine and Biology Society Conf., September 1-4, 2005

Xiao Y., Lin J., Boric-Lubecke O. and Lubecke V. M., "Frequency Tuning Technique for Remote Detection of Heartbeat and Respiration Using Low-Power Double-Sideband Transmission in Ka-Band", IEEE Trans. Microwave Theory and Techniques, vol. 54, pp. 2023 - 2032, May 2006

Zhou Q., Liu J., Host-Madsen A., Boric-Lubecke O., Lubecke V., "Detection of multiple heartbeats using Doppler radar", Proc. IEEE Int'l Conf. on Acoustics, Speech, Signal Processing (ICASSP), vol. 2, 2006, pp. II-1160–II-1163

Part 2

Application Scenarios and Case Studies

10

Mobile Web Application Development to Access to Psychiatric Electronic Health Records

Isabel de la Torre Díez, Míriam Antón-Rodríguez
and Francisco J. Díaz-Pernas
University of Valladolid
Spain

1. Introduction

Mobile communication systems in clinical routine have the potential to greatly improve communication, facilitate healthcare information access (e.g. to Electronic Health Records (EHRs)), and increase the quality of patient attention (Ammenwerth, et al., 2000). Even more important with the advantage of mobility in the pocket, patients and physicians are able to carry with them their personal health records as they move across states or countries. Mobile health management seeks to extend the benefits of mobility to patients who are geographically mobile (Chan, 2000), but the development and use of mobile devices in health care is still rare; studies evaluating prototypes have revealed that the acceptance of such tools was rather low, although physicians principally would like to use a mobile EHR system (Reusss, et al., 2004). Mobile EHRs with high usability as outlined here would make a substantial contribution to reach this aim. Moreover, the development of mobile medical information systems is having significant impact on remote medical monitoring, home healthcare, outpatient service, and patient safety making healthcare more flexible and convenient. Mobile medical care services are gradually spreading in hospitals and with the maturity of mobile technology, the time has come for employing mobile healthcare in different school-based health centers (Jen, 2009).

In this context, EHRs system contains information about the type of treatment that a patient has received from a healthcare provider, such as the patient's medical history, etc. They are not just record-keeping tools but also play an important role in quality improvement and data exchange (Esper, et al., 2010). One major barrier to the adoption of such systems is the concern that EHRs may take longer for physicians to use than paper-based systems (Pizziferri, 2005). But, as the authors showed, EHRs did not require additional physician time during a primary care clinic session. Moreover, an EHR is a fundamental part of health information technology and its use is growing quickly. It can be defined as a set of relevant patient data stored in digital format that allows adequate medical assistance delivered to the patient even in different places and scenarios (Furuie, et al., 2007). It can be organized either on a document-based backbone, or on a structured database system. EHRs system fall under the purview of health informatics. It is a combination of computation, computer science and medical record keeping. In recognizing the advantages of EHRs, health information systems are being rapidly deployed. Some recent technological advances have enabled the introduction of an important number of e-health applications in healthcare computing (Hung and Zhang, 2003). Moreover, EHRs are increasingly being implemented by care providers in order to streamline processes and improve quality of care (Edwards, et al., 2008). Some potential advantages of an EHR over a traditional paper-based patient record involve: distributed and simultaneous access, fast information retrieval, better quality, high availability, higher confidence, etc. (Furuie, et al., 2007). In spite of these advantages, there are several barriers to their adoption such as training, costs, complexity and lack of a national standard for interoperability (Gans, et. al, 2006).

Hence, a crucial question is the standardization, it is a very important aspect to exchange health information as it allows the integration of different healthcare services and it facilitates clinical trials. There are several international organizations concerned with EHR standardization, and the Health Level 7 (HL7) authority is influencing in this process. Its development has also been of great benefit in telemedicine applications. The standard proposed by HL7 is employed for many different medical environments. It is the XML-based international standard more commonly-held for storing and exchanging EHRs. HL7 Document is intended to be the basic unit of a document-oriented EHR. According to HL7 standard, there are mobile clinical information systems which use HL7 to integrate the patient data (Choi, et al., 2006). In May 2005, Clinical Document Architecture (CDA) Release 2 became an ANSI-approved HL7 Standard. A CDA document is a defined as a complete information object that can include text, images, and other multimedia contents (Dolin, et al., 2006). Extensive use of HL7/CDA standard is very desirable for all fields present in medicine (Marcheschi, et al., 2004).

Moreover, EHRs systems are subjected to security and privacy issues. This is crucial in EHRs since they involve very important private data, as important as banking information. Slamanig & Stingl (2010) defined security and piracy objectives and explain that they play an important role in the context of Web-based EHRs. Since it is considered that current deployed solutions present clear weaknesses in terms of security, it is explained that a holistic system, whose functionalities cover all the aspects of EHRs, can overcome the drawbacks of already existing solutions. Many studies conclude that in order to obtain the full potential of EHRs, patients should be able to access them anywhere and anytime (Sadan, 2001). This can be achieved by making EHRs portable, turning them into Personal Health Records (PHRs); a solution is to keep PHRs in portable storage media, such as USB flash drives. This portability adds an additional mobility feature whose security needs to be covered; it is necessary to prevent the data from being exposed.

In this paper, we present a mobile Web application, EHRmobile, to store and exchange EHRs in the Psychiatric field. It has been built using Java Servlet and Java Server Pages (JSP) technologies. Its architecture is triple-layered and EHRs are stored in the open-source XML database, eXist 1.2.6, according to HL7/CDA Release 2 standard. We chose this database according to the results shown in (De la Torre, et al., 2010a). EHRmobile verifies the standards related to privacy and confidentiality. Nowadays, the application has been tested by specialists from Fundación Intras, Spain, managing records from 87 patients with cognitive disabilities from Castilla y León (Spain).

The remainder of this paper is organized as follows. Section 2 presents related works, Section 3 describes the methodology to develop the platform, Section 4 focuses on the results achieved (EHRmobile platform), and Section 5 presents conclusions and future work.

2. Related works

Accessing to EHRs through mobile devices provides a number of advantages both for health centers and clinical staff, and for patients. Among these advantages are: accessing to patients' information in real time (from wherever and whenever), resource savings, improving the information management, and reducing the delay in health care. In the field of mental health, there are important epidemiological studies releasing relevant information about types and rates of the more frequent disorders. However, a significant number of people with mental diseases remain unnoticed due to the incorrect identification of the symptomatology, the resistance to seek either help or information regarding these services, among others. Mobile technologies can offer their full potential for helping people with cognitive problems and their supporting staff.

Healthcare organizations are increasingly implementing EHRs and other related health information technology. Even in organizations which have long adopted these computerized systems, their employees continue to rely on paper to complete their work (Saleem, et al., 2009). EHR systems have a great potential to improve safety, quality and efficiency in medicine. Previous studies addressing this issue have been done in primary care (Lo et al., 2007).

Before launch effort on developing a system, we performed a deep analysis about web-based EHR systems in specialties like pediatrics (Ginsburg, 2007), urgency (Amouh, et al., 2005), oncology (James, et al., 2001), etc. In the telematic system for oncology, they used a data warehouse as EHR server however the authors did not present an EHR standardization process. Information system for emergency department has been implemented by prototyping a web-based application which makes use of the XML-based openEHR standard. There are other web applications, like CareWeb™, using the HL7 standard (Halamka, et al., 1999). Becker & Sewell (2004) presented an EHR system, InfoDOM, based on web technologies. Siika et al. (2005) described the development and structure of an EHR system for patients with Human Immunodeficiency Virus (HIV) in Kenya. Cho & Park (2003) developed an EHR system based on the Korean beta version of the International Classification for Nursing Practice (ICNP). The system was evaluated by 20 nurses and 57 patients, in 2 Korean hospitals. Karagiannis et al. (2007) implemented a web-based EHR system (pEHR) that was proven by 22 physicians and 150 patients of 3 European hospitals. The system was developed to meet the needs of patients with a congenital heart disease, Parkinson or type 2 Diabetes. Sharda et al., (2006) studied the use of discharge summaries by psychiatrists with experts being given two hypothetical emergency care scenarios with narrative discharge summaries and being asked to verbalize their clinical assessment. The narratives were presented in a more structured form. Other EHRs systems are: PHIMS and CipherMe. PHIMS is a web-based repository of patient health information, which provides interfaces for storing structured and categorized patient information (Kim, 2006). CipherMe architecture enables individual entities to store private information about themselves and to manage access to selected items by other parties (Hansen, 2006). Other authors designed and developed a template based system, called Julius. This system was integrated with existing EHR systems (Chen, 2007). The system has been implemented, tested and deployed to three health care units in Stockholm, Sweden. In the application OpenSDE, authors have expanded the traditional row modeling methodology with additional columns to allow structured representation of medical narrative (Los, 2004). In the EHRs system context, Electronic Medical Records (EMRs) are currently being implemented in psychiatric hospitals throughout Europe (Boyer, et al., 2009a; Boyer, et al., 2009b; Boyer, et al., 2011).

Taking a look at the international scenario, it can be determined that EHRs are not equally adopted in all countries. Whereas the United States and Canada are the most advanced countries in EHRs integration, in other such as Spain EHRs are not that widespread (Dorr, et al., 2007; Srinivasan, et al., 2007; Cheong, et al., 2009). The authors of the present work accomplished a web-system for ophthalmological EHRs and medical images management, TeleOftalWeb (De la Torre, et al., 2010a; De la Torre, et al., 2010b). This system is in used in the the Institute of Applied Ophthalmobiology (Instituto de Oftalmobiología Aplicada, IOBA) of the University of Valladolid, Spain. TeleOftalWeb complies with the Health Level 7-Clinical Document Architecture Release 2.0 (HL7-CDA) standard for EHRs storage.

Mobile applications offer a chance to improve health services. Most healthcare providers offer mobile service for their medical staff; and few healthcare providers supply mobile service as part of their outpatient service (Jen, et al., 2007). Nowadays there are few applications integrating mobile communications with EHRs. Velde & Brobbel (2001) developed a mobile information system intended for cardiology field. Shyu et al. (2006) performed a mobile EHR system for the family medicine department in the National Taiwan University Hospital (NTUH) from Taiwan. Chan (2000) examines the important need to implement mobile health management systems providing continuous health care delivery even while an individual is on the move. In senSAVE project, authors developed a mobile system for monitoring vital parameters. The user interface and the interaction were specifically adapted to the needs of the elderly. In this paper they described the development of the system and the outcome of an evaluation (Lorenz & Oppermann, 2009).

In Spain, the Health Department (Conselleria de Sanitat) from the Community of Valencia allows the opportunity to access to the personal health record through its website, downloading the record updated and ciphered. Hence, patients can be better assisted out of the region. Nevertheless, some barriers still exist to achieve the extended use of this kind of systems: many EHR systems are still in a consolidation phase; information is not shared among different health systems. There is uncertainty in issues related to security and data protection.

3. Methodology

3.1 System overview

EHRmobile is a mobile Web system for performing a complete management of EHRs of patients with mental disabilities providing two different ways of access depending on the device in use, a desktop web and a mobile web. It includes the capability of interoperability with other systems thanks to the use of the standard HL7/CDA Release 2, specifically the version provided by the Department of Health from Castilla y León (Spain) (Consejería de Sanidad, 2010). Fig. 1 shows the schema of the EHRmobile system. It has got three layers: presentation, business and database.

- **Presentation layer.** This layer includes the graphic interface utilized by the user to access the system through the browser. The type of device used is detected to provide the appropriate design and features, when accessing the system either via PC or mobile device. Accessing from a PC allows the complete management of the system, while accessing from a mobile device provides functionalities for browsing and updating clinical data along with additional features related to the terminals used, and always prioritizing information security and privacy. For example, accessing from PC, it is possible to add new EHRs, search in them, update, and delete them. Using a mobile device, data can be consulted, updating those needed, always interacting with a user-friendly interface, considering the possibilities of the device.

- **Business layer.** This layer accomplishes the processing required for attending the user requests, hence, it includes all the system logic, completely developed under JSP using Apache Tomcat 6.0 Web server. This layer has been divided into different modules according to their functionalities:

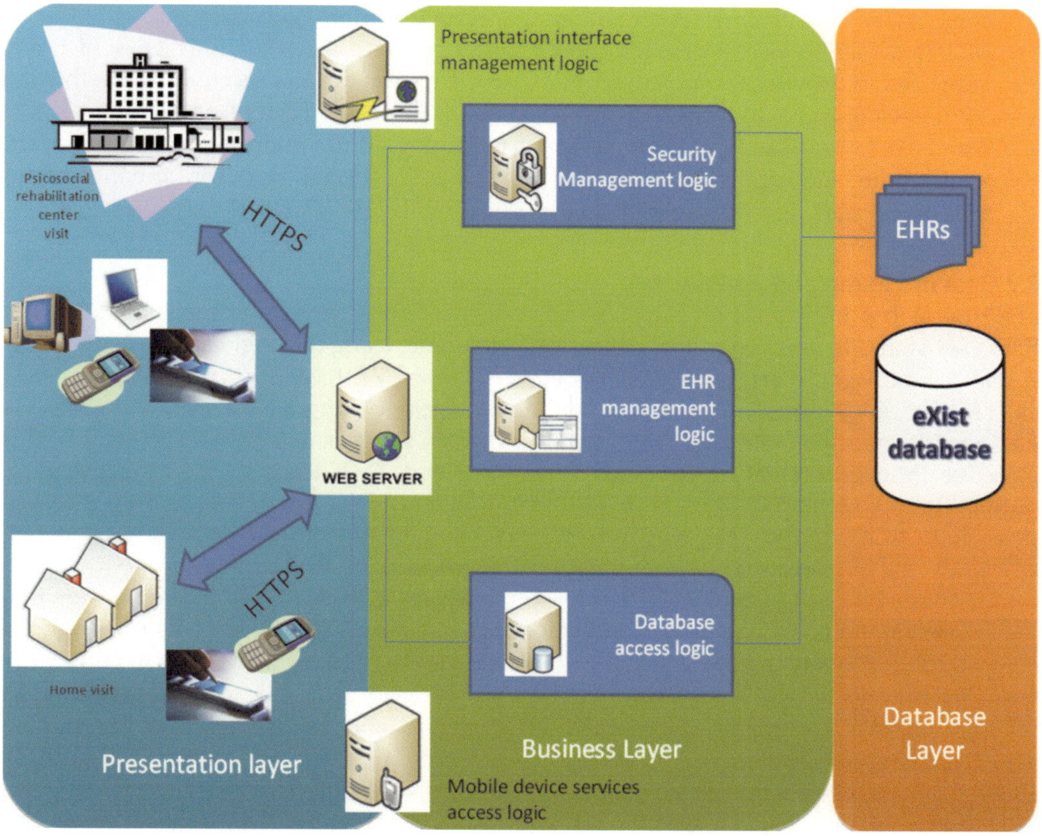

Fig. 1. Shema of EHRmobile.

- Security management logic: Among the security measures taken are in this platform are: user identification determining a privilege level within the system, securing the communication established within the system, physical security. Personal identification is performed every time when trying to access the system, providing information according to the privilege level assigned to each user by Fundación Intras. In order to provide communications security we use OpenSSL, which implements the Secure Socket Layer (SSL) protocol. All the system communications use the Hypertext Transfer Protocol over Secure Socket Layer (HTTPS) protocol which includes a SSL based ciphering.
- Presentation interface management logic: It undertakes the task of detecting the device requesting access to the system in order to show the interface better fitting its features. As it was previously said, detecting the device is not only important at design level providing a more compact and light web to the mobile terminal, but also at a functionality level, as from a desktop browser it is possible to access to the entire application, allowing inserting new EHRs, delete them, and administration the system.

- EHR management logic: It is the module in charge of standardizing the EHRs observing the standard HL7/CDA.
- Database access logic: It is the module in charge of performing the database (eXist) accessing. Database includes all the information required about patients such as: anamnesis, clinical observation, medication, and clinical appraisal. Moreover, it contains data about clinical staff and system administration information.
- Mobile device services access logic: As HTML5 standard is not yet finished, which it is supposed to provide a complete accessing to the mobile devices services. Meanwhile, to complete the access to the camera, we used Adobe® Flash®, JQuery, and JSP.

- **Database layer.** This layer is in charge of managing all the information in a persistent way, storing and supplying the data to the business layer. It includes information about the clinical staff, and the complete EHRs following the HL7/CDA Release 2 standard.

3.2 Data modeling and architecture

EHRmobile has been built on Java Servlet and Java Server Pages (JSP) technologies. The EHRs are stored in an open source native XML database, using the engine eXist 1.2.6. In Fig. 2, the web manager interface for eXist database is shown. We have different collections such as "records" and "users". One of the main advantages of using a XML native database is data format interoperability and the interface for data input is determinant to achieve this objective (Mabanza, et al., 2006). Combining Java and XML leads to the attractive dual portability of code and data (Fan, et. al, 2005). Wherever Java programs can run, it is also possible to access to the XML files, this enables Java and XML information to interoperate efficiently and effectively on different platforms (Fedyukin, et. al, 2002).

Furthermore, HL7/CDA uses XML and has three different levels of granularity as shown in Table 1, where each level iteratively adds more markups to clinical documents, although the clinical content remains constant at all levels (Eichelberg, M, et. al, 2006). A HL7/CDA structure may include texts, sounds, pictures and all kind of multi-media contents; it can refer to external documents, procedures, observations, and acts. It includes information about authors, authenticators, custodians, participants, patients, and so on (Treins et al. 2006). The HL7/CDA used format in EHRmobile is shown in Fig. 3.

CDA specification prescribes XML markup for CDA Documents: CDA instances must valid against the CDA Schema and may be subject to additional validation. Its development methodology is a continuously evolving process that looks forward to carry out specifications that facilitate interoperability between different healthcare systems. There is a Document Type Definition (DTD), CDA Level One, for all types of clinical documents. A HL7-CDA document is comprised of a header, referred to as the CDA Header, and a body, which at CDA Level One is referred to as the CDA Level One Body. A CDA Level One schema is shown in Fig. 4. CDA Level One is specified by three components:

- **CDA Header.** It identifies and classifies the document and provides information on the document authenticator, the patient, the encounter, provider and other service actors. Document-related information includes the id, set id, version, type, and various timestamps. The id element uniquely identifies the specific clinical document. The type and version elements identify the clinical document template. Encounter data include the id, code, timestamps, service location and local header. The id and code elements uniquely identify the relevant encounter and its type in the regional network, while attribute-value pairs in the local header facilitate interoperability with the EHR system (Paterson, et al., 2002)..

- **CDA Level One Body.**
- **Reference Information Model (RIM) data type DTD.** RIM data type DTD is an XML implementation of the abstract data type specification. It used by both the CDA and the HL7 Version 3 message specifications.

CDA R1	CDA Level One
	CDA Level Two
	CDA Level Three
CDA R2	Unconstrained CD specification
	CDA specification with section-level templates applied
	CDA specification with entry-level templates applied

Table 1. Levels of document granularity in CDA R1 and CDA R2.

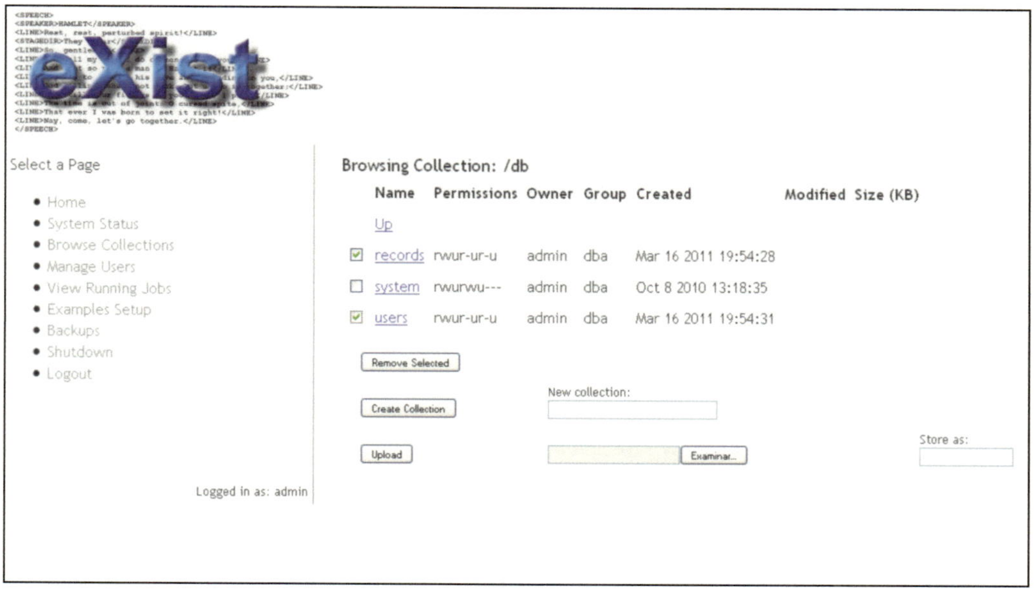

Fig. 2. Web manager interface in eXist database in EHRmobile application.

```
<?xml-stylesheet type="text/xsl" href="cda.xsl"?>
<ClinicalDocument xmlns="urn:hl7-org:v3" xmlns:voc="urn:hl7-org:v3/voc"
    xmlns:xsi="http://www.w3.org/2001/XMLSchema-instance"
    xsi:schemaLocation="urn:hl7-org:v3 xsd/CDA.xsd">
    <typeId root="2.16.840.1.113883.1.3" extension="POCD_HD000040"/>
    <id root="8694706b-7f87-4928-b190-85ab95ef700b" extension="2406538"/>
    <code code="28634-4" codeSystem="2.16.840.1.113883.6.1" codeSystemName="LOINC"
        displayName="OID de LOINC a nivel mundial"/>
    <title>INFORME GENERAL DE ALTA</title>
    <effectiveTime value="200802221250"/>
    <confidentialityCode code="N" codeSystem="2.16.840.1.113883.5.25"/>
    <languageCode code="es-ES"/>
    <recordTarget>
        <patientRole>
            <id root="91e8b514-6eea-48e6-86ce-63cfce67a96b" extension="56864"/>
            <addr>
                <streetAddressLine>FERMOSELLE</streetAddressLine>
                <city>CALLE GENERAL SANJURJO</city>
                <state>ZAMORA</state>
                <postalCode>49220</postalCode>
            </addr>
            <patient>
                <realmCode code="5/140665/4" codeSystem="6fdf0743-4fd5-4921-9a34-
24298b2941eb"
                    codeSystemName="OID de la tarjeta sanitaria a nivel comunitario"/>
                <name>
                    <given>ANTONIO</given>
                    <family>DE LA TORRE</family>
                    <family>PUENTE</family>
                </name>
                <administrativeGenderCode code="F" codeSystem="2.16.840.1.113883.5.1"/>
                <birthTime value="19440708"/>
            </patient>
            <providerOrganization>
                <id extension="0501" root="aea19799-c1a4-4a6b-a7c6-5ba778e2d29c"/>
                <name>Complejo Asistencial de Zamora</name>
                <telecom value="980548200"/>
                <telecom value="980512838"/>
                <addr>
                    <streetAddressLine>Avda. Requejo, 35</streetAddressLine>
                    <city>Zamora</city>
                    <state>Zamora</state>
                    <postalCode>49022</postalCode>
                </addr>
            </providerOrganization>
        </patientRole>
    </recordTarget>
    <author>
        <time value="200802221240"/>
    </author>
    <component>
        <structuredBody>
            <component>
                <section>
                    <code code="yyyyMMddHHmmss" codeSystem="HL7DATE" codeSystemName="Fecha"
                        displayName="Fecha ingreso"/>
                    <title>Fecha ingreso</title>
                    <text>20/01/2009 12:00</text>
                </section>
            </component>
            <component>
                <section>
                    <code code="yyyyMMddHHmmss" codeSystem="HL7DATE" codeSystemName="Fecha"
                        displayName="Fecha alta"/>
                    <title>Fecha alta</title>
                    <text>22/02/2009 00:00</text>
                </section>
            </component>
            <component>
                <section>
                    <code code="08675-1" codeSystem="LN"
                        codeSystemName="OID de LOINC a nivel mundial" displayName="Anamnesis"/>
                    <title>Anamnesis</title>
                    <text>Texto por defecto</text>
                </section>
            </component>
        </structuredBody>
    </component>
</ClinicalDocument>
```


Fig. 3. A part of EHR in CDA format in EHRmobile application.

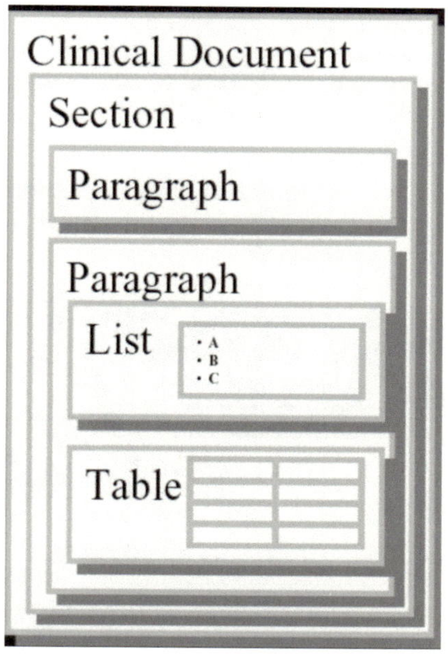

Fig. 4. CDA level one.

Fig. 5 shows the application architecture. The system is platform-independent thanks to the use of XML and Java technologies. XPath and XUpdate languages are used in communication with the used native XML database. XPath is employed to find information in an XML document. XUpdate makes heavy use of XPath for selecting a set of nodes to modify or remove them. The Java servlet inserts the record into the eXist database. It stores and indexes collections of XML documents both in native and mapped forms for highly efficient querying, transformation, and retrieval (Staken, 2001).

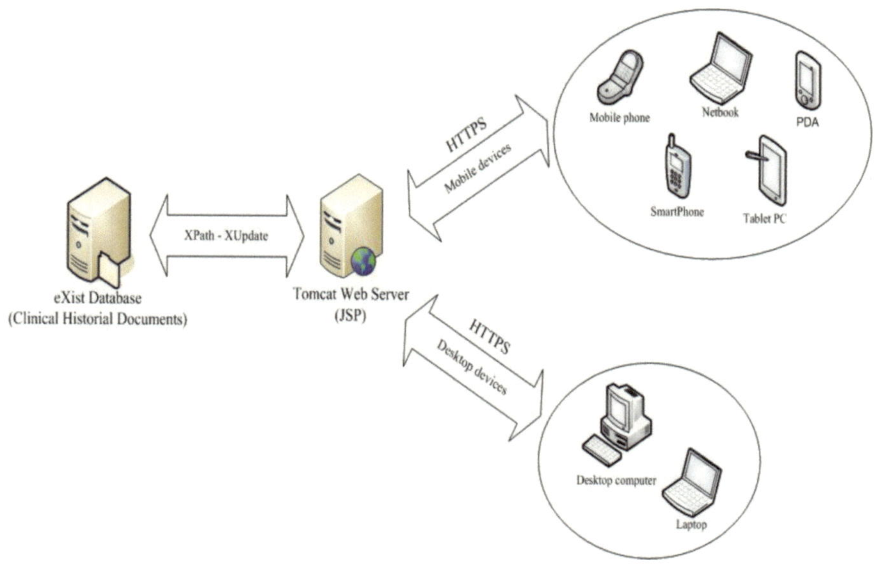

Fig. 5. EHRmobile Architecture.

4. Results

In this section, we present EHRmobile application (desktop and mobile version).

4.1 EHRmobile application

Fig. 6 (a) shows the interface to access to EHRmobile application from desktop version and Fig. 6 (b) from mobile version. All users have to introduce the login and password. The interface includes the following parts:

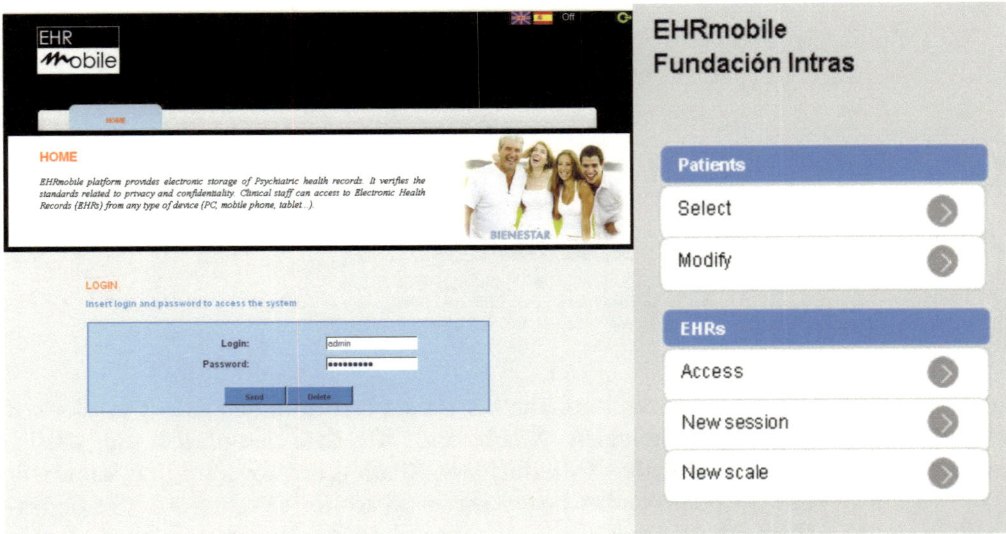

Fig. 6. (a) View from desktop version of platform. (b) View from mobile version of the platform.

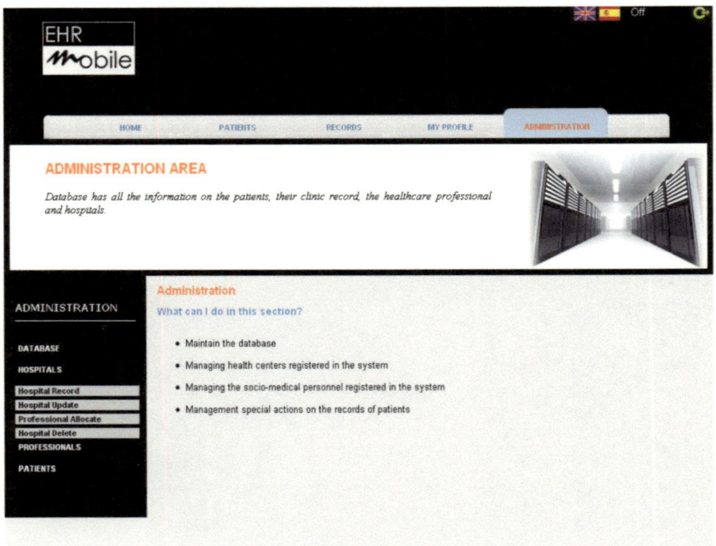

Fig. 7. Home view from desktop version of platform, manager profile.

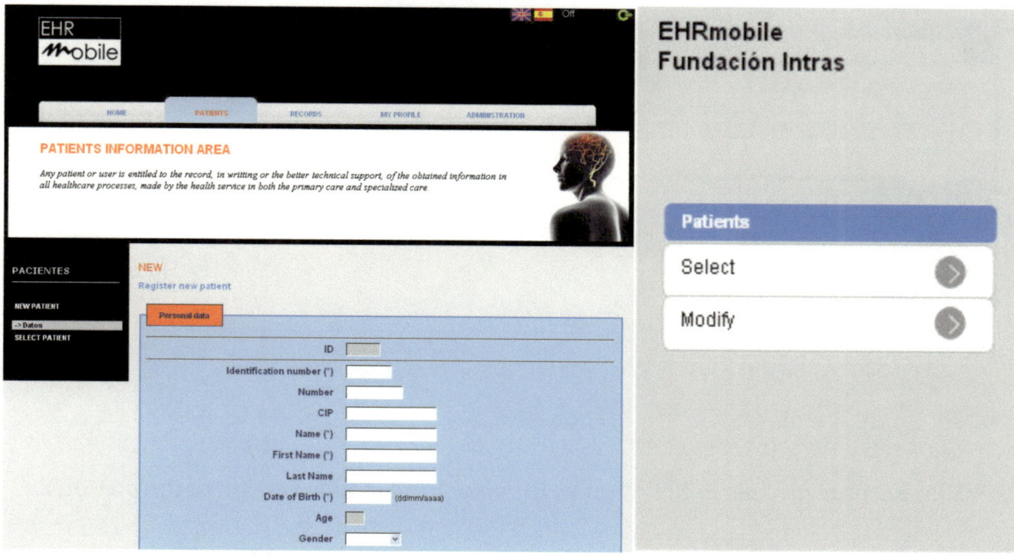

(a) (b)

Fig. 8. (a) Patients module in EHRmobile. (b) View from mobile version of EHRmobile.

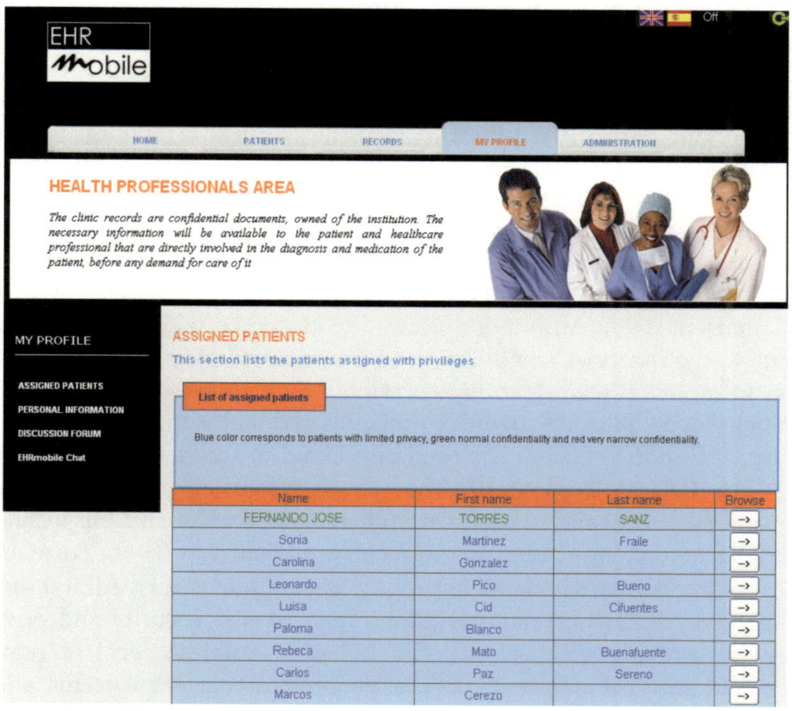

Fig. 9. My profile in EHRmobile.

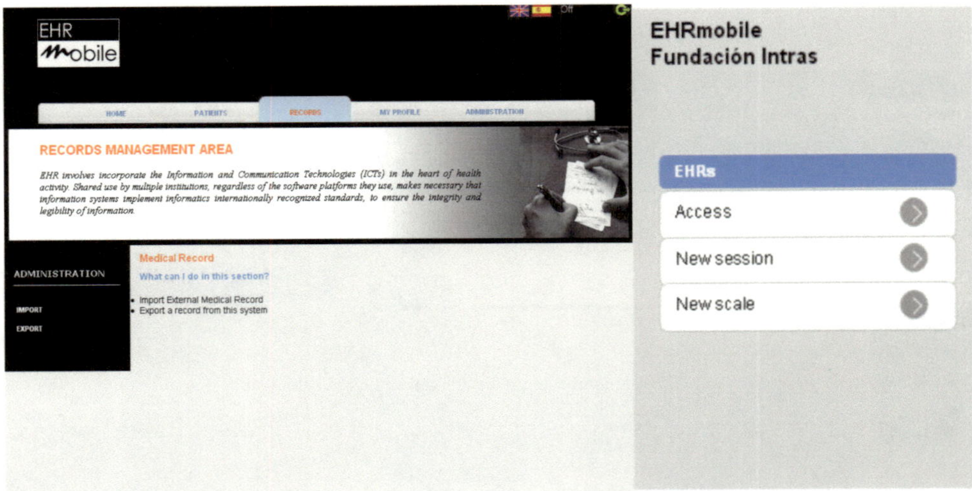

(a) (b)

Fig. 10. (a) Records module in EHRmobile. (b) View from mobile version of the platform.

5. Conclusions and future work

Nowadays, applying mobile technologies to health assistance may open new possibilities: better access to relevant information, counseling and cooperation among health professionals, and patient care assistance at home. However, these new facilities must inexorably include security and privacy information issues. Furthermore, the use of EHR management systems, specifically framed in the mental health field which suffers from an ever-expanding perspective, can mean an important support for improving both the treatment quality of these patients and the work quality of the socio-sanitary staff. EHRs will be an important part of the future of medical practice. Behavioral health treatment demands certain additions to the capabilities of a standard general medical EHRs system. An efficient and effective EHRs system will greatly assist the overall clinical enterprise in a number of important areas (Lawlor & Barrows, 2008). The employment of EHRs will contribute to continuity of care across organizations for the growing number of elderly and chronically ill people who need continuous nursing care after an episode of hospitalization (Helleso & Lorensen, 2005). An important number of people with mental diseases remain unnoticed due to the incorrect identification of the symptomatology, the resistance to seek either help or information regarding these services, etc. Mobile technologies can offer a full potential for helping people with cognitive problems and their supporting staff.

In this chapter, EHRmobile system has been developed to access to EHRs in Psychiatry by using HL7/CDA Release 2 standard. The whole system is implemented using open technologies and free software. It has been built on Java Servlet and JSP technologies. We employed eXist 1.2.6 database according to results published in (De la Torre, et al., 2010a, 2010b). It verifies the standards related to privacy and confidentiality. All transactions in the systems are secure. All EHRs systems require a high level of security and privacy control because they can provide great accessibility (whether wireless, local or remote) to the patients' personal medical information. The majority of current systems address these implications in a different form, and even different countries apply their unique policy to their respective e-Health systems. EHRs need to be robust without any open issue;

moreover, EHRs contain data that may decide the life of a person in a critical situation. Since people can attend different hospitals and suffer unpredictable illnesses, EHRs need to be available anywhere and anytime, but that implies more security and privacy.

In summary, we have developed a mobile Web application to store and share Psychiatric EHRs by using HL7/CDA. Our application tries to solve some of the barriers to the EHRs adoption in this speciality. It has several distinct advantages over paper health records. The records are continuously updated and are available concurrently for use everywhere. Nowadays, the system is on a trial basis with the final user (Fundación Intras), managing records from 87 patients with cognitive disabilities from Castilla y León (Spain). The possibility of accessing to the updated information of the patients in the house calls means an important benefit for the Fundación Intras's staff and so, for its patients. Nevertheless, some issues have emerged, like the accessibility to the system from a mobile device, as a usual complaint is to have to type the URL accessing the system and, then, the patient's name. At this point, we pretend to incorporate the QR codes to give access to the patient's information. Moreover, we are working in the process to get from the XML documents to PDF printable documents and statistics from the system.

The future extension of the system will include the integration with Gradior, the rehabilitation system used by Fundación Intras and a great deal of associated centers, so as the data about the patient and his/her rehabilitation sessions.

6. Acknowledgments

This research has been partially supported by the Department of Health, Government of Castile and Leon (Spain) under the project GES39/VA05/10 and the Spanish Ministry of Science and Innovation under the project TIN2010-20529.

7. References

Ammenwerth, E., Buchauer, A., Bludau, B., and Haux, R. (2000). Mobile information and communication tools in the hospital. International Journal of Medical Informatics, 57, pp. 21-40.

Amouh, T. et al. (2005). Versatile Clinical Information System Design for Emergency Departments. IEEE Transactions on Information Technology in Biomedicine, 9(2), pp. 174-183.

Becker, M.Y. and Sewell, P. (2004). Cassandra: flexible trust management, applied to electronic health records. Proceedings of 17th IEEE Computer Security Foundations Workshop, pp. 139-154.

Boyer, L., Renaud, M.H., Baumstarck-Barrau, K., Fieschi, M., Samuelian, J.C. (2009a) Establishment of an electronic medical record in a psychiatric hospital: evolution of professionals' perceptions. L'Ence´phale.

Boyer, L., Renaud, M.H., Limousin, S., Henry, J.M., Cai¨etta, P., Fieschi. M., et al. (2009b). Perception and use of an electronic medical record system by professionals of a public psychiatric hospital. L'Ence´phale, vol. 35, pp. 454–60.

Boyer, L., Baumstarck-Barrau, R., et al. (2011). Validation of a professionals' satisfaction questionnaire with electronic medical records (PSQ-EMR) in psychiatry.European Psychiatry, vol. 26, pp. 78–84.

Chan, A. (2000). WWW_smart card: towards a mobile health care management system, International Journal of Medical Informatics, 57, pp. 127–137.

Chen, R., Enberg, G. and Klein, G. (2007). Julius--a template based supplementary electronic health record system, BMC Medical Informatics and Decision Making, pp. 7-10.

Cheong, N.Y. et al. (2009). Improving Korean Service Delivery System in Health Care: Focusing on National E-health System. International Conference on eHealth, Telemedicine, and Social Medicine, pp. 263-268.

Cho, I. and Park H. (2003). Development and evaluation of a terminology-based electronic nursing record system. Journal of Biomedical Informatics, 36(4), pp. 304-312.

Choi, J., Yoo, S., Park, H. and Chun, J. (2006) MobileMed: A PDA-Based Mobile Clinical Information System, IEEE Transactions on Information Technology in Biomedicine, vol. 10, 3, pp. 627-635.

Consejería de Sanidad, Junta de Castilla y León (2010). Estándares de integración HL7. http://www.salud.jcyl.es/sanidad/cm/empresas/tkContent?idContent=500929 &locale=es_ES&textOnly=false. Last visited: November, 2010.

De la Torre-Díez, I. et al. (2010a). Choosing the most efficient database for a Web-based system to store and exchange Ophthalmologic Health Records. Journal of Medical Systems. (In press). DOI: 10.1007/s10916-009-9422-2.

De la Torre-Díez, I. et al. (2010b). Performance evaluation of a Web-based system to exchange Electronic Health Records using queueing model (M/M/1). Journal of Medical Systems. (In press). DOI: 10.1007/s10916-010-9555-3.

Dolin, R.H., Alschuler, L., Boyer, S., Beebe, C., Behlen, F.M., Biron, P.V., and Shabo, A. (2006). HL7 Clinical Document Architecture, Release 2, Journal of the American Medical Informatics Association, 13(1), pp. 30-39.

Dorr, D. et al. (2007). Informatics Systems to Promote Improved Care for Chronic Illness: A Literature Review. Journal of the American Medical Informatics Association, 4,, pp. 156-163.

Edwards, P.J., Moloney, K.P., Jacko, J.A., Sainfort, F. (2008). Evaluating usability of commercial electronic health record: A case study. International Journal of Human-Computer Studies, 66(10), pp. 718-728.

Eichelberg, M., Aden T., Riesmeier J., Dogac A., Laleci G. (2006) Electronic Health Record Standards - A Brief Overview, 4th International Conference on Information and Communications Technology (ICICT 2006), Cairo, Egypt

Esper, G.J., Drogan, O., Henderson, W.S., Becker, A., Avitzur, O., Hier, D.B. (2010). Health Information Technology and Electronic Health Records in Neurologic Practice. Neurologic Clinics, 28 (2), pp. 411-42.

Fan, R. Ceded, L., Toser, O. (2005), Java plus XML: a powerful new combination for SCADA systems, Computing & Control Engineering Journal, 16, pp. 27-30.

Fedyukin, I., Reviakin, Y.G., Orlov, O.I., Doarn, C.R., Harnett, D.M. and Merrell, R.C. (2002). Experience in the application of Java Technologies in telemedicine," eHealth International, 1(3), pp. 1-6.

Furuie, S.S., Rebelo. M.S., Moreno, R.A., Santos, M., Bertozzo, N., Mota, G., Pires, F.A. Gutierrez, M.A (2007). Managing Medical Images and Clinical Information: InCor's Experience. IEEE Transactions on Information Technology in Biomedicine, 11(1), pp. 17-24.

Gans, D., Kralewski, J., Hammons, T. and Dowd, B. (2006). Medical groups' adoption of electronic health records and information systems. Health affairs (Project Hope), 24(5), pp. 1323-1333.

Ginsburg, M. (2007). Pediatric Electronic Health Record Interface Design: The PedOne System. Proceedings of the 40th Hawaii International Conference on System Sciences, pp. 1-10.

Halamka, J. D. et al. (1999). CareWeb™, a web-based medical record for an integrated health care delivery system. International Journal of Medical Informatics, 54, pp. 1–8.

Hansen, I.B. (2006). CipherMe: personal Electronic Health Records in the hands of patients-owners, Proceedings of the 1st Distributed Diagnosis and Home Healthcare (D2H2) Conference, pp. 148-151.

Helleso, R., Lorensen, M. (2005). Inter-organizational continuity of care and the electronic patient record: A concept development. International Journal of Nursing Studies, 42(7), pp. 807-822.

Hung, K. and Zhang, Y. (2003) Implementation of a WAP-Based Telemedicine System for Patient Monitoring. IEEE Transactions on Information Technology in Biomedicine, vol. 7, 2, pp. 101-107.

James, A. et al. (2001). A Telematic System for Oncology Based on Electronic Health and Patient Records. IEEE Transactions on Information Technology in Biomedicine, 2(1), pp. 16-17.

Jen, W.Y., Chao, C.C., Hung, M.C., Li, YC., Chi, Y.P. (2007). Mobile information and communication in the hospital outpatient service. International Journal of Medical Informatics, 76(8), pp. 565-574.

Jen, W.Y. (2009). Mobile healthcare services in school-based health center, International Journal of Medical Informatics, vol. 78, pp. 425-434.

Kaplan HI, Sadock BJ. (1998). Clinical examination of the psychiatric patient. Synopsis of psychiatry. 8th ed. Baltimore, Maryland: Williams and Wilkins, pp. 240–74.

Karagiannis, G. E. et al. (2007). Web-based personal health records: the personal electronic health record (pEHR) multicentred trial. Journal of Telemedicine and Telecare, 13, 32-34.

Kim, E.H. (2006). Web-based Personal-Centered Electronic Health Record for Elderly Population," Proceedings of the 1st Distributed Diagnosis and Home Healthcare (D2H2) Conference, pp. 144-147.

Lawlor, T., Barrows, E. (2008). Behavioral Health Electronic Medical Record. Psychiatric Clinics of North America, 31(1), pp. 95-103.

Lo, HG., Newmark, L.P., Yoon, C., Volk, L.A., Carlson, V.L., Kittler, A.F., Lippincott, M., Wang, T. and Bates, D.W. (2007). Electronic Health Records in Specialty Care: A Time-Motion Study, Journal of the American Medical Informatics Association, 14(5), pp. 609-615.

Lorenz, A, Oppermann, R. (2009).Mobile health monitoring for the elderly: Designing for diversity, Pervasive and Mobile Computing, 5, pp. 478-495.

Los, R., van Ginneken, A.M., de Wilde, M. and. van der Lei, J. (2004). OpenSDE: Row Modeling Applied to Generic Structured Data Entry, Journal of the American Medical Informatics Association, 11, pp. 162-165.

Mabanza, N., Chadwick, J., & Rao, G.S.V.R. (2006). Performance Evaluation of Open Source Native XML databases. University of Fort Hare, Alice, South Africa.

Marcheschi, P., Mazzarisi, A., Dalmiani, S. and Benassi, A. (2004) HL7 clinical document architecture to share cardiological images and structured data in next generation, Computers in Cardiology, pp. 617-620.

Paterson, G.I., Shepherd, M., Wang, X., Watters, C., Zitner, D. (2002) Using the XML-based Clinical Document Architecture for Exchange of Structured Discharge Summaries. In Proceedings of the 35th Hawaii International Conference on System Sciences, pp. 119-128.

Pizziferri, L. (2005). Primary care physician time utilization before and after implementation of an electronic health record: A time-motion study, Journal of Biomedical Informatics, 38, pp. 176-188.

Reusss, E., Menozzi, M., Büchi, M., Koller, J., Krueger, H. (2004). Information access at the point of care: what can we learn for designing a mobile CPR system?, International Journal of Medical Informatics, vol. 73, pp. 363-369.

Sadan, B. (2001). Patient data confidentiality and patient rights. International Journal of Medical Informatics, 62, pp. 41–49.

Saleem, J.J., Russ, A.L., Justice, C.F., Hagg, H., Ebright, P.R., Woodbrigde, P.A., Doebbeling, B.N. (2009). Exploring the persistence of paper with the electronic health record. International Journal of Medical Informatics, 78(9), pp. 618-628.

Sharda, P., Das, A.K., Cohen, T.A., Patel, V. (2006). Customizing clinical narratives for the electronic medical record interface using cognitive methods. International Journal of Medical Informatics, 75(5), pp. 346-368.

Shyu, F. et al., (2006). Context-based Model for Mobile Electronic Medical Records. Proceeding of the eighth international conference on e-Health networking , application and services, 140-146.

Siika, A. M. et al. (2005). An electronic medical record system for ambulatory care of HIV-infected patients in Kenya. International Journal of Medical Informatics, 74(5), pp. 345-355.

Slamanig, D., Stingl, C. (2010) Electronic Health Records: An Enhanced Security Paradigm to Preserve Patient's Privacy. Communications in Computer and Information Science, 52(4), pp. 369-380.

Srinivasan, G. et al. (2007). Personal Health Record (PHR) in a Talisman. International Conference on e-Health Networking, Application and Services, pp. 277-279.

Staken, K. (2001). Introduction to Native XML Databases. Retrieved November 15, 2010, from http://www.xml.com

Treins, M., Curé, O., Salzano, G. (2006) On the interest of using HL7 CDA release 2 for the exchange of annotated medical documents, Proceedings of the 19th IEEE Symposium on Computer-Based Medical Systems (CBMS'06), pp. 524-532

Velde, E.T. et al. (2001). Application of Handheld Computers for Mobile Access to a Cardiology Information System. Computers in Cardiology, 28, 157-160.

11

Clinical Psychology and Medicine for the Treatment of Obesity in Out-patient Settings: the TECNOB Project

Gianluca Castelnuovo[1,2], Gian Mauro Manzoni[1,3], Stefania Corti[1], Paola Cuzziol[1,2], Valentina Villa[1] and Enrico Molinari[1,2]

[1] *Istituto Auxologico Italiano IRCCS, Psychology Research Laboratory Ospedale San Giuseppe, Verbania*

[2] *Department of Psychology, Catholic University of Milan, Milan*

[3] *Department of Psychology, University of Bergamo, Bergamo*

Italy

1. Introduction

In 2005, about 1.6 billion adults (above 15 years of age) were estimated to be overweight, whereas about 400 million people were obese. Obesity is a condition with such an increasing prevalence that it can be defined as a global epidemic. In 2015, approximately 2.3 billion adults will be overweight and more than 700 million will be obese (WHO, 2006). Obesity increases the risk of many health complications such as cardiovascular diseases, some types of cancer, osteoarthritis, hypertension, dyslipidemia, and hypercholesterolemia, and is associated with early death (Flegal, Graubard, Williamson, & Gail, 2005; Whitlock, et al., 2009). Obesity is a strong risk factor for the development of type 2 diabetes (Klein, et al., 2004a, 2004b). Indeed, as BMI (Body Mass Index) increases, the risk of developing type 2 diabetes increases in a "dose-dependent" manner (Colditz, et al., 1990; Must, et al., 1999). The prevalence of type 2 diabetes is 3–7 times higher in obese than in normal-weight adults, and those with a BMI >35 are 20 times more likely to develop type 2 diabetes than those with a BMI between 18.5 and 24.9 (Field, et al., 2001; Mokdad, et al., 2003).

Obesity-related medical complications weigh heavily on public health care costs and developing effective interventions for substantially reduce weight, maintain weight loss and prevent or manage associated diseases like type 2 diabetes in cost-effective manner is a priority.

Stand-alone and combined treatment options (dietetic, nutritional, physical, behavioral, cognitive-behavioral, pharmacological, surgical) are available, but clinical practice and research have shown significant difficulties with regard to availability, costs, treatment adherence and long-term efficacy (Weinstein, 2006). These procedures imply high costs both for the obese individuals and the public health system, overall within an enduring care setting. Indeed, the main challenge in the treatment of obesity is to maintain weight loss in the long term (Hill, Thompson, & Wyatt, 2005). Most overweight and obese individuals regain about one third of the weight lost with treatment within 1 year, sometimes even before the end of the intervention, and they are typically back to baseline in 3 to 5 years (Jeffery, et al., 2000; Katan, 2009; Wing, Tate, Gorin, Raynor, & Fava, 2006). Similarly, few

patients with diabetes go on taking their prescribed medication entirely as intended (Dale, Caramlau, Docherty, Sturt, & Hearnshaw, 2007; Donnan, MacDonald, & Morris, 2002).
Continuous and cost-effective approaches that can reach a large number of obese individuals are thus needed. A new promising method for granting continuity of care to wide populations of patients at low costs is telemedicine and its more specific branches called "e-therapy", "telecare" and "e-health": information and communication technologies (ICT) used in order to exchange information useful for the diagnosis, treatment, rehabilitation and prevention of diseases (Eysenbach, 2001; Pagliari, et al., 2005). Telecare can be carried out with tools such as web-sites, e-mail, chat lines, videoconference, telephone and mobile phones (Castelnuovo, Gaggioli, Mantovani, & Riva, 2003). As already indicated in several studies (Cline & Wong, 1999; Goulis, et al., 2004; Jeffery, et al., 2003; Maglaveras, et al., 2002; Rice, 2005) and in various reviews (Neve, Morgan, Jones, & Collins, 2009; Saperstein, Atkinson, & Gold, 2007; Weinstein, 2006), behavioral treatments delivered through the internet (web-site and e-mail) may be valid alternatives to reduce expensive and time-consuming clinical visits.

2. Clinical telepsychology and telemedicine for obesity

Nowadays Clinical Psychology has found a lot of different applications in traditional clinical settings (public and private hospitals, clinics, services, laboratories, etc.) and innovative clinical settings (remote outpatients' clinics, tele-health and e-health based settings). Medicine alone could be "a soul without psychology" (TIME magazine, Dec. 24, 1956) and so "in these times there is no medical area without a corresponding field in Clinical Psychology: psycho-cardiology, psych-oncology, psycho-geriatrics are only three examples of this significative spread of psychology into the clinical settings, traditionally limited to a bio-medical source" (p.1, Castelnuovo, 2010).
The Internet offers a novel delivery tool in clinical psychology for weight loss and weight loss maintenance interventions, with the potential to offer long-term intervention at a low cost, in comparison to traditional face-to-face treatments.
A recent systematic review has underlined the evidence on the effectiveness of internet-based interventions for weight loss and maintenance enhanced by professional feedback (Manzoni, Pagnini, Corti, Molinari, & Castelnuovo, 2011). Moreover, although Internet programs with counseling from a human therapist may make treatment more effective than automated e-counseling, developing technologies make virtual counselors possible.
Unfortunately studies that have been conducted up to date on this issue are very heterogeneous and furthermore no study has compared an internet based program with a "real" control group (Manzoni, et al., 2011).
About the cost of treatment delivery, only 2 studies of the 26 reviewed assessed cost-effectiveness of an internet-based intervention. Telemedicine applications for obesity would take into account the saving of additional costs through elimination of travel costs and travel time (Manzoni, et al., 2011; Rojas & Gagnon, 2008).
Up to now Internet and Telemedicine have offered a novel tool for weight loss and weight loss maintenance interventions with the potential to improve long-term intervention at low cost, in comparison to traditional face-to-face treatments (Ekeland, Bowes, & Flottorp, 2010; Khaylis, Yiaslas, Bergstrom, & Gore-Felton, 2010).
Khalys and colleagues identified five components that are considered crucial in facilitating weight loss in technology-based interventions (Khaylis, et al., 2010):

1. SELF-MONITORING: the process in which individuals regulate and keep track of their own behaviors and changes.
2. COUNSELOR FEEDBACK AND COMMUNICATION: the feedback from a professional therapist regarding goals, progress, and results.
3. SOCIAL SUPPORT: the group treatment modality that could be the preferred setting in behavioral weight-loss interventions.
4. STRUCTURED PROGRAM: the structured technology-based weight-loss interventions programs including principles of behavior therapy and change.
5. INDIVIDUALLY TAILORED PROGRAM: the interventions that have to be individually tailored to each participant characteristic

3. An application of telemedicine with clinical psychology in the treatment of obesity in out-patient settings: the TECNOB project

In order to determine which features of telemedicine and internet-based interventions are critical in a cost-effective approach, TECNOB project has been developed.

TECNOB (TEChNology for OBesity) Project is a comprehensive two-phase stepped down program enhanced by telemedicine for the medium-term treatment of obese people seeking intervention for weight loss (Castelnuovo, et al., 2011; Castelnuovo, et al., 2010). Its core features are the hospital-based intensive treatment (1-month), that consists of diet therapy, physical training and psychological counseling, and the continuity of care at home using new information and communication technologies (ICT) such as internet and mobile phones. The effectiveness of the TECNOB program compared with usual care (hospital-based treatment only) will be evaluated in a randomized controlled trial (RCT) with a 12-month follow-up. The primary outcome is weight in kilograms. Secondary outcome measures are energy expenditure measured using an electronic armband, glycated hemoglobin, binge eating, self-efficacy in eating and weight control, body satisfaction, healthy habit formation, disordered eating-related behaviors and cognitions, psychopathological symptoms and weight-related quality of life (Castelnuovo, et al., 2011; Castelnuovo, et al., 2010).

During the in-patient phase, participants attend an intensive four-week hospital-based and medically-managed program for weight reduction and rehabilitation. All patients are placed on a hypocaloric nutritionally balanced diet tailored to the individual after consultation with a dietitian (energy intake around 80% of the basal energy expenditure estimated according to the Harris-Benedict equation and a macronutrient composition of 16% proteins, 25% fat and 59% carbohydrates). Furthermore, they receive nutritional counseling provided by a dietitian, brief psychological counseling provided by a clinical psychologist and have physical activity training provided by a physiotherapist. Nutritional rehabilitation program aims to improve and promote change in eating habits and consists of both individual sessions (dietary assessment, evaluation of nutrient intake and adequacy, nutritional status, anthropometric, eating patterns, history of overweight, readiness to adopt change) and group sessions (45 minutes each twice a week) including: information on obesity and related health risks, setting of realistic goals for weight loss, healthy eating in general, general nutrition and core food groups, weight management and behavior change strategies for preventing relapse) (Castelnuovo, et al., 2011; Castelnuovo, et al., 2010).

Psychological counseling is provided once a week both individually and in group setting. Individual sessions, lasting 45 minutes each, are mainly based on the cognitive-behavioral approach described by Cooper and Fairburn and emphasize the techniques of self-monitoring, goal setting, time management, prompting and cueing, problem solving, cognitive restructuring, stress management and relapse prevention. Group sessions (small groups of 5/6 persons), lasting 1 hour each, focus on issues such as motivation to change, assertiveness, self-esteem, self-efficacy and coping. Developing a sense of autonomy and competence are the primary purposes of the in-hospital interventions. Patients are afforded the skills and tools for change and are supported in assigning positive values to healthy behaviors and also in aligning them with personal values and lifestyle patterns (Castelnuovo, et al., 2011; Castelnuovo, et al., 2010).

Physical activity takes place once a day except for week-end and consists of group programs (20 individuals) based on postural gymnastics, aerobic activity and walks in the open. Patients with specific orthopedic complications carry out individual activities planned by physiotherapists and articulated in programs of physical therapy, assisted passive and active mobilization and isokinetic exercise.

In the last week of hospitalization, just before discharge from the hospital, participants allocated to the TECNOB program are instructed for the out-patient phase. Firstly, they receive a multisensory armband (SenseWear® Pro3 Armband), an electronic tool that enables automated monitoring of total energy expenditure (calories burned), active energy expenditure, physical activity duration and levels (METs). Patients are instructed to wear this device on the back of the upper arm and to record data for 36 hours every two weeks in a free-living context. The Armband holds up to 12 days of continuous data which the outpatients are instructed to download into their personal computer and to transmit online to a web-site specifically designed for data storing. Outpatients are also told that they can review their progress using the SenseWear® 6.1 Software which analyzes and organizes data into graphs and reports. Secondly, participants are instructed to use the TECNOB web-platform, an interactive web-site developed by TELBIOS S.P.A. (http://www.telbios.it) (see Figure 1 and 2).

The TECNOB web-platform supports several functions and delivers many utilities, such as questionnaires, an animated food record diary, an agenda and a videoconference virtual room. In the "questionnaires" section, patients submit data concerning weight and glycated hemoglobin. In the "food record diary" participants submit actual food intake day by day through the selection of food images from a comprehensive visual database provided by METEDA S.P.A. (http://www.meteda.it). The same procedure is also possible through a software called METADIETA (Meteda s.p.a.) previously installed on the outpatients' mobile phones before discharge. Through the mobile phones outpatients maintain the contact with the dietitian who regularly sends them SMS containing syntax codes that METADIETA, the software previously installed into the outpatients' mobile phones, uses in order to visually display the food choices (frequency and portions) outpatients have to adhere according to dietary prescriptions (see Figure 3 and 4).

By this way, outpatients can keep a food record diary allowing comparisons between current eating and the recommended hypocaloric diet along the whole duration of the program. The "agenda" allows the patients to remember the videoconference appointments with the clinicians and the days when to fill in the questionnaires. Moreover, the patients can use the "memo" space to note down any important event occurred to him/her in the previous week/month. The clinical psychologist has thus the opportunity to discuss with the outpatients about the significant events reported in the "memo" space during the videoconference sessions and cognitively reconstruct dysfunctional appraisals in functional ways. Finally, outpatients are instructed to use the videoconference tool (see Figure 5).

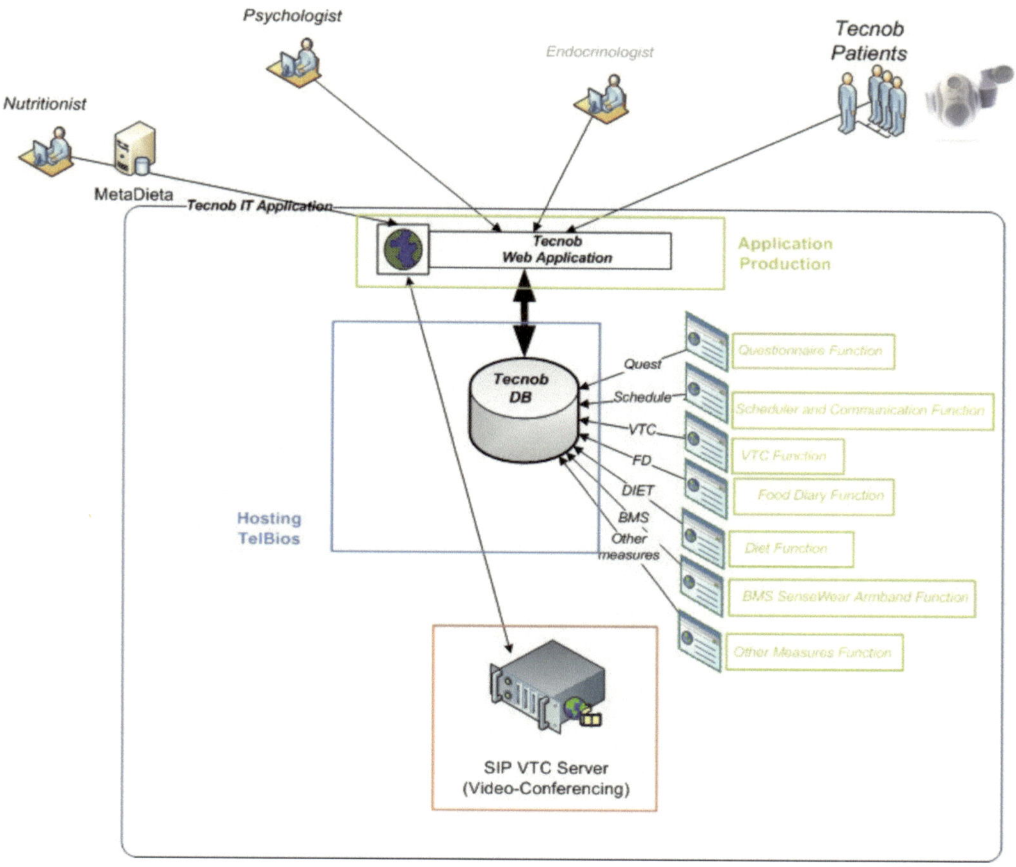

Fig. 1. The TECNOB Telemedicine Platform (devoloped by TELBIOS http://www.telbios.it)

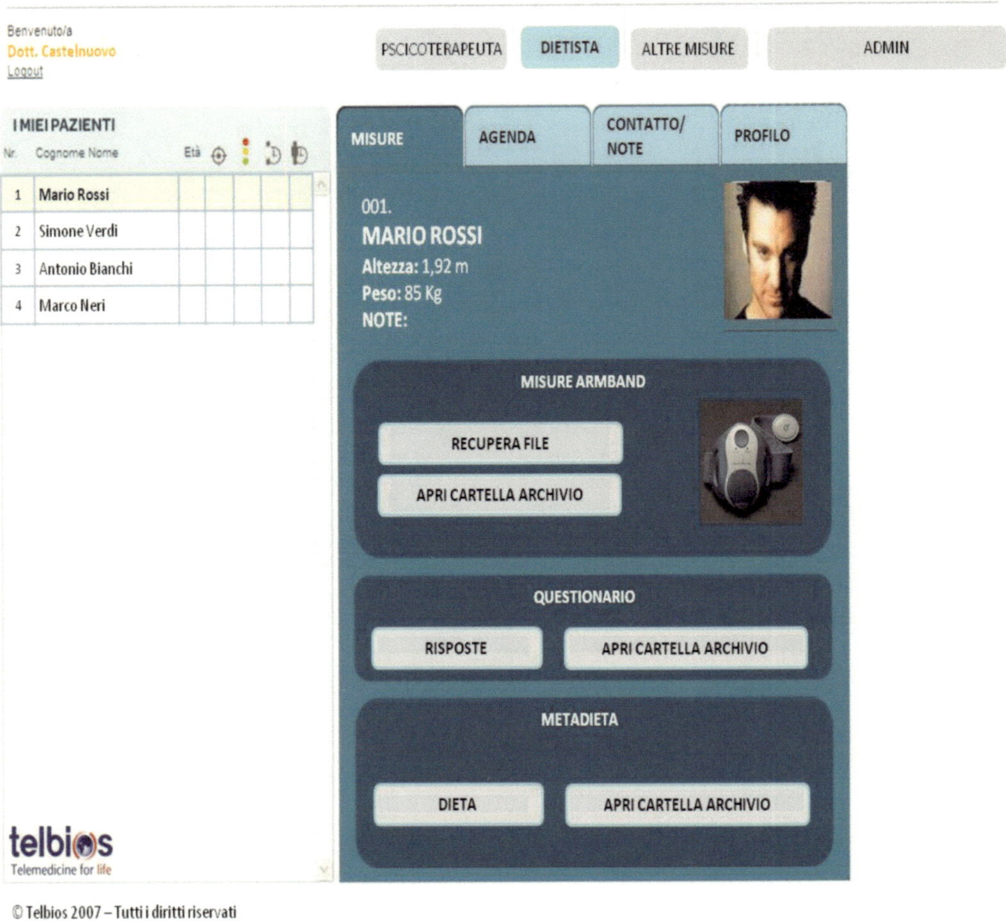

Fig. 2. A screenshot of the TECNOB web-platform with the ARMBAND application (devoloped by TELBIOS http://www.telbios.it)

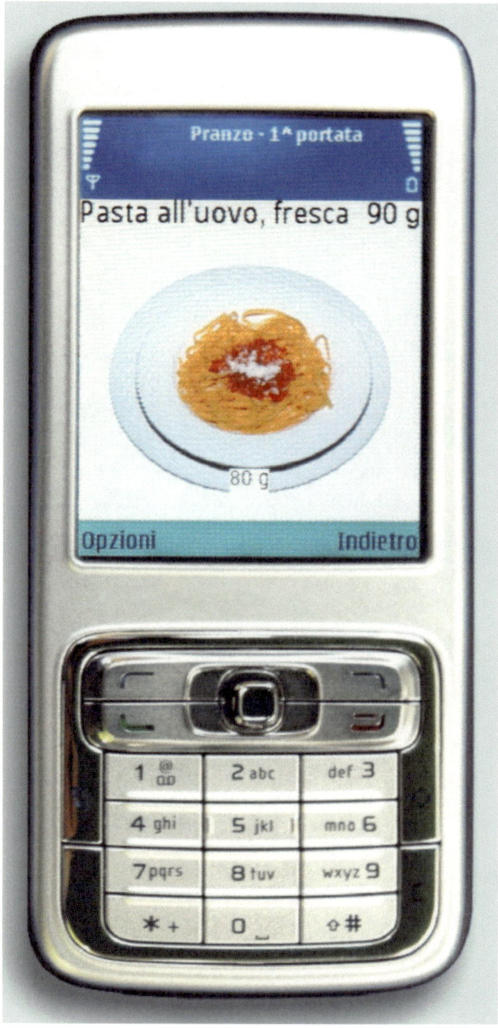

Fig. 3. A screenshot of the METADIETA application for mobile phones (devoloped by METEDA http://www.meteda.it)

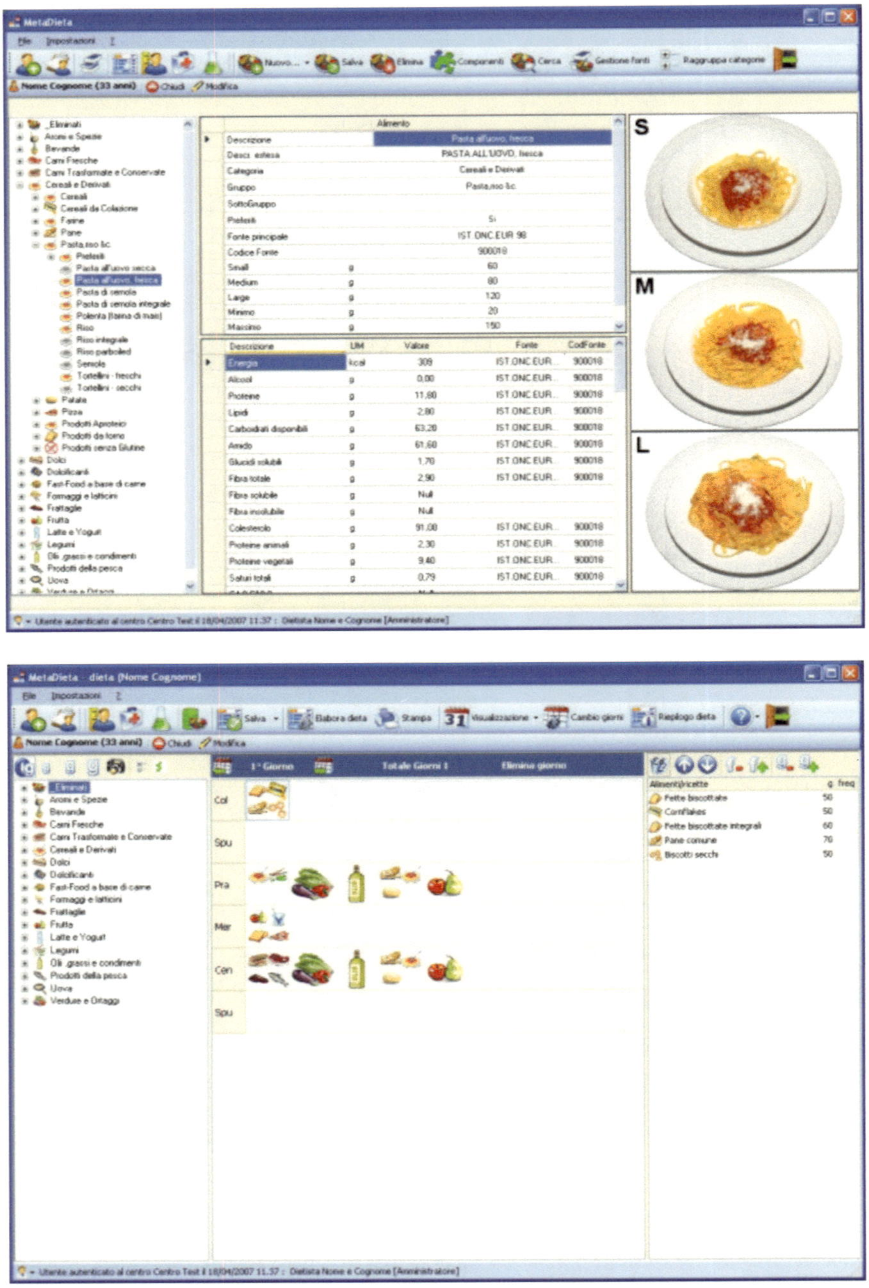

Fig. 4. Two screenshots of the METADIETA application to manage the diet (devoloped by METEDA http://www.meteda.it)

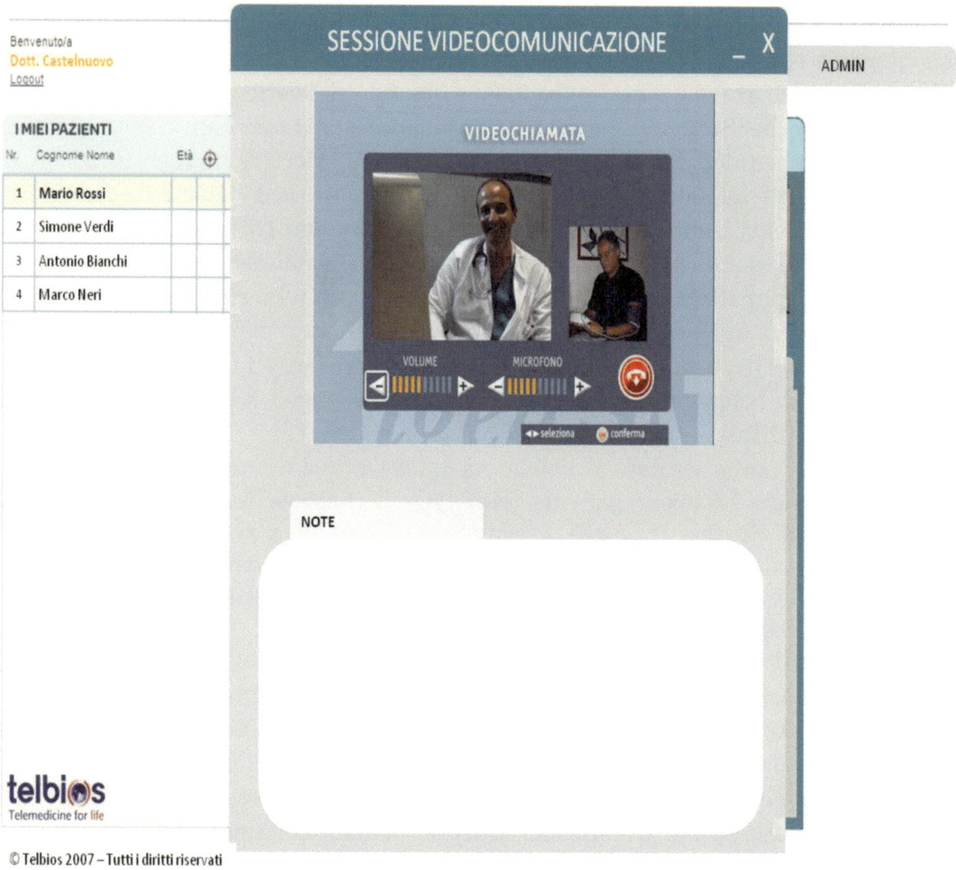

Fig. 5. A screenshot of the TECNOB web-platform with the VIDEOCONFERENCE application (devoloped by TELBIOS http://www.telbios.it)

Thanks to this medium, they receive nutritional and cognitive-behavioral tele-counseling with the dietitian and the clinical psychologist who attended the patients inside the hospital. In particular, just after discharge, participants have 6 videoconference contacts with both clinicians along 3 months. From the 3rd to the 6th month sessions are scheduled every 30 days and then even more spaced up to an interval of 60 days. During tele-sessions, clinicians (psychologist and dietitian) test the outpatients' progress, their mood, the maintenance of the "good alimentary and physical activity habits", the loss/increase of weight and ask about critical moments, especially those ones reported on the "memo" web-space. In particular, tele-sessions with the clinical psychologist aim to consolidate strategies and abilities acquired during the in-patient phase, to improve self-esteem and self-efficacy, to support motivation, to prevent relapse and to provide problem-solving and crisis counseling. On the other hand, dietitian assesses adherence and compliance to dietary therapy with a special focus on normal eating behavior, sufficient fluid intake, hunger and fullness regulation, appropriate eating/etiquette (pace and timing of meals), slow rate of eating, and addresses critical points such as plateau in weight loss or lack of readiness to improve dietary habits (Castelnuovo, et al., 2011; Castelnuovo, et al., 2010).

In addition to videoconference, outpatients can further contact clinicians by e-mail. Indeed, each patient is given the possibility to join his clinician beyond the established videoconference contacts in case of urgency or emergency. According to the e-message's content, clinicians choose the most appropriate format for delivering feedback among e-mail or telephone. In order to avoid excessive dependence and to contain costs, a maximum number of 1 not scheduled contact a week is established a priori. Great relevance is given to the clinicians-patient relationship as an important medium and vehicle of change. After discharge, out-patients begin to experience the autonomy and competence to change they develop during the in-patient phase and inevitably face resistances and barriers. Thanks to videoconferences, outpatients are supported by the clinicians who attended them during the in-hospital phase in exploring resistances and barriers they experience and in finding functional pathways to cope. Furthermore, out-patients are helped to experience mastery in terms of the health behavior change that needs to be engaged (Castelnuovo, et al., 2011; Castelnuovo, et al., 2010).

Some preliminary results are now available. As indicated in a recent paper (Castelnuovo, et al., 2011), at present 72 obese patients with type 2 diabetes have been recruited and randomly allocated to the TECNOB program (n=37) or to a control condition (n=39). However, only 34 participants have completed at least the 3-month follow-up and have been included in this ad interim analysis. 21 out of them have reached also the 6-month follow-up and 13 have achieved the end of the program.

The first ad interim analysis of the data from the TECNOB study has not revealed any significant difference between the TECNOB program and a control condition in weight change at 3, 6 and 12 months. Within-group analysis showed significant reductions of initial weight at all time-points but not at 12-month follow-up (Castelnuovo, et al., 2011). The median percentage of initial weight loss for the whole sample was -5,1 kg (-6,6 to -3,7) at discharge from the hospital. Completers analysis of data collected at 6 and 12 months showed that participants regained back part of the weight loss and the difference between weight at baseline and at 12-month follow-up was no more statistically significant. Notably, sample sizes at 6 and 12 months are small (n=21 and n=12 respectively) due to the ongoing status of the study and these results may be unreliable (Castelnuovo, et al., 2011).

These ad interim findings did not support the effectiveness of the TECNOB protocol over a control condition. Notably, this kind of data analysis (ad interim analysis) is underpowered and results we obtained may be unreliable, in particular at 6 and 12 months. However, we gained a significant insight into an important component of the study design, i.e. the hospital-based program. The effect that such uncontrolled factor has on weight loss was very high and probably overwhelmed the effect of the TECNOB intervention. Hence, much statistical power is necessary to enhance the chance to detect the effect of the TECNOB program: the hospital-based program has a very high effect in the first months after discharge but such effect may reduce in the long term. A 12-month follow-up is probably sufficient to detect the TECNOB effect over and above the weakened effect of the hospital-base program (Castelnuovo, et al., 2011). Study is still on-going and complete results will be published in the next years.

4. Acknowledgment

This chapter is related to the TECNOB Project (Technology for Obesity Project) supported by the "Compagnia di San Paolo" private foundation. Our technological partners are TELBIOS (http://www.telbios.it) and METEDA (http://www.meteda.it).

5. References

Castelnuovo, G. (2010). No medicine without psychology: the key role of psychological contribution in clinical settings. [Original Research Article]. *Frontiers in Psychology for Clinical Settings, 1*.

Castelnuovo, G., Gaggioli, A., Mantovani, F., & Riva, G. (2003). From psychotherapy to e-therapy: the integration of traditional techniques and new communication tools in clinical settings. *Cyberpsychol Behav, 6*(4), 375-382.

Castelnuovo, G., Manzoni, G. M., Cuzziol, P., Cesa, G. L., Corti, S., Tuzzi, C., et al. (2011). TECNOB Study: Ad Interim Results of a Randomized Controlled Trial of a Multidisciplinary Telecare Intervention for Obese Patients with Type-2 Diabetes. *Clinical Practice and Epidemiology in Mental Health, 7*, 43-50.

Castelnuovo, G., Manzoni, G. M., Cuzziol, P., Cesa, G. L., Tuzzi, C., Villa, V., et al. (2010). TECNOB: study design of a randomized controlled trial of a multidisciplinary telecare intervention for obese patients with type-2 diabetes. *BMC Public Health, 10*, 204.

Cline, A. D., & Wong, M. (1999). New frontiers in using telemedicine for nutrition intervention. *J Am Diet Assoc, 99*(11), 1442-1443.

Colditz, G. A., Willett, W. C., Stampfer, M. J., Manson, J. E., Hennekens, C. H., Arky, R. A., et al. (1990). Weight as a risk factor for clinical diabetes in women. *Am J Epidemiol, 132*(3), 501-513.

Dale, J., Caramlau, I., Docherty, A., Sturt, J., & Hearnshaw, H. (2007). Telecare motivational interviewing for diabetes patient education and support: a randomised controlled trial based in primary care comparing nurse and peer supporter delivery. *Trials, 8*, 18.

Donnan, P. T., MacDonald, T. M., & Morris, A. D. (2002). Adherence to prescribed oral hypoglycaemic medication in a population of patients with Type 2 diabetes: a retrospective cohort study. *Diabet Med, 19*(4), 279-284.

Ekeland, A. G., Bowes, A., & Flottorp, S. (2010). Effectiveness of telemedicine: a systematic review of reviews. *Int J Med Inform, 79*(11), 736-771.

Eysenbach, G. (2001). What is e-health? *J Med Internet Res, 3*(2), E20.

Field, A. E., Coakley, E. H., Must, A., Spadano, J. L., Laird, N., Dietz, W. H., et al. (2001). Impact of overweight on the risk of developing common chronic diseases during a 10-year period. *Arch Intern Med, 161*(13), 1581-1586.

Flegal, K. M., Graubard, B. I., Williamson, D. F., & Gail, M. H. (2005). Excess deaths associated with underweight, overweight, and obesity. *JAMA, 293*(15), 1861-1867.

Goulis, D. G., Giaglis, G. D., Boren, S. A., Lekka, I., Bontis, E., Balas, E. A., et al. (2004). Effectiveness of home-centered care through telemedicine applications for overweight and obese patients: a randomized controlled trial. *Int J Obes Relat Metab Disord, 28*(11), 1391-1398.

Hill, J. O., Thompson, H., & Wyatt, H. (2005). Weight maintenance: what's missing? *J Am Diet Assoc, 105*(5 Suppl 1), S63-66.

Jeffery, R. W., Drewnowski, A., Epstein, L. H., Stunkard, A. J., Wilson, G. T., Wing, R. R., et al. (2000). Long-term maintenance of weight loss: current status. *Health Psychol, 19*(1 Suppl), 5-16.

Jeffery, R. W., Sherwood, N. E., Brelje, K., Pronk, N. P., Boyle, R., Boucher, J. L., et al. (2003). Mail and phone interventions for weight loss in a managed-care setting: Weigh-To-Be one-year outcomes. *Int J Obes Relat Metab Disord, 27*(12), 1584-1592.

Katan, M. B. (2009). Weight-loss diets for the prevention and treatment of obesity. *N Engl J Med, 360*(9), 923-925.

Khaylis, A., Yiaslas, T., Bergstrom, J., & Gore-Felton, C. (2010). A review of efficacious technology-based weight-loss interventions: five key components. *Telemed J E Health, 16*(9), 931-938.

Klein, S., Sheard, N. F., Pi-Sunyer, X., Daly, A., Wylie-Rosett, J., Kulkarni, K., et al. (2004a). Weight management through lifestyle modification for the prevention and management of type 2 diabetes: rationale and strategies. A statement of the American Diabetes Association, the North American Association for the Study of Obesity, and the American Society for Clinical Nutrition. *Am J Clin Nutr, 80*(2), 257-263.

Klein, S., Sheard, N. F., Pi-Sunyer, X., Daly, A., Wylie-Rosett, J., Kulkarni, K., et al. (2004b). Weight management through lifestyle modification for the prevention and management of type 2 diabetes: rationale and strategies: a statement of the American Diabetes Association, the North American Association for the Study of Obesity, and the American Society for Clinical Nutrition. *Diabetes Care, 27*(8), 2067-2073.

Maglaveras, N., Gogou, G., Chouvarda, I., Koutkias, V., Lekka, I., Giaglis, G., et al. (2002). Communication infrastructure in a contact center for home care monitoring of chronic disease patients. *Proc AMIA Symp*, 479-483.

Manzoni, G. M., Pagnini, F., Corti, S., Molinari, E., & Castelnuovo, G. (2011). Internet-Based Behavioral Interventions for Obesity: An Updated Systematic Review. *Clinical Practice and Epidemiology in Mental Health, 7*, 19-27.

Mokdad, A. H., Ford, E. S., Bowman, B. A., Dietz, W. H., Vinicor, F., Bales, V. S., et al. (2003). Prevalence of obesity, diabetes, and obesity-related health risk factors, 2001. *JAMA, 289*(1), 76-79.

Must, A., Spadano, J., Coakley, E. H., Field, A. E., Colditz, G., & Dietz, W. H. (1999). The disease burden associated with overweight and obesity. *JAMA, 282*(16), 1523-1529.

Neve, M., Morgan, P. J., Jones, P. R., & Collins, C. E. (2009). Effectiveness of web-based interventions in achieving weight loss and weight loss maintenance in overweight and obese adults: a systematic review with meta-analysis. *Obes Rev.*

Pagliari, C., Sloan, D., Gregor, P., Sullivan, F., Detmer, D., Kahan, J. P., et al. (2005). What is eHealth (4): a scoping exercise to map the field. *J Med Internet Res, 7*(1), e9.

Rice, C. A. (2005). Prevention: the most economical way to manage diabetes. *Nurs Econ, 23*(6), 327-329.

Rojas, S. V., & Gagnon, M. P. (2008). A systematic review of the key indicators for assessing telehomecare cost-effectiveness. *Telemed J E Health, 14*(9), 896-904.

Saperstein, S. L., Atkinson, N. L., & Gold, R. S. (2007). The impact of Internet use for weight loss. *Obes Rev, 8*(5), 459-465.

Weinstein, P. K. (2006). A review of weight loss programs delivered via the Internet. *J Cardiovasc Nurs, 21*(4), 251-258; quiz 259-260.

Whitlock, G., Lewington, S., Sherliker, P., Clarke, R., Emberson, J., Halsey, J., et al. (2009). Body-mass index and cause-specific mortality in 900 000 adults: collaborative analyses of 57 prospective studies. *Lancet, 373*(9669), 1083-1096.

WHO (2006). Definition and Diagnosis of Diabetes Mellitus and Intermediate Hyperglycemia. *Report of a WHO/IDF consultation.*

Wing, R. R., Tate, D. F., Gorin, A. A., Raynor, H. A., & Fava, J. L. (2006). A self-regulation program for maintenance of weight loss. *N Engl J Med, 355*(15), 1563-1571.

12

The Role of Standard 12-lead ECG in a Telecardiology Consultation Service

Kjell Nikus[1], Vesa Virtanen[1], Samuel Sclarovsky[2] and Markku Eskola[1]
[1]Heart Center, Department of Cardiology, Tampere University Hospital, Tampere,
[2]Tel Aviv University, Tel Aviv,
[1]Finland
[2]Israel

1. Introduction

Electrocardiography (ECG), introduced in 1902 by Einthoven, is the most commonly used procedure for the diagnosis of heart disease. It is a frequently performed procedure by internists and family practitioners as well as by emergency department physicians and cardiologists. As a record of electrical activity of the heart, it is a technology that provides information not readily obtained by other methods. The 12-lead ECG has numerous potential clinical uses. It serves as the criterion standard for noninvasive diagnosis of arrhythmias and conduction disturbances, and occasionally it is the only marker for the presence of heart disease. Prior studies have shown that misinterpretation of the ECG can lead to inappropriate diagnoses and clinical decisions.

Telecardiology is one of the oldest applications in telemedicine, and has been largely applied during the last 10-20 years. Telecardiology encompasses a wide variety of applications and is one of the fastest-growing fields in telemedicine. Telecardiology in some fields such as emergency and chronic care undoubtedly improves the quality of health care and helps to contain rising costs. ECG consultations between general practitioners and specialists encompass a wider spectrum of clinical entities, including non-urgent patient care.

An internet-based telecardiology centre for ECG consultations was established in 2008. The centre provides physicians with comprehensive ECG consultations, including description of the ECG findings, case urgency, need for further examinations, and recommendations for therapeutic strategy, like changes in medication or need for hospital admission. The service was initially provided by a separate enterprise, which in 2010 was incorporated into the Tampere University Hospital Heart Centre, a tertiary cardiologic referral centre.

In this chapter, the patient material from the consultation service is presented, including age, sex, and estimated case urgency. The ECG findings are classified into clinical categories, like suspected acute coronary syndrome, and arrhythmias. Consultation response delays and technical aspects are reported, as well as recommendations provided by the cardiology experts.

The potential benefit of an ECG consultation service, which provides clinical recommendations, is discussed. There are quite a few challenges with the introduction of a new consultation model. Many physicians are unaware of their limitations and believe that they can interpret ECGs well. Physicians may prefer telephone contact instead of an internet-based consultation service. Advantages and disadvantages of different consultation models are discussed; also cost issues are discussed.

2. Telemedicine

Telemedicine is the provision of healthcare services, through use of information and communication technology, in situations where the health care professional and the patient, or two health care professionals, are not in the same location. It involves the secure transmission of medical data and information, through text, sound, images, or other forms needed for the prevention, diagnosis, treatment and follow-up of patients (Saxena et al., 2003). Despite the potential of telemedicine, its benefits and the technical maturity of the applications, the use of telemedicine services is still limited, and the market remains highly fragmented. Integrating new types of services in healthcare services is a challenging task (Commission of the European Communities: COM(2008)689). Privacy and security related aspects are also major components of building trust and confidence in telemedicine systems. Interoperability and standardisation in telemonitoring are crucial to allow widespread use of the technologies. The societal and economic benefits from wider use of telemedicine are potentially huge. At the present moment, they are far from being fully appreciated or achieved (Edwards et al., 2008; Hämäläinen et al., 2008).

3. Telecardiology

Telecardiology is one of the oldest applications in telemedicine, and has been largely applied during the last 10-20 years (Hailey et al., 2004). Telecardiology encompasses a wide variety of applications. Over 200.000 patients worldwide are being managed via remote implantable electronic cardiovascular device monitoring to facilitate the recognition of abnormal device behaviour and verify the patient's immediate physiological response to the many programmable therapies the devices offer (Jung et al., 2008). Data collected in several completed and ongoing studies strongly suggest that this new technology will make important contributions, particularly with respect to the facilitation of device follow-ups, enhancement of patient safety and quality of life, and lowering of medical costs. Continuous home monitoring of vital parameters like weight, blood pressure and heart rate, using external telemedicine devices, can improve outcomes in heart failure patients (Cleland et al., 2005; Goldberg et al., 2003; Louis et al., 2003).

Telecardiology applications can be categorized as pre-hospital, in-hospital and post-hospital (Scalvini & Glisenti 2005). Coronary artery disease provides an ideal target for telehealth intervention because of its great and increasing financial cost, and the overrepresentation of heart disease in rural and remote communities (Hooper et al., 2001). The major purpose of pre-hospital 12-lead ECG diagnosis is the early detection of acute myocardial infarction with ST-segment elevation and the communication of that information to the receiving emergency physician before the arrival of the patient (Terkelsen et al., 2005). Transmission of prehospital 12-lead ECG directly to the attending cardiologist's mobile telephone decreased door-to-device time by >1 hour when patients with ST-elevation myocardial infarction were transported directly to invasive centres, bypassing local hospitals (Sejersten et al., 2008). Ambulance transport was safe despite longer transport times. On the other hand, long transport times may allow the catheterization suites more preparation time. The telephone display showed sufficient resolution for ECG interpretation.

In-hospital telecardiology is used between small hospitals in rural regions and main hospitals (Zaliunas et al, 2009). Telemedicine here has the potential to improve access to echocardiography diagnoses in the intensive care unit, emergency room and newborn nursery (Sekar & Vilvanathan, 2007). Post-hospital applications include teleconsulting between general practitioners and specialists, home telenursing for chronic cardiac diseases and the diagnosis of arrhythmias (Goh et al., 2006; Scalvini et al., 2006).
Publications related to telecardiology surveillance of coronary care unit monitoring data outside hospital are scarce and mostly deal solely with technical aspects (Nikus et al., 2009).

4. Electrocardiology

The 12-lead ECG has been used in clinical medicine since the early 1900s as a first-line diagnostic tool in studying both acute and chronic cardiac diseases. The ECG is a noninvasive, relatively inexpensive diagnostic test that provides important information regarding not only the heart, but also non-cardiac events impacting the cardiac system.
Numerous studies have compared cardiologists and non-cardiologists in their ability to recognize ECG changes. A review of the literature showed a wide variety in skills among various specialities (Mele, 2008). Non-cardiologists were in disagreement with the cardiologist reference interpretations from 4 % to 64 % of the time, depending on the specific abnormality in question. Salerno et al suggested that up to one third of ECG interpretations have some error when compared to the expert reference (Salerno et al., 2003). The authors estimated that up to 11 % resulted in inappropriate management, e.g. anticoagulation for non-existent atrial fibrillation; close to 1 % had significant adverse outcomes or potentially preventable death. A screening study from 49 general practices in central England showed that many primary care professionals cannot accurately detect atrial fibrillation on an ECG, and interpretative software is not sufficiently accurate to circumvent this problem, even when combined with interpretation by a general practitioner (Mant el, 2007). Twenty per cent of cases of atrial fibrillation were missed by the general practitioners, and the probability that a positive diagnosis was correct was only 41 %.
There is wide variability in ECG over-reading, in part because of lack of standards for certifying individuals to over-read ECGs. According to a position statement by the American College of Cardiology and the American Heart Association, all ECGs should be over-read either by cardiologists or ECG-tested physicians (Kadish et al., 2001). The statement has good scientific background, but it is difficult to implement in many countries. Hongo and Goldschlager proposed telemedicine as a possible solution to improve ECG diagnostics (Hongo & Goldschlager, 2004). In an editorial, they discussed the difficulties of automated computer analysis to assess cardiac rhythm and concluded that physicians should become less reliant on computerized interpretations. A system with on-call ECG reading service that accepts tracings by fax or via electronic mail to handheld devices was suggested. ECGs performed in an outpatient setting could be sent for centralized interpretation that would then be returned to an office "in-box". The authors predict that this approach would ensure that ordering physicians, as a matter of routine, review finalized ECG interpretations and take responsibility for patient follow-up.
Correct ECG interpretation is extremely important in patients with a suspicion of acute coronary syndrome. Vijayaraghavan et al investigated ECG interpretation on site with core laboratory interpretation in acute coronary syndrome patients, focusing on ST elevation (Vijayaraghavan et al., 2008). Overall concordance between the core-lab and on site

interpretation was 62 % and the calculated kappa 0.49, indicating modest agreement. In an editorial referring to this article, Brady and O'Connor state that the physician receiving the ECG in the suspected acute coronary syndrome patient must be an expert in ECG interpretation (Brady & O´Connor, 2008). Studies have shown consistently high rates of agreement between the emergency physician and the cardiologist (Kuhn et al., 1992; Todd et al., 1996). However, at least in our country, patients with suspected acute coronary syndromes are likely to be treated by inexperienced junior doctors. This highlights the importance of the possibility to consult a specialist through telemedicine.

5. Tele-ECG consultation

In teleconsultation a representative of health care personnel approaches an expert in a remote place for advice. In the *Real time interactive mode* the patient is present with an attending physician or paramedical personnel and a specialist is present at a remote center. In the *Store-and-forward mode* all relevant information is transmitted electronically to the specialist, who generates a report within hours or days. The latter model is typical for teleradiology.

Molinari et al studied the role of telecardiology in reducing unnecessary hospital admissions of patients with suspected life-threatening cardiac events, evaluated by general practitioners. One hundred general practitioners in remote rural areas in Italy sent a trans-telephonic 12-lead ECG, mostly from the patients' home to a cardiologist on 24/7 duty (Telemedicine Institute, Genoa) (Molinari et al., 2002). The general practitioners used transportable ECG equipment. Before teleconsultation, the general practitioners recorded their own opinion (based on clinical evaluation only) about the presence of a cardiac event. Following transmission of the ECG, this opinion was compared with that of the cardiologist. In total there was agreement between the general practitioner and cardiologist about the presence of a cardiac event in 316 of the patients (69%) and disagreement in 140 patients (31%). This represents a specificity and sensitivity of the general practitioners' diagnosis of 76% and 47%, respectively. For 84 of 134 patients judged as having a cardiac event by the general practitioner, telecardiology avoided hospitalization. On the other hand, telecardiology identified a cardiac event in 56 of 322 patients judged as not having a cardiac event by the general practitioner. The authors concluded that telecardiology is a useful tool to reduce unnecessary hospitalizations in patients with suspected life-threatening cardiac events. The system presented seems to be useful in countries and regions with frequent use of home visits by physicians.

Investigators have reported their experiences with ECG transmission by patients to a telemedicine center. Chiantera et al compared two models of assistance (telecardiology versus usual care) for patients discharged after acute coronary syndrome in the assessment of angina pectoris (Chiantera et al., 2005). Two hundred patients were randomized either to telecardiology or to usual care. Patients randomized to usual care underwent a control visit 15 and 30 days after discharge. In the telecardiology group, the patients were provided with a portable device by means of which a 12-lead ECG could be recorded and transmitted to the service centre by fixed or mobile telephone. ECGs were sent either for symptoms, or as routine at 4 weeks follow-up. The service offered by the telemedicine institution was available 24 h per day. Early hospital readmission in the first month occurred in 16 patients (7 in the telecardiology Group and 9 in the usual care group). The authors concluded that telecardiology slightly reduced hospital readmissions and better identified true angina pectoris.

Experiences from the Shahal organization in Israel pointed to considerable cost savings by trans-telephonic ECG transmission by the service subscribers thanks to shorter delays from anginal symptom onset to call for medical help. In the majority of calls, an ambulance transport could be avoided (Roth et al., 2006).

6. Real time interactive tele ECG

Procardia Medical Center in Israel provides large volume on-line internet-based tele-ECG consultations to health care professionals around the country (unpublished data reported by one of the authors, Professor Samuel Sclarovsky, director of telemedicine at Procardia). Planning of a tele-ECG consultation service in Tampere University Hospital started in the mid-2000s. Basically, the logistics of the system should enable treating physicians to consult cardiology specialists about ECG-related medical topics, and get a swift response. The cardiologist should also give medical advice about additional tests needed, need for change in medication, patient urgency etc. In other words, the system should not provide technical ECG analysis only. In addition, the system should be easy to use, technically robust and adequately secure for the handling of patient data. Finally, the system should enable interactivity through messages in addition to the consultation requests and responses.

It was decided that the most urgent cases should not be handled through the telecardiology consultation service, because clinical decisions should be made within minutes in acute cardiac urgencies. The Heart Center at Tampere University Hospital provides telecardiology consultation service 24/7/365 for acute ST-elevation myocardial infarction patients. In that system, the ECGs are sent by fax or mobile phone to a handheld communicator and clinical decisions are made by telephone contact between the cardiologist on duty and the treating physician or emergency medical personnel. Delays from the first ECG to arterial puncture and to first device are well within recommendations from international guidelines (article published in Finnish).

7. Telecardiology pilot

During the planning phase for the tele-ECG service, a pilot study was performed in 2007. In the pilot, the Tampere University Hospital Heart Center provided tele-ECG consultation service for one health centre and for the emergency department of a regional hospital. The 12-lead ECGs were immediately stored at these 2 remote units into a digital ECG archive (GE Muse database), with immediate access for the cardiologist to the recordings and, if available, to previous recordings for comparison. The Personal Information Repository (PIR) document service was used in delivering consultation requests, responses and other related documents. The architecture of the PIR document service and the experiences from the pilot have been described in a previous article (Lähteenmäki et al., 2009). In a questionnaire, usability of the service was evaluated. Health care personnel estimated possible benefits for the patients as high. No major technical problems were encountered.

Based on the pilot phase, literature reviews and multidisciplinary planning, a telecardiology service company in close association with the Heart Centre was established. A business plan pointed to possibilities for the company to show positive results, providing the consultation service would be largely implemented in health centres in different parts of our country. In addition, other telecardiology applications were planned.

7.1 The consultation system

During the final planning phase, the PIR document service was replaced by an internet homepage-based consultation system. Physicians from the health care units, who participate in the telecardiology service, typically general practitioners, have user names and passwords to enter the consultation program. A structured form is filled in and sent to the telecardiology centre. Arrival of a consultation request will alert the cardiologist by an SMS to a mobile phone. The cardiologist opens the consultation program by user name and password. Most health centres in the Pirkanmaa Hospital district store the ECGs digitally into the GE Muse database, from which the ECGs can be analyzed by the cardiologists in the hospital. Alternatively, the ECGs can be sent as a fax or as a scanned document.

The customers only pay a standard fee per consultation, no annual fee or payment for information and communication technology services exists. A small market analysis directed to potential customers indicated that pricing is dependent on case urgency. Doctors were ready to pay €20-40 if the expert response would be given within 2 days, but €40-60 for short response times.

7.2 Cardiology expertise

For the first year of the study period, from June 2009 to May 2010, there was tele-ECG service from 8:00 to 20:00 Monday to Friday. Service was provided as real-time interactive consultation; responses were sent within 30 minutes from the arrival of the consultation request and the ECG. From June 2010 on, responses are provided within 4 hours as part of the Heart Centre cardiology consultation service.

7.3 The heart center

The Tampere University Hospital is the only central hospital in the Pirkanmaa Hospital District, which has about 481.000 inhabitants. The Tampere University Hospital Heart Center is a tertiary cardiology and cardiac surgery referral centre for the neighbouring hospital districts. Heart Center Co. began its operations as a process-based organization dedicated to cardiac patients in 2004 when it merged with Tampere University Hospital's cardiac, cardiothoracic and cardiac-anesthesiology operations. In 2005, the Heart Center was made into its own financial unit and in 2007 Heart Center Co. began serving the public as a corporation. Close to 20 cardiologists work in the Heart Centre.

7.4 Customers

By the end of the study period, 23 customers had signed a written agreement for telecardiology service. The majority are health centres within the Pirkanmaa Hospital District. Sales and marketing aimed at reaching agreements with health care providers, municipal and private, all around our country. Challenges met during the sales and marketing process will be covered in the Discussion.

8. Study results

8.1 ECG consultation volume and response time

In total, 505 ECG consultations were handled during the study period from June 2009 to the end of February 2011. The first consultation request was sent in June 2009. During the first 3 months, only a few consultations were handled. From September 2009 on, the number of consultations per month varied from 16 to 54. The maximum number was reached in

February 2010, 8 months after the introduction of the service. In June 2010 there was a drop in the number of consultations, and after that the maximal number of consultations per month was 27. When comparing the period of real-time interactive consultation service, excluding the first 3 months, to the period of a longer response time ("store-and-forward model"), the mean number of consultations per month were 35 (min 16 - max 54) and 21 (min 16 – max 27). Both periods represent 9 months.

There was wide variation in the number of consultations per customer. The highest volume, 91 requests, was provided by a health centre, which was involved already in the telecardiology pilot phase. Different time points for signing agreements for the service explains some of the variation between the customers.

For response time, only time from arrival of the consultation request was studied. This overestimates the response time as the ECG, if sent by fax, typically arrives later than the request. As expected, when comparing two 9 months periods, the response times were shorter during the first period with on-line consultation service. From the arrival of the consultation request, 52% of the responses were sent within 30 minutes and 75% within 45 minutes during the first 9 month period. During the second 9 month period, the corresponding numbers were 13% and 24%, respectively.

8.2 Consultation requests and responses

The reasons for consulting the telecardiologist are presented in Table 1. The treating physician did not always indicate a specific reason for consultation. In that case, patients are categorized as "pathological ECG". This category also includes cases, where the treating physician did not specify his or her interpretation of the ECG findings, but only indicated that the finding was abnormal. As mentioned, the consultation service is not intended for patients with acute myocardial infarction, neither for cases with acute coronary syndrome, where acute hospitalization is clearly indicated. This is also stated on the consultation form. In patients with accidental findings of Q waves without signs of acute coronary syndrome and in cases where the clinical picture is atypical, consultation is recommended.

In Table 2 the main ECG findings are presented. Only one classification per patient is used and the analysis was done by one of the authors (KN). Clinical importance was used when classifying the findings. For example, myocardial ischemia was considered as the main finding although first degree AV-block was present. On the other hand, if the patient's actual problem was arrhythmia, the category extrasystole was used, although a patient had ECG signs of left ventricular hypertrophy. The largest group, "miscellaneous" consists of many ECG findings, like left or right frontal axis shift and fragmented QRS complex. Also 5 cases with pre-excitation with delta waves, and 2 with electrode misplacement were included in this group. Due to the hierarchical classification, the numbers under-estimate the actual prevalence of the different subgroups of ECG findings.

In Table 3, the first-line recommendations by the cardiologist are presented. Again, only one recommendation per patient is presented. For example, if the cardiologist recommended a control ECG before definite decision about actions needed, the category ECG control was indicated. In case of suggested ECG control within hours, or laboratory tests, like troponin, the cardiologist usually presented alternatives for further measures in the consultation request, depending on the test results. This was considered as time saving, as the treating physician would not have to send additional consultation requests for the same patient.

Reason for consulting	N (%)
Arrhythmia	174 (35)
Myocardial ischemia or infarction	131 (25)
Pathological ECG	114 (23)
Conduction disturbance	42 (8)
Prolonged QT	26 (5)
Pacemaker	8 (2)
Perimyocarditis	10 (2)

Table 1. Reasons for consulting the cardiologist.

ECG findings	N (%)
ECG pathology, miscellaneous	107 (21)
Conduction disturbance	84 (17)
Normal ECG	84 (17)
Tachyarrhythmia	74 (15)
Left ventricular hypertrophy	41 (8)
Extrasystole	39 (8)
Myocardial ischemia	33 (6)
Ectopic atrial rhythm	19 (4)
Myocardial infarction (old or recent)	17 (3)
Short PQ interval	7 (1)

Table 2. Main ECG findings during the study period.

Recommendation	N (%)
No measures needed	105 (21)
Change of medication	95 (19)
Cardiology consultation, non-urgent	93 (18)
Holter	70 (14)
Stress test	36 (7)
Control ECG	34 (7)
Urgent hospitalization	33 (7)
Blood tests	26 (5)
Cardiology consultation, urgent	13 (2)

Table 3. First line recommendations to the treating physician by the telecardiologist.

Figure 1 shows the age distribution of the patients. The youngest patient was 2 years and the oldest 96 years old. The mean age was 60 years. There were slightly more males (n=263, 52 %) than females (n=242, 48 %).

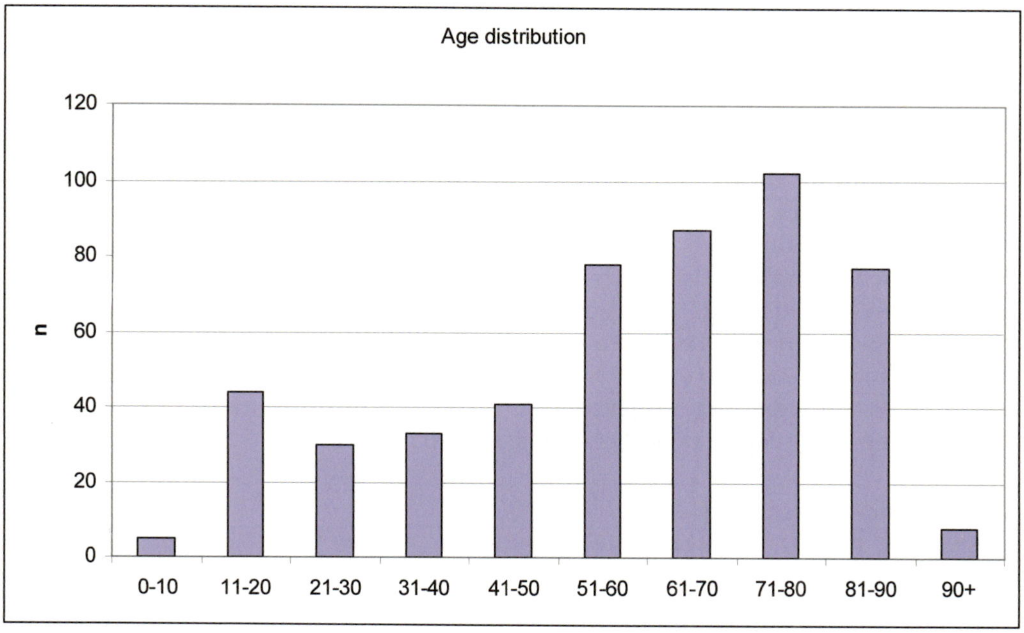

Fig. 1. Age distribution of the study patients

8.3 Technical aspects

Detailed analysis of the technical performance of the consultation system has not been done so far. In general, the system was well-functioning. In five patients, the cardiologist was not able to read the ECG and/or the consultation request due to technical problems. In these cases, the cardiologist responded based on the clinical data and the ECG analysis made by the treating physician.

The fax system poses the greatest challenge to the consultation system. The technical quality of the faxed ECGs is sometimes poor. Also, one has to check for possible height (mV) or length (ms) distortion in the faxed ECGs. Sometimes, fax transmission is slow and it may be difficult for the cardiologist to know how soon after the arrival of the consultation request to check with the treating physician whether the ECG has been faxed or not.

9. Discussion

9.1 Real time interactive tele-ECG consultation

It is apparent that a real time interactive tele-ECG consultation service has a number of advantages. This is also supported by experiences elsewhere as reported by one of the authors (SS). The treating physician gets an expert opinion about the ECG findings, and possible actions needed, based on the findings, while the patient is in the doctor's office or in the emergency department. In some cases, potentially life-threatening conditions can be identified. In many more cases medication can be modified. Also, indications for additional tests, like holter, stress tests and echocardiography can be better appreciated by a specialist than by a general practitioner. In a small pilot study, we found that planned referrals for cardiology consultations could be avoided by the telecardiology consultation service (Lähteenmäki et al, 2009). In many cases, the physician wants a second opinion from a specialist before making treatment decisions, and that is possible through the consultation service.

Compared to traditional telephone consultation, exact documentation of the consultation process is a clear advantage of our telecardiology consultation service. The consultation requests and responses with their exact timing are stored. It is well known that telephone consultations are not always documented in the patient files, although this should be done. At least in our country, there are no studies to show how frequently documentations are left out. Related to patient security, when the system is built on user name and password, it is possible to identify individuals, who have entered the system.

Our system enables interactivity through messages. Both the medical professional asking for advice and the expert may add comments or questions related to a specific consultation through the internet-based system. For example, the expert may ask for additional clinical data. Messages are used rather frequently in our consultation service. Messages may also aid in avoiding misunderstandings between the two parts.

9.2 Telemedicine processes

The planning phase of our telecardiology service to a large part dealt with telemedicine processes. Telemedicine service platforms are typically focused to limited telemedicine areas and measurement devices. The Personal Information Repository (PIR) document service provides a generic platform with the objective to support an extremely wide spectrum of different applications in the field of telemedicine (Lähteenmäki et al, 2009). Application specific support is obtained by specific components, which can be easily connected by using open interfaces. During the planning phase of our telecardiology service, the proposed document-based approach was assessed as attractive in many respects. The HL7 CDA R2 document model used is an international standard, which is widely being adopted for Electronic Patient Record (EPR) systems. This provides potential for semantic interoperability between the telemedicine system and other patient information resources. On the other hand, the document-based approach allows complete recording of the service process (in the form of a document archive) at both the customer and the service provider side. By adding digital signatures to the documents, non-repudiation of all interactions can be achieved. However, interoperability remains a challenge also with this service. There is only limited support for integration with other systems. Improvement in this respect is needed as centralised health information archives ("national EPRs") are being established in many countries, including Finland. The national EPRs are providing standard interfaces through which health information can be inserted and accessed, along with the consent provided by patient.

The pilot phase showed that a cardiac consultation service is useful even without full integration with the EPR. In the pilot, the EPR could be opened in another window while providing the consultation response. On the other hand, the necessary texts could be moved to the EPR by using the clipboard. Both the Heart Centre cardiologists and the physicians of the remote units considered the benefits of the consultation service to be high. In the consultation cases, cardiology diagnostics and medication could be refined and guidance for patient logistics was provided. The pilot comprised thirty consultations. In ten patients, there was a recommendation for change in medication. In five cases, the patient was sent to the emergency department of the Tampere University Hospital, in two of the cases, the physician who asked for consultation had not identified case urgency. It was estimated that in five cases, a planned consultation to cardiologist was avoided thanks to telemedicine consultation, although the pilot process did not involve exact appreciation of how the handling of patients was affected. In four cases, non-urgent referral to a cardiologist was recommended. In most of these cases, the treating physician had planned to send the patient to a specialist. In two patients, an arrhythmia was identified: one necessitated change of medication, and one was potentially fatal (ventricular tachycardia). Two cases with silent myocardial infarction and one with unrecognized acute ischemia were noted. The physicians participating in the pilot considered it feasible to use a commercial consultation service when available.

The PIR document service was replaced by an internet homepage based telecardiology service model in the final part of the planning phase. Although the PIR document service has potential advantages in a comprehensive telemedicine service with different types of telemedicine applications, an internet-based system was considered easier to maintain for the simpler model of consultations between health care professionals. For example, new program versions are easy to introduce, as no changes are needed locally in the health care organizations involved in the service.

9.3 Challenges

Based on our experience, there are many challenges with a telecardiology ECG consultation service. In our country, the biggest challenge is to make the service profitable. During the sales and marketing process, potential customers liked the system, but at the end preferred to consult specialists in their own region. One reason for this was that the local specialist service was considered as free of charge. Hence, the telecardiology consultation system was considered as expensive. Actually, regional systems proved to cost about the same or were more expensive, at least as reported by the local authorities. Pricing of the telecardiology service was accommodated to the prevailing pricing level of telephone consultations in our country. Also, experiences from a market analysis and form the pilot study were exploited when the pricing level was determined. Transparency was also sought for by charging only for the consultation with no annual fee or payment for ICT services.

It was appreciated already in the planning phase that regional consultation systems have certain advantages over a system, where the consultation response is provided from a central organization. It seemed, though, that regional and central hospitals would not be able to provide specialist service with response times comparable with the telecardiology service. The cardiology speciality in Finland is invasive. Hence, many cardiologists are busy in catheterization suites during routine working days. In many regions, ECG interpretation as a consultation service is probably provided by specialists in internal medicine familiar with cardiology. The level of ECG interpretation skill of internists has not been studied in our country.

In the Finnish health care system, local authorities provide primary health care (www.kunnat.fi). Municipal public-health work is the foundation of the Finnish health system. Local authorities run about 172 health centers. Alongside municipal health care, there is an occupational health service system, financed by employers and the State, which is responsible for much of the health care for the workforce. There is also a relatively extensive system of private medical services, partly financed by the sickness insurance system. Hospitals run by joint municipal authorities provide 95 per cent of all specialist medical care; the remaining 5 per cent is provided by the private sector. Every local authority is required by law to be a member of a joint municipal authority administering a hospital district. There are 20 hospital districts in all.

One can also see the Finnish health care system as rather fragmented with small units deciding about how to organize specialist consultations. As all actors in the field have their own budgets, it is many times difficult to appreciate total savings with new innovations. Also, decisions about what ECG equipment to use and how the ECGs are stored are decided by the local authorities. In the health centers in the Pirkanmaa hospital district area, there are ECG machines from many different companies. For that reason, ECGs have to be transmitted either by fax or as scanned documents to the specialist in the telecardiology service.

9.4 ECG analysis

In Finland, there are no specific competence requirements for physicians who interpret ECGs. The way of documenting ECG findings varies, as there are no strict recommendations. Typically, possible pathological findings are documented as part of the patient records, or the finding is stated as normal. A more structured way of reporting findings could improve the level of ECG analysis. ECG interpretation is incorporated in the medical studies, but in practice, the skills are far from sufficient in the beginning of the career as a practicing physician. As previously discussed, many studies have shown that non-cardiologists fare worse than cardiologists in ECG interpretation, and that false interpretation may result in even fatal events. Many physicians are unaware of their limitations and believe that they can interpret ECGs well. This is probably one reason for not using the consultation system.

A tele-ECG consultation system has the potential to serve as a learning environment. Actually, this could be one reason for diminishing consultation volumes in our study. One does not need to ask the specialist many times about a particular ECG pathology. The best for the patient should, of course, always be what medical professionals are striving for.

Outsourced health care also proved to be a challenge for our consultation service. In many places in our country, health care service is partly outsourced. A large pool of younger physicians is responsible for the acute and to some part also for elective, patient care in health centers. Information about the existing consultation service and user name and password handling proved to be very challenging, and these physicians rarely used our service.

9.5 Potentials for ECG consultation in non-urgent situations

In urgent cases, the value of telecardiology service consists of better patient outcome and more optimal usage of resources. There is much potential to be gained in the individual case. In non-urgent cases, the diagnostic and prognostic information contained in the ECG is clinically important in many cases, although the benefits of correct interpretation are not as evident as in the acute situations. However, the volume of ECG recordings is much larger in non-urgent situations, and the superiority of expert interpretation compared to non-cardiologist analysis is evident. From the standpoint of the treating physician, the need for consultation may arise from different scenarios. It is not unusual to have accidental ECG findings during regular controls for chronic disease like diabetes. General practitioners and specialists in occupational medicine may not have the knowledge to either make a correct diagnosis from the ECG or to draw the right clinical conclusions from the unexpected findings. Many times, patients who seek for acute or subacute symptoms do not fit into established guidelines for patients care. The symptoms may be atypical, the ECG findings difficult to interpret and the laboratory tests may not provide definite answers concerning the disease process. Also in risk evaluation before surgery or fitness programs, pathological ECG findings may set in motion a process, where the telecardiologist has a central role.

9.6 ECG screening

Ashley et al. performed a literature review related to the use of ECG as a screening tool for cardiovascular disease for large populations (Ashley et al, 2001). They found that no study directly approached the question, so no direct answer to whether ECG screening is useful or not is available. However, the authors suggested that high-risk asymptomatic people in middle age should undergo a screening ECG. They justified their conclusion by specific ECG findings, especially left ventricular hypertrophy, new Q waves, atrial fibrillation, and ST-segment depression, which may affect patient prognosis. ECG left ventricular hypertrophy is a well recognized risk factor for cardiac death. Left ventricular hypertrophy is potentially reversible with antihypertensive therapy with potential for improved prognosis. In the Losartan Intervention For Endpoint Reduction in Hypertension (LIFE) study, less-severe ECG left ventricular hypertrophy by Cornell product and Sokolow-Lyon voltage criteria during antihypertensive therapy was associated with lower likelihoods of cardiovascular morbidity and mortality, independent of blood pressure lowering and treatment modality in persons with essential hypertension. Hence, antihypertensive therapy targeted at regression or prevention of ECG left ventricular hypertrophy may improve prognosis (Okin et al, 2004). Ashley et al. in their review article stressed that clinicians should have a low threshold for performing a screening ECG in patients with known predisposing conditions for ECG left ventricular hypertrophy (age, hypertension, obesity, stature, and glucose intolerance).

Atrial fibrillation is the most prevalent sustained cardiac arrhythmia in adults, affecting > 1% of general population and up to 10% of those aged > 80 years. Atrial fibrillation is commonly associated with structural heart disease and is a major cause of significant cardiovascular morbidity and mortality. Individuals who have not been properly anticoagulated remain at risk of stroke which may result from thromboembolic phenomena. Portable devices may help in recognizing episodes with paroxysmal atrial fibrillation through telemedicine. However, it seems equally important to improve the ECG diagnosis of this particular arrhythmia from 12-lead ECG. As pointed out earlier, diagnosis of atrial fibrillation is not optimally diagnosed by primary care professionals, even with the aid of interpretative software (Mant el, 2007). A telecardiology consultation service has the potential to improve diagnostic quality as part of a screening program.

Q waves noted on screening ECGs are important as markers for unrecognized cardiac disease. Estimates regarding the proportion of actual infarctions that go unrecognized, the syndrome of painless myocardial infarction, vary, but the average is between 15% and 30%, increasing with age (Nadelmann et al., 1990). Study data suggests that for the age group 40 to 59, even 1 silent myocardial infarction in 100 patients could be identified by routine screening (Ashley et al, 2001). On the other hand, false positive myocardial infarction diagnosis by the treating physician, may result in unnecessary anti-thrombotic and anti-ischemic medication.

9.7 Findings from the study

Our study indicates that the real time interactive consultation model (within about half an hour) is superior to a system with delayed response. The number of consultations dropped after the response time was prolonged. This came as no surprise, as one of the main ideas with the service was to provide a specialist response with the patient still in the doctor's office or in the emergency department. Rapid response time enables the physician to immediately inform the patient about diagnostic tests, change of medication etc. Otherwise the doctor and the patient need to be in contact through telephone or mail.

The reason for delaying the response time was to a large part economical. In a nation-wide perspective, the sales and marketing process did not result in enough customers within reasonable time. It was not considered profitable to provide the service via a separate company dedicated mainly to ECG consultations. The consultations were incorporated into the Heart Centre's cardiology consultation service.

As expected, electrophysiological problems constituted a large part of the consultation requests. Arrhythmias, conduction disturbances, including AV-block and sick sinus syndrome, pacemaker ECGs and prolonged QT represent half of the reasons for consultation. Modern pacemaker technology with different technical solutions from different companies represents a great challenge for ECG interpretation by non-cardiologists (Figure 2). General practitioners who see patients with a suspicion of pacemaker dysfunction will ask a cardiologist for advice in the vast majority of cases.

The group with suspected myocardial ischemia was large taking into account that clear acute coronary syndrome cases are not included in the telecardiology service. However, less than half of the cases with a suspicion of ischemia were classified as ischemic by the ECG expert. We think that there is potential for cost savings here, as a considerable proportion of patients with suspected ischemia did not need immediate hospitalization according to the tele-cardiologist. However, cost issues were not part of the study protocol.

Regional guidelines and logistic systems both for acute ST-elevation myocardial infarction and non-ST elevation acute coronary syndrome were established already quite a few years ago in our hospital district. Only 3 patients with acute ST-elevation myocardial infarction were encountered in the study. In these cases, the treating physician was contacted per telephone to speed up the therapeutic process. Fourteen patients showed "silent" myocardial infarction; new pathological Q waves without a diagnosis of myocardial infarction.

Normal ECG was found in 17 % of the cases. In these instances, the treating physician was uncertain whether findings represented normal variants or needed further investigations. Benign early repolarization was often encountered, and was classified as a normal variant (Figure 3). In many cases, it was evident from the consultation request that the automated ECG analysis had alerted the physician about possible pathology. One typical case was ectopic atrial rhythm, which may be difficult to diagnose for inexperienced interpreters (Figure 4). We had 39 cases (8 %) with consultations related to extrasystoles. The number may seem high as the diagnosis often is easy. However, our system always includes clinical interpretation of the ECG findings, not only ECG diagnostics. Therefore, it is evident that treating physicians send consultation requests to get advice about handling of the patients.

The distribution of first-line recommendations (Table 3) show that, at least primarily, the patients' treatment could continue in the referring unit, not in specialist care. If the health care unit provided stress tests and holters, which is the typical case, no referral to specialist care was recommended in 73 % of the cases. In 18 % of the cases, a non-urgent cardiology consultation was recommended. The main reason for this was rule-out of organic heart disease by echocardiography. It is well known that some ECG findings are associated with organic heart disease. For example, the S1S2S3 pattern may be a normal variant, but it may also indicate pulmonary artery hypertension. Left bundle branch block may be a primary intraventricular conduction defect, or it may be secondary to structural heart disease. Left axis deviation is typical for increased left ventricular mass in hypertensive heart disease. Children with left axis deviation should undergo further cardiology evaluation.

Not surprisingly, the age group 71 – 80 years was the largest. Patients with coronary artery disease, heart failure, atrial fibrillation, sick sinus syndrome and AV-block typically belong to this age group in many countries. The wide age variation also mirrors the wide spectrum of patients treated in the health centers.

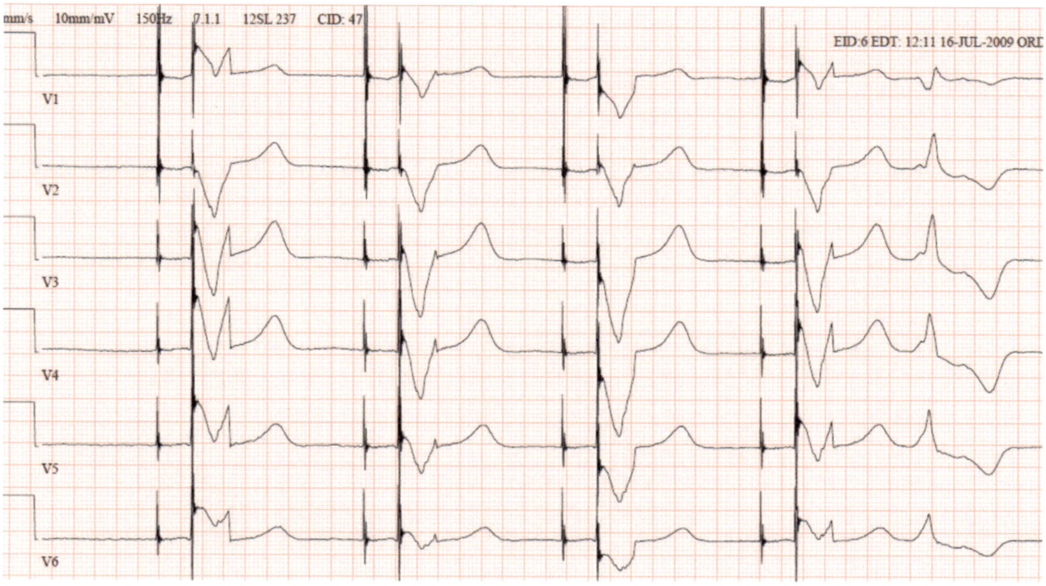

Fig. 2. Normal dual chamber pacing with atrial and ventricular pacemaker spikes. ECG recorded at 50 mm/sec.

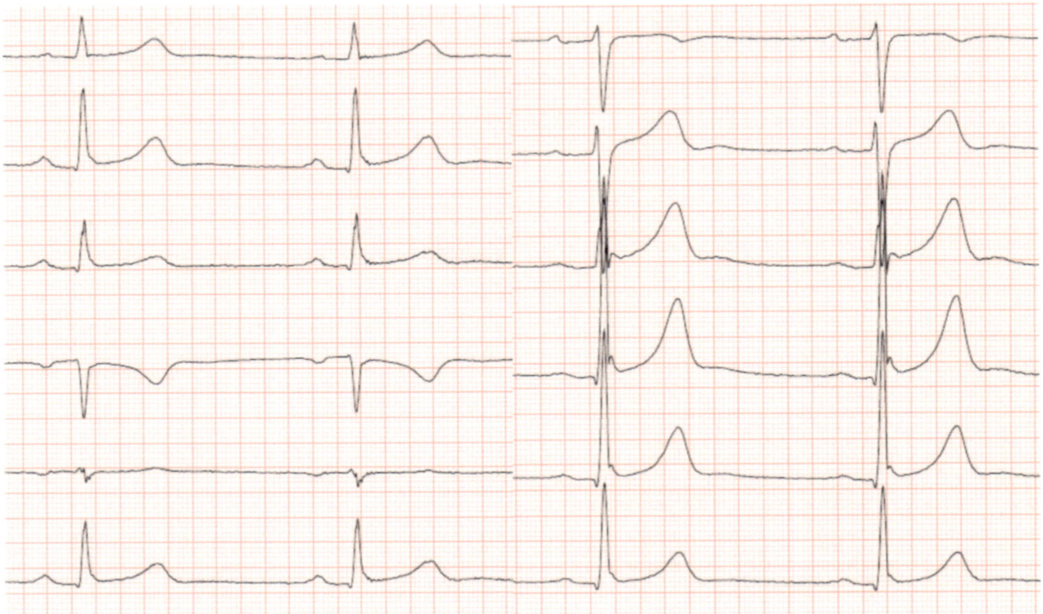

Fig. 3. Typical early repolarization findings in a 22 year old male patient with atypical chest pain. The J point is elevated with ST segment elevations and prominent T waves in many leads. Leads V3-V5 show the most prominent changes. ECG recorded at 50 mm/sec. Extremity leads I, II, III, aVR, aVL, aVF to the left and chest leads V1-V6 to the right.

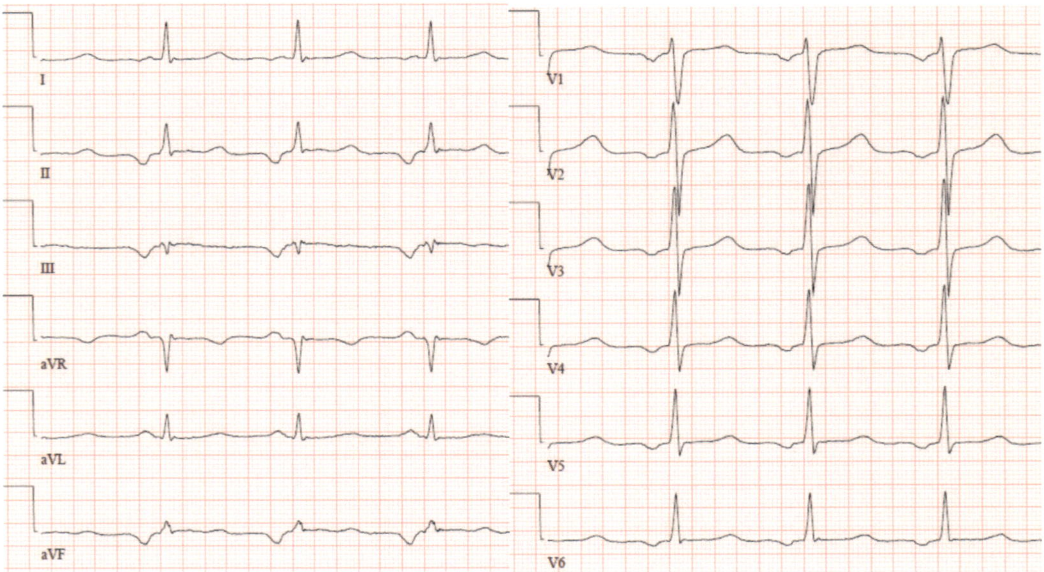

Fig. 4. Ectopic atrial rhythm in a 59 year old female. The P waves are negative in leads II, III and aVF, and in all the precordial leads. Lead aVR shows positive P waves. ECG recorded at 50 mm/sec.

10. Conclusions

We have presented our experiences with a tele-ECG consultation system in Finland. The system was created as a user-friendly, low-cost alternative to traditional specialist consultation. We believe that there is a place for telemedicine also in this field. However, many obstacles were encountered during the process. Success of a real time interactive consultation model probably depends on many factors, like the structure of the health care organization, systems of reimbursement and ECG equipment.

11. References

Ashley EA, Raxwal V, & Froelicher V. (2001). An evidence-based review of the resting electrocardiogram as a screening technique for heart disease. *Progress in Cardiovascular Diseases.* Vol.44, No.1, pp. 55-67, ISSN 0033-0620

Brady WJ, & O'Connor RE. (2008). Interpretation of the electrocardiogram: Clinical correlation suggested. *European Heart Journal.* Vol.29, No.1, pp.1-3, ISSN 0195-668X

Chiantera A, Scalvini S, Pulignano G, Pugliese M, De Lio L, Mazza A, Fera MS, Bussolotti L, Bartolini S, Guerrieri L, Caroselli A, & Giovannini E. (2005). Role of telecardiology in the assessment of angina in patients with recent acute coronary syndrome. *Journal of Telemedicine and Telecare.* Vol.11, Suppl 1, pp. 93-94, ISSN 1357-633X

Cleland JG, Louis AA, Rigby AS, Janssens U, Balk AH, TEN-HMS Investigators. (2005). Noninvasive home telemonitoring for patients with heart failure at high risk of recurrent admission and death: The trans-European network-home-care management system (TEN-HMS) study. *Journal of the American College of Cardiology.* Vol.45, No.10, pp. 1654-1664, ISSN 1558-3597

Edwards J, Handler TJ, Shaffer V, & Lovelock J. (2008). Hype cycle for telemedicine. *Gartner Industry Research Report.* Pub. 25 June 2008. ID number G00157397

Goh KW, Kim E, Lavanya J, Kim Y, & Soh CB. (2006) Issues in implementing a knowledge-based ECG analyzer for personal mobile health monitoring. *Conference Proceedings IEEE Engineering in Medical and Biology Society.* 1:6265-6268, New York, NY, ISSN 1557-170X

Goldberg LR, Piette JD, Walsh MN, Frank TA, Jaski BE, Smith AL, Rodriguez R, Mancini DM, Hopton LA, Orav EJ, Loh E; WHARF Investigators. (2003). Randomized trial of a daily electronic home monitoring system in patients with advanced heart failure: The weight monitoring in heart failure (WHARF) trial. *American Heart Journal.* Vol.146, No.4, pp. 705-712, ISSN 0002-8703

Hailey D, Ohinmaa A, & Roine R. (2004). Published evidence on the success of telecardiology: A mixed record. *Journal of Telemedicine and Telecare.* Vol.10, Suppl 1, pp. 36-38, ISSN 1357-633x

Hongo RH, & Goldschlager N. (2004). Overreliance on computerized algorithms to interpret electrocardiograms. *American Journal of Medicine.* Vol.117, No.9, pp. 706-708, ISSN 0002-9343

Hooper GS, Yellowlees P, Marwick TH, Currie PJ, & Bidstrup BP. (2001). Telehealth and the diagnosis and management of cardiac disease. *Journal of Telemedicine and Telecare*. Vol.7, No.5, pp. 249-256, ISSN 1357-633X

Hämäläinen P, Reponen J, & Winblad I. (2008) eHealth of Finland. *Chech point 2008*, Report 1/2009, Gummerus. Jyväskylä, Finland 2009

Jung W, Rillig A, Birkemeyer R, Miljak T, & Meyerfeldt U. (2008). Advances in remote monitoring of implantable pacemakers, cardioverter defibrillators and cardiac resynchronization therapy systems. *Journal of Interventional Cardiology and Electrophysiology*. Vol.23, No.1, pp. 73-85 ,ISSN 1540-8183

Kadish AH, Buxton AE, Kennedy HL, Knight BP, Mason JW, Schuger CD, Tracy CM, Winters WL Jr, Boone AW, Elnicki M, Hirshfeld JW Jr, Lorell BH, Rodgers GP, Tracy CM, & Weitz HH; American College of Cardiology/American Heart Association/American College of Physicians-American Society of Internal Medicine Task Force; International Society for Holter and Noninvasive Electrocardiology. (2001). ACC/AHA clinical competence statement on electrocardiography and ambulatory electrocardiography: A report of the ACC/AHA/ACP-ASIM task force on clinical competence (ACC/AHA committee to develop a clinical competence statement on electrocardiography and ambulatory electrocardiography) endorsed by the international society for holter and noninvasive electrocardiology. *Circulation*. Vol.104, No.25, pp. 3169-3178, ISSN 0009-7322

Kuhn M, Morgan MT, & Hoffman JR. (1992). Quality assurance in the emergency department: Evaluation of the ECG review process. *Annals of Emergency Medicine*. Vol.21, No.1, pp. 10-15, ISSN 1097-6760

Louis AA, Turner T, Gretton M, Baksh A, & Cleland JG. (2003). A systematic review of telemonitoring for the management of heart failure. *European Journal of Heart Failure*. Vol.5, No.5, pp. 583-590, ISSN 1388-9842

Lähteenmäki J, Leppänen J, Kaijanranta H, Nikus K, Veijonen T, Laakko T, & Nummiaho A. (2009). Document-based service platform for telemedicine applications. *eHealth International Journal*. Vol.5, No.1, pp. 10-17, Open access

Mant J, Fitzmaurice DA, Hobbs FD, Jowett S, Murray ET, Holder R, Davies M, & Lip GY. (2007). Accuracy of diagnosing atrial fibrillation on electrocardiogram by primary care practitioners and interpretative diagnostic software: analysis of data from screening for atrial fibrillation in the elderly (SAFE) trial. *British Medical Journal*. Vol.335, No.7616, pp. 380-386, ISSN 0959-8138

Mele P. (2008). Improving electrocardiogram interpretation in the clinical setting. *Journal of Electrocardiology*. Vol.41, No.5, pp. 438-439, ISSN 0022-0736

Molinari G, Reboa G, Frascio M, Leoncini M, Rolandi A, Balzan C, & Barsotti A. (2002). The role of telecardiology in supporting the decision-making process of general practitioners during the management of patients with suspected cardiac events. *Journal of Telemedicine and Telecare*. Vol.8, No.2, pp. 97-101, ISSN 1357-633X

Nadelmann J, Frishman WH, Ooi WL, Tepper D, Greenberg S, Guzik H, Lazar EJ, Heiman M, & Aronson M. (1990). Prevalence, incidence and prognosis of recognized and unrecognized myocardial infarction in persons aged 75 years or older: The Bronx

Aging Study. *American Journal of Cardiology*. Vol.66, No.5, pp. 533-537, ISSN 0002-9149

Nikus K, Lähteenmäki J, Lehto P, & Eskola M. (2009). The role of continuous monitoring in a 24/7 telecardiology consultation service--a feasibility study. *Journal of Electrocardiology*. Vol.42, No.6, pp. 473-480, ISSN 0022-0736

Okin PM, Devereux RB, Jern S, Kjeldsen SE, Julius S, Nieminen MS, Snapinn S, Harris KE, Aurup P, Edelman JM, Wedel H, Lindholm LH, & Dahlöf B; LIFE Study Investigators. (2004). Regression of electrocardiographic left ventricular hypertrophy during antihypertensive treatment and the prediction of major cardiovascular events. *Journal of the American Medical Association*. Vol.292, No.19, pp. 2343-9, ISSN 0098-7484

Roth A, Korb H, Gadot R, & Kalter E. (2006). Telecardiology for patients with acute or chronic cardiac complaints: The 'SHL' experience in Israel and Germany. *International Journal of Medical Information*. Vol.75, No.9, pp. 643-645

Salerno SM, Alguire PC, & Waxman HS. (2003). Competency in interpretation of 12-lead electrocardiograms: A summary and appraisal of published evidence. *Annals of Internal Medicine*. Vol.138, No9, pp. 751-760, ISSN 0003-4819

Saxena SC, Kumar V, & Giri VK. (2003). Telecardiology for effective healthcare services. *Journal of Medical Engineering Technology*. Vol.27, No.4, pp. 149-159, ISSN 1752-6418

Scalvini S, & Glisenti F. (2005). Centenary of tele-electrocardiography and telephonocardiography - where are we today? *Journal of Telemedicine and Telecare*. Vol.11, No.7, pp. 325-330, ISSN 1357-633X

Scalvini S, Capomolla S, Zanelli E, Benigno M, Domenighini D, Paletta L, Glisenti F, & Giordano A. (2005). Effect of home-based telecardiology on chronic heart failure: Costs and outcomes. *Journal of Telemedicine and Telecare*. Vol.11, Suppl 1, pp. 16-18, ISSN 1357-633X

Scalvini S, Zanelli E, Paletta L, Benigno M, Domeneghini D, De Giuli F, Giordano A, & Glisenti F. (2006). Chronic heart failure home-based management with a telecardiology system: A comparison between patients followed by general practitioners and by a cardiology department. *Journal of Telemedicine and Telecare*. Vol.12, Suppl 1, pp. 46-48, ISSN 1357-633X

Sejersten M, Sillesen M, Hansen PR, Nielsen SL, Nielsen H, Trautner S, Hampton D, Wagner GS, & Clemmensen P. (2008). Effect on treatment delay of prehospital teletransmission of 12-lead electrocardiogram to a cardiologist for immediate triage and direct referral of patients with ST-segment elevation acute myocardial infarction to primary percutaneous coronary intervention. *American Journal of Cardiology*. Vol.101, No.7, pp. 941-946, ISSN 0002-9149

Sekar P, & Vilvanathan V. (2007). Telecardiology: Effective means of delivering cardiac care to rural children. *Asian Cardiovascular & Thoracic Annals*. Vol.15, No4, pp. 320-323, ISSN 0218-4293

Terkelsen CJ, Lassen JF, Nørgaard BL, Gerdes JC, Poulsen SH, Bendix K, Ankersen JP, Gøtzsche LB, Rømer FK, Nielsen TT, & Andersen HR. (2005). Reduction of treatment delay in patients with ST-elevation myocardial infarction: Impact of pre-hospital diagnosis and direct referral to primary percutanous coronary intervention. *European Heart Journal*. Vol.26, No.8, pp. 770-777, ISSN 0195-668x

Todd KH, Hoffman JR, & Morgan MT. (1996). Effect of cardiologist ECG review on emergency department practice. *Annals of Emergency Medicine*. Vol.27, No1, pp. 16-21, ISSN 0196-0644

Vijayaraghavan R, Yan AT, Tan M, Fitchett DH, Georgescu AA, Hassan Q, Langer A, Goodman SG; Canadian Acute Coronary Syndromes Registry Investigators. (2008). Local hospital vs. core-laboratory interpretation of the admission electrocardiogram in acute coronary syndromes: Increased mortality in patients with unrecognized ST-elevation myocardial infarction. *European Heart Journal*. Vol.29, No1, pp. 31-37, ISSN 0195-668X

Zaliunas R, Benetis R, Vanagas G, Slapikas R, & Vainoras A. (2009). Implementation of international transtelephonic ECG platform for patients with ischemic heart disease. *Medicina (Kaunas)*. Vol.45, No2, pp 104-110, ISSN 1648-9144

13

Tele Oncology for Cancer Care in Rural Australia

Sabe Sabesan[1,3] and Sean Brennan[2,3]
[1]*Departments of Medical Oncology and* [2]*Radiation Oncology*
Townsville Cancer Centre, The Townsville Hospital
Townsville, Queensland
[3]*School of Medicine and Dentistry, James Cook University*
Townsville, Queensland
Australia

1. Introduction

Rural cancer patients in Australia and other countries with significant rural populations face difficulties with accessing various sub specialist services mainly because of shortage of health care work force and long travel distances to access these services(Underhill et al,2009). Partly as a result, their survival is lower than their urban counterparts(Campbell et al,2001; Australian Institute of Health and Welfare,2010; Sabesan and Piliouras,2009).

To improve equity of access and quality of life, clinics and treatment centres should be located closer to homes in rural towns. Currently, there are several models of care exist to address some of the issues as follows(Underhill et al,2009): (1) medical oncologists travel to larger rural towns and chemotherapy is administered there. Frequency of these visits range between weekly to three monthly intervals; (2) patients travel to larger centres for consultation and return to their home towns to receive their chemotherapy; (3) patient's travel to major towns to see the specialists and to receive chemotherapy. These models are often inadequate, expensive and cause problems for patients, specialists as well as rural doctors who would ultimately care for these patients.

There are several problems with the first model. This is only suitable for larger towns with higher patient loads. In between specialist visits, patients who are sick would be transferred to major centres to be treated by the specialists or managed by rural doctors without direct supervision by the specialists who initiated the treatment. It also causes disruption to the routine of specialists who already have a significant work load and a waiting list at their home sites.

Problems faced by patients and families under the second and third models are numerous(McGrath, 2000). They often travel long distances for shorter consultations. They often have to relocate to major centres for extended periods for investigation and treatment which results in significant disruption to family and work routine and incurs significant out of pocket expenses. Patients having chemotherapy face another challenge in that they often travel back long distances after chemotherapy regimens that can make them nauseous. In

addition, these models are expensive because of cost of travel and accommodation for patients and their families and specialists.
This calls for alternative ways of consulting and treating patients from smaller rural centres. Care of cancer patients using videoconferencing is an attractive model to satisfy this call. This technology allows patients, doctors, health workers like nurses and other allied health practitioners and family members to see each other while discussing management options unlike telephone consultations. Centres with established teleoncology services include Kansas, USA; British Columbia, Canada ; Townsville, Australia and many others around the world(Doolittle et al,2001;Taylor et al' 2007; Sabesan et al, 2009).

2. Models of teleoncology outreach care

Technologies in telemedicine like videoconferencing can be used for various purposes in cancer care. These include 1. Discussion between health care professionals about cases in multidisciplinary meetings, 2. Consultation of patients by allied health professionals, 3. Consultations by medical oncologists, radiation oncologists, palliative care physicians and haematologists for ambulatory patients and inpatients in rural hospitals.

2.1 Townsville Cancer Centre model

Townsville Cancer Centre, a comprehensive cancer centre, is located in Townsville in Queensland, Australia and is the tertiary referral centre for a population of 650,000 in the North Queensland. Over the last four years to improve the rural access to specialist medical oncology services, department of medical oncology of the Townsville Cancer Centre has been using videoconferencing technology to oversee the management of medical oncology patients from rural and remote towns of the Townsville and Mt Isa Health Service Districts, approximate area of 1200 x 1200 kms. Initially patients were seen face to face for the first consultation, with subsequent video link consultations and treatment performed in Mt Isa or in alternative nearby towns. In the last 12 months the role of videoconferencing in the Townsville Cancer Centre has expanded, with patients now managed exclusively via videoconferencing from the first consultation to treatment and follow up.
Videoconference consultations are conducted on a weekly basis and patients are allocated a time slot in routine medical oncology clinics, although urgent cases are seen anytime. Prior to initial consultations, informed consent is obtained from patients and individuals declining to be seen via video link would be given the option of travelling to Townsville. In Mt Isa, at the receiving end of the video link, patients and their support persons are joined by a chemotherapy competent nurse, senior medical officer, and allied health workers. Patients are examined by the attending doctors during consultations. If a patient has had a recent CT scan (computer tomography) then physical examination is not performed, except for checking vital signs. Treatment decisions and chemotherapy regimes are decided by the medical oncologists and are administered in Mt Isa by chemotherapy competent nurses, supervised by the local medical team. Any dose modifications are made by the specialists and patients needing urgent chemotherapy for aggressive disease receive their chemotherapy in Mt Isa without delay. Patients who are severely unwell, due to their primary diagnosis or due to treatment adverse effects, are seen more frequently via video link while they are in patients, with the option of transfer to the Townsville Hospital. For other towns in the health services district, where administration of intravenous chemotherapy is not feasible, a nurse and sometimes doctors accompany the patients and

families during consultations. Recently radiation oncology and haematology consultations have commenced on videoconferencing using this model.

3. Benefits of teleoncology

Telemedicine offers many advantages for patients , their families and rural health workers. Benefits observed by the Townsville Cancer Centre between Jan 2007 and Nov 2010 are described below. Data was extracted from the oncology information system of the Townsville Cancer Centre.

3.1 Ability to provide consultations to patients at their home towns

Since the inception of the project, 150 patients have been consulted resulting in 609consultations. Demographic details are described in table 1 and 2. Of the 77 new patients seen, all were seen for a first new patient consultation via videoconferencing. 60 patients were seen at least once in person when they travelled to Townsville for other medical or social reasons.

Tele Oncology Centres (distance from Townsville)	**Number of Patients**	**Number of Consultations**
Mt Isa(900 km)	123	517
Proserpine/Bowen(275 km)	16	43
Hughenden(385 km)	02	11
Winton(599 km)	04	21
Doomadgee(1200 km)	01	03
Palm Island	01	01
Gulf of Carpantaria(740-1200 km)	04	14
Total	150	609
Gender -Male	69	
-Female	81	
Ethnicity- Indigenous	17	
- Non indigenous	133	
First consultation on videoconference	77	
Seen face to face prior to videoconference	73	

Table 1. Demographic details of patients attending teleoncology clinics

Cancer types	Number of patients	Curative intent	Palliative intent
Breast	55	28	27
Colorectal	31	10	21
Lung	33	00	33
Upper GI Malignancy(stomach, esophagus & pancreas)	13	01	12
Genitourinary malignancy (Testis, prostate, bladder & kidney)	08	02	06
Melanoma	05	02	03
Ovarian cancer	03	03	00
Invasive mole	01	01	00
Mesothelioma	01	00	01
Total	150	47	103

Table 2. Cancer types of patients attending teleoncology clinics

Gulf of Carpentaria comprises a cluster of remote rural and indigenous towns in North West Queensland. This area is frequently cut off from rest of Queensland during wet season and travel by road for face to face consultations are not feasible during this period.

3.2 Ability to provide urgent medical care at their home towns

8 patients required urgent consultation and all were seen via videoconferencing within 24 hours. Table 3 describes the clinical nature of these patients. Prior to the videoconferencing these patients would have required transfer to Townsville hospital for assessment. Of these 8 patients, 2 required transfer to palliative care in Mt Isa after discussion with the family and patient. Treatment was initiated for the remainder within 48 hours. No inter hospital transfers occurred since the project began.

Cancer type	patients	Chemotherapy	palliation
Extensive stage small cell	3	2	1
Non small cell lung	2	2	0
Metastatic Head and neck	1	0	1
Metastatic colon cancer	1	1	0
Invasive mole	1	1	0
Total	8		

Table 3. Clinical nature of patients consulted urgently

3.3 Accommodating indigenous needs

17 indigenous patients were consulted and treated under this model of care. 12 patients were accompanied by 4 or more extended family members for consultations and treatments accommodating cultural family norms.4 were accompanied by their spouses. One patient was accompanied by a traditional healer. Table 3 describes the nature of cancer and the treatment received by indigenous patients.

3.4 Ability to provide cancer treatments closer to patients' homes

81 patients received chemotherapy in Mt Isa. Table 5 shows various chemotherapy regimens and number of cycles administered. Since the project began, no patient has travelled to Townsville for chemotherapy.

Type of cancer	patients	Active treatment	palliation
Breast cancer	3	2 Chemotherapy, 1 hormonal agent	0
Small cell lung cancer	3	2 pts chemotherapy,	1
Non small cell lung cancer	5	2 chemotherapy, 1 targeted agent,	2
Oesophageal cancer	2	1 chemotherapy	1
Metastatic Head& neck cancer	1	none	1
Rectal cancer	1	chemotherapy	0
Metastatic colon cancer	1	chemotherapy	0
Ovarian cancer	1	3 lines of chemotherapy	0
Total	17		

Table 4. Clinical nature of indigenous patients attending teleoncology clinics

Regimens	Number of patients	Median number of cycles(range)
Breast cancer		
TAC	6	6(2-6)
TC	3	4(4)
AC	2	4(4)
Taxol/gemcitabine	3	8(6-8)
FEC100-Taxotere	3	6(6)
Colorectal cancer		
XELOX	8	6(1-13)
FOLFOX	2	10(10-12)
Fluorouracil	3	24weeks
Xeloda	3	8(1-8)
Lung cancer		
Carboplatin /Taxol	6	6(3-6)
Carboplatin/Vinorelbine	4	4(2-4)
Carboplatin/Gemcitabine	8	4(3-6)
Carboplatin/etoposide	5	6(2-8)
Ovarian cancer		
Carboplatin/Taxol	3	6(6)
Germ cell tumour		
BEP	1	4(4)
Invasive mole		
Methotrexate infusion	1	2(2)
Others	20	
Total	81	

Abréviations: T-docetaxel, A-Adriamycin, C-cyclophosphamide.

Table 5. Chemotherapy regimens supervised via telemedicine.

3.5 Discussion

Results from analysis of our project demonstrate that provision of equitable cancer care to the rural and remote towns and indigenous patients can be achieved using videoconferencing. The model facilitates equitable and immediate access to medical oncology specialist services and allows reviews on an urgent basis within 24 hours without the need for costly inter hospital transfers and inherent delays in transfer. Disturbance to family and work routine is minimised, Inter hospital transfer costs are reduced and disruption to health systems and patients and their families is minimised. Under our model, immediate consultation is possible, with investigation initiated and treatment commenced within 48 hours.

The system is simple to operate and efficient in its ability to dial into different towns in one sitting allowing greater geographical access than that allowed by attending a limited number of prescribed peripheral clinics. Feedback regarding investigations and post treatment assessments are possible without delays incurred by clinic schedules.

17 indigenous patients and their families from Mt Isa, Lake Nash, Doomadgee and Mornington Island were seen in clinics. Special attention to cultural norms and community involvement in patient care is facilitated by allowing patients to remain located within their immediate communities whilst accessing specialist advice and management. On average, indigenous patients were accompanied by 4-6 family members. Explaining to the family members about the illness and clarifying questions from community members contributed significantly to patient care. Improved treatment acceptance and compliance is observed. Attendance of local traditional healers with patients at their consultation offers the opportunity of education and acknowledgement of cultural values. An unanticipated potential opportunity has developed from many separate families asking questions regarding the causes of cancer and in particular smoking related malignancy. An educational component to extended families during the interview could be incorporated into video linked clinics in addition to the patient focus.

A major benefit of this system is the ability to treat patients with chemotherapy closer to their homes. Mt Isa provides all solid tumour chemotherapies, both oral and intravenous, whilst smaller towns can safely supervise oral agents. Since the project began, no patients from Mt Isa had to travel to Townsville for chemotherapy. A further advantage is that patients may be reviewed immediately for complications and appropriate advice discussed with the physician responsible at the remote centre.

Initial challenges to the successful implementation of the project were overcome with staff training on relevant technology. Hearing and visual impairment in patients presented no greater impediment to successful communication than it did in face to face clinics. Accompanying nurses, doctors and patient family members ensured the correct message was passed on to the patients.

The benefits this project offered to rural patients has resulted in clinicians from other departments within Townsville Cancer Centre (including Radiation Oncology, Haematology and Palliative Care) introducing the technology in selected rural patient consultations. The model has potential wide applicability within medicine. Adoption of the model will require specific tailoring to the unique needs of the medical subspecialty clinicians and their patients.

In conclusion, medications have changed, health technology has advanced but the way we deliver health care services has not changed over the last 100 years. Videoconferencing is an alternative and /or complimentary technology to enhance the rural access not only to specialist oncology services but also for all fields of medicine and could become part of day to day business of all departments involved in care of rural patients. This would be one of the first few steps in closing the gap between rural and urban health outcomes and indigenous and non indigenous health outcomes, not only in Australia but also in many other countries with significant rural population.

4. Measurement of outcomes

In addition to the overall benefit of teleoncology described above, it is useful also to measure and document other outcomes to promote this model of care among other health workers and patients. They include level of patient and health workers satisfaction, safety of chemotherapy supervision and delivery and cost effective analysis.

4.1 Satisfaction of patients and health care workers

4.1.1 Introduction

Studies executed with smaller patient numbers suggest both patients and physicians are satisfied with videoconference consultations. A regional cancer centre in Victoria Canada compared satisfaction levels between 60 sequential patients, 30 consulted via videoconferencing, and 30 seen face to face(Weinerman et al;2005). Results demonstrated patients were very satisfied with teleconsultation, particularly as it saved travel time. However, the oncologist involved in this study was reported to feel that video consultation was less effective. Another study from British Columbia also revealed a high level of satisfaction, with greater than 90% of the patients involved in agreement with the highest offered positive questionnaire options(Taylor et al;2007). The consulting physicians in this study demonstrated slightly less satisfaction, with 80% or more cumulative agreement. One question however scored lower for both the patients and physicians and concerned the absence of a physical examination by specialists. Our aim was to examine the level of satisfaction among patients and health workers in relation to the Townsville model.

4.1.2 Methods

At Townsville Cancer Centre(TCC), a questionnaire based survey was conducted by telephoning patients, following informed consent (Sabesan et al;2011),. Questionnaires addressed the following: (a) demographic details (age, gender, educational level, difficulties with hearing and vision, cancer types, (b) type of consultation (new vs reviews) and (c) 16 statements regarding satisfaction levels in various aspects of telemedicine(figure 1). Responses to each statement were recorded on a 5 point Likert scale with 5 indicating strong agreement, 3 agreement and 1 strong disagreement. Question 17 allowed patient suggestions for future improvement of the service.
The first 13 questions were extracted from the study discussed earlier by Taylor *et al*, (2007), for ease of future comparisons between Townsville and British Columbia models, with town name changes as necessary. The last 3 questions were added to assess overall satisfaction and safety. These 3 questions were not validated but piloted on a smaller sample before use in the main study. Q17 was added to obtain further qualitative input regarding this model of care . Interviews were conducted in 2007/8 in the first consecutive 27 patients, when the service began, and in 2009/10 in 28 consequent patients, after the service was fully established.

Perspective of health workers:

This study collected responses from a range of 18 health care workers who accompanied patients during videoconferencing sessions, including: 5 registered nurses, 9 doctors (2 resident medical officers, 4 senior medical officers, 2 registrars, 1 physician), 1 breast care nurse, 1 social worker and 2 indigenous health workers. Since there are no validated questionnaires to assess the views of the health workers in relation to teleoncology, open ended questions were asked to explore the following themes: (1) safety of chemotherapy delivery, (2) comparison between face-to-face and videolink, (3) major benefits for patients, (4) benefits staff, (5) potential problems that could arise for this model of care, and (6) medico legal concerns. This study was approved by the ethics committees of the Townsville and Mt Isa Hospitals.

1. I could talk to the specialist easily and openly.
2. I felt I could ask my specialist questions.
3. I did not feel that anything important was missed during my visit with my doctor.
4. I understood what the specialist told me.
5. I felt that the doctor and the nurse answered all my questions and concerns.
6. I felt the specialist was able to understand my situation and provide satisfactory care.
7. I felt my privacy and confidentiality were preserved during my first visit with my doctor.
8. I felt it is important for the specialist to examine me.
9. It is important to have the local doctor or nurse with me when my specialist is consulting.
10. I would rather travel to Townsville to
11. I had no difficulty seeing and hearing the doctor through the video link system.
12. I would rather video consult with my doctor now than have to wait for a few weeks to see him/her in person.
13. I felt that being able to video consult with my doctor was convenient and/or saved me time and money.
14. I was able to develop a friendly relationship with my specialist.
15. I am getting satisfactory care from the specialist on video link with the help of doctors and nurses locally.
16. I was able to take medications safely after the consultation with the specialist
17. Anything you feel important that we need to address to improve?

Fig. 1. Statements regarding patient satisfaction

4.1.3 Results

Between June 2007 and June 2010, 113 patients were seen in the telehealth clinic. A total of 55 patients were approached, 27 from the first period and 28 from the second period. 2 patients from the first period and 3 patients from the second period declined for personal reasons. Demographic details of the consenting patients were summarised in table 6. Subjective hearing and vision impairment were reported in 4% of the patients, who were able to complete consultations with the help of their families and accompanying nurses and doctors. The majority of consultations were for pre-chemotherapy visits and routine follow up after being seen initially face-to-face in Townsville. All 8 patients seen for their initial consultation belonged to the second period, after which all patients were cared for without being seen face-to-face first.

Patient satisfaction survey:

A response of the patients to the questionnaire statements is shown on figure 2. Except for questions 8 and 9, the majority of the responses were in agreement or stronger agreement with the score of 3 or more on the Likert scale. For Question 8, which refers to the need for a specialist physical examination, 76% of the patients thought it was necessary, though they were examined by local doctors or had imaging scans. For Question 9, which refers to the need for local doctors and nurses to accompany them, 24% were in agreement. In Q10 22% were willing to travel to TSV rather than attending the videoconference but were happy to have chemotherapy in Mt Isa. Nine of these patients were from the initial period. In contrast to this in Q12 over 82% preferred to receive care via the videolink than travel to a larger centre for a consultation.

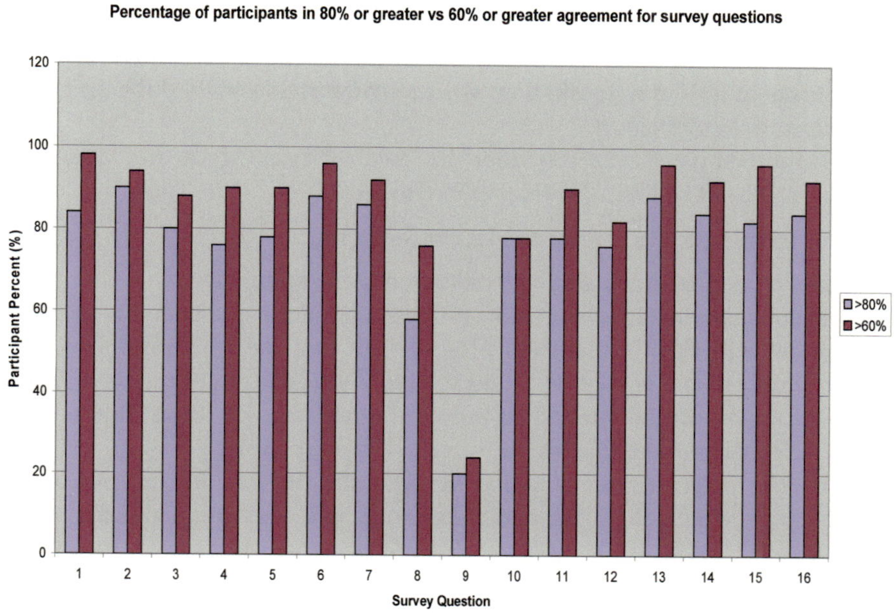

Fig. 2. Responses to satisfaction statements by patients

Age	Mean 58y(range 28-83)	
Total number participating	50 patients	
Gender	Male Female	24% 76%
Educational level	University TAFE High school Less than high school	20% 10% 46% 24%
Hearing and vision impairment		10%
Cancer type	Breast Colorectal Lung Other	42% 18% 10% 30%
Prognosis	Curable Incurable	30% 70%
Type of visit	New Pre chemotherapy Follow up	8% 48% 44%

Table 6. Demographic details of participating patients

Views of the health workers are collated under corresponding themes as follow.

Safety of chemotherapy delivery

1. It is safe as long as procedures are followed and events documented properly,
2. Mutual trust between local doctor and specialist is important and specialist have to be vailable and contactable easily,
3. If patients are too complicated, they could be flown to Townsville,
4. Since health workers are present during consultations and hearing the discussions and instructions, there would be less chance of communication break down.
5. Since we go to TSV for up skilling, we are comfortable with skills and feel safe in administering chemotherapy.
6. Since chemotherapy scripts are done by medical oncologists and they follow the patients up. It can't be less safer than in face to face.

Comparison between face to face and videoconferencing

1. Consultation on videoconferencing looks smooth and spontaneous,
2. Rapport and relationship is easily established, since patients are in their own environment with family members present with local health workers accompanying them, they are relaxed enough to be engaged in discussion regarding their illness.
3. Of course rapport would depend on personalities of the specialists. But here, I can not see any difference between face to face and videoconferencing,
4. I can't believe how effective it is. Face to face still the best for rapport but falls just behind. But patients seem to like it and the conversation is natural and smooth.

Major benefits for patients

1. Less travel for patients
2. Complex services are available locally including chemotherapy delivery
3. Less disturbance to family life,
4. Convenient for patients,
5. Saves money for system and patients
6. Excellent innovation, if it is replicated everywhere, Angel care flight advertisements would need to be modified,
7. Patients appreciate it and expect it and community can not afford to not embrace this technology.

Benefits for doctors, nurses and allied health workers

1. Continuing education,
2. Ready support by specialists,
3. It is like having staff medical oncologist in our town,

Potential problems that could arise for this model of care

1. Coordination is important for smooth running,
2. Minor hearing difficulties could arise, but attending team members could fill in the gaps
3. Doctors with lack of communication skills will find it difficult to engage with patients and would need specific training.
4. Technical difficulties could be frustrating but easily rectified these days.

Medico legal concerns

1. Since patients are seen in a team setting and discussions are documented, no difference between face to face and video link. It may even be safer via videolink because in face to face, patients are seen without other health workers present.
2. Since medical oncologists are involved in all aspects of the care with close follow up, risk of litigation would be similar to that of face to face.
3. Because we follow the procedures and policies that are ratified by the hospital, no cause for concern.

4.1.4 Discussion

Based on favourable patient satisfaction and positive health care workers responses, this study further strengthens the argument for implementing videoconferencing as part of routine medical oncology clinics. Our study evaluates a model of care where chemotherapy regimes and dosing decision is part of the telehealth service, unlike models where videolink is mainly employed for consultations and reviews.

Main themes receiving approval were the following; ease of communication and ability to form rapport, ability to save time and money as the result of reduced travel, medication safety, and the opportunity to receive specialist services closer to home. Of the participating 50 patients, more than 80% were in agreement with satisfaction statements except for Questions 8, 9, and 10. The first 7 Qs relate to the quality of consultations and satisfaction levels proved high. Question 15 examines the overall perceived satisfaction of the medical oncology service, including videoconferencing and local administration of treatment, and demonstrated 96% in agreement with the satisfaction statement, and 82% in stronger agreement. Interestingly Q8 scored highly, indicating patients' desire for physical examination by the medical oncologists. However this appeal reduced once the results of imaging investigations were discussed during consultations. We expected patients to find it important for local doctors and health workers to participate in the videoconferencing yet our results indicated otherwise. However, we believe it is important for the health workers to join patients during consultations since local health care workers have the ability and opportunity to facilitate and fill in the gaps of communication between specialists and patients. In addition, health workers also gain educational benefits for themselves. It is somewhat unexpected that 22% of the patients would rather travel to Townsville than videoconference however the majority were from the first period when the service was in its initial stage. In the later cohort, when our model was operating smoothly, only 2 patients preferred to travel.

Results of our survey are not dissimilar to other surveys indicating overall satisfaction with this model of care(Weinerman et al, 2005; Taylor,2007). Major benefits include travel time saved and improved access to specialist services. The need for physical exam continues to be a concern among the few studies that examined this aspect of care. In a Kansas study 9 of the 22 patients expressed concern about the role of the nurse as a proxy for the doctor in performing certain parts of the physical examination(Mair et al,2000). In the British Columbia study 35% of participants showed the same concern and yet when the physical exam was performed by the specialist within 60 days, no change in treatment decision was reported(Taylor et al,2007). Our study reported 76% of the participants proposed it was necessary, despite examination by local doctors. Unlike the Kansas study, where a nurse was the examiner, the patients are examined by a senior medical officer. In the future this concern could be alleviated by case-by-case explanations at the time of consent demonstrating why an examination by the medical specialist is not required.

After the initial set up period, following adequate training of staff and development of work instructions, technical difficulties were minor and infrequent. The speed and clarity of videoconferencing has greatly improved with advanced technology, simplifying installation and day to day operation.
Satisfaction levels of health care staff involved in videoconferencing have not clearly been established in literature. Currently available study populations include only the specialists and local doctors and study numbers are small, preventing statistically significant conclusions. Similarly our health care worker cohort consisted of few nurses, social workers, and indigenous health workers. Nevertheless this model of care is seemingly welcomed and appreciated by rural health workers due to the benefits to the patients and their treating teams. Unlike many face-to-face consultations, where the specialist consult only with patients and their support persons, in this model medical staff accompanying the patients receive ongoing case-based education and support from the specialists. This study revealed no concerns with litigation and in reality all our videoconference patients are seen personally by medical oncologists, unlike major teaching centres where a significant proportion of patients are seen by trainees with instructions handed down from the specialist following a verbal handover. The risk of litigation, therefore, would be not higher than face-to-face consultations.
Despite being the second largest study focused on this model of care in oncology, our participants' number was still limited. Telehealth is commonly used for smaller rural towns, where patient numbers are small, and consequently randomised controlled studies are unrealistic and subgroup analysis is not meaningful. While we had 2 cohorts, overall responses were similar in terms of satisfaction, with less participants in the second group querying the need of specialist physical examination. This illustrates improved acceptance and satisfaction over time.
In conclusion patients and health workers approve of this model of care due to its many benefits to rural and remote patients. Videoconferencing allows oncology patients to be cared for closer to home without costly long distance travel. From our experience we believe this technology can be complementary to any models of care in looking after rural and remote patients, in all fields of medicine. Since the results of patient satisfaction surveys are consistent and rural health workers approve of this model, telehealth could become a part of standard practice.

4.2 Safety of chemotherapy and medication administration

4.2.1 Introduction and methods

Currently there are no studies in the literature examining the safety of supervision of chemotherapy administration at remote sites via videoconferencing. Therefore a prospective and retrospective chart audits in Townsville and Mt Isa hospital were conducted in patients between January 2007 and November 2010 to examine side effects and admission rates. Results of this audit were to be compared with data from Townsville hospital chemotherapy unit using t-test on SPSS version17.

4.2.2 Results

81 patients received a total 431 cycles of chemotherapy in that time period. 13 patient admissions occurred, 12 patients for treatment related complications and 1 for a

methotrexate infusion in Mt Isa. Reasons for admission included neutropenic sepsis (6 patients), bowel obstruction or diarrhoea (2 patients), pulmonary embolism (1 patient), cardiac arrest(1patient) and pain (2 patients). One patient died after one cycle of capecitabine from severe pneumonia. This patient was on long term prednisone for chronic obstructive pulmonary disease. One patient with gastric cancer suffered a cerebro vascular accident after 4 cycles of EOX (epirubicin,oxaliplatin and capecitabine). Xelox (oxaliplatin and capecitabine) regimen had to be ceased after one cycle in one patient because of severe anaphylactic reaction to oxaliplatin. Rates of side effects were similar to the rates in Townsville ($p = 0.108$).

4.2.3 Conclusion

Our data shows that, using videoconferencing, it is safe to supervise chemotherapy administration by chemotherapy competent nurses at remote sites. It would prudent to document side effects in a prospective manner to enhance the validity of these results. It is also important to ensure that the staffing levels, competencies and training and infrastructure are adequate for achieving and maintaining safety at remote sites.

4.3 Cost effectiveness

4.3.1 Introduction and methods

Cost effective analysis of telemedicine in cancer care is reported only in few studies(Doolittle et al,1997). Along with these studies, many other studies in telemedicine reveal savings to the health systems and families by embarking on telemedicine(Smith et al, 2003;Stalfors et al,2005;Smith et al,2007). All these studies compare cost of out patient clinics or multidisciplinary meetings performed via telemedicine with face to face consultations and fail to include other factors that could potentially increase the financial benefits of telemedicine. Cost effective analysis incorporating many other factors was performed in our center and the methods and results are described below(Thaker and Sabesan,2010).

Data on teleoncology clinics between March 2007 and May 2010, run by TCC between Townsville medical oncology and its satellite centers (Mt Isa, Proserpine, Hughenden, Doomadgee and Winton) was gathered from the Oncology Information Management system.

Crowe's model was used to calculate cost effectiveness which includes project establishment, equipment, maintenance, Communication and Staffing costs (Crowe,1998). Benefit was calculated based upon following factors: prevention of air/road travel and accommodation of patients and relatives from satellite centres to Townsville, prevention of urgent air transfer of patients and prevention of visits of specialists to these centres.

4.3.2 Results

Total of 409 consultations were performed for 110 patients over a period of 38 months from Townsville cancer centre to five satellite centers. Cost of travel, air medical retrieval and accommodation vary between towns depend on distance and road services. During flood, only available mode of transport is by air for some rural towns. For the purpose of this analysis, cheapest available travel cost was used, but in reality, in most cases fares are two to three times higher due to last minute requirements.

Total cost of telemedicine taking into account most of the clinical and technical factors is tabulated in table 7 and the expenses prevented is tabulated in table 8.

Four patients from Mt Isa were consulted urgently on the day of referral or within 24 hours during the period of analysis. These cases would have required transfer to Townsville

Cancer Centre prior to the commencement of the tele oncology services. Our calculations allow for only one escort to accompany patients when they travel to Townsville and does not allow for ideal circumstances. For example, many indigenous patients and some non indigenous patients were accompanied by more than 5 family members and friends during tele consultations. If the government has to pay for travel and accommodation for all the family members, then the expense would be even greater. These calculations do not include out of pocket expenses incurred by patients and families. Other factors like sick leave for patient and a family member, loss of income resulting from long travel and overnight stay would further add to the financial strain faced by patients.

Type of cost	Cost per centre	Cost for all centres for three years	Total
Project establishment	6000	6000 X 6	36000
Equipment	23,726	23,726 X 6	142,356
Maintenance	3558 per centre per year	3558 X 6 X 4	85392
Communication	0.00	0.00	0.00
Staffing	50,000 per year for all centres	50,000 X 4	200,000
Total cost over four years			463,748 AUD

Table 7. Total cost of telemedicine

Description of expenses prevented		Total
Return travel cost for patient and one relative to Townsville	Mt Isa: 516 X 2X 600 $ = 619,200 Proserpine: 40 X 2 X 150 $ = 12000 Hughenden: 11 X 2 X 260 $ = 5720 Winton: 21 X 2 X 320 $ = 13440 Doomadgee: 3 X 2 X 1150 $ = 6900 Normanton: 8 X 2 X 480 $ = 7680 Mornington Island: 4 X 2 X 580= 4640 $ Palm Island: 1 X 2 X 110 = 220 $ Karumba: 1 X 2 X 480 = 960 $	670,760 AUD
Overnight accommodation at Townsville	100 $ X 605	60500
Urgent Aero Medical Retrieval of four patients from Mt. Isa	13,100 $ X 4	52,400
Specialist/Registrar travel once a week for three years	500 $ X 48 X 3	72,000
Total savings over four years		855,660 AUD

Table 8. Expenses prevented by telemedicine.

Another analysis reveals that the cost is higher during establishment period and the savings become greater with time. For example, total cost was 113,006 AUD (Australian dollar) in the first year and the savings was 82820 AUD. In the second year, running cost was 53,554 AUD and saving was 180,320 AUD. In the third year, as many other centres were open, total cost was 229,399 AUD while the benefit was 188,420 AUD. In 2010, running cost was 67,789 AUD and the benefit was 404,100 AUD.

4.3.3 Conclusion

It is clear that teleoncology is cost effective to the patients and the health systems. It seems that the cost is higher than the benefit at the establishment phase because of capital investment and the benefit becomes greater with expansion of services to many other centres with increase in number of consultations and other clinical services like urgent reviews and preventing inter hospital transfers.

5. Factors to consider before embarking on teleoncology

Many factors need to be considered and issues addressed prior to establishing tele oncology clinics in order to avoid conflicts in the future(Sabesan et al,2010). Most of these factors are related to models of care, funding issues, staff level and competencies and service level agreements between provider and receiver of these services. These are discussed below.

5.1 Models of care

It is important to decide on the model of care at the outset that determines the requirements for the clinics. Technical and staffing requirements to provide comprehensive and complex services would differ from that of basic and limited services as discussed below.

5.2 Staff level and competencies

This aspect of telehealth depends on the extent of the services provided via videoconferencing. To provide a comprehensive cancer care including chemotherapy delivery, chemotherapy competent nurses, chemotherapy waste disposal mechanisms, medical officers to supervise and deal with acute complications, administrative support officers to coordinate services and allied health workers are necessary at the receiving end. If simple chemotherapy regimens are administered in rural towns, it would be unrealistic to expect chemotherapy competent nurses and oncology pharmacists in small rural towns. Tele nursing and tele pharmacy could be alternatives. If the service is limited to consultations and short reviews, however, then there may not be a need for a multidisciplinary team. It is important that attendance of rural doctors is not requested unnecessarily given the lack of medical workforce and their clinical work load in rural towns.

Pathology turn around time is another factor to consider and for most chemotherapy regimens, turn around time of 24-48 hours should be adequate. Lastly, oncologists and administrative support officers are needed to run these services at the providing end. When these specialists are busy at their home site, it might be more convenient to have smaller weekly clinics than larger clinics at less frequent intervals. This also allows patients and rural health workers to have regular personal contacts with specialists.

5.3 Equipment

Main issues for consideration are clarity of the images and sound. But the type of technology required depends on the model of care and the purpose of the clinics. For example, if the purpose of the consultation is to discuss issues, then a videophone or internet based systems like skype is adequate. If the clinic is to talk, examine patients and show scans, then a different system with remote control capacity and duovideo systems would be necessary. For example, Queenland health in Australia uses Tandberg 990 codecs and Sony Bravia 32 inch LCD monitors. The codec can be connected to a computer, to show radiology images to the patients. Standard bandwidth for consultations is 256 kbps over IP(internet protocol). Once every one involved is trained on how to operate the technology, consultations would be faster and smoother.

5.4 Medico legal issues and service level agreements

These are usually related to patient consent, documentation of decision making and safety of administration of toxic chemotherapy. Queensland Health's patient consent form, which the patients sign prior to the tele oncology consultations, is designed to protect staff and patients participating in telehealth clinics and use of the Telehealth Patient Information brochure helps ensure that consent is informed. Documentation is similar to that required for an outpatient consultation. Drugs are prescribed by medical oncologists or other oncologists and then checked by nurses and pharmacists as per hospital policies. Adhering to these precautions, we have demonstrated that it is safe to administer and supervise chemotherapy for most cancers in Mt Isa using this technology.

Service level agreements between providers and receivers need to include discussions regarding ownership and allocation of responsibilities when patients become acutely ill. Hospital policies on admission process and care of the admitted patients should be determined early to avoid conflicts over responsibility for the admitted patients. In Mt Isa, patients are admitted under senior medical officers and resident physicians when patients have chemotherapy. The treating specialists can also review inpatients via videoconference. Issues related to funding and remuneration for services are matter for hospitals and health departments to sort out.

5.5 Inability of the specialist to perform a physical examination

This issue can be overcome by having a doctor sitting with patients during consultations and perform physical examination when necessary. If a patient has had recent CT scans of visceral organs, then a physical examination is not always needed. It is also important to explain to patients why physical examination by specialists is not always required. In studies by Mair et al and Taylor et al, nearly one third of the patients were concerned about lack of physical examination by specialists but when physical examinations were performed within 60 days by the specialists, no change in management was made (Taylor et al, 2007).

6. Conclusion

In conclusion, we have demonstrated that telemedicine is an excellent tool for addressing the issue of lack of access to specialist services among rural, remote and indigenous communities. Ability to give urgent medical advice also reduces the need for inter hospital transfers and resulting unexpected and sudden relocation of family members to major centres. Other social benefits for the patients are many. This model of care also allows the specialists to care for many towns in one setting without wasting time on travel. Patients seem to appreciate and accept this model of care and health workers find it beneficial for professional reasons. Level of rapport formed between specialist and patients is difficult to measure, though the overall patient satisfaction is high. Safety is always a concern in medicine and we have shown that it is safe to supervise chemotherapy using videoconferencing. Teleoncology seems to be cost effective for the patients and the health systems. By embarking on telemedicine, valuable funds could be used for infrastructure development instead of wasting on travel. We could also contribute to the climate change agenda by significantly reducing travel.

7. Future

Use of telemedicine in the future is not going to be limited to ambulatory care alone. When patient are admitted to the in patient facilities in rural towns, further support to the local medical and nursing staff could be given via this technology. With enthusiasm among doctors in medical and radiation oncology, palliative care and haematology, this model of care could be applied across all the sub specialities in cancer centres as part of core business to create a concept of "cancer centres in cyber space". Education for rural and remote communities on smoking prevention and other life style issues are not usually the focus of many tertiary cancer centres mainly because of lack of access to these communities. Telemedicine could facilitate regular educational events, in an interactive format, to these isolated communities. Lastly allied health consultations and nursing interventions could be achieved via videoconferencing. One attractive idea is chemotherapy administration by non chemotherapy competent nurses in remote communities, supervised and mentored by chemotherapy competent nurses from tertiary centres using videoconferencing. It would be a dream come true, when the entire medical oncology services including patient consultations, chemotherapy delivery and follow up are one day provided to remote and indigenous patients using telemedicine.

8. Acknowledgement

We thank our operational director Liza Tomlinson, Townsville Hospital's telehealth facilitator Barbara Van Houts and medical oncology administrative support officers Patricia Grady, Mary Urquhart, Michelle Toombes and Kellie Poole for making this model of care a success.

9. References

Australian Institute of health and welfare and Australasian society of cancer registries. (2010)Cancer in Australia: in brief, *Cancer series*. No 59, Cat No CAN 55, Canerra: AIHW, ISSN: 1039-3307

Campbell NC, Ellis A, Sharp L et al. (2010). Rural and urban differences in stage at diagnosis of colorectal and lung cancers. *Br J Cancer*, 84,910-914.

Crowe, B. (1998). Cost effectiveness analysis of telemedicine. *J Telemd and telecare*, 4(supp 1), 14-17, ISSN: 1357-633X

Doolittle, G. C. (2001). Telemedicine in Kansas: the successes and the challenges. *Journal of Telemedicine & Telecare*, 7 Suppl 2, 43-6, ISSN: 1357-633X

Doolittle, G. C., A. Harmon, et al. (1997). A cost analysis of a tele-oncology practice. *Journal of Telemedicine & Telecare*, Suppl 1, 20-2, ISSN: 1357-633X

Mair, F., P. Whitten, et al. (2000). Patients' perceptions of a telemedicine specialty clinic. *Journal of Telemedicine & Telecare,* 6(1), 36-40, ISSN1357-633X

McGrath, P. (2000). Post treatment support for patients with haematological malignancies: findings from regional, rural and remote Queensland. *Australian Health Review,* 23(4), 142-149.

Sabesan, S, Van Houts, B. Parkinson C. (2010). Factors to consider when starting up a medical oncology videolinked clinic." *Aust J Rural Health,* 18, 89-90, ISSN: 1440-1584

Sabesan S, Piliouras. P... (2009). Disparity in cancer survival between urban and rural patients: how can clinicians help reduce it?" *Rural and Remote Health,* 9(online):1146.Available from http://www.rrh.org.au

Sabesan S, Varma S., Nel P.(2009). Letter to the editor-Telemedicine across the ages." *Medical Journal of Australia,* 190(12), 719, ISSN: 1326-5377

Sabesan S, Simcox K, Marr I (2011) Medical oncology clinics via videoconferencing: An acceptable tele health model for rural patients and health workers. Internal Medicine Journal(accepted for publication) april 2011)

Smith, A. C., Scuffham P et al. (2007). The costs and potential savings of a novel telepaediatric service in Queensland.*BMC Health Services Research,* 7,35.

Smith, A. C., Youngberry K et al. (2003). The family costs of attending hospital outpatient appointments via videoconference and in person. *Journal of Telemedicine and Telecare,* 9(Suppl.2), 58-61.

Stalfors, J., Bjorholt I et al. (2005). A cost analysis of participation via personal attendance versus telemedicine at a head and neck oncology multidisciplinary team meeting. *Journal of Telemedicine & Telecare,* 11*(4), 205-10.*

Taylor M, Saltman D et al. (2007). The use of telemedicine to care for cancer patients at remote sites. *Journal of Clinical Oncology,* Part I. Vol 25, 18S(June 20),Abstract:6538, ASCO Annual Meeting Proceedings Chicago,USA.

Thaker D, Sabesan S.(2010).Cost effective analysis of videolinked medical oncology clinics: Townsville experience, *Asia-pac J clin oncol* ,6(suppl.2),140,abstract 160,Proceedings of the Clinical oncology society of Australia ASM, Melbourne, Australia.

Underhill C, Bartel R,Goldstien D et al. (2009). Mapping oncology services in regional and rural Australia. *Aust J Rural Health,* 17, 321-329.

Weinerman, B., den Duyf J, et al. (2005). Can subspecialty cancer consultations be delivered to communities using modern technology?--A pilot study. *Telemedicine Journal & E-Health,* 11(5),608-15.

14

Telemedicine in the Diagnosis and Management of Congenital Heart Disease

Brian McCrossan and Frank Casey
Department of Paediatric Cardiology
Royal Belfast Hospital for Sick Children
Northern Ireland

1. Introduction

Several telemedicine applications have become well established in paediatric cardiology but there is potential for improvement in and expansion of existing programmes and opportunities for new applications. This chapter shall discuss why telemedicine has an important role to play in paediatric cardiology, examine current applications from fetus to adult, including the evidence base and suggest what future steps may be taken to promote the use of telemedicine in paediatric cardiology. We shall also consider what equipment and personnel are necessary for successful tele-cardiology. However, before examining the role of telemedicine in paediatric cardiology, it is first important to understand what congenital heart disease is and how it presents to clinicians.

1.1 What is congenital heart disease

Congenital heart disease can be defined as "a structural abnormality of the heart or intrathoracic great vessels that is actually or potentially of functional significance."(Mitchell et al., 1971) The generally accepted incidence of congenital heart disease is between eight and nine per 1,000 live-born babies and this has remained consistent over several decades. (Ferencz and Neill, 1992; Royal College of Physicians, 2009) The combined incidence of moderate and severe forms of CHD is approximately 6 per 1,000 live births.(Hoffman and Kaplan, 2002) This is perhaps a more reliable and more important statistic as it accounts for babies with structural congenital heart defects that will require treatment. CHD is the most prevalent group of major congenital defects and contributes to at least 5 - 10% of neonatal deaths.(Ferencz and Neill, 1992; Wilkinson and Cooke, 1992)

1.1.1 How congenital heart disease presents

Congenital heart disease may present with a range of symptoms and clinical findings and may present at any age. However, there is certainly a trend towards earlier and even fetal diagnosis.

Symptoms: There is a wide range of cardio-respiratory and even neurological symptoms attributable to heart disease such as cyanosis, shortness of breath, syncope, presyncope and palpitations. It is increasingly common for significant CHD to be diagnosed before the patient experiences any symptoms.

Signs: It is also common for CHD to be diagnosed following the detection of an abnormal clinical sign during a routine clinical assessment or evaluation for an unrelated problem. (Table 1.1)
Imaging: Congenital heart disease may be diagnosed during routine echocardiographic screening in babies and fetuses with risk factors for CHD.

	Presentation	Urgency	Potential for telemedicine
Antenatal	Suspected CHD on routine anomaly scan Risk factor for CHD	Non-urgent	Support sonographers Streamline antenatal screening
Neonate	Cyanosis Murmur Clinical shock Abnormal femoral pulses Risk factor for CHD	Usually an emergency	Immediate diagnosis or exclusion of CHD Institute potentially life-saving therapy Decide upon need for transfer
Infant & Child	Murmur Tachypnoea Hepatomegaly Abnormal femoral pulses Failure to Thrive	Usually less urgent	Virtual clinics could help reconfigure workload for paediatric cardiologists

Table 1. How congenital heart disease presents and the potential for telemedicine to support district general hospitals within a clinical network.

1.2 Why is paediatric cardiology suited to telemedicine

The single biggest reason why paediatric cardiology is suited to telemedicine is that it is a highly specialised field of medicine with a small cadre of professionals. Care is concentrated in a few regional centres. Therefore, large distances separate the patient and non-specialist from expert advice. However CHD presents, it is unlikely that a non-specialist will be confident in making a definitive diagnosis, counselling parents or instituting specific treatment without verification from a paediatric cardiologist. Fortunately, all forms of CHD can be diagnosed by a specialist using a combination of clinical examination, including stethoscopy, ECG, Chest X-Ray and echocardigraphic images i.e. on the analysis of data. These data are suitable for digitisation and electronic transmission and so used in telemedicine.(Dowie et al., 2009) Babies with significant CHD may present to a hospital with on-site paediatric cardiology but considering only 13 hospitals in England and Wales have this facility compared with the 184 DGHs providing acute paediatric care, most will present to post-natal wards, neonatal units and emergency departments without on-site paediatric cardiology expertise. (Workforce Review Team, 2009)
Telemedicine can potentially support paediatricians faced with the predicament of a sick, cyanosed newborn baby with a suspected duct dependent CHD. Duct dependent lesions are a subgroup of severe CHD in which the circulation to either the lungs or body is dependent upon patency of the ductus arteriosus. This usually closes within the first 72 hours of life. In babies with duct dependent CHD, closure of the ductus arterious heralds the onset of severe symptoms. If not treated urgently duct dependent CHD is invariably fatal. The main differential diagnosis in this life-threatening scenario is persistent pulmonary hypertension of the newborn. The treatment of the two conditions is very different. Tele-

echocardiography interpreted by a paediatric cardiologist can offer timely diagnosis, institution of appropriate therapy and expedite or avoid transfer to a paediatric cardiology centre.(Finley et al., 1997; Casey, 1999; Mulholland et al., 1999) Antenatal diagnosis of CHD is chiefly reliant upon an abnormality being suspected by a sonographer at a DGH, with very limited experience and knowledge of CHD, during routine anomaly scanning. Telemedicine may offer support to these radiographers. Telemedicine may also facilitate a rationalisation of paediatric cardiology outreach clinics.

Paediatric cardiologists hold outreach clinics at a number of DGHs within their region, travelling on a half day or full day once a month or once every two or three months. Lower thresholds for referring asymptomatic children with clear cut innocent murmurs for "a second opinion" have swollen outreach clinics.(Dowie et al., 2009)(Dowie et al., 2009) Further pressures have been placed on service provision because of the need to comply with guidelines recommending screening of babies with various syndromes and family screening of certain inheritable conditions. Thus the paediatric cardiologist may be away from the tertiary unit on average at least once a week. Whilst an excellent service is provided at the outreach clinic, it does not seem to be efficient from the tertiary unit's perspective.(Qureshi, 2008) It is understood that most patient's first port of call will be their DGH. Therefore it is important to foster confidence and competence in managing children with CHD. On the other hand, patients with a clinical problem requiring a paediatric cardiology opinion that cannot wait for the next outreach clinic, need transferred to the tertiary centre for a specialist opinion.

A recent innovation has been the curriculum for paediatricians with special expertise in cardiology. Several posts have been appointed in DGHs throughout the UK.(Royal College of Paediatrics and Child Health, 2009) The role of the paediatrician with special expertise in cardiology is to unload some of the outpatient work currently being done by the tertiary centres (e.g. evaluation of children with asymptomatic murmurs or chest pain), to be the link person for children with CHD followed up at that DGH and to be competent at performing 2-D echocardiography. These paediatricians will need to be supported by the relevant tertiary centre. One of the key methods of providing this support could be via telemedicine links.

Congenital cardiac surgery for children for England is currently provided across 11 centres. Each tertiary centre serves several DGHs staffed by paediatricians. A tertiary congenital cardiology service is provided by cardiac surgeons, specialising in congenital cardiac surgery, and paediatric cardiologists. The role of telemedicine in diagnosing and excluding CHD has been recognised at a national level in the UK. Various models of care have been debated leading to a number of recommendations including the establishment of telemedicine links between DGHs and the tertiary unit in order to have echocardiograms interpreted by paediatric cardiologists at all hours, all the year round. (Qureshi, 2008)

A proposed restructuring of paediatric cardiology services in the UK would reduce the number of paediatric cardiology surgical centres from eleven to six.(National Health Service, Specialsed Services, 2011) Several tertiary care centres will therefore need to significantly reorganise their working practices and become part of a large network of hospitals across a wide area (Figure 1). This development, which is likely to be adopted in other countries, is proposed in order to further centralise expertise and hopefully improve outcomes for patients. However, this may disadvantage paediatric cardiologists working in non-cardiac centres and further isolate paediatricians in DGHs. The shared care of patients with CHD, between tertiary non-surgical cardiac centres and the quaternary surgical centres, will necessitate excellent communication and case conferences. CHD case conferences are based around imaging data. It is easy to see that reliable telemedicine links between the various hospitals within this network will be essential.

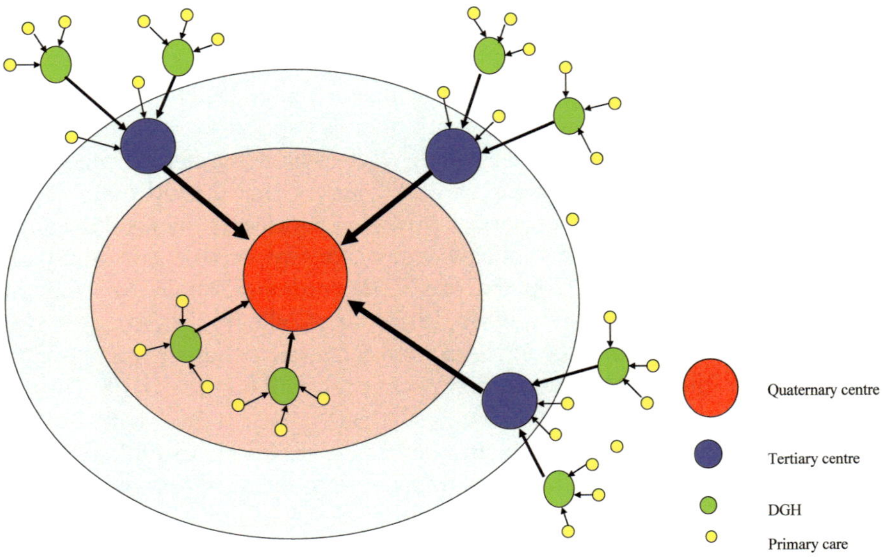

Fig. 1. The complex web of a managed clinical network

In summary, congenital heart disease is potentially lethal. Its diagnosis is reliant upon interpretation of audio and visual data by a small number of experts, concentrated in a few tertiary units. Telemedicine seems to be the ideal tool to provide support to the non-specialist thereby promoting access to specialist advice and improving patient care.

1.3 History of telecardiology

Theoretically, telemedicine has been in existence since the inception of the telephone. It is a commonly held belief that Alexander Graham Bell was working on ideas to benefit the hearing-impaired when he invented the telephone in 1875.(Boettinger, 1977) In 1906, Einthoven presented his first attempts at transmitting ECGs via telephone lines.(Einthoven, 1906) The modern cardiac ambulance still utilises this application to decide upon the emergency treatment of acute myocardial infarction. In 1910 descriptions of how auscultatory sounds from a stethoscope could be amplified and similarly transmitted appeared. Apart from remote evaluation of ECGs, further developments in tele-cardiology did not materialise as the technology was not available and the clinical need not established. However, there was evidently some public interest (Figure 2).

In the 1980's telemedicine grew steadily with developments in transmission technologies such as T-1 and ISDN and the fact that there was "something worth showing." Developments in medical imaging during the 1980's (e.g. echocardiography) increased diagnostic reliance on investigations whose interpretation requires an expert, usually located in a specialist centre. The first report of tele-echocardiography appeared in the 1980's but telecardiology did not really take off in a big way until the mid 1990's with the availability of cheaper, reliable ISDN lines and commercially available, affordable videoconferencing codecs.(Finley et al., 1989) Telecardiology has since branched out from tele-echocardiography to other applications. In the noughties tele-homecare and remote monitoring have become the key growth areas in tele-cardiology. Research and published articles have appeared alongside each application and helped drive the field forward.

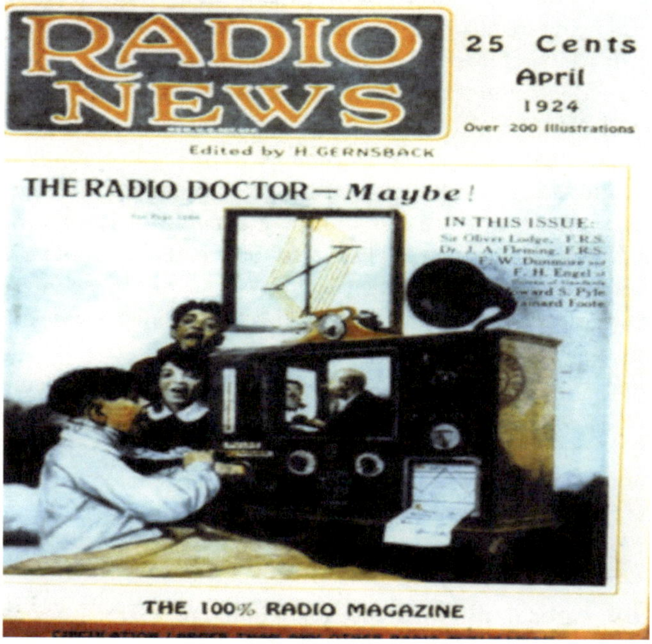

Fig. 2. Cover of Radio News magazine from April 1924 prophesising the potential role of telemedicine.

1.4 Overview of evidence available in paediatric tele-cardiology

There is a substantial body of research to support the feasibility of many applications of telecardiology in both paediatric and adult populations. There is much less good quality evidence demonstrating its clinical utility and cost-effectiveness. Most of the evidence is from small or uncontrolled studies. This is particularly difficult in paediatric cardiology because the numbers of patients involved are necessarily smaller than adult studies. However, there are larger scale randomised control trials in tele-homecare. There is now robust evidence advocating a role for telemonitoring and structured telephone support for patients with chronic heart failure. This will be discussed in more detail later in this chapter. There is also evidence suggesting that remote monitoring of pacemakers and implantable cardiac defibrillators is reliable, safe, that it may improve patient satisfaction and reduce costs. Large randomised control trials are ongoing which should hopefully clarify the role of remote monitoring in this patient group.(Burri and Senouf, 2009)

1.5 What is needed to carry out telecardiology?

The most important point to consider is: what is required from the proposed service? This should dictate the format, equipment and personnel involved. Do not start up a telecardiology service just because a particular piece of equipment comes into your possession.

1.5.1 Hardware

Videoconferencing equipment: There is not much difference from other areas of telemedicine in terms of the equipment needed. A videoconferencing codec is required at both sending and receiving ends. PC based codecs with an attached webcam were formerly favoured as they were much cheaper than purpose built, commercially available videoconferencing machines. However, through the noughties competition between the various videoconferencing companies led to significant improvements in protocols and software resulting in vastly improved videoconferencing codecs at much more affordable prices. Truly mobile videoconferencing units are now commercially available in the form of high spec web cams. This latest development is promising but has not been evaluated yet in telecardiology. Mobile phone technology is capable of facilitating many store and forward telemedicine applications e.g. simple physiological parameters and even chest-xray and ECGs. However, 3G connections are not routinely capable of facilitating medical quality videoconferencing. Mobile phones screens are also too small to conduct a video-consultation which includes a visual examination of the patient. Whatever videoconferencing equipment is employed there should be the facility to record consultations, especially those involving diagnostic imaging.

Cardiology equipment: This depends on the application. For tele-echocardiography, a standard cardiac ultrasound machine should have the requisite outputs (VGA, BNC or Phono) which will permit transmission of the echocardiographic image data to the codec. Tele-stethoscopy and tele-homecare may require more specific equipment which shall be detailed later in the chapter.

1.5.2 Network

Telecardiology grew particularly with the availability of ISDN lines which were much cheaper than what was previously available. However, in comparison with internet transmission, ISDN lines are very expensive. The majority of tele-echocardiography research has been conducted using ISDN lines and it is generally agreed that 384Kbps (ISDN6) is a satisfactory bandwidth.(Houston et al., 1999) Although no research has been conducted on this point, it is our experience that transmission of grey scale images such as cardiac angiograms requires a higher bandwidth, in the region of 1MBps. Many hospitals are part of healthcare organisations with wider computer networks affording large bandwidths for internet based videoconferencing. Thus, echocardiographic and other diagnostic images maybe transmitted at bandwidths close to 2MB. Telemedicine equipment maybe plugged into any network point in the hospital. This seems ideal for inter and intra-hospital telecardiology. However, it is still our experience that dedicated ISDN lines are the most reliable network. This advantage must be weighed against the cheaper, more flexible and higher bandwidth internet alternative. Undoubtedly the current is in favour of internet transmission.

Tele-homecare is much more fluid than inter-hospital telecardiology. Because each link is dedicated to one patient, the cost per patient is much greater than for a dedicated inter-hospital link. For home videoconferencing, ISDN links can be utilised and have the advantage of a guaranteed bandwidth but have to be installed for each home and are expensive. Whereas home broadband is already installed in many homes and in some developed countries up to two-thirds of households have internet connections with more having the availability. Home broadband connections have improved considerably in the past 10 years with larger bandwidths routinely available. Although home broadband suffers from the problem of "contention" there are methods of "tagging" a routers packages to give them priority traffic thereby protecting the bandwidth and videoconference quality. Therefore, home broadband is now the preferred network for conducting hospital - home videoconferences.(Horrigan, 2009)

1.5.3 Personnel

Again the question of what your telemedicine service is hoping to achieve dictates the personnel that should be involved.

Inter-hospital tele-echocardiography: Two sets of personnel are required. At the sending end, a health professional is required to relay the clinical information to the receiving end. This should be the most senior doctor available. At the receiving end, a senior paediatric cardiologist is required to interpret the clinical history and transmitted images and formulate a management plan. This should preferably be a consultant but a senior trainee may also be permissible. A health professional is also required to acquire echocardiographic images.

Published literature is divided into studies where an adult cardiac sonographer has performed the echocardiogram and those where a paediatrician has acquired the images.(Finley et al., 1997; Mulholland et al., 1999; Tsilimigaki et al., 2001; Sable et al., 2002; Widmer et al., 2003) There are arguments in favour of either method. One of the major obstacles to performing tele-echocardiography is the lack of personnel who can use a cardiac ultrasound machine. It requires quite a lot of practice to become familiar with the controls not to mention how and where to position the probe in order to acquire images. An adult cardiac sonographer may not perform echocardiograms on neonates but they are very proficient at using a cardiac ultrasound machine and the standard probe positions are common to both paediatric and adult echocardiography. Therefore, little guidance is required from the paediatric cardiologist. This method is well suited to a store and forward protocol. However, many DGHs do not have out-of-hours cardiac sonographer cover which could limit tele-echocardiography to a nine to five, Monday to Friday service which acute medicine most certainly is not.

Alternatively, the attending paediatrician / neonatologist could receive some training in performing echocardiography and acquire the relevant images for the tele-consultation. This requires more patience and input from the paediatric cardiologist in terms of directing the paediatrican which way to position the probe and pointing out the relevant cardiac structures as they come into view. Therefore, real-time telemedicine is much better suited to this method. With the paediatrician performing the echocardiogram, there is now the possibility of a 24 hours a day, seven days a week telemedicine service which is obviously preferable. It also provides opportunities to educate and re-enforce good practice. However, it is important that scanning skills are refreshed. For these reasons, we prefer the paediatrician to be actively involved in performing the echocardiogram as opposed to adult cardiac sonographers but acknowledge that there are advantages to the latter.

Tele-stethoscopy: The drive behind tele-stethoscopy is to produce remote paediatric cardiology out-patient clinics. These have been successfully set-up in neurology, ENT and Dermatology to name but a few. (Patterson, 2001)(Levin and Warshaw, 2009)(Dorrian et al., 2009)A consultant paediatric cardiologist is required at the receiving end as he/ she has to ultimately take responsibility for the consultation. At the sending end, a nurse could be trained to take a history and perform an ECG (if necessary), then direct the camera for a visual examination followed by placing the tele-stethoscope in the requisite positions for

auscultation. This telemedicine application does not necessarily require a doctor at the transmitting end. However, this would be a rare and excellent opportunity for continuing professional development.
Tele-homecare: In the home, only the parent/ primary carer along with the patient are required. However, it is useful for primary care staff such as the health visitor or community children's nurse to be occasionally present. This allows the non-specialist to see what the paediatric cardiologist focuses on during a consultation and fosters good working relations. It is important that tele-homecare delivered by the tertiary unit does not undermine the primary care team. In the hospital, the tele-consultation should be taken by a health professional experienced in paediatric cardiology and familiar with each patient's diagnosis and history. This may be a paediatric cardiology trainee or an experienced nurse such as a cardiac liaison nurse. It is important that the consultant paediatric cardiologist is kept informed of developments with his/ her patients and is supportive of the staff involved in the tele-homecare programme.

1.6 Economic evaluation

The area most neglected in telecardiology research is economic analysis. There have been even fewer economic analyses of telemedicine applications in paediatric cardiology. The Royal Brompton Hospital, London, have published a series of articles whose main interest has been economic evaluation of a paediatric telecardiology service. This service encompasses real-time and store and forward telemedicine for fetal tele-echocardiography, neonatal tele-echocardiography and paediatric cardiology outpatient services. Using Bootstrapping analysis, costs were calculated for the first six months after the initial telemedicine consultation. Across all four hospitals with in the telemedicine network, the mean cost of implementing and running the telemedicine service is higher at each time interval than conventional referral. However, owing to the large standard deviation, these differences are not statistically significant. This analysis of the full range of paediatric tele-cardiology services is valuable. However, the amalgamation of services evaluated, the different populations involved (fetuses, neonates and children) and the different telemedicine formats employed make it difficult to elicit generalisable conclusions. For any paediatric cardiology centre considering embarking on a telemedicine programme it is perhaps more helpful to individually assess the separate components of a tele-cardiology service. To this end, the Brompton group describe an economic evaluation of their experience of a fetal tele-cardiology service. The authors conclude that the telemedicine assessment was more costly than a face-to-face examination in London ($p < 0.001$). However, using bootstrapped analysis, the telemedicine service becomes cost neutral at 14 days and six months. This study allows the reader to make more definite conclusions as to what the costs and savings of providing a similar fetal tele-cardiology service in their own region.(Dowie et al., 2007; Dowie et al., 2008; Dowie et al., 2009) The only other economic evaluation relating to paediatric cardiology reported in the literature is a cost minimisation study of a paediatric cardiology telemedicine network in Quebec, Canada. Whilst the authors describe this study as a cost-effectiveness analysis, no cost per health outcome is presented. This study suggests that telemedicine care is more expensive than conventional care.(Sicotte et al., 2004)
However enthusiastic telemedicine initiatives begin many are not sustained. One of the reasons for the short term nature of telemedicine projects is a lack of long-term funding which is partly due to sparse quantitative evidence including cost analyses.(Smith et al.,

2007) Previous studies reporting feasibility and diagnostic accuracy have included cost analysis as a secondary outcome.(Mulholland et al., 1999; Sable et al., 1999) However, these cost analyses were methodologically flawed, being cost-minimisation studies based on small scale, start-up programmes.

Another criticism of cost analyses involving telemedicine projects is that they are based upon start up programs where the initial burst of interest and activity decreases the unit cost of a teleconsultation. (Roine et al., 2001)Telemedicine cost analyses have been criticised for being small scale, short term pragmatic evaluations. In a systematic review of cost effectiveness studies in telemedicine, Whitten et al concluded that there is no good evidence that telemedicine is cost effective.(Whitten and Cook, 1999) In fact there have been very few cost-effectiveness studies because by definition this requires measuring a cost per unit of health outcome e.g. QALY. Most cost analysis to date have been cost minimisation studies which are out of favour and not likely to persuade health authorities to fund telemedicine services.

Payment for telemedicine consultations remains problematic. In our healthcare model (UK National Health Service) there is no mechanism in place for the regional unit to receive payment for each remote consultation. However, it maybe possible to build telemedicine services into the job plan of specialists in recognition of time undertaken in remote consultations. This is not a satisfactory situation. Other healthcare organisations, for example in the USA, have the potential to charge the referring institution a fee for each telemedicine consultation. Up to 12 states in the USA now mandate that health care plans cover telemedicine.

In summary, despite the presence of many paediatric cardiology telemedicine programmes, there is really very little evidence supporting its use from an economic perspective. This seems paradoxical as one of the founding hopes of telemedicine was that it would be cost-effective. In reality, the main problem with economic evaluation of paediatric tele-cardiology is a lack of well conducted studies!

2. Telemedicine applied to specific cardiology situations

2.1 Telemedicine in fetal cardiology

There are a number of features of fetal cardiology that appear to make telemedicine an attractive proposition:

2.1.1 The clinical imperative

1. Fetal cardiology is a highly centralized subspeciality with even fewer specialists than paediatric cardiology.
2. Patients often travel large distances (up to 160 km in Northern Ireland) to attend a fetal cardiology clinic. The distance between home and the specialist centre is even greater in larger countries. In Quebec, 34% of mothers referred to a fetal cardiology service travel more than 100km.(Cloutier and Finley, 2004)
3. The summary of fetal cardiology literature demonstrates that timely, antennal diagnosis of CHD is important for improving outcomes for fetus and family by facilitating: parental counselling, elective delivery at an appropriate centre, parental choice in terms of termination and permitting fetal intervention in terms of pharmacotherapy for dysrhythmias and catheter intervention for severe complex lesions.(Bonnet et al., 1999; Allan, 2000; Tworetzky et al., 2001; Gardiner, 2008)

4. The vast majority of fetuses with CHD are born from pregnancies without a recognisable antenatal risk factor. Obviously, formal evaluation by a fetal cardiologist cannot be offered to every single pregnancy. Therefore, in order to maximise antenatal detection of CHD, greater proficiency, from the non-specialist, is required at confirming normality and identifying pathology.

In the UK, the most practicable method of promoting antenatal detection of CHD is by improving cardiac evaluation during the routine anomaly scan. Previous studies have demonstrated the benefit and relative ease with which more detailed imaging of the heart may be incorporated into routine anomaly scanning.(Stumpflen et al., 1996) However, such reports often reflect working practices immediately after the introduction of a training program. As the teaching study from Hunter et al demonstrated, there is a danger that if support from paediatric cardiology is not ongoing then the initial efficacy of training may diminish.(Hunter et al., 2000) Telemedicine has the potential to facilitate earlier diagnosis of CHD by offering increased and quicker access to specialist opinion. Telemedicine may also support sonographers' education and training.

Fetal cardiology is predominantly a speciality of medical imaging as physical examination of the fetal cardiovascular system is obviously not possible and fetal catheter and surgical interventions are limited to a handful of centres worldwide. As is well documented, telemedicine lends itself to areas where medical imaging is crucial to diagnosis.(Casey, 1999) It may be suggested that performing fetal tele-echocardiography is much the same as tele-echocardiography in neonates but fetal echocardiography is significantly different from neonatal echocardiography:

1. The fetal heart is smaller and beats faster which may exacerbate motion artefact.
2. The fetus is surrounded by the mother so that ultrasound has to travel through more tissue impacting on image quality.
3. The fetus may move.
4. The fetus may be in a disadvantageous position e.g. back up.

Experience of telemedicine in fetal cardiology is still in its infancy. The fetal cardiology telemedicine programs that are currently active appear to have developed from centres with a major interest in telemedicine and fetal medicine.Whilst an acceptable bandwidth (384kbps) has been established for neonatal tele-echocardiography. This is not the case with fetal tele-echocardiography. Therefore, research is required in this area.

2.1.2 Evidence for fetal tele-cardiology

Despite a potential role for telemedicine in fetal cardiology, there are very few studies investigating its potential. Only one study is reported to date that investigates the feasibility and acceptability of performing remote, real-time 2-D fetal echocardiography. Sharma et al performed a study in two phases. Phase one was a laboratory study, investigating the effect of bandwidth on image quality and overall adequacy of scan. Sixty-four fetal echocardiograms were performed and randomly assigned to transmission across 128, 384 and 768 kbps and recorded on Super VHS videotape for subsequent review. Six studies were excluded due to the presence of CHD. Of the 58 real-time studies interpreted, 15 / 58 were transmitted across 128 kbps, 21 across 384 kbps and 22 across 768 kbps. The image quality was felt to be significantly poorer at 128 kbps. At 128 kbps, the mean Likert score was 1.1/5 compared with 3.1 / 5 at 384 kbps ($p < 0.01$) and 3.4 / 5 at 768 kbps ($p < 0.01$). There was no significant difference in perceived image quality in transmission across 384 kbps compared with 768 kbps ($p = 0.08$). Similarly, there was no significant difference in the adequacy of studies transmitted across 384 kbps compared with 768 kbps. In this first phase, Sharma et al conclude that 384 kbps is an adequate bandwidth for the identification of normal heart structures.(Sharma et al., 2003)

In the second phase of the study, 34 fetal echocardiograms were successfully transmitted and interpreted in real-time. In four cases (11%) technical problems prevented transmission. The fetal echocardiogram was performed by a fetal cardiac sonographer or a paediatric cardiology fellow with experience in fetal echocardiography. This was compared with a video recording of the study made at the transmitting site. Mothers were followed up with a face-to-face fetal echocardiogram if a concern was identified on the transmitted fetal echocardiogram. In order to evaluate patient satisfaction, a questionnaire was completed by all 34 expectant mothers and a control group of 195 patients referred from peripheral hospitals to the regional fetal cardiology clinic. There was no significant difference in the completeness of each study between the tele-fetal echocardiogram and the recorded fetal echocardiogram. CHD was identified correctly in two transmitted fetal echocardiograms with a third case of CHD being suspected but only confirmed on direct fetal echocardiography.

The satisfaction survey results were very positive. In all nine questions, the mean patient satisfaction score indicated high levels of satisfaction with the telemedicine consultation. In eight questions there was no significant difference in patient satisfaction between the telemedicine and control groups. In addition, only 6% of patients stated that they felt uncomfortable talking to the doctor across the tele-link and only 3% felt it was difficult to ask questions.

In this important study, the authors conclude that transmission of fetal echocardiograms across 384 kbps is feasible and adequate for the interpretation of screening fetal echocardiograms. Community acceptance of telemedicine screening and counselling is not adversely affected by a lack of direct personal contact with the specialist.

Whilst this study is valuable there are some limitations. The majority of transmitted fetal echocardiograms were not followed up with a face-to-face fetal echocardiogram which is the gold standard. The proportion of fetuses with CHD was small in this cohort. Therefore, the diagnostic accuracy of the telemedicine process was not adequately assessed. The fetal echocardiograms were performed by an operator already skilled in fetal echocardiography. This may falsely enhance the adequacy and quality of the fetal echocardiogram being transmitted. It is suggested that most difficulties in interpreting echocardiograms transmitted via a tele-link are related to image acquisition rather than transmission (Cloutier, 2000). Eleven per cent of studies were terminated due to technical difficulties. A routine clinical service would be significantly limited if 11% of consultations were aborted due to technical difficulties.

There are also reports of telemedicine facilitating 3-D fetal echocardiography by spatio-temporal image correlation (STIC) and datasets transmitted across an ADSL link. STIC is a relatively new approach for clinical assessment of the fetal heart. It is an easy technique for acquiring data from the fetal heart (a single, automatic volume sweep) and produces a 4D cine sequence.(Michailidis et al., 2001) A group from Chile conducted a similar study STIC transmitted across an ADSL connection with bandwidths of 300 and 600 kbps. In total fifty scans were transmitted from two peripheral hospitals to the regional centre. On average complete fetal echocardiograms could be interpreted in 92%.(Vinals et al., 2005) However, these isolated studies have not been followed up in the literature.

In a study conducted in our own department we evaluated fetal echocardiography, performed by sonographers with little training in fetal cardiology, but guided by a fetal cardiologist and transmitted in real-time across ISDN 6 (Figure 3). The remote consultation concluded with a videoconference in which the fetal cardiologist explained the diagnosis and answered any questions from the prospective parents. This fetal-telecardiology consultation was compared with the subsequent "face-to-face" fetal cardiology consultation at the regional centre. Sixty-eight fetal tele-echocardiograms were performed and followed-up. The diagnostic accuracy was very high ((κ - statistic = 0.89, sensitivity = 0.92, specificity = 0.98, ppv = 0.92, npv = 0.98) (Figure 4). Sonographers were very positive regarding their involvement in the study and reported significantly improved levels of confidence in performing fetal echocardiography. A significant positive feature of real-time fetal tele-echocardioghraphy is the continued support provided to radiographers performing fetal anomaly scans in DGHs. Patients were very positive about the telemedicine process and were equally satisfied with the remote consultation as the face-to-face consultation. Patients were equally satisfied with each consultation but consistently replied that they would prefer to have the fetal cardiology consultation performed at the local hospital facilitated by a tele-link rather by a face-to-face consultation at the regional centre. (McCrossan, 2009)

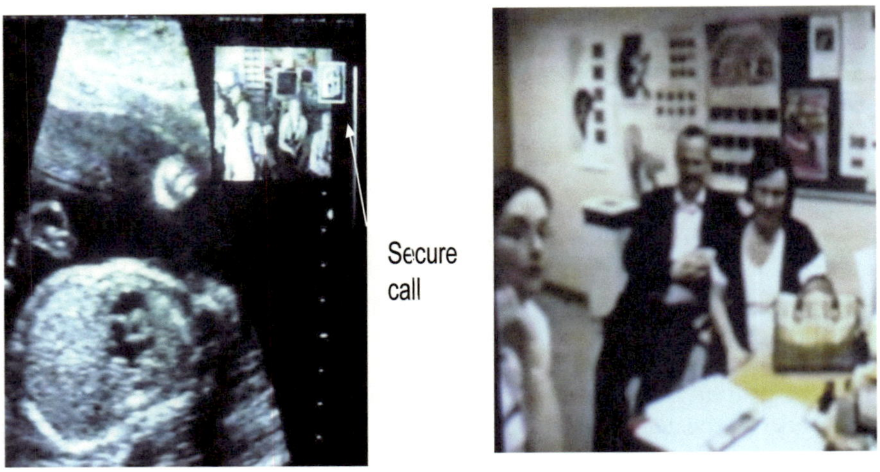

a) b)

Fig. 3. What is seen by the paediatric cardiologist a)Live guidance of fetal echo,
b) Counselling parents

During the study it was noted that the received fetal echocardiographic images were of poorer quality following an upgrade in the ultrasound scanner. This did not appear to affect diagnostic accuracy. With the superior imaging, this deterioration in received picture quality was probably due to excess data being transmitted down the 384kbps connection with resulting package loss and pixellation. This problem would likely be reduced if a larger bandwidth was employed. Extensions to inter-hospital networks make this a realistic option. Alternatively SDSL links (2MBps) can be installed at much cheaper rates than corresponding ISDN bandwidths.

The introduction of a remote fetal cardiology service would have attendant costs which are not offset by savings in inter-hospital transfers. However, the possible establishment of a "one-stop-shop" for "high-risk" pregnancies in which the routine fetal anomaly scan is followed by a remote fetal echocardiogram confidently identifying all relevant cardiac structures (55% in this cohort) could potentially be cost neutral, relieve pressure on the regional unit and present time and cost savings to the patient. Ultimately the aim of future work should be aimed towards the establishment of a regional fetal tele-echocardiography service.

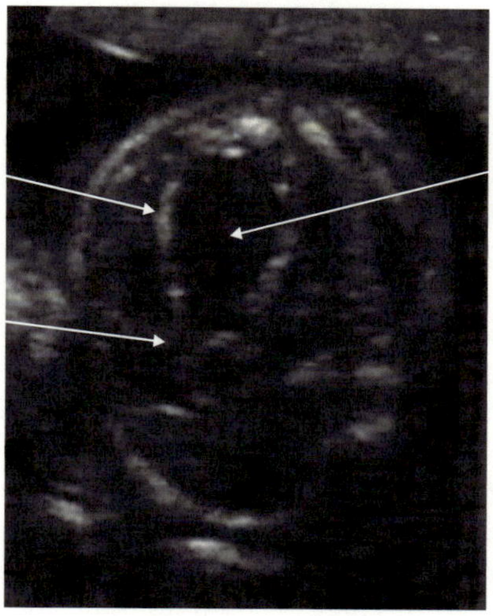

Fig. 4. Example of severe congenital heart disease accurately diagnosed via tele-link in this study.

2.2 Tele-echocardiography in paediatrics

The main application of telemedicine in paediatric cardiology to date has been remote diagnosis of congenital heart disease by the transmission of echocardiograms from DGH to specialist. There are many articles in the literature confirming the effectiveness of this telemedicine application.(Finley et al., 1997; Mulholland et al., 1999; Sable, 2003; Widmer et al., 2003; Grant et al., 2010)(Tsilimigaki et al., 2001)

2.2.1 Clinical imperative

1. It can be challenging to confidently rule out CHD in the differential diagnosis of a critically ill newborn baby. In these cases, paediatricians often find it difficult to confidently exclude CHD.
2. Many such babies present at DGHs with no paediatric cardiology support on site.
3. The treatment of CHD can be very different from that of other life-threatening conditions. Therefore making the correct diagnosis can be life-saving.
4. Sick newborn babies without CHD maybe cared for very well at the DGH and should be spared a potentially hazardous medical transfer.

2.2.2 Evidence for neonatal tele-echocardiography

The literature demonstrates that neonatal tele-echocardiography is feasible and reliable. High diagnostic accuracy is reproducible with live guidance by a paediatric cardiologist.(Mulholland et al., 1999; Sable et al., 1999; Widmer et al., 2003; Grant et al., 2010) Store and forward formats have also been utilised but in this situation the paediatric cardiologist must be confident that the echocardiographer will obtain a detailed and complete echocardiographic study. If the echocardiographer is capable of performing such a study it is questionable whether further interpretation is necessary. More recent studies also demonstrate that tele-echocardiography helps avoid potentially risky transfers of sick newborn babies between hospitals.(Grant et al., 2010) Most importantly, neonatal tele-echocardiography has become accepted as an integral part of many regional paediatric cardiology services across the world.

The value of telemedicine in continuing professional development has been well documented if not fully researched.(Casey, 1999; Sable, 2002) Our experience of the educational benefit of real time transmission of echocardiograms has been very positive. Having performed echocardiograms under the guidance of a paediatric cardiologist, paediatricians report an improvement in their ability to interpret echocardiograms and have been observed to gain confidence in echocardiography. We believe that real-time, live guidance of the paediatrician by the paediatric cardiologist has advantages compared to a "store and forward" protocol, in both acquiring quality images and in providing an educational support. Often the inexperienced sonographer obtains images that they believe are not adequate. However, it is a difficulty interpreting the images that is the major contributing factor to poor image acquisition. During the videoconference, the paediatric cardiologist is able to highlight relevant structures as they appear and describe what manoeuvres are necessary to view other structures.

There is an important caveat to tele-echocardiography. In a small number of cases major CHD will be suspected following the transmitted scan but a definite diagnosis cannot be established. These cases highlight the importance of recognising the limitations of telemedicine. If there is a clinical suspicion of major CHD that cannot be confidently diagnosed or excluded, following a tele-echocardiogram, then transfer to a regional unit for hands-on assessment should not be delayed.

Ideally, we envisage a hub and spoke model for the provision of paediatric cardiology with tele-echocardiography acting as a valuable aid in supporting a paediatrician with special expertise in cardiology.

Economic analysis

As discussed previously, economic analysis of telemedicine applications is lacking and this holds true for neonatal tele-echocardiography. However, a study performed at our own institution demonstrates clearly that neonatal tele-echocardiography is cost-saving for each DGH within the telemedicine network. Although there are significant start-up costs for each hospital, these are outweighed by the savings made from avoiding expensive inter-hospital transfers as a result of the remote consultation. This study was conducted over an eight year period and suggests that telemedicine services can continue to be cost saving beyond the initial enthusiasm surrounding a new service. Northern Ireland is a small geographical area, therefore the potential saving for larger regions is even greater.(Grant et al., 2010)

One of the main barriers to increased use of telemedicine is the initial start up cost. Running costs for ISDN 6 lines are also significant. As predicted, the cost of videoconferencing codecs suitable for transmission of echocardiograms has decreased significantly over the past 10 years. More recently, the possibility of using the internet as a means of transmission has been explored with some success. This maybe achieved through a healthcare organisation's wide area network or by installing individual internet links such as an SDSL connection (Up to 2MBps). Our experience of ADSL (in its current provision) is that the variable bandwidth is not suitable for tele-echocardiography. As comparable internet links are much less expensive than ISDN lines, switching to internet connections will only help the economic argument in favour of telemedicine.

Payment for telemedicine consultations remains problematic. In our healthcare model (UK National Health Service) there is no mechanism in place for the regional unit to receive payment for each remote consultation. However, it maybe possible to build telemedicine services into the job plan of specialists in recognition of time undertaken in remote consultations. This is not a satisfactory situation. Other healthcare organisations, for example in the USA, have the potential to charge the referring institution a fee for each telemedicine consultation. Up to 12 states in the USA now mandate that health care plans cover telemedicine. This seems a more sustainable approach to telemedicine and should be possible in any healthcare organisation as payments are routinely made between health boards for face-to-face medical consultations.(Macios, 2010) This seems a more sustainable approach to telemedicine and should be possible in any healthcare organisation as payments are routinely made between health boards for face-to-face medical consultations.

2.3 Tele-homecare in paediatric cardiology

2.3.1 Background

Paediatric cardiology has changed dramatically over the past twenty years. Improvements in diagnostic imaging and innovations in surgical technique along with intensive care, have revolutionised the prognosis for children with major congenital heart disease.(Laussen, 2001; McElhinney and Wernovsky, 2001)(Laussen, 2001; McElhinney and Wernovsky, 2001)(Laussen, 2001; McElhinney and Wernovsky, 2001) In particular children with complex CHD, typified by single ventricle physiology, now have the possibility of life beyond the neonatal period.(Marino, 2002) However, such patients are not "cured" but receive long-term palliation in the form of a staged surgical programme over several years.

Parents often state that the most anxious and stressful period is not around the time of diagnosis or even surgery but actually the day they take their baby home for the first time. Parents feel very reassured by the presence of nursing staff and the 24 hour availability of medical expertise which is only possible in hospital.(Holmes, 1996)

The clinical imperative

1. Patients with severe congenital heart disease require particularly careful follow-up in early infancy and it seems logical that home support / monitoring could potentially contribute to the quality of care delivered.
2. At discharge there may be ongoing clinical issues which may not require medical attention but are an added stress to parents e.g. feeding difficulties, ongoing cyanosis and inter-current viral infections. In this setting, it is understandable that parents are extremely anxious and in want of support and reassurance.
3. It is recommended that tele-home care be targeted at conditions that require close monitoring, clinical assessment and early intervention to avoid adverse events such as hospitalization or emergency visits.(Dellifraine and Dansky, 2008)
4. Paediatric cardiology is a highly specialized and centralized field of medicine. The paediatric cardiology team who have been involved in the daily management of these patients are ideally placed to monitor the patient's progress and deal with any problems as they arise.

2.3.2 Evidence for tele-homecare in paediatric cardiology

The group of congenital cardiac lesions that have attracted most interest over the past 15 years have been those which fall within the umbrella term - "hypoplastic left heart syndrome." In HLHS, there is severe under development of some or all left heart structures.(Dhillon and Redington, 2002) Until relatively recently, surgical intervention was not widely available. However, it is now exceptional for babies with HLHS not to be offered surgical intervention. This usually takes the form of staged surgical palliation culminating in a total cavo-pulmonary anastomosis with a systemic right ventricle. The first stage is the Norwood procedure, performed during the early neonatal period, with the second stage occurring during mid-infancy.(Bove et al., 2004; Sano et al., 2004; Stasik et al., 2006) Although modifications to the Norwood procedure have been associated with a reduction in early mortality, there remains a significant attrition rate between the first and second stages.(Forbess, 2003) This group of patients could particularly benefit from additional monitoring and support following discharge from hospital.

A group from Wisconsin, USA, postulated that patients at risk of inter-stage mortality could be identified by a deterioration in their physiological status. A daily home programme of measuring arterial oxygen saturations and weight was combined with a protocol guiding the need for hospitalisation. There was significantly less mortality observed during the 15 month intervention period compared with the preceding 50 month control period (0% vs 16%, $p = 0.039$).(Ghanayem et al., 2003; Ghanayem et al., 2004; Ghanayem et al., 2006)

We conducted a randomised control trial of a home support programme facilitated by videoconferencing compared with telephone support and a control group for babies with major CHD. With the assistance of a videoconferencing company, we installed commercially available, portable videoconferencing systems in the patients' homes and included pulse oximetry when clinically indicated. ISDN lines were initially utilised but this was switched to an ADSL connection during the latter half of the study. Regular remote consultations were conducted in both intervention groups (Figure5). The results of this study demonstrated that home support delivered by videoconferencing is feasible, reliable, sustainable and superior to telephone support in terms of reducing parental anxiety. Moreover, videoconferencing home support was associated with significantly reduced health service utilisation and may possibly be cost-saving.(Morgan et al., 2008; McCrossan, 2009) Our institution has secured government funding to incorporate videoconferencing home support into the post-discharge care for a subset of babies with major CHD.

2.3.3 Tele-homecare in adult cardiology

There is a wide array of tele-care projects and services available. In adult cardiology, most tele-monitoring services are centred around the regular transmission of vital parameters (Blood pressure, heart rate, respiratory rate and weight) from home to hospital. There are many tele-homecare systems specifically designed for this purpose. Variations in the patient's observations outside set limits trigger a response from the hospital which may involve changing medication etc. Other services are based upon structured telephone support which is usually nurse led. Web-based patient education often forms a component of tele-health services.

There is good and increasing evidence that tele-homecare can be an effective method of health care delivery. A recent meta-analysis of all home based telehealth research indicated a moderate positive effect on health outcomes (mean weighted effect size = 0.5, $p<0.01$). Sub-analysis revealed particular benefits in patients with mental health illness and chronic adult heart disease but no significant effect in diabetes mellitus.(Dellifraine and Dansky,

2008) The potential for tele-homecare in the management of chronic obstructive pulmonary disease has also been highlighted and trials are now in process.(McKinstry et al., 2009; Lewis et al., 2010) Home monitoring is now established as an adjunct to the ongoing management of specific adult cardiac populations: e.g. chronic heart failure, hypertension and implantable cardiac defibrillators / pacemakers.(Clark et al., 2007)(Cleland et al., 2005)(Heidbuchel et al., 2008)(Raatikainen et al., 2008; Parati et al., 2009) This has culminated in a Cochrane review confirming that telephone support and tele-monitoring programmes for patients with congestive heart failure are effective in reducing the risk of all-cause mortality and CHF-related hospitalisations. Furthermore such programmes improve quality of life and reduce costs.(Inglis et al., 2011)

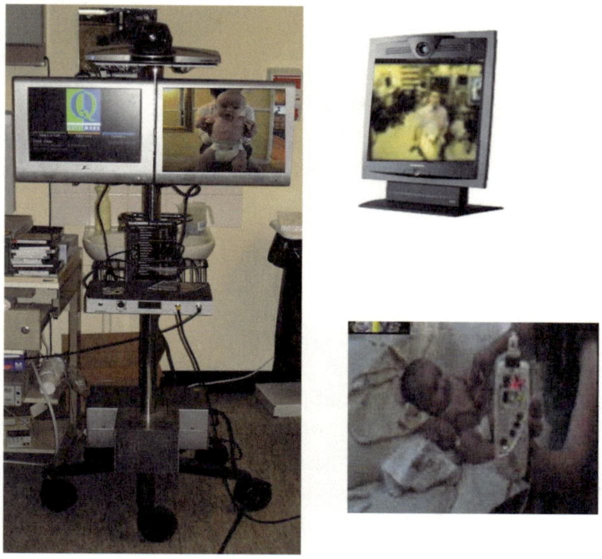

Fig. 5. Telemedicine hardware needed for hospital-home videoconferencing. What the doctor sees and what the family sees

Following the accumulation of good quality evidence, government funding has been forthcoming. The EU has invested more than €650 million in funding tele-health and telecare initiaves.(Celler et al., 2007) Unsurprisingly, tele-homecare projects are the main growth area in telemedicine within cardiology. In the context of current healthcare models, this is set to continue.

2.3.4 Future

There is a strong case for conducting similar research trials in other paediatric sub-specialties e.g. ex-preterm infants, chronic respiratory and neurological patients. The central premise is common: complex, vulnerable patients scattered across a wide geographical area who are likely to benefit from regular, direct input from the tertiary care team. The scope of home monitoring could also be increased to include ECG monitoring for patients with dysrhythmias and patients requiring INR monitoring for warfarin. A significant proportion of a cardiac liaison nurse's workload could be facilitated by a telemedicine home support mechanism. Such a scheme could potentially reorganise the role of the cardiac liaison nurse and provide more efficient use of resources. Advances in home broadband links in terms of quality, geographical coverage and cost will facilitate more ambitious tele-homecare programmes with the potential to improve patient care.

2.4 Tele-stethoscopy

2.4.1 Clinical imperative

1. Innocent murmurs are very common during childhood. Whilst definitive studies have proved elusive, the estimated prevalence in developed countries is approximately 50%. However, congenital heart disease diagnosed following the detection of a murmur after infancy is rare in comparison. Approximately 2% of patients with a murmur presenting after 12 months old have CHD.(O'Rourke, 2004)
2. Paediatric cardiology outpatient clinics are over subscribed and there is limited capacity for extra clinics at a regional unit.
3. Outreach clinics are an important aspect of a regional service but take the paediatric cardiologist away from the tertiary unit.

As there are only a small number of paediatric cardiologists this can be a significant consideration in terms of providing senior cover at the tertiary centre. It is possible that remote consultations could be substituted for face-to-face consultations. Alternatively telemedicine may streamline referrals. In both situations the auscultatory findings are paramount.

2.4.2 The role of auscultation in paediatric cardiology outpatients

Traditionally, clinical examination has been the primary method of assessing children referred for evaluation of an asymptomatic murmur. Prior to the advent of 2-D echocardiography, reliable, non-invasive imaging of the heart was not possible. With improvements in computer software, enabling superior 2-D imaging, colour flow mapping, Doppler measurements, and the increased availability of ultrasound scanners, comes the temptation to routinely employ echocardiography. However, there is good evidence that clinical examination alone is highly sensitive and specific.

The question is: *who* should perform this assessment? There are numerous studies in the literature examining the roles of the non-specialist and paediatric cardiologist in the initial evaluation of children with asymptomatic cardiac murmurs. The available literature suggests that non-specialists are better than they think at detecting congenital heart disease achieving good levels of specificity. However, they are much less confident at excluding congenital heart disease. (Rushforth and Wilson, 1992) The result is a high volume of referrals of patients with innocent murmurs. Anecdotally, this lack of confidence in distinguishing innocent from significant murmurs has increased over the past 30 years.(Noonan, 1999) The reasons for this may be due to concerns over malpractice, greater availability of sophisticated investigations and a misperception that echocardiography is necessary to rule out pathology.(Danford et al., 1993) Therefore we have a situation where there is a highly centralised service with limited capacity in which the key feature of the consultation is auscultation. Sound waves may be captured, processed and transmitted for evaluation at a distance. The key question is: can heart sounds be reliably sampled and transmitted for accurate interpretation at a remote location?

2.4.3 The evidence for tele-stethoscopy

Although remote stethoscopy was reported as early as 1973, the first significant study, appeared in the 1990s. In an elegant study, Belmont et al demonstrated that real-time tele-stethoscopy was accurate and clinically useful (κ > 0.6) for detecting murmurs, distinguishing specific murmurs (innocent, pathological, vibratory, diastolic aortic, diastolic pulmonary) and diagnosing congenital heart disease (κ = 0.63). Interestingly, Belmont found that remote stethoscopy's accuracy suffered in younger children (κ = 0.29). Consequently, Belmont et al conclude that remote stethoscopy provided accurate, dependable detection of congenital heart disease but only in children five years old and above. The feasibility and accuracy of real-time tele-stethoscopy have been supported by further studies including research at our own institution.(McConnell et al., 1999; Grant, 2006)(McCrossan, 2009)

Alternatively, tele-stethoscopy maybe achieved using a store and forward protocol. Digital stethoscopes are capable of sampling and recording heart sounds which can then be e-mailed to the paediatric cardiologist along with the history and additional clinical findings. Several studies, using this technique, have been published which demonstrate similarly high levels of accuracy in differentiating innocence from pathology i.e. the need for further investigation in the form of echocardiography.(Dahl et al., 2002; Finley et al., 2006)(Mahnke et al., 2008)

Although the Belmont study suggested that tele-stethoscopy was significantly less accurate in children under 5 years, more recent reports in the literature and our own experience do not support this claim. We would suggest that children three years and over are suitable for tele-stethoscopy i.e. the pre-school child with a murmur.

There are arguments in favour of both real-time and store and forward protocols in the application of tele-stethoscopy. Real-time stehoscopy requires more elaborate telemedicine equipment which has historically been bespoke PC-based systems. Such home-built systems are temperamental and difficult to replicate. However, there are now better quality, commercially available tele-stethoscopy systems which are more user friendly (Figure 6). Real-time tele-stethoscopy is more time consuming and requires greater co-ordination. However, the audio-visual contact with the patient and parent is probably beneficial in terms of reassuring parents. There is also the opportunity to repeat auscultation and perform respiratory and positional manoeuvres which may tease out the character of a murmur. Whilst this is possible with store and forward sampling, not every aspect of auscultation is performed with every consultation. The course of a clinical examination is influenced by what the clinician believes is the differential diagnosis on first hearing the murmur / heart sounds. Therefore, either a large number of samples are recorded for each patient, which must increase the number of inadequate samples, or a limited number of samples are recorded which may leave the paediatric cardiologist wishing that he/ she could have another listen. However, there is an undeniable advantage to sitting in an office, reading the history / examination, viewing the ECG / CXR and then listening to a few audio files compared with setting up and co-ordinating a remote clinic. For this reason, the future of tele-stethoscopy, as a clinical tool for out-patient referrals, is likely to rest with the store-and-forward technique.

Adult cardiology does not have the same need for tele-stehoscopy as paediatric cardiology. Ischaemic heart disease rather than structural defects comprise the bulk of the workload so murmurs do not have equivalent significance. Additionally, most DGHs have adult cardiology specialists with access to echocardiography. However, there are reports of real-time tele-stethoscopy from an Italian group which they believe should be useful in the setting of tele-homecare. Fragrasso et al employed a commercially available, purpose built videoconferencing tele-stethoscopy system. They report that cardiac and respiratory auscultation was accurate and valuable. (Fragasso et al., 2007)

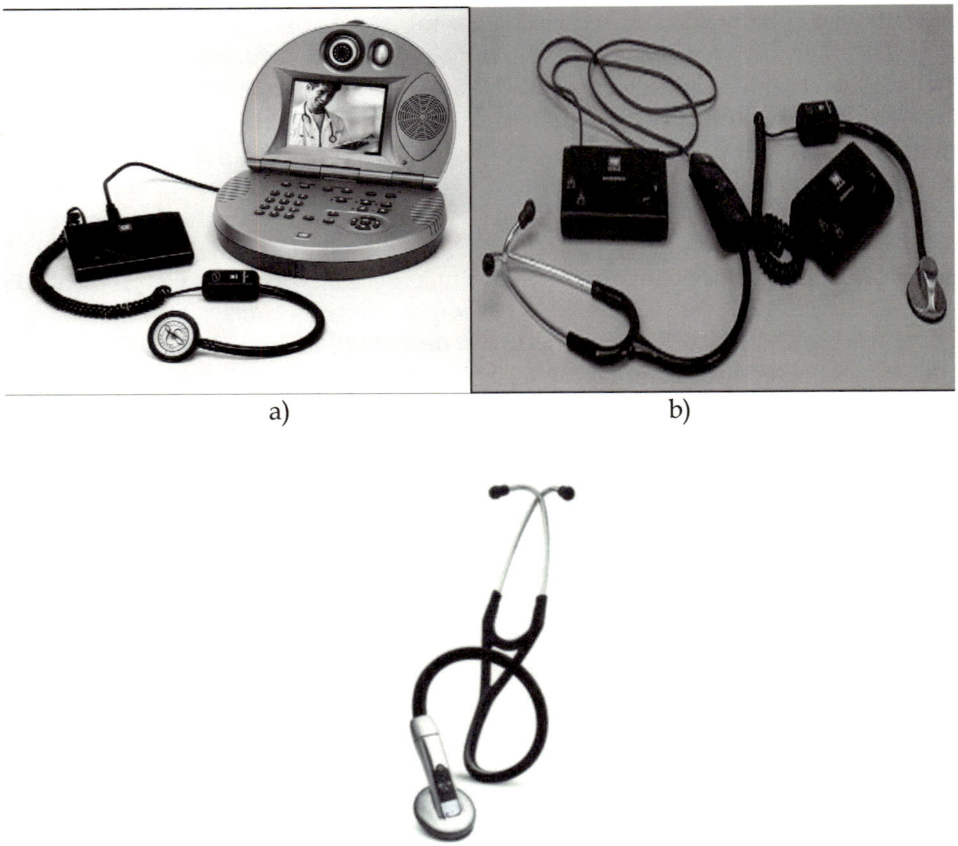

a) b)

c)

Fig. 6. (a and b) Commercially available tele-stehthosopy system from Aethra and (c) Digital stethoscope

3. Conclusions

The research presented in this thesis demonstrates that telemedicine may be applied across multiple common paediatric cardiology scenarios: from fetus, to neonate, to infant to child; and from home, to outpatient clinic. A wide range of clinical data, including visual examination, auscultatory sounds, physiological parameters and echocardiographic images, may be transmitted in real-time across telemedicine links facilitating accurate diagnosis, effective decision making and promoting access to specialist opinion. Telemedicine is an acceptable process to both health professionals and the public. It is associated with high levels of parental satisfaction. Telemedicine applications are shown to impact on patient managent and reduce health service utilisation with the net effect of keeping patients and their families closer to home. Established telemedicine programmes may continue to be cost saving beyond the initial start-up phase. Internet transmission is likely to improve significantly in the future and is economically more sustainable compared with ISDN.

In this chapter I have not addressed the issue of who takes legal responsibility for the patient following the telemedicine consultation. Despite almost 20 years of experience of

telemedicine in paediatric cardiology, there are no agreed guidelines concerning professional responsibility. Currently, it is likely that all physicians involved take responsibility for their own professional conduct in relation to the patient. To date there have been no cases of medical negligence resulting from telemedicine consultations in the UK. This may conceal out of court settlements. (Avienda Telemedicine Consultancy, 2007)
The main recommendation from this chapter is for clinicians (for only clinicians can make telemedicine work) to consider whether areas of their clinical practice are negatively affected by distance separating themselves from either patients or colleagues. If so telemedicine may facilitate more effective and efficient use of resources and improve patient care.

4. Acknowledgements

The authors would like to acknowledge the advice and support of Questmark Ltd in conducting research at the Royal Belfast Hospital for Sick Children

5. References

Allan, L., 2000, Antenatal diagnosis of heart disease, *Heart* (British Cardiac Society), vol. 83, no. 3, p. 367.

Avienda Telemedicine Consultancy, Personal Communication, 2007.

Boettinger, H. M., 1977, *The Telephone Book*, Croton-on-Hudson, New York, Riverwood Publications.

Bonnet, D., A. Coltri, G. Butera, L. Fermont, J. Le Bidois, J. Kachaner, and D. Sidi, 1999, Detection of transposition of the great arteries in fetuses reduces neonatal morbidity and mortality, *Circulation*, vol. 99, no. 7, p. 916-918.

Bove, E. L., R. G. Ohye, and E. J. Devaney, 2004, Hypoplastic left heart syndrome: conventional surgical management, Seminars in thoracic and cardiovascular surgery. *Pediatric cardiac surgery annual*, vol. 7, p. 3-10.

Burri, H. and D. Senouf, 2009, Remote monitoring and follow-up of pacemakers and implantable cardioverter defibrillators, *Europace : European pacing, arrhythmias, and cardiac electrophysiology : journal of the working groups on cardiac pacing, arrhythmias, and cardiac cellular electrophysiology of the European Society of Cardiology*, vol. 11, no. 6, p. 701-709.

Casey, F. A., 1999, Telemedicine in paediatric cardiology, *Archives of Disease in Childhood*, vol. 80, no. 6, p. 497-499.

Celler, B. G., N. H. Lovell, and J. Basilakis, 2007, The business case for home telecare: a comparative analysis between the USA, Europe and Australasia, *Conference proceedings : Annual International Conference of the IEEE Engineering in Medicine and Biology Society.IEEE Engineering in Medicine and Biology Society.* Conference, vol. 2007, p. 6152.

Cloutier, A., 2000, Distance diagnosis in pediatric cardiology: a model for telemedecine implementation, *Telemedicine Today*, vol. 8, no. 3, p. 20-21.

Cloutier, A. and J. Finley, 2004, Telepediatric cardiology practice in Canada, *Telemedicine journal and e-health : the official journal of the American Telemedicine Association*, vol. 10, no. 1, p. 33-37.

Dellifraine, J. L. and K. H. Dansky, 2008, Home-based telehealth: a review and meta-analysis, *Journal of telemedicine and telecare*, vol. 14, no. 2, p. 62-66.

Dhillon, D. and A. N. Redington, 2002, Hypoplastic Left Heart Syndrome, *in* Anderson, R. H., E. J. Baker, F. J. Macartney, M. L. Rigby, E. A. Shinebourne, and M. Tynan, eds., *Paediatric cardiology*, Edinburgh, Churchill Livingstone, vol. 2, p. 1191-1192-1211.

Dorrian, C., J. Ferguson, K. Ah-See, C. Barr, K. Lalla, M. van der Pol, L. McKenzie, and R. Wootton, 2009, Head and neck cancer assessment by flexible endoscopy and telemedicine, *Journal of telemedicine and telecare,* vol. 15, no. 3, p. 118-121.

Dowie, R., H. Mistry, T. A. Young, G. C. Weatherburn, H. M. Gardiner, M. Rigby, G. V. Rowlinson, and R. C. Franklin, 2007, Telemedicine in pediatric and perinatal cardiology: economic evaluation of a service in English hospitals, *International Journal of Technology Assessment in Health Care,* vol. 23, no. 1, p. 116-125.

Dowie, R., H. Mistry, T. A. Young, R. C. Franklin, and H. M. Gardiner, 2008, Cost implications of introducing a telecardiology service to support fetal ultrasound screening, *Journal of telemedicine and telecare,* vol. 14, no. 8, p. 421-426.

Dowie, R., H. Mistry, M. Rigby, T. A. Young, G. Weatherburn, G. Rowlinson, and R. C. Franklin, 2009, A paediatric telecardiology service for district hospitals in south-east England: an observational study, *Archives of Disease in Childhood,* vol. 94, no. 4, p. 273-277.

Einthoven, W., 1906, Le telecardiogramme, *Archives Internationales de Physiologie, de Biochimie et de Biophysique,* vol. 4, p. 132-133-164.

Ferencz, C. and C. A. Neill, 1992, Cardiovascular malformations: prevalence at livebirth. *in* Freedom, R. M., L. Benson, and J. Smallhorn, eds., *Neonatal Heart Disease,* London, Springer-Verlag, p. 19-29.

Finley, J. P., D. G. Human, M. A. Nanton, D. L. Roy, R. G. Macdonald, D. R. Marr, and H. Chiasson, 1989, Echocardiography by telephone--evaluation of pediatric heart disease at a distance, *The American Journal of Cardiology,* vol. 63, no. 20, p. 1475-1477.

Finley, J. P., G. P. Sharratt, M. A. Nanton, R. P. Chen, P. Bryan, J. Wolstenholme, and C. MacDonald, 1997, Paediatric echocardiography by telemedicine--nine years' experience, *Journal of telemedicine and telecare,* vol. 3, no. 4, p. 200-204.

Forbess, J. M., 2003, Pre-stage II mortality after the Norwood operation: addressing the next challenge, *The Journal of thoracic and cardiovascular surgery,* vol. 126, no. 5, p. 1257-1258.

Gardiner, H. M., 2008, In-utero intervention for severe congenital heart disease, Best practice & research. *Clinical obstetrics & gynaecology,* vol. 22, no. 1, p. 49-61.

Ghanayem, N. S., G. M. Hoffman, K. A. Mussatto, J. R. Cava, P. C. Frommelt, N. A. Rudd, M. M. Steltzer, S. M. Bevandic, S. S. Frisbee, R. D. Jaquiss et al, 2003, Home surveillance program prevents interstage mortality after the Norwood procedure, *The Journal of thoracic and cardiovascular surgery,* vol. 126, no. 5, p. 1367-1377.

Ghanayem, N. S., J. R. Cava, R. D. Jaquiss, and J. S. Tweddell, 2004, Home monitoring of infants after stage one palliation for hypoplastic left heart syndrome, Seminars in thoracic and cardiovascular surgery. *Pediatric cardiac surgery annual,* vol. 7, p. 32-38.

Ghanayem, N. S., J. S. Tweddell, G. M. Hoffman, K. Mussatto, and R. D. Jaquiss, 2006, Optimal timing of the second stage of palliation for hypoplastic left heart syndrome facilitated through home monitoring, and the results of early cavopulmonary anastomosis, *Cardiology in the young,* vol. 16 Suppl 1, p. 61-66.

Grant, B., G. J. Morgan, B. A. McCrossan, G. E. Crealey, A. J. Sands, B. Craig, and F. A. Casey, 2010, Remote diagnosis of congenital heart disease: the impact of telemedicine, *Archives of Disease in Childhood,* vol. 95, no. 4, p. 276-280.

Hoffman, J. I. and S. Kaplan, 2002, The incidence of congenital heart disease, *Journal of the American College of Cardiology,* vol. 39, no. 12, p. 1890-1900.

Holmes, A., 1996, The role of the cardiac liaison nurse, *Paediatric nursing,* vol. 8, no. 1, p. 25-27.

Horrigan, J., 2009, Home Broadband Adoption 2009, <http://www.pewinternet.org/~/media/Files/Reports/2009/Home-Broadband-Adoption-2009.pdf> Accessed 30/03/2011, 2011.

Houston, A., K. McLeod, T. Richens, W. Doig, S. Lilley, E. Murtagh, and N. Wilson, 1999, Assessment of the quality of neonatal echocardiographic images transmitted by ISDN telephone lines, *Heart (British Cardiac Society)*, vol. 82, no. 2, p. 222-225.

Hunter, S., A. Heads, J. Wyllie, and S. Robson, 2000, Prenatal diagnosis of congenital heart disease in the northern region of England: benefits of a training programme for obstetric ultrasonographers, *Heart (British Cardiac Society)*, vol. 84, no. 3, p. 294-298.

Laussen, P. C., 2001, Neonates with congenital heart disease, *Current opinion in pediatrics*, vol. 13, no. 3, p. 220-226.

Levin, Y. S. and E. M. Warshaw, 2009, Teledermatology: a review of reliability and accuracy of diagnosis and management, *Dermatologic clinics*, vol. 27, no. 2, p. 163-76, vii.

Macios, A., 2010, Payment for Telemedicine Gaining Momentum, <http://www.medscape.com/viewarticle/725115> Accessed 725115, 2011.

Marino, B. S., 2002, Outcomes after the Fontan procedure, *Current opinion in pediatrics*, vol. 14, no. 5, p. 620-626.

McCrossan, B. A., 2009, The Role of Telemedicine in Paediatric cardiolog, p. 135-136-197.

McElhinney, D. B. and G. Wernovsky, 2001, Outcomes of neonates with congenital heart disease, *Current opinion in pediatrics*, vol. 13, no. 2, p. 104-110.

Morgan, G. J., B. Craig, B. Grant, A. Sands, N. Doherty, and F. Casey, 2008, Home videoconferencing for patients with severe congential heart disease following discharge, *Congenital heart disease*, vol. 3, no. 5, p. 317-324.

Mulholland, H. C., F. Casey, D. Brown, N. Corrigan, M. Quinn, B. McCord, J. Rogers, and B. G. Craig, 1999, Application of a low cost telemedicine link to the diagnosis of neonatal congenital heart defects by remote consultation, *Heart (British Cardiac Society)*, vol. 82, no. 2, p. 217-221.

Michailidis, G. D., J. M. Simpson, C. Karidas, and D. L. Economides, 2001, Detailed three-dimensional fetal echocardiography facilitated by an Internet link, *Ultrasound in obstetrics & gynecology : the official journal of the International Society of Ultrasound in Obstetrics and Gynecology*, vol. 18, no. 4, p. 325-328.

Mitchell, S. C., S. B. Korones, and H. W. Berendes, 1971, Congenital heart disease in 56,109 births. Incidence and natural history, *Circulation*, vol. 43, no. 3, p. 323-332.

National Health Service, Specialsed Services, 2011, Safe and Sustainable- A New Vision for Children's Congenital Heart Services in England: Consultation Document. , p. 5.

Patterson, V., 2001, How best to organise acute hospital services? Realtime teleneurology can help small hospitals, *BMJ (Clinical research ed.)*, vol. 323, no. 7324, p. 1306.

Qureshi, S. A., 2008, Requirements for Provision of Outreach Paediatric Cardiology Service, p. 1-17.

Roine, R., A. Ohinmaa, and D. Hailey, 2001, Assessing telemedicine: a systematic review of the literature, *CMAJ : Canadian Medical Association journal = journal de l'Association medicale canadienne*, vol. 165, no. 6, p. 765-771.

Royal College of paediatrics and Child Health, 2009, Cardiology training for paediatric SpRs. March 2005. <www.rcph.ac.uk/publications/education_and_training_documents/cardiology_for_paeds_march2005.pdf> Accessed 11/29, 2007.

Royal College of Physicians, 2009, Consultant physicians working with patients. The duties, responsibilities and practice of physicians in general medicine and the specialties - Paediatric cardiology, <http://www.rcplondon.ac.uk/pubs/contents/39318d3e-4efb-49d6-994b-761892064f03.pdf> Accessed 04/01, 2009.

Sable, C., T. Roca, J. Gold, A. Gutierrez, E. Gulotta, and W. Culpepper, 1999, Live transmission of neonatal echocardiograms from underserved areas: accuracy, patient care, and cost, *Telemedicine journal : the official journal of the American Telemedicine Association*, vol. 5, no. 4, p. 339-347.

Sable, C. A., S. D. Cummings, G. D. Pearson, L. M. Schratz, R. C. Cross, E. S. Quivers, H. Rudra, and G. R. Martin, 2002, Impact of telemedicine on the practice of pediatric cardiology in community hospitals, *Pediatrics*, vol. 109, no. 1, p. E3.

Sable, C., 2002, Digital echocardiography and telemedicine applications in pediatric cardiology, *Pediatric cardiology*, vol. 23, no. 3, p. 358-369.

Sable, C., 2003, Telemedicine applications in pediatric cardiology, *Minerva pediatrica*, vol. 55, no. 1, p. 1-13.

Sano, S., K. Ishino, H. Kado, Y. Shiokawa, K. Sakamoto, M. Yokota, and M. Kawada, 2004, Outcome of right ventricle-to-pulmonary artery shunt in first-stage palliation of hypoplastic left heart syndrome: a multi-institutional study, *The Annals of Thoracic Surgery*, vol. 78, no. 6, p. 1951-7; discussion 1957-8.

Sharma, S., I. A. Parness, S. A. Kamenir, H. Ko, S. Haddow, L. G. Steinberg, and W. W. Lai, 2003, Screening fetal echocardiography by telemedicine: efficacy and community acceptance, *Journal of the American Society of Echocardiography : official publication of the American Society of Echocardiography*, vol. 16, no. 3, p. 202-208.

Sicotte, C., P. Lehoux, N. Van Doesburg, G. Cardinal, and Y. Leblanc, 2004, A cost-effectiveness analysis of interactive paediatric telecardiology, *Journal of telemedicine and telecare*, vol. 10, no. 2, p. 78-83.

Smith, A. C., P. Scuffham, and R. Wootton, 2007, The costs and potential savings of a novel telepaediatric service in Queensland, *BMC health services research*, vol. 7, p. 35.

Stasik, C. N., S. Gelehrter, C. S. Goldberg, E. L. Bove, E. J. Devaney, and R. G. Ohye, 2006, Current outcomes and risk factors for the Norwood procedure, *The Journal of thoracic and cardiovascular surgery*, vol. 131, no. 2, p. 412-417.

Stumpflen, I., A. Stumpflen, M. Wimmer, and G. Bernaschek, 1996, Effect of detailed fetal echocardiography as part of routine prenatal ultrasonographic screening on detection of congenital heart disease, *Lancet*, vol. 348, no. 9031, p. 854-857.

Tsilimigaki, A., S. Maraka, T. Tsekoura, V. Agelakou, A. Vekiou, C. Paphitis, and V. Thanopoulos, 2001, Eighteen months' experience with remote diagnosis, management and education in congenital heart disease, *Journal of telemedicine and telecare*, vol. 7, no. 4, p. 239-243.

Tworetzky, W., D. B. McElhinney, V. M. Reddy, M. M. Brook, F. L. Hanley, and N. H. Silverman, 2001, Improved surgical outcome after fetal diagnosis of hypoplastic left heart syndrome, *Circulation*, vol. 103, no. 9, p. 1269-1273.

Vinals, F., L. Mandujano, G. Vargas, and A. Giuliano, 2005, Prenatal diagnosis of congenital heart disease using four-dimensional spatio-temporal image correlation (STIC) telemedicine via an Internet link: a pilot study, *Ultrasound in obstetrics & gynecology : the official journal of the International Society of Ultrasound in Obstetrics and Gynecology*, vol. 25, no. 1, p. 25-31.

Whitten, P. S. and D. J. Cook, 1999, School-based telemedicine: using technology to bring health care to inner-city children, *Journal of telemedicine and telecare*, vol. 5 Suppl 1, p. S23-5.

Widmer, S., R. Ghisla, G. P. Ramelli, F. Taminelli, B. Widmer, L. Caoduro, and A. Gallino, 2003, Tele-echocardiography in paediatrics, *European journal of pediatrics*, vol. 162, no. 4, p. 271-275.

Wilkinson, J. L. and W. I. Cooke, 1992, Cardiovascular disorders, *in* Roberton, N. R. C., ed., *Textbook of Neonatology*, London, Churchill Livingstone, p. 559-603.

Workforce Review Team, 2009, Workforce summary - Paediatric Cardiology, <http://www.wrt.nhs.uk/index> Accessed 04/01, 2009.

15

Telemedicine for Managing Patients on Oral Anticoagulant Therapy

Sophie Testa, Oriana Paoletti, Anke Zimmermann, Laura Bassi and Emilia Cancellieri
Haemostasis and Thrombosis Center, A.O. Istituti Ospitalieri, Cremona Italy

1. Introduction

Telemedicine system is defined as the use of tele-communications to support health care with the purpose to facilitate the interaction between patient and health care provider and to achieve improved treatment results and lower treatment costs. This approach, currently spreading, is becoming a useful mean to ensure home health care, remote patient monitoring and disease management. Furthermore, telemedicine can support educational and training programs for patients and health care providers. Technological innovation in medical care and introduction of telecommunication technologies in medical practice have led to the development of telemedicine programs in many medical specialities. The principal aims of a telemedicine system applied to clinical practice are to improve health care and social assistance. The concept of telemedicine in Oral Anticoagulant Therapy (OAT) management grows from the necessity to improve interactions between patients and health care providers and, at the same time, to enhance management system. The increase of communication requests among different subjects can be facilitated through the elaboration of data networks between the Anticoagulation Clinic (AC), general practitioner or other peripheral districts and patients. Telemedicine systems for OAT have been developed during the last few years with the aim to decentralize in the health territorial care units the activity of ACs, improving the quality of life of the patients living far from the AC site and maintaining the same clinical quality levels. A telemedicine system for anticoagulated patients should be structured through net supported programs (intra and internet) to collect and elaborate clinical data, connected among hospital divisions, health care peripheral districts and patients. A digital format to collect clinical data, an electronic medical record, communication tools to connect patients and peripheral health care and a global quality control system are mandatory requirements to set up a telemedicine system. All communications, including clinical data, laboratory controls, alerts, prescriptions and recommendations have to be available in real time through a bi-directional connection. The telematic organization could develop different types of solutions for different types of patients in OAT population. For example:

- independent patient, who lives far away from the Clinic but can reach a peripheral district (Hospice, General Practitioner and so on);
- home patient not independent;

- totally independent patient.

From a general point of view, new web telematic organizations can provide several advantages in comparison with standard treatments, with the principal aim to improve patient management, as , for, example:

- direct communication between districts and AC;
- good or improved clinical quality (time spent in the therapeutic range and major complications);
- improvement in patient's satisfaction and in their quality of life;
- continuing medical record update;
- time gained by staff;
- possibility to manage different antithrombotic drugs (heparins and new oral anticoagulant agents).

2. Antivitamin K antagonists

In this chapter we will refer to OAT considering only Anti-vitamin K antagonists (AVK). The new oral anticoagulant drugs, very recently approved, are prescribed only in few countries all over the world and insufficient information on types of management are available at present. AVK are very effective drugs in many clinical conditions such as deep venous thrombosis, pulmonary embolism, atrial fibrillation, prostheses heart valve, myocardial infarction and cardioembolic ischemic stroke. AVK as oral anticoagulation therapy (OAT) are life-saving therapies that can effectively prevent cardioembolic strokes related to atrial fibrillation and heart valve replacements, treat venous thromboembolism, with a relative low risk of major bleeding complications. Because of their characteristics, still at present, AVK are under/and sub-optimal used and consequently their maximum efficacy is not still reached in the real world patient population. As well known, the major incidence of thromboembolic or haemorragic events occurs when the prothrombin time (PT), expressed as the international normalized ratio (INR), is out of the therapeutic range. Therefore effectiveness and safety of OAT increase when a good control of anticoagulation level is guaranteed. For this reason, a correct use of AVK requires a careful clinical and laboratory monitoring, as well as specific competences for managing the possible complications and/or emergencies (Ansell et al., 2008). The risk of thrombosis increases with age and the progressive ageing of the population causes a constant increase of patients who need OAT as consequence. For this reason, during the last 15 years, patients on AVK are constantly increasing and results coming from unofficial data show about 1.000.000 patients in Italy, with a prevalence that is 1.6% of the total population (Fig. 1). Vitamin K antagonists determine their anticoagulant effect by interfering with the metabolism of vitamin K. In Italy two different types of coumarins are available, warfarin (Coumadin) and acenocoumarol (Sintrom) which differ because of their half-life, that is longer for warfarin (36-42 vs 12-16 hours), the most prescribed drug in Italy at present. Warfarin has high bioavailability and is rapidly absorbed from the gastrointestinal tract; the maximal blood concentration is reached 90 minutes after oral administration. Coumarins in the blood are bound to plasma proteins (principally albumin) and accumulated in the liver, where they act through the inhibition of vitamin K epoxide reductase enzyme (Fig. 2).

The high inter and intra-individual biological variability is one the main problem in AVK management, principally due to genetic conditions, drug absorption, drug interferences, diet and co-morbidities (Feero, Guttmacher, 2011). On this basis many anticoagulation clinics (AC) have been set up in Italy, operating in the framework of the Italian Federation of Anticoagulation Clinics (FCSA) (Fig. 3).

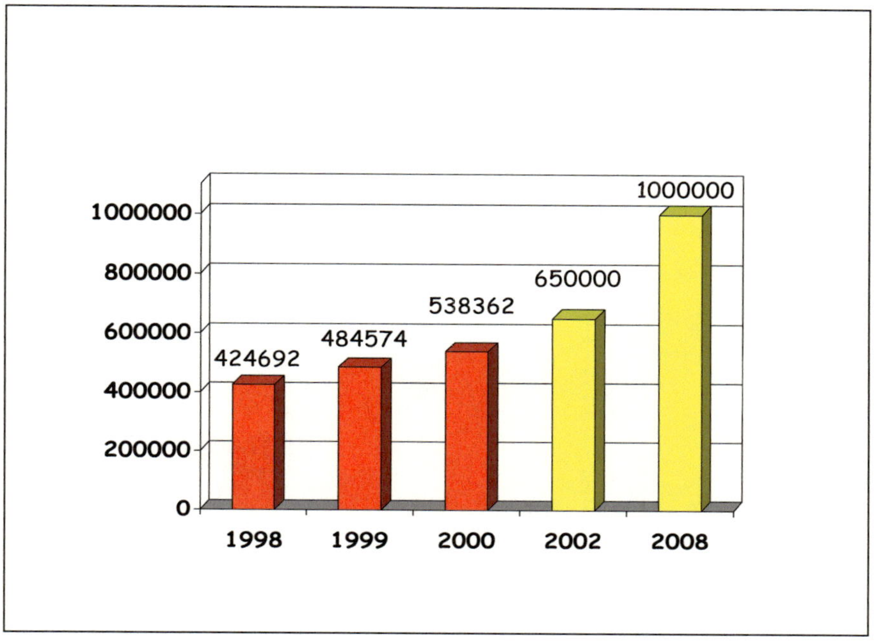

Fig. 1. Increase of patients on AVK in Italy

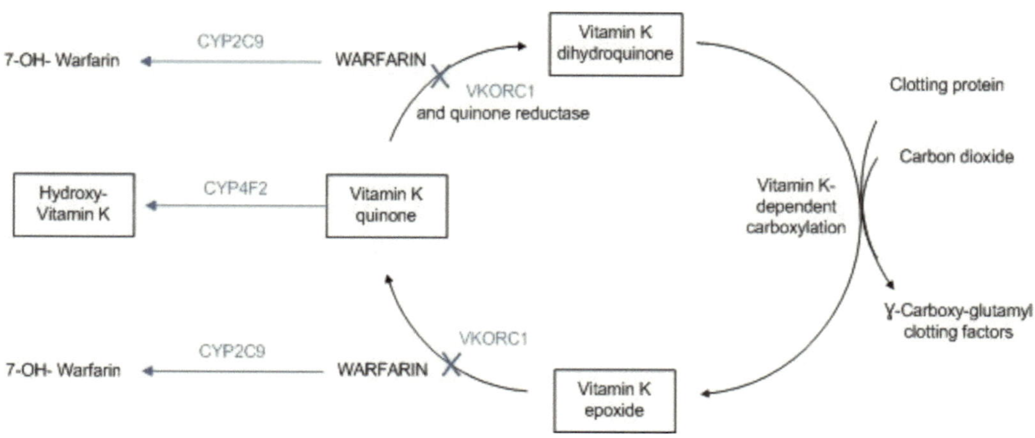

Fig. 2. Warfarin and vitamin K cycles

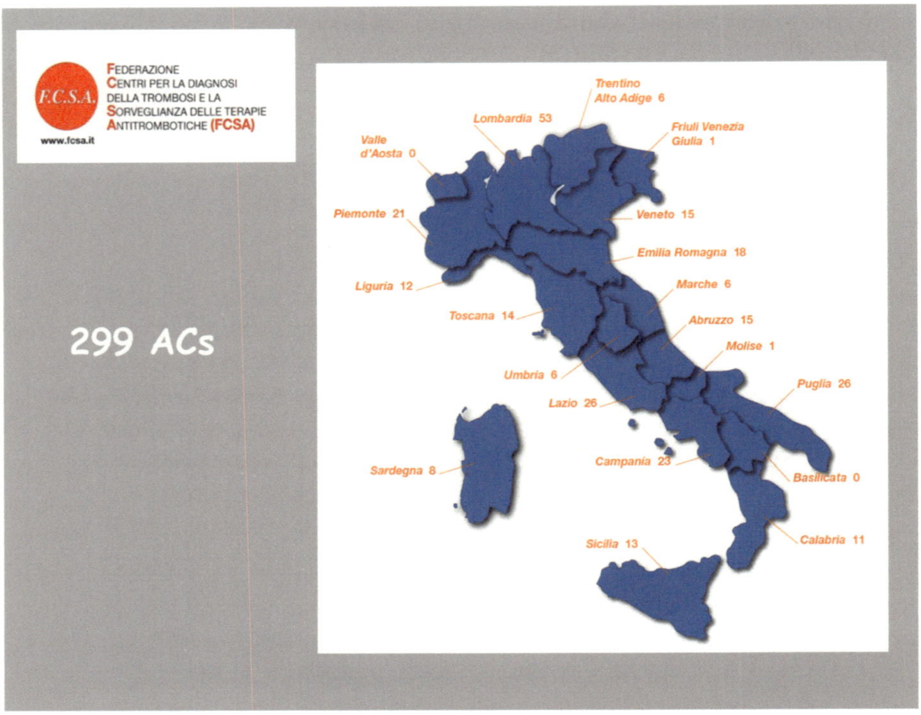

Fig. 3. Italian Federation of Anticoagulation Clinics (FCSA): ACs distribution

Compliance of patients that require long-term therapy is a crucial problem and represents an important factor of variability of both quality of treatment and patient management. In fact, as shown in literature, patients on chronic therapy omit about 40% of their daily medications and 10-26% of the patients on chronic OAT are not compliant (Barcellona et al., 2002). As a consequence, poor compliance is associated to bad quality treatment. Educational courses for patients (indications for treatment, risk and benefit, problem in drug administration, dietary behaviour, interactions with other drugs and intercurrent disease) and for health territorial care units can improve patient's compliance (Barcellona et al., 2002). Telemedicine systems can empower educational programs with the aim to improve drug adherences, increase interactions between OAT patients and health care organizations. Taking into consideration economical and clinical advantages provided by AC, compared to other types of management (see paragraph 3.3), the decentralization into peripheral health units using telemedicine systems, represents an effective evolution of the management strategies.

3. Model of management

3.1 Type of management

As for all pharmacological treatments even for AVK, three crucial points should be considered to define not only the correct drug indications but also risks and advantages. In synthesis before starting anticoagulation we should answer to the following questions:

- is OAT indicated on that clinical condition ? (= treatment effectiveness);
- is there an increase of benefit compared to OAT risk? (= treatment safety);

- which is the appropriate management model ?(= type of patient management).

The growth of OAT population recorded in the past twenty years is undoubtedly related to many factors, including the organization of Anticoagulation Clinics (AC) and the standardisation of laboratory methods, which has allowed to perform clinical trials in order to demonstrate OAT efficacy and safety (Bussey et al., 1989). These studies have supplied a better knowledge of therapeutic indications, optimal anticoagulation levels (therapeutic ranges), risk of haemorrhagic and thrombotic complications, pharmacological interference and the importance of a specialistic management (Charney et al., 1988). However, in daily clinical practice OAT is still underused because often considered by the medical class itself as a therapy that can be hardly managed, laborious and potentially dangerous for the patient, and a certain number of patients self-prescribe without specific training with serious risks for their health. We can consider 4 different management models: 1) routine medical care (RMC), 2) AC, 3) patient self testing and 4) patient self management. The four models for OAT control are variously developed in different countries. The model prevailing in the United States is the Usual Care (UC), in which patients refer directly to their own general practitioner or specialist; the INR is determined in external laboratories or in general practitioner's consulting room through portable monitors. In countries such as England, Holland, Italy and Spain, Anticoagulation Clinics (AC) are developed. ACs can interact with the general practitioners on various levels, according to their competence. In particular, ACs have been set up in Italy in order to:

- determine the appropriate clinical indications for anticoagulant treatment;
- determine the laboratory tests necessary for pharmacological monitoring;
- prescribe the anticoagulation regimen based on the results of the laboratory tests;
- define intervals for regular anticoagulation controls;
- evaluate any potential pharmacological interference;
- take care of patients undergoing surgical interventions or invasive procedures;
- manage the patients during intercurrent diseases;
- hold training courses and educational programs for patients and healthcare providers.

Several studies have shown that anticoagulation management is crucial to ensure quality of treatment and, among different types of management, Anticoagulation Clinic (AC) results in better clinical control compared with routine medical care (RMC) (Bussey et al. 1996; Chiquette et al. 1998).

3.2 Patient self testing and patient self management

New technologies applied to INR testing determined the development of portable coagulometers. Portable monitors are small, handy instruments, easy to transport and allow PT/INR testing with a drop of whole blood. The widespread use of portable monitors in clinical practice allowed the development of point of care testing, shifting the analytical phase from the laboratory to patient with considerable advantage in terms of convenience and comfort for the patient. Those systems are very useful to manage patients at home or at peripheral health care units (nursing homes, groups of general practitioners, health communities), simplifying and improving OAT management. OAT self monitoring through portable coagulometers has the potential advantage to be easy to use for the patient or caregivers and potentially improve patient's quality of life (Tripodi et al. 1993). There are several ways for using portable coagulometers that we can summarize as self-testing (PST) and self-management (PSM). With PST the patient autonomously monitors his/her own

PT/INR using portable coagulometer, living OAT decision to AC. Self-testing therefore offers the patient the opportunity of increasing test frequency (Watzke et al., 2000). With PSM the patient not only monitors his/her own PT/INR but also self-prescribes drug dosage. As shown in literature self-testing and self-management leads to a significant 50% reduction in thromboembolism and 13% reduction in major haemorrhage, compared to RMC (Fitzmaurice et al., 2005; Sawicki et al., 1999). A recent Cochrane review analyzed 18 randomized trials, including 4723 patients, to compare PSM vs RMC and confirmed an advantage for self-management in thrombotic and haemorrhagic complications (RR for thrombosis=0.47; RR for bleeding=0.56) (Garcia-Alamino et al., 2010). We have to highlight that just a few number of patients, highly selected, has been enrolled in these studies and a real clinical advantage of self-management compared with ACs hasn't been demonstrated (Garcia-Alamino et al., 2010; Cromheecke et al., 2000). Several experiences of OAT management in peripheral health units, involving general practitioners and nursing homes, coordinated by ACs through telemedicine system, have been started in the last years. Aim of these projects, as example of virtual "coagulation clinic", is to facilitate the anticoagulant treatment, improving management quality, reducing risk of complications due to inadequate monitoring, with a continuos update of clinical data recording.

3.3 Cost analysis of different management strategies

In the last few years, we observed an increased interest in define and control health care costs. First Anglo-Saxon countries, in particular the United States, assessed the costs of different anticoagulation management, comparing the specialist system (AC) with non specialist system (general medical care, including all physicians who manage patients on OAT–RMC) (Elston-Lafata et al., 2000). Although several studies have been published on bleeding and thrombotic complications on OAT, only few of them have been focused on the evaluation of differences between the two management models (RMC/AC) (Bussey et al. 1996). It should be noted that most of the available data derived from studies on controlled population managed by Anticoagulation Clinics, making it difficult to determine the true incidence of complications in other management models. In the ISCOAT study, the most large, prospective Italian investigation study, including a cohort from 34 ACs, the incidence of major bleeding complications was 1.25 for 100 patient-years, whereas the incidence of thromboembolic events was 3.5 for 100 patient-years (Palareti el al., 1997). Literature analysis showed that patients on RMC had a 2-fold increase (2.5 vs 1.25% patient-years) and 3-fold increase (10.5 vs 3.5% patient-years) of bleeding and thromboembolic risks, respectively, compared to patients followed by AC (Palareti et al., 1996; Palareti et al., 1997) (Tab. 1).

COMPLICATION	RMC (PERCENT P-Y)	AC (PERCENT P-Y)	OR (CI= 95%)
Major bleeding	2.5	1.25	0.49 (0.31-0.76)
Thrombosis	10.5	3.5	0.22 (0.13-0.37)

Table 1. Risk of major bleeding and thrombotic complication in RMC versus AC

The final result of the analysis, regarding cost of complications (elaborated on the basis of the economic values calculated for diagnosis related groups -DRG- of the Lombardy Region in Italy) and the cost of management in ACs, showed an advantage for ACs (366,1 € vs 688,5

€). In conclusion AC reduces risk of complications and allow to save 322 € per patient per year. The superiority of this anticoagulation management model is due to several reasons, the most important of which probably are the accurate laboratory control of PT/INR, a structured network for the management of emergencies and major and minor complications and a general system that guarantees education, communication and patient's follow-up continuously. For all these reasons ACs currently represent the reference standard for OAT management and all new management systems, such as patient self testing (PST) and patient self management (PSM), must be compared to ACs to define their global quality (Tab. 2, Tab. 3, Tab. 4). In summary:

- RMC is less expensive, but less effective and safe;
- AC represents a very good model in term of quality of management, but it's more expansive compared with RMC;
- PSM is effective and safe, but it can be applied only in nearly 25 % of the patient population , highly selected and trained;
- PST represents the best model (increase in Time spent in Range-TTR, but no differences in clinical events compared with AC), but it is the most expensive. It represents an opportunity to increase frequency of testing.

	OD (95% CI)	P
RMC/AC	0.53 (0.29-0.98)	0.03
RMC/PST	0.19 (0.09-0.39)	<0.01
RMC/PSM	0.57 (0.32-1.03)	0.04
AC/PST	0.36 (0.17-0.75)	0.002
AC/PSM	1.07 (0.58-1.98)	0.07
PST/PSM	2.2 (1.04-4.72)	0.02

Table 2. Time spent in range: comparison among different types of OAT management

Economical variables	RMC (€ PT/Y)	AC (€ PT/Y)	PST (€ PT/Y)	PSM (€ PT/Y)
Laboratory monitoring	65.7	65.7	250	250
AC management	---	147.3	147.3	---
Warfarin	30.4	30.4	30.4	30.4
Total	96.7	243.4	331.7	280.4

Table 3. Cost comparison among different management strategies

	RMC	AC	PSM	PST
CLINICAL QUALITY	+	++++	++++	++++
TTR	+	+++	+++	++++
ACCESSIBILITY	++++	++	+	++
COSTS	+	++	+++	++++

Table 4. Summary of the characteristics of the different management models

4. Telemedicine applied to Anticoagulation Clinic

4.1 Anticoagulation Clinic

Taking into account both economic and clinical advantages provided by an AC, and also the logistic problems, a reorganization plan could be necessary. The most frequent difficulties that an AC could face are the following:

- strong increase in the number of patients within the AC, mainly on long-term treatment, without a concomitant development of structures and increase of health care personnel;
- difficulty for many patients living far from the AC location in reaching the hospital clinic as well as the lack of any AC in the peripheral areas;
- discomfort of patients (and their relatives) due to overcrowding and lack of public transportation;

A telemedicine system offers the opportunity to empower the daily activity, decentralizing the management into peripheral health units, using informatic support and bi-directional web connection (Gardiner et al., 2006). In particular the aims of a telemedicine reorganization could be summarized as follow:

- reduce the number of patients referring daily to the AC, decentralizing in peripheral health units;
- maintain the same quality levels defined as the time spent in the therapeutic range and number of complications;
- reduce patient's discomfort;
- increase the total number of patients with OAT indications, creating a network that reaches home and remote patients;
- send therapy prescription in real time, through the direct communication between the Anticoagulation Clinic and peripheral districts;

Telemedicine reorganizations give opportunities to peripheral health units to provide the following services:

- Anticoagulation testing performed with portable coagulation analysers, assessing the prothrombin time (PT) expressed as international normalized ratio (INR);
- Quality control of the portable coagulation analyzers;
- Clinical evaluation of patients (concomitant disease, changes in the drug regimen, administration of new drugs, potential surgical interventions, planning of specialist visits) through the administration of a medical history questionnaire;
- Real-time data transmission to the AC.

Bi-directional connection between AC and peripheral districts allow two different management levels: 1) treatment prescription and patient management centralized in AC; 2) treatment prescription and patient management performed in peripheral health units, referring to AC in case of complications, over/under treatment, surgery, bridging. The AC has also organizing and epidemiological functions. The AC should ensure clinical validation of the data received, transmission of therapeutic measures and clinical advices, patient management in case of complications and in case of any other clinical condition interfering with treatment. Through a telemedicine system AC can provide healthcare to both home monitored patients and self-managing patients. Home monitored patients, defined as patients who cannot leave home due to serious physical illness, documented disease or advanced age, are managed by trained staff using mobile monitoring units connected with AC. These equipments can perform INR measurement and transmit the clinical data to the AC from the patient's home setting, in order to receive indications for appropriate therapy and urgent medical advice. Self-testing patients, defined as stable and trained patients, directly communicate with AC using a telemedicine device installed at home. These patients are able to perform PT INR on portable monitors and receive therapy prescription from the AC through the web.

4.2 Portable monitor quality control

In peripheral health units, INR measurement from capillary blood specimens could be performed by portable monitors in a quality assurance global system (Marco et al., 2000). The PT/INR determination from venous blood specimens, performed in AC's laboratory, could be considered as the reference system. Taking as reference system PT/INR performed on central laboratory, the assessment of agreement should be always evaluated both for single patients and for the global accuracy. In general, quality control procedures are performed on all portable monitors to assess accuracy and efficacy and, because of no standardized recommendations are available, some predefined criteria have to be established. Based on current guidelines for laboratory QC the following items can be applied:

- PM suitabily: a) precision calculated on normal plasma pool, repeated 10 times, acceptable if CV < 5%; b) accuracy, evaluated on 10 pathological specimens with INR < 4.0, accettable if INR differences < ± 0.5.
- Intra-assay precision: each PHU elaborates monthly the Lewej-Jennings cards. Internal QC, provided by the company, is performed at the beginning of each session and every 20 samples. A CV between ± 20% is considered acceptable.
- Quaterly accuracy to assess the agreement between analytical instruments: every 3 months PT values from 3 venous blood samples of patients with capillary whole blood PT values in the low (2.0-3.0), intermediate (3.0-4.0) and high (> 4.0) INR range are compared. Differences ≤ 0.5 INR are considered acceptable. In case of discrepancies between capillary and venous PT values of more than ± 0.5, the portable monitor is replaced. The choice of this cut-off value derived from the fact that a higher value would require remarkable adjustments in the therapeutic regimen.
- External quality assessment (NEQAS): it considers both laboratory data and clinical treatment, to assess the accuracy of the global therapeutic management (Kitchen et al., 2006).

4.3 Staff training

All the staff involved in the global patient management (physicians, laboratory technicians, nurses) has to be trained through specific educational programs and updating sessions as for example, recommended by the Italian Federation of Anticoagulation Clinics (FCSA). The program should include educational courses on OAT, dedicated courses on the use of portable monitors and training on computer programs (Sawicki et al., 1999). Specific manuals for patients, physicians and nurses should be structured. Periodic evaluations should be planned, reviewing all procedures and discussing results and problems.

4.4 Telemedicine global quality assessment

A quality assessment plan should be available to control and monitor a telemedicine health care system. A system for automatically flagging and providing information on the results has to be structured specifically. In detail a telemedicine system for anticoagulated patients requires alerts on the following indicators:

- control of coagulation testing;
- time spent in therapeutic range for patient managed in AC versus peripheral health units;
- number of controls for patients/year/peripheral health unit;
- number of bleeding and thromboembolic complications (percent patient-years);
- increase in patient attendance at the medical services provided by the peripheral health units resulting in a better distribution of workloads;
- waiting times for access/blood drawing;
- waiting times for therapeutic prescription;

A patient's satisfaction questionnaire has to be structured.

5. A telemedicine Anticoagulation Clinic: An example of web organization

In Italy from the beginning of 2001, some AC started telemedicine projects in different areas, interesting the following cities: Bologna, Cremona, Merano, Parma, Perugia. Even if these organizations differ in some aspects, like type of software used and level of management, the general principle and aims are common. As an example we describe the experience of the Cremona Hospital. Cremona AC started its activity 20 years ago and in 2011 is managing about 4494 patients. In 2002 a project intended to define criteria for decentralizing the management of OAT patients in suburban health districts, through a telemedicine system, bi-directional connected was elaborated. Principal aims were to create a web organization in order to improve the quality of life of the patients living far from the AC site, maintaining the same clinical quality level. All procedures adopted are on controlled certified quality program. The INR is determined on capillary blood through portable monitors and the AC receives INR results with anamnestic questionnaire. Electronic medical record includes information upload on general clinical conditions, diet intake and drug co-medication, INR and other laboratory data, general compliance and drug adherence, significant clinical events such as hospitalizations, surgery and invasive procedures. These data, collected in peripheral health care units (Nursing Homes, Groups of General Practitioners (GPs) and other hospitals of the area), are sent in real time to the AC, in order to share bi-directionally all clinical records. Moreover, AC is able to manage home patients (who can not leave their home due to serious physical problems, diseases in progress, old age) through mobile units and totally independent patients who directly communicate through the web connection system with the AC (Fig. 4).

11 peripheral health care units (2 Nursing Homes and 9 GP's peripheral health units) and 20 self-testing patients are currently connected for a total number of 1393 patients, i.e. 31% of

the total number of patients. 106 GPs and 22 nurses underwent training courses. As regard clinical quality indicators, no differences in time spent in the therapeutic range were observed between AC and GP's units, while Nursing Homes showed, as expected because of sub-acute illnesses, the lower TTR (TTR AC=73%; TTR GP's units=73.4%; TTR Nursing Homes=66%) (Tab. 5). No differences in major (haemorrhagic and/or thrombotic) complications were observed (Tab. 6).

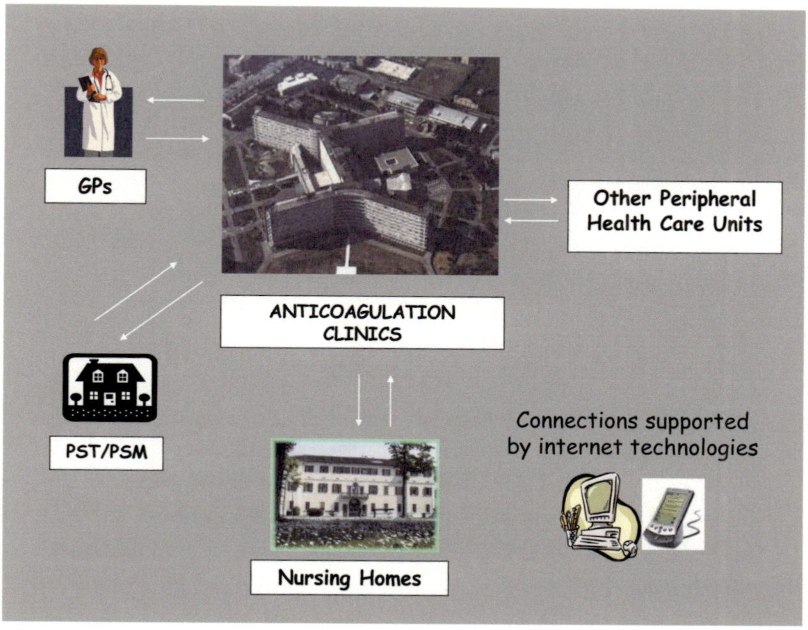

Fig. 4. A model of web organization

	% IN RANGE	% UNDER RANGE	% OVER RANGE	INR > 4.5 (%)
AC	73.7 %	21.5	4.8	0.2
GPs	73.4 %	21.3	5.3	0.2
Nursing Homes	66 %	24.2	9.8	0.6

Table 5. Time spent in range: comparison between AC and Peripheral Health Units

EVENTS	AC	Peripheral Units
MAJOR BLEEDING (percent p/y)	1.1 %	1.0 %
THROMBOSIS (percent p/y)	2.8 %	2.5 %
MINOR BLEEDING (percent p/y)	4.5 %	3.1 %

Table 6. Clinical Quality 2010

All patients express their satisfaction, showing a general improvement in their quality of life. The development of this telemedicine organization facilitates patient access and reduces waiting times for patients and their relatives as well as improves global quality of clinical assistance. The bi-directional informatic system used in this project is planned to set up the anticoagulated patient's clinical record that is constantly updated and already structured to manage new anticoagulant drugs (Fig. 5).

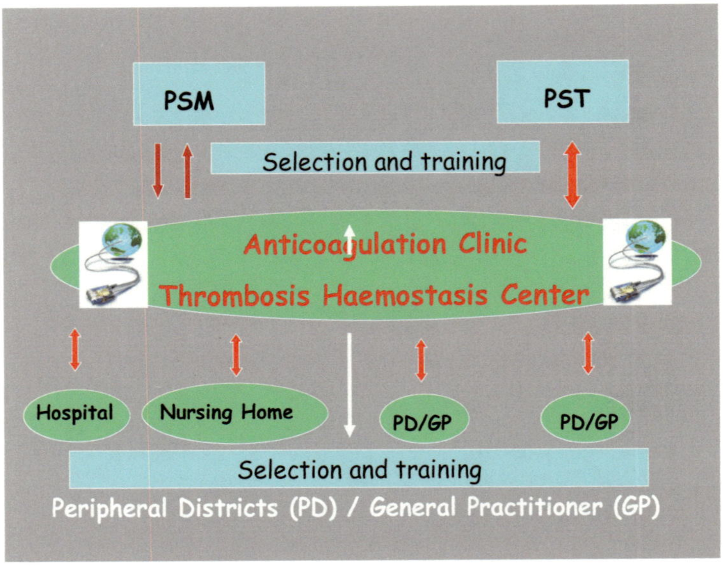

Fig. 5. Bidirectional connection between AC and peripheral districts

6. Limits in telemedicine development

Several barriers can limit the development of telemedicine in health care system. Major difficulties are represented by differences among different countries and regions, due to legal, cultural and organizational problems. Informatic evolution technologies should solve problems in connectivity among different health care structures. Furthermore, the lack of clear regulations for telemedicine development still represents a limit, increasing the rate of uncertainty. A telemedicine system have to guarantee a strict surveillance to avoid the potential lack of data and all unauthorized accesses. Health care telemedicine systems should be validated by experts, easy to use, flexible and adaptable in different clinical conditions. Training for all health care staff on new technologies have to be provided before starting up telemedicine management. Clinical protocols and all procedures have to be shared and formally approved, waiting for institutional regulations.

7. Conclusion

One of the major problem in anticoagulation management is represented not only by the increasing number of OAT patients as a result of ageing, but also by the extension of clinical indications and choice of the best management strategies to assure effectiveness and safety. Telemedicine systems are technologies that allow the development of new management models in different medical fields (Klonoff, 2009). Telemedicine applied to anticoagulated patients offers several advantages, both for organization as well as for improving communications. Decentralize clinical activity through a telemedicine system give the opportunity to redistribute patient population into different health care areas, whose medical services could be otherwise underused, and to facilitate accessibility to health care services for an increased number of patients, empowering management strategies. At the same time the web creates the opportunity to export quality procedures and competences outside specialized centres, increasing communications, not only between physician and patient, but also between different medical specialties. Telemedicine organizations are opportunities to improve health care and patient's quality of life through a capillary distribution of medical assistance, supporting physicians in the application of good clinical practice in anticoagulation management and in providing the following actions :

- properly define indications
- avoid treatment in patients who have major controindications
- stop therapy when advantages are less than risks
- identify drug and food interactions
- provide educational courses for patients and relatives
- determine a proper periodical control of anticoagulation level
- prescribe the right daily drug dose
- manage complications
- define protocols for patients undergoing invasive procedure or surgery
- periodically verify clinical and analytical performances

Telemedicine systems should help physicians to ensure the above mentioned items in order to give the best quality of management and avoid malpractice. The mainstay of this model relies on its extreme flexibility and that it can be adopted by either nursing care facilities, such as nursing homes, or healthcare facilities equipped with a medical staff, than by hospitals or groups of general practitioners. Moreover, it may help patients who cannot attend AC because of work-related reasons or remote location (patients on self-testing or self-management) or for those who cannot leave their homes because of chronic illness. As regard clinical quality, telemedicine system provide a very high quality comparable to the best standard and it can allow a reduction of health care costs through a more effective patient management compared to RMC. The service's accessibility represents probably the best advantage, giving to all patients the opportunity to be managed with a good clinical quality. Telemedicine represents an improvement in equity of health care and should be empowered by the government of different countries (Clark et al., 2010). The bidirectional computer connection allow peripheral health units to directly communicate with References structures, like AC or other specialists, creating electronic clinical chart constantly updated. Because of anticoagulant drugs are changing in the last few years and will rapidly change in the next future, through the introduction of new antithrombotic drugs, telemedicine could help the management. Informatic connections represent the starting point of a telemedicine system that will enable healthcare providers to monitor patients either on OAT or treated with new classes of anticoagulants (low molecular weight heparins, fondaparinux, idraparinux, dabigatran, rivaroxaban, apixaban or other new oral factor II or factor X inhibitors, etc). Probably, the new-generation antithrombotic drugs will need different types of management compared with AVKs, with a less frequent clinical and laboratory control. Nevertheless it will be necessary to follow up and record patient's data to guarantee the strict quality control on adherence, compliance, time in the therapeutic range, incidence of intercurrent diseases, adverse events and complications. Telemedicine can also support, in the next future, phamacovigilance procedures, usefull to improve knowledge on all new drugs (adverse events, major and minor complications, potentially dangerous drug interactions). However, notwithstanding these advantages due to telemedicine organizations, periodical clinical evaluations will be mandatory in order to assess any disease progression or changes in individual bleeding/thromboembolic risks. For these reasons a direct interactive communication between general practitioners and medical specialists is necessary and a telemedicine model will prove to be very useful, facilitating contacts and reporting. Health Authorities should promote telemedicine development with the aim to favour web organization for anticoagulation among different structures and specialists like Anticoagulation Clinics, General Practitioners or others. A web telemedicine organization have to assure the adoption of certification procedures to guarantee the quality of management and pharmacovigilance reports for the different anticoagulant drugs. The advantage of a web organization can be summarized as following:

- accessibility for a higher number of patients to a high quality management system;
- integration among different specialists and health structures
- continuing medical record update;
- possibility to manage patients on different antithrombotic drugs.

The web give the possibility to rapidly increase connections modulating the management in relation to different molecules, assuring clinical control for all patients.

It's advisable the empowerment of telemedicine strategies in routine clinical practice, through informatic programs suitable for each type of anticoagulant and patient, to favour a global management.

8. References

Ansell J, Hirsh J, Hylek H, Jacobson A, Crowther M, Palareti G. (2008). Pharmacology and management of the Vitamin K Antagonists: American College of Chest Physiscians Evidence-Based Clinical Practice Guidelines (8th edition). *Chest,*133:160S-198S

Barcellona D, Contu P, Marongiu F. (October 2002). Patient education and oral anticoagulant therapy. *Haematologica,* vol 87 (10), pp. 1081-1086

Bussey HI, Rospond RM, Quandt CM, Clark GM. (1989) The safety and effectiveness of long-term warfarin therapy in an anticoagulation clinic. *Pharmacotherapy,* Vol. 9, pp. 214-219

Bussey HI, Chiquette E, Amato MG. Anticoagulation clinic care versus routine medical care: a review and interim report. *Journal of Thrombosis and Thrombolysis* 1996; 2: 315-9

Charney R, Leddomado E, Rose DN, Fuster V. (1988). Anticoagulation clinics and the monitoring of anticoagulant therapy. *International Journal of Cardiology,* Vol. 18, pp. 197-206

Chiquette E, Amato MG, Bussey HI. (1998). Comparison of an anticoagulation clinic with usual medical care. *Archives of Internal Medicine,* 158: 1641-7

Clark PA, Capuzzi K, Harrison J. (November 2010). Telemedicine: medical, legal and ethical perspectives. *Medical Science Monitor,* vol 30, issue 16 (12), pp. RA261-272

Cromheecke ME, Levi M, Colly LP, de Mol BJ, Prins MH, Hutten BA, Mak R, Keyzers KC, Buller HR. (2000). Oral anticoagulation self-management and management by a specialistic anticoagulation clinic: a randomized cross-over comparison. *Lancet,* Vol. 356, pp. 97-102

Elston-Lafata J, Martin SA, Kaatz S, Ward RE. (2000). The cost effectiveness of different management strategies for patients on chronic warfarin therapy. *Journal of General Internal Medicine,* 15: 31-37

Feero W.G, Guttmacher AE. (2011). Genomic and Drug Response. *New England Journal of Medicine,* 364;12:1144-53

Fitzmaurice DA, Gardiner C, Kitchen S, Mackie I, Murray ET, Machin SJ; British Society of Haematology Taskforce for Haemostasis and Thrombosis. (October 2005). An evidence-based review and guidelines for patient self-testing and management of oral anticoagulation.*British Journal of Haematology,* vol. 131(2): pp. 156-165

Fitzmaurice DA, Murray ET, McCahon D, Holder R, Raftery JP, Hussain S, Sandhar H, Hobbs FD. (Novembre 2005). Self management of oral anticoagulation: randomised trial. *British Medical Journal,* Vol. 5, No. 331(7524):1057.

Garcia-Alamino JM, Ward AM, Alonso-Coello P, Perera R, Bankhead C, Fitzmaurice D, Heneghan CJ. (April 2010). Self-monitoring and self-management of oral anticoagulation. *Cochrane Database Systematic Review,* Vol. 14, No 4: CD003839

Gardiner C, Williams K, Mackie IJ, Machin SJ, Cohen H. (2006). Can oral anticoagulation be managed using telemedicine and patient self-testing? A pilot study. *Clinical and Laboratory Haematology,* Vol. 28, pp. 122-125

Kitchen S, Kitchen DP, Jennings I, Woods TA.L, Walker ID, Preston FE. (2006) Point-of-care International Normalized Ratios: UK NEQAS experience demonstrates necessity for proficiency testing of three different monitors. *Thrombosis and Haemostasis,* Vol. 96, No. 5, pp. 590-596

Klonoff DC. (July 2009). Using Telemedicine to improve outcomes in diabetes - An emerging Technology. *Journal of Diabetes Science and Technology,* Vol 3, No. 4, pp. 624-628

Marco F, Sedano C, Bermudez A, Lopez-Duarte M, Zubizzarreta A. (2000). Improving methods to assess therapeutic quality control of treatment with oral anticoagulants. *Thrombosis and Haemostasis,* Vol. 84, pp. 921-922

Palareti G, Leali N, Coccheri S, Poggi M, Manotti C, D'Angelo A, Pengo V, Erba N, Moia M, Ciavarella N, Devoto G, Berrettini M, Musolesi S, on behalf of the ISCOAT (Italian Study on Complications of Oral Anticoagulant Therapy) Study Group. (1996). Bleeding complications of oral anticoagulant treatment: an inception-cohort, prospective collaborative study (ISCOAT). *Lancet,* Vol. 348, pp. 423-428

Palareti G, Manotti C, D'Angelo A, Pengo V, Erba N, Moia M, Ciavarella N, Devoto G, Berrettini M, Poggi M, Legnani C, Musolesi S, Coccheri S on behalf of the ISCOAT (Italian Study on Complications of Oral Anticoagulant Therapy) Study Group. (1997). Thrombotic events during oral anticoagulant treatment: results of the inception-cohort, prospective collaborative ISCOAT study. *Thrombosis and Haemostasis,* Vol. 78, pp.1438-1443

Sawicki PT, Working Group for the Study of Patient Self-Management of Oral Anticoagulation. (1999). A structured teaching and self-management program for patients receiving oral anticoagulation: a randomized controlled trial. *JAMA;* Vol. 281, pp. 145-150.

Tripodi A, Arbini AA, Chantarangkul V, Bottega D, Mannucci PM. (1993). Are capillary whole blood coagulation monitors suitable for the control treatment by international normalized ratio? *Thrombosis and Haemostasis*, Vol. 70, pp. 921-924

Watzke HH, Forberg E, Svolba G. (2000). A prospective controlled trial comparing weekly self-testing and self-dosing with the standard management of patients on stable oral anticoagulation. *Thrombosis and Haemostasis*, Vol. 83, pp. 661-665

16

Telemedicine for Chronic Digestive Diseases: A Systematic Qualitative Review

Sandra M. Quezada[1] and Raymond K. Cross[1,2]
[1]*University of Maryland School of Medicine*
Department of Medicine, Division of Gastroenterology and Hepatology
[2]*Veterans Affairs Maryland Health Care System*
USA

1. Introduction

According to 2004 statistics from the National Digestive Diseases Information Clearinghouse, digestive diseases affect 60-70 million people in the United States, resulting in 105 million ambulatory visits and 13.5 million hospitalizations. The cost burden associated with these diseases is high. It is estimated that direct and indirect medical costs related to digestive diseases are $98 billion and $44 billion, respectively. Chronic digestive diseases make up a significant proportion of these disorders, including but not limited to celiac disease, chronic constipation, chronic pancreatitis, cirrhosis, Crohn's disease, gastroesophageal reflux disease, irritable bowel syndrome, ulcerative colitis, and viral hepatitis.

Telemedicine has been used successfully in chronic conditions such as asthma, diabetes, and congestive heart failure. In patients with asthma, telemedicine improves symptoms, decreases use of quick relief inhalers, improves adherence with self-action plans, improves quality of life and patient knowledge, and decreases urgent care visits (Joshi *et al*, 2005). In diabetes, telemedicine reduces glycosylated hemoglobin levels (Quinn *et al*, 2009). Telemedicine improves quality of life, and decreases hospitalizations and costs in congestive heart failure (Roth *et al*, 2004).

Telemedicine has proven to be a feasible and well accepted method of treatment delivery in the field of gastroenterology as well. A systematic review of scientific publications was performed in order to identify all studies conducted examining the application of telemedicine in digestive diseases. Database searches in MEDLINE, the Cochrane Controlled Trials Register, and Web of Science Conference Proceedings Citation Index were done with the following search terms: telemedicine, gastroenterology, inflammatory bowel disease, ulcerative colitis, Crohn's disease, gastroesophageal reflux disease, hepatitis C, hepatitis B, chronic liver disease, cirrhosis, constipation, irritable bowel syndrome, microscopic colitis, celiac disease and chronic pancreatitis. This search yielded telemedicine studies conducted in one of three disease states: inflammatory bowel disease with a specific focus in ulcerative colitis, irritable bowel syndrome, and chronic viral hepatitis C. In this chapter, we will review the use of telemedicine for these chronic digestive diseases and the effect of telemedicine on access to care, disease activity, education, and quality of life.

2. Inflammatory bowel disease

Many of the telemedicine studies in digestive diseases focuses on the chronic disease model of inflammatory bowel disease (IBD). IBD is comprised of ulcerative colitis (UC) and Crohn's disease (CD), two inflammatory conditions of the intestines that affect approximately 1.4 million Americans, with that number evenly split between the two conditions (Crohn's and Colitis Foundation of America [CCFA], 2010). Symptoms of UC and CD can be quite debilitating, most commonly including diarrhea (which can be bloody) and abdominal pain. Typically, symptoms are chronic and characterized by periods of remission interrupted by exacerbations.

Effective medical therapy for induction and maintenance of remission exists for both UC and CD; however, the relatively young age at diagnosis, potential for medication side effects, and the long-term need for medication to maintain remission can result in decreased adherence, which places patients at risk for exacerbations of disease (Kane *et al.*, 2003). Also, patient miscomprehension can lead to decreased medication adherence (Sewitch, *et al.*, 2003) and delays in seeking medical care with associated adverse outcomes.

Several studies have evaluated the use of telemedicine in the IBD population. One pilot study assessed the acceptance of a home telemanagement system (HAT) in ten patients with IBD (Cross *et al.*, 2006). This study utilized a HAT system developed for patients with asthma and other chronic respiratory diseases (Finkelstein *et al*, 2001 as cited in Cross *et al*, 2006). IBD HAT is comprised of three components: a patient home unit, a decision support server, and a web-based clinician portal as depicted in Figure 1.

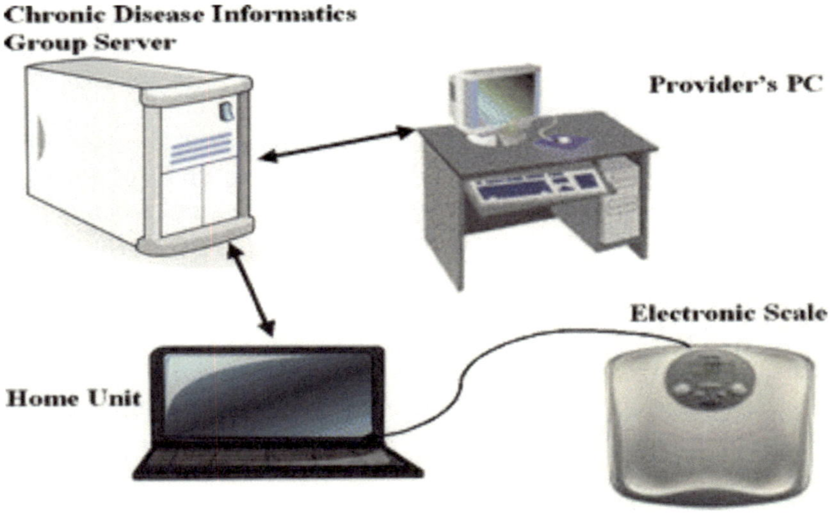

Fig. 1. Model of the home telemanagement system for inflammatory bowel disease

The patient home unit includes an electronic weight scale connected to a laptop computer via a serial port for self-testing. The laptop computer contains a symptom diary, side effect inventory, adherence check, and assessment of body weight. Patients answer questions directly using the laptop; weight is assessed after audio prompts from the laptop. Individualized patient data is entered into the secure web portal; information collected includes contact information, medication prescriptions, HAT testing schedules, and disease history. Clinicians use the web portal to customize medication and side effect profiles.

Furthermore, a clinical alert system is customized for each patient based on responses to the symptom diary, medication side effect questions, self-reported adherence, and body weight. Once self-testing is completed, patients received an IBD-related educational prompt in the format of a "tip of the day"; the following week, patients are asked a question about the tip. Patients cannot advance in the educational curriculum unless they answer the question correctly. The results of self-testing are submitted telephonically and are available for review immediately on the secure web server.

Five participants in this study were diagnosed with CD and five were diagnosed with UC. The mean disease duration was 15 years. Participant average age was 47 years. Ninety percent of participants were Caucasian, with mean years of education of 15 years. All reported excellent English proficiency. Thirty percent reported limited knowledge of IBD. Two participants had never used a home computer and one had never used the Internet.

All participants found the self-test procedures to be uncomplicated and reported no difficulty using the computer or answering the symptom diary and side effect questions. Ninety percent reported no difficulty with using the weight scale. All patients felt the self-testing procedures took very little time and felt it would result in very little to no interference with their daily activities. Thirty percent would feel significantly or moderately safer while using this system. Seventy percent of participants reported that testing up to four times per week was feasible; all participants felt that weekly testing was realistic.

Based on their results, the authors concluded that patients with IBD accepted IBD HAT technology and that use of IBD HAT was feasible in the IBD population.

A follow-up analysis was performed to assess acceptance and feasibility of the home telemanagement system among 34 participants with IBD (Cross & Finkelstein, 2007). After an initial 40 minute training period, participants were asked to complete weekly self-testing for six months. Disease activity, quality of life and IBD knowledge were assessed at baseline and at six months. Seven participants were excluded, due to either lack of adherence with home installation of the system or lack of a telephone line. Overall, weekly adherence to self-testing over the 6 month study was 91%. Once again, participants reported that IBD HAT was easy to use and did not interfere with their daily activities. In addition, use of IBD HAT positively impacted participants' satisfaction with their IBD care, as 86% reported receiving excellent care after use of IBD HAT as compared with 65% of participants at baseline. Similarly, 71% reported having their needs met at the end of the six months as compared with 57% at baseline. Ninety percent reported that they were quite satisfied with their IBD care at 6 months compared with 70% initially. Patient knowledge also improved significantly after using the IBD HAT educational curriculum.

While this study was not powered to detect significant differences in disease activity and disease-specific quality of life, the authors reported strong trends toward improvement in these factors, as measured by the Harvey Bradshaw Index (HBI) for CD activity (a modified HBI was utilized for UC) (Harvey & Bradshaw, 1980, as cited in Cross & Finkelstein, 2007) and the Short Inflammatory Bowel Disease Questionnaire (SIBDQ) for disease-specific quality of life (Irvine *et al*, 1996, as cited in Cross & Finkelstein, 2007).

Qualitative interviews were performed for 23 of the participants (Castro *et al.*, 2006). Feedback from participants was categorized into one of three topics: 1) content of the system components, 2) interface between the system and the user, and 3) process of using the system. Participants reported that the greatest benefit of IBD HAT was the increased sense of empowerment and control over their IBD care as compared with regular monitoring. This resulted in improved patient satisfaction and outcomes. Overall, the authors concluded that use of IBD HAT over 6 months was feasible and that patient acceptance of the technology was high.

An abstract from the Digestive Diseases Week (annual conference of the American Gastroenterological Association) in May 2010 presented data on a prospective, randomized, controlled, pilot study, performed to evaluate the effectiveness and applicability of a novel telemedicine system in an IBD clinic (Krier *et al.*, 2010). Newly established patients were randomized into one of two groups: 1) a remote clinical encounter via telemedicine with an IBD provider (located 33 miles away) or 2) a conventional in-person encounter with an IBD provider. The telemedicine system consisted of two standard Apple computers running a secure protocol between the subspecialist and the participant. Fifteen participants were enrolled (8 with UC, 7 with CD). Eighty percent of participants were men, with a median age of 60 years and median disease duration of 7 years. Participant experience was rated using the Ware Specific Visit Standard Questionnaire (1 = excellent, 5 = poor). Participants in both groups rated their clinic experience highly (1.2 ± 0.4 in the telemedicine group versus 1.1 ± 0.4 in the conventional group). Both remote and in-person clinic visits were of similar duration (58 minutes in the telemedicine group versus 53 minutes in the conventional group). High ratings on the technical and informational quality of the telemedicine sessions were reported from the providers involved. The authors concluded that telemedicine can be used successfully to increase access to quaternary care in large health care systems, resulting in patient satisfaction similar to face-to-face clinical encounters.

In summary, the above studies demonstrate that patients with IBD reported a high level of acceptance of telemedicine as a means of receiving care. Telemedicine positively impacted participants' perception of their care and gave them a sense of empowerment, as it encouraged them to actively participate in their disease management. The relatively low numbers of participants in the initial studies limited the ability of the investigator's to evaluate for differences in disease activity, quality of life, or utilization of health care resources. However, the results supported the need for further investigation in this field with larger sample sizes of patients with IBD.

2.1 Ulcerative colitis

As noted earlier, IBD is comprised of two distinct disease entities UC and CD. While the two disease processes are similar, important symptomatic and prognostic distinctions exist between the two. For example, while both CD and UC cause diarrhea, the diarrhea in UC tends to be bloody, while in CD it is not. In addition, CD can be complicated by intestinal stricture, fistula formation, and perianal disease involvement. Thus, measuring symptoms and disease activity of both diseases collectively misrepresents the unique symptomatic characteristics of each. Telemedicine has been studied primarily in the UC population.

In 2009, Cross *et al*. tested the feasibility and acceptance of telemedicine in ten patients with UC (Cross *et al*, 2009), with certain modifications to the IBD HAT system described previously (Cross *et al*, 2007). First, questions in the symptom diary were altered to be specific for UC. The UC symptom diary consists of 14 questions which assessed overall well being, functional status, bowel symptoms, systemic symptoms, and extraintestinal manifestations of UC. Responses were scored from a minimum of one to a maximum of five, yielding an overall minimum score of 14 and maximum score of 51. An alert was generated for a score of 25 or higher. Subscores from 4 to 15 were also generated for a group of questions felt to be critically important that dealt with overall well-being, number of liquid stools per day, nocturnal awakening, and amount of visible blood in bowel movements. In this instance a subscore of 8 or more generates an alert to the provider. Total and sub-score thresholds can be individualized for each participant to increase or decrease sensitivity. Likewise, the alert system was altered to coincide with the new symptom diary.

Action plans at the end of each self-testing session were developed for participants. Based on scores generated from the UC symptom diary, participants receive self-action or action plans in one of three categories: 1) Green zone, for patients with no to mild symptoms, 2) Yellow zone, for patients with moderate symptoms, or 3) Red zone, for patients with severe symptoms. Each severity zone lists several actions that providers can choose for participants to initiate as part of their self-management plan. These action plans can also be modified by the provider on the web portal as needed. Lastly, an electronic messaging system was added to the HAT system for UC (UC HAT) so that participants can communicate with the medical center. The messaging center allows for both automated and free text messaging.

Attitudinal surveys were done to pre-test the UC HAT system. Pre-testing yielded similar results in the UC population compared to the overall IBD population. All participants felt that using the computer and self-testing system was not complicated, and nine of the ten participants reported no difficulty in using the weight scale or in answering the symptom diary and side effect questions. Seven participants reported that they would feel safer using UC HAT, and eight felt it was important that the IBD center physicians monitored their results. Participants also expressed a sense of improved communication, knowing the provider would be informed of their flares immediately. This improved communication, along with an increased sense of self-awareness, resulted in participants feeling empowered. Some participants reported that the self-testing process could replace clinic visits, although one participant stated that "certain things would be best discussed in person". There was some negative feedback about the UC HAT system as well. One participant felt the system was not tailored to him or her, and another felt that the system inaccurately overestimated the severity of his or her symptoms. Overall, the investigators felt that the UC HAT system was well received in this population and anticipated that its use would result in improved clinical outcomes as compared with routine care in patients with UC.

Subsequently, Cross *et al.* designed a randomized controlled trial to test the hypothesis that the UC HAT system would decrease disease activity, increase quality of life, and improve medical adherence compared with best available care (Cross *et al.* 2011). Forty-seven participants with UC were randomized to receive either home telemanagement with the UC HAT system (25 participants) or best available care (22 participants). Participants in the UC HAT group underwent self-testing weekly. Participants in the best available care group underwent routine and as needed clinic and telephone follow up, received educational fact sheets about IBD and received self-action plans without reinforcement. Disease activity was measured by the Seo Index (Seo *et al*, 1992, as cited in Cross *et al.* 2011) and disease-related quality of life was measured by the Inflammatory Bowel Disease Questionnaire (IBDQ) (Guyatt *et al.*, 1989, as cited in Cross *et al.* 2011).

Sixty-four percent of the participants were women, and 66% were Caucasian. At baseline, 27% of participants in the best available care group used immune suppressants compared to 56% in the UC HAT group (p=0.05). Further, IBDQ scores at baseline were lower in UC HAT participants compared to the best available care group. During the trial, 8 participants withdrew in the UC HAT arm compared to 1 in the best available care arm. There was no difference in disease activity scores or remission rates between the treatment groups at 4, 8 and 12 months. After adjustment for baseline quality of life, disease activity scores decreased 12 points from baseline in the UC HAT arm (p=0.08) compared to 1 point in the best available care arm (p=0.84). IBDQ scores increased in the UC HAT arm and remained stable in the best available care arm, though these differences were not significant at any time point post baseline. However, after adjustment for baseline disease knowledge, UC HAT participants were noted to have a 16-point improvement in quality of life scores from baseline compared to the best available care group (p=0.04). Adherence was low in both groups at baseline; adherence improved in both groups over 12 months. No significant differences in adherence were noted between groups. These results suggest that telemedicine may decrease disease activity and increase quality of life in patients with UC despite the finding that self-reported adherence did not improve in the UC HAT group. The high attrition rate in the UC HAT arm was concerning; it is possible that a different telemedicine system, such as a web-based design, would improve retention rates in future trials.

A randomized controlled trial in Denmark and Ireland was conducted to assess UC patients' use of web-based home telemanagement (Elkjaer *et al.*, 2010). Patients with mild-to-moderate UC were randomly assigned to either a web-group with disease-specific education and self-treatment or a control group that received standard care for 12 months. Outcomes of interest included feasibility of the telemanagement approach and its influence on participants' medication adherence, UC knowledge, quality of life, safety, and health care costs. Exclusion criteria included use of infliximab and immune suppressant therapy, narcotic dependence, previous IBD surgery or likelihood of surgery during the study period, 2 or more flares per year requiring high-dose steroid therapy, pregnancy, and breastfeeding.

This study used the "Constant Care" website (http://www.constant-care.dk). Each participant was given a unique username and password. Prior to using the website, all participants in the web-group, and their relatives, were given educational training with a 1.5-hour slide presentation on IBD etiology, pathology, anatomy, medical and surgical treatments, disease course, adherence, nutrition, mortality risk, colorectal cancer chemoprevention, pregnancy, and breastfeeding. Participants and family members also underwent a 1.5-hour training session in using the Constant Care website. Guidelines for indications on when to call the provider included having greater than six stools per day, daily rectal bleeding, rectal bleeding occurring between relapses, fever >37.5 degrees Celsius, heart rate >90 beats per minute, severe abdominal pain, symptoms persisting more than eleven days despite escalation of therapy, unexplained weight loss, and/or for any doubts or questions regarding the study.

Disease-specific quality of life was measured on the website with the SIBDQ, and the Simple Clinical Colitis Activity Index (SCCAI) was used to assess disease activity (Walmsey *et al.*, 1998, as cited in Elkjaer *et al.*, 2010). Symptoms were categorized in a similar manner as in the UC HAT study; quiescent-to-mild symptoms appeared as a green traffic light, moderate symptoms appeared as a yellow light, and highly active symptoms appeared as a red light. During symptom flare, participants were instructed to log onto the system daily to complete the SCCAI until their symptoms entered the green zone. Entry frequency was then reduced to once weekly until 4 weeks after the initial relapse. The SIBDQ was to be completed at the beginning and end of each relapse. Once in remission, participants were to log into the system once monthly until the next relapse occurred. If symptoms were entered such as rectal bleeding, 3 or more bowel movements daily, or nighttime bowel movements, the system recommended initiation of 4 gm daily or more of 5-aminosalicylic acid (5-ASA) treatment for a total of 28 days. Participants were given the option to extend this treatment period by an additional 28 days if remission into the green zone was not achieved.

Participants could also choose additional topical 5-ASA treatment and prednisolone, based on previous maximal extent of disease and participants' prior treatment experience.

All participants were to have study visits at baseline, six months, and 12 months. During each of these visits participants were asked to complete a series of questionnaires, including the SCCAI, SIBDQ, Crohn's Colitis Knowledge Score (CCKNOW) (Eadan JA *et al.*, 1999, as cited in Elkjaer *et al.*, 2010), SF-36 (Ware *et al.*, 2002, as cited in Elkjaer *et al.*, 2010), Hospital Anxiety and Depression Scale (Zigmond & Snaith, 1983, as cited in Elkjaer *et al.*, 2010), and Compliance Questionnaire. The Compliance Questionnaire was developed at Herlev Hospital in Denmark, and it included 5 questions on the following topics: ease of access to prescription, ability of relapse recognition, following the medical doctor's advice, ability to self-initiate acute treatment, and adherence to 5-ASA treatment.

In total, 333 participants, aged 18-to-69 years, from both Danish and Irish sites were randomized. Of these, 135 participants completed the 12-month follow-up visit. The control group was predominantly female (70% in control group vs. 51% in web-based group) and older (median age of 48 years in the control group compared with 41 years in the web group). Otherwise, there were no significant differences between the two randomized groups in terms of age at diagnosis, disease duration, disease extent, 5-ASA medication history, smoking status, marital status, education, or occupation.

In the Danish arm of the study, there were no differences in 5-ASA adherence, as measured by medication refills from the e-prescription pharmacy database, between the web and control participants (68% vs. 69% respectively refilled at least 80% of their medication, p=NS). The web group demonstrated significantly higher adherence to four weeks of acute treatment compared to controls (73% vs. 42%, $p = 0.003$). There were significantly greater improvements in web group participants in IBD knowledge, disease-specific quality of life ($p = 0.04$), general health ($p = 0.009$), vitality ($p = 0.03$), and emotional ($p < 0.0001$) and social functioning ($p = 0.002$) as compared with the control group. Half of all participants experienced at least one flare of symptoms during the study period, with no difference in flare rates between the web and control groups. However, relapses were significantly shorter in the web group compared to the control group (18 days vs. 77 days, $p < 0.0001$). There was otherwise no difference between the groups in disease activity scores as measured by the SCCAI, or in the rate of hospitalizations.

There were a few differences seen in the Irish arm of the study. Medication adherence to four weeks of treatment was significantly greater in the web group compared to controls (73% vs. 29%, $p = 0.03$). There were no differences between study groups in terms of IBD knowledge or disease-specific quality of life. The web group demonstrated improved mental health ($p = 0.01$), physical functioning ($p = 0.03$), and social functioning ($p = 0.02$) compared to controls. The web group experienced a higher frequency of relapses; however, these were shorter than the relapses experienced by controls (30 days vs. 70 days, $p < 0.03$).

A cost analysis revealed that UC-related acute visits were higher in the control group compared to the web group (107 vs. 21 visits, $p < 0.0001$). There were also fewer routine visits in the web group. Conversely, there were a significantly higher number of emails (86) and phone calls (21) from web participants than from controls (7 emails and 17 phone calls).

Fecal calprotectin was measured in both the Dutch and Irish arms of the study to serve as an objective measure of inflammation. Overall, a lower proportion of web group participants had an elevated fecal calprotectin level compared to controls.

Overall, 88% of participants in the web group preferred telemedicine to conventional care. Participants felt empowered by the ability to initiate treatment using the web-guided solution and safe with the option of a web-based follow-up with their provider. The authors proposed that a web-based treatment strategy such as this could reduce patients' dependency on doctors as well as mitigate health care costs. However, like the study by Cross *et al.*, this study also had a high attrition rate over one year of follow up.

In summary, telemedicine is well accepted by patients with IBD, including patients with UC. Longitudinal use of these systems seems feasible; however the high attrition rates reported in both randomized, controlled trials raises concerns about long term adherence to telemonitoring systems. In addition to showing high rates of patient acceptance and feasibility, available studies have demonstrated improvements in clinical outcomes. The quasiexperimental study by Cross *et al.* reported decreased disease activity, improved quality of life, and increased knowledge after use of IBD HAT for 6 months. Similarly, both randomized controlled trials of telemedicine for UC showed improvements in disease activity as measured by disease activity indices or fecal calprotectin levels and improvements in quality of life. However, flare rates were increased in the European study. Despite the higher rate of flares in the telemedicine arm, the length of flares was less in the telemedicine group. Despite improvements in disease activity, adherence was not consistently better in the telemedicine arms in either study, except in the acute treatment phase of the study by Elkjaer *et al.* Quality of life improved in the telemedicine arms of both studies and utilization of health care resources was less in the telemedicine group in the European study (although email and phone calls increased in the telemedicine group). Therefore, the evidence thus far in IBD and UC, demonstrates a positive effect of telemedicine on clinical outcomes. Further studies are needed to confirm these results and to study the CD population. Further, larger studies are needed to explore subgroups that might particularly benefit from telemedicine, specifically patients with decreased access to care, a history of nonadherence, poor social support, more severe disease (moderate to severe IBD), patients with active disease vs. disease in remission, and patients initiating new drug therapy. Lastly, the financial impact of telemedicine on IBD care, positive or negative, needs to be explored.

3. Irritable bowel syndrome

Irritable bowel syndrome (IBS) is chronic, functional gastrointestinal condition characterized by chronic intermittent abdominal pain associated with an alteration in bowel movements. The change in bowel movements can be in frequency (diarrhea or constipation) or a change in stool formation (liquid stools, hard stools, unusual stool shapes). Patients often have associated bloating and worsening of symptoms during stress. IBS differs from IBD in that there is no inflammatory component, and endoscopy and biopsy results are normal Nonetheless, the chronic symptoms of IBS can be quite distressing to patients, decrease quality of life, and result in a high rate of work absenteeism.

A German group set out to investigate whether an open-access Internet-based questionnaire on gastrointestinal symptoms and quality of life could be used to collect data from patients with IBS (Enck *et al.*, 2006). To accomplish this, investigators created an abbreviated symptom questionnaire modified from the IBS Rome II modular questionnaire, a validated questionnaire for IBS (Drossman *et al*, 2000, as cited in Enck *et al.*, 2006). This was done to reduce estimated completion time from 30 minutes to 5 minutes. They also used a validated 22-item general quality of life questionnaire that took 10 minutes to complete. Both questionnaires were available online over a 43-month period. A total of 5,256 individuals completed the questionnaires, with an average of 100 respondents per month. Data from 850 individuals were excluded due to incomplete responses. Two thirds of respondents were women. The mean age of participants was 38 years. The investigators determined that among all respondents, 61% met criteria for the diagnosis of IBS. Verification of the diagnosis of presumed participants with IBS was not performed. A commentary on this study was published two years later by Muth and Switzer in the *European Journal of Gastroenterology* that identified concerns with its validity (Muth & Switzer, 2008). They argued that while Enck's group used a validated questionnaire to assess quality of life, the questionnaire had been validated for pen-and-paper use only. Muck and Switzer also commented on the abbreviated survey tool used to assess gastrointestinal symptoms. While the survey had content validity since it was based on the standard Rome criteria for the diagnosis of IBS, the impact of having reduced items on this questionnaire was not assessed. In addition, it was unclear in what language the tools were administered. Nevertheless, Enck *et al.* did demonstrate that completion of an IBS and quality of life instrument electronically was feasible in an IBS population.

While the previous study solely aimed to examine the role of the Internet in data collection, a randomized control trial was performed in Sweden to investigate whether cognitive behavior therapy delivered via the Internet could be effective in managing patients with IBS (Ljotsson *et al.*, 2010). Eighty-five self-referred participants were recruited to participate in the trial between May 2008 and July 2008. Self-referrals were generated from several online Swedish discussion forums for patients with IBS, a major newspaper article, and a Stockholm clinic that specialized in IBS care. Only patients with a diagnosis of IBS confirmed by Rome criteria were included in the study. Exclusion criteria included: a) initiation of symptoms after age 50, b) blood in the stool without history of hemorrhoids, c) diarrhea-predominant IBS without colonoscopic evaluation, d) rapid weight loss not explained by diet, e) nocturnal symptoms causing sleeplessness, and f) less than 2 years of IBS symptoms. Participants were also excluded if they had any previous history of IBD, celiac disease, or lactose intolerance. The GI Symptom diary (Blanchard, 2001, as cited in Ljotsson *et al.*, 2010) was used to measure symptom severity and the Irritable Bowel Syndrome Quality of Life Instrument (Patrick *et al*, 1998, as cited in Ljotsson *et al.*, 2010) for disease-specific quality of life, respectively. These questionnaires were used for pre- and post-intervention testing.

A total of 83 participants completed pre-testing then were randomized to either the treatment or control group. The 42 participants assigned to the treatment group received a 10-week cognitive behavioral therapy (CBT) protocol, which consisted of a five-step self-help manual presented on printer-friendly web pages. The five steps in the CBT manual guided participants through a series of mindfulness exercises in which they were encouraged to be immediately aware of their gastrointestinal symptoms, thoughts, feelings, behaviors, and impulses. The fifth step covered a series of exposure exercises, in which participants were to experience situations that would likely provoke symptoms such as eating trigger foods or attending a meeting with tight clothes that would provoke pain. They were encouraged to use mindfulness exercises during these exposure exercises. Participants in the treatment group had access to an online discussion forum to discuss the treatment with other participants and to communicate with a graduate psychology student trained in CBT over the course of the treatment period.

The 43 participants randomized to the control group were placed on a waiting list for CBT. The authors gave control participants access to a separate online discussion forum and allowed participants to contact a psychology student. However, the student did not provide

CBT-based advice for treatment of IBS symptoms. After completing post-testing, participants in the control group were then invited to cross over into the treatment arm to receive CBT.

In the treatment group, 74% of participants reached the fifth step in the CBT manual. Four participants never completed the first step. Participants in the treatment group reported significant improvement in abdominal pain, bloating, flatulence, and IBS-specific quality of life. Effects on diarrhea, constipation, nausea, or belching were small or insignificant. Small but significant improvements in depressive symptoms and gastrointestinal symptoms were observed in the control group from baseline.

There were several limitations to the study. First, since participants were self-referred, it is possible that participants were not representative of the IBS community (better educated, higher motivation, etc.). Second, the precise role of telemedicine on the improved outcomes in this study is not known as the control group did not receive CBT in any form. A comparison arm of patient treated with conventional CBT would have been useful. Nevertheless, this study provided evidence that the Internet is a viable method of delivery of CBT for a select IBS population. Further studies on this delivery method, as well as on the content of treatment delivered, are warranted.

In summary, there are limited studies available on the use of telemedicine for patients with IBS. The data available demonstrates that patients with IBS can complete web-based questionnaires and that therapy using a web-based system is feasible and effective in a select IBS patient population. Whether other forms of IBS therapy (medical therapy or other forms of psychotherapy) can be delivered electronically to improve outcomes is not known at this time. Further, it is not clear that telemedicine for IBS improves outcomes compared to standard of care or best available care. Lastly, the ability of telemedicine to decrease health care costs in IBS has not been assessed.

4. Chronic hepatitis C infection

Chronic hepatitis C virus (HCV) infection is another chronic disease process in the field of gastroenterology in which telemedicine has been studied. As the incidence and prevalence of HCV infection rises in the United States, access to care becomes a barrier in providing adequate treatment. According to the Centers for Disease Control, HCV infection is the most common chronic blood-borne infection in the United States; approximately 3.2 million persons are chronically infected. Anti-viral treatment reduces the risk of disease progression to cirrhosis and liver cancer, both potentially fatal outcomes of this infection. Liver transplantation remains a limited and costly option, and is only applicable in the final stages of disease. Telemedicine consulting with videoconferencing has been described as a method to connect practitioners in the rural setting and in correctional facilities with gastroenterologists and hepatologists at tertiary care facilities in order to improve access to care and anti-viral therapy.

The first description of this type of telemedicine application emerged in 1994. The University of Alberta was identified as the center for a nation-wide, free-physician consultation service in which practitioners in rural areas across Canada were given immediate access to a gastroenterologist by phone, fax, or email (Rafuse, 1994). The project was designed to offer consultation on the treatment and management of hepatitis. Although expectations were high about the positive impact of this project on hepatitis patient outcomes in Canada, no qualitative or quantitative data were published revealing the effect of this particular intervention.

Nine years later, an abstract presented at the 2003 Digestive Diseases Week conference entitled *"Application of Telemedicine in the Management of Chronic Hepatitis C in Texas Prisons"* summarized the experience of applying telemedicine in the treatment of HCV in the correctional setting (Lau, Fehmi, & Sifuentes, 2003). Upon screening, correctional facility physicians discussed patient laboratory results and medical conditions with hepatologists via telemedicine prior to initiation of anti-viral treatment. Regular telemedicine clinics were scheduled during the treatment period to review laboratory results and medication side effects. 470 patients completed six months of therapy, with 52% of patients being Caucasian, 18% African American, and 30% Hispanic. Among those with genotype 1 virus, 33% demonstrated treatment response as compared with 71% with non-genotype 1 HCV. The presenters concluded that telemedicine was an effective means of managing the treatment of chronic HCV in the correctional health system given that these response rates were comparable with those in the general community.

That same year the University of California, Davis (UCD) published a cohort study describing patient and provider acceptance of their telemedicine program created to aid in the management of patients with HCV (Rossaro *et al*, 2003). The UCD telemedicine program encompassed a large referral network of over 60 sites throughout the state of California. Telecommunication methods used through this program included T1, frame relay and the Integrated Services Digital Network. Relevant clinical information such as laboratory testing, imaging, and liver biopsy reports were required to be sent for review by the specialist prior to each hepatology consultation. Primary care providers were invited to participate during the consultation, often performing the physical exam as instructed by the specialist, which added a distance learning component to the consultation. In some situations, a "patient exam" camera was used to magnify details, such as skin changes consistent with liver disease like spider angiomata or palmar erythema.

After each telemedicine consultation, patients and providers completed a satisfaction survey. Both parties indicated if they would choose to continue using the telemedicine service or return to standard care. The authors did not disclose how many surveys were sent, but 22 patient surveys and 20 provider surveys were returned from 5 clinics. Satisfaction was scored on a 5-point scale that ranged from 1 representing "Poor" to 5 representing "Excellent." Overall satisfaction scores were high among patients and providers, with mean scores ranging from 4.7 to 4.95 for items such as overall satisfaction with the system, ability to understand consultant recommendations, and quality of the audio and video signal from the telemedicine equipment. All patients indicated they would prefer to continue using telemedicine in the future, and all providers also reported they would recommend use of telemedicine services in the future. This is another example where telemedicine offered the opportunity to improve access to specialized care for the treatment of HCV to patients in rural areas and correctional facilities, while providing educational opportunities for primary care providers.

In 2007, the UCD group published a follow-up quasi-experimental study, comparing the impact of multi-point videoconferencing versus standard lecturing to primary care providers (Rossaro *et al* 2007). Participants included primary care physicians, nurse practitioners, physician assistants, and registered nurses. Prior to the educational intervention, participants completed a single page questionnaire, documenting certain demographic information such as their total number of HCV patients seen, year of graduation from professional training, and attendance at Continuing Medical Education

(CME) conferences within the previous 6 months. The outcome of interest in this study was improved knowledge of the history, diagnosis, and treatment of hepatitis C, measured by a quiz administered before and after the educational intervention. This quiz was based on a review of current literature and guidelines for the treatment of hepatitis C. The investigators hypothesized that telemedicine conferencing would yield knowledge outcome measures comparable with traditional teaching methods.

A board certified gastroenterologist delivered the educational intervention with identical outlines and slide materials for both the standard teaching and the videoconferencing groups. To ensure consistency of teaching, the same individual delivered the intervention for both study groups. One hundred and seventy-five providers from 14 different sites met criteria to be included in the study. There were no statistically significant differences between study groups in terms of background, training, experience, or recent CME attendance. Most providers were in practice over 10 years since graduation from professional training, and more than half had seen 10 or fewer patients with hepatitis C.

In both study groups, pre-testing knowledge scores did not differ significantly between the three disciplines of training, but there was a significantly higher level of pre-test knowledge in the standard teaching group as compared with the videoconferencing group ($p < 0.05$). While an improvement in HCV knowledge was seen in all learners in both groups, a statistically greater improvement in knowledge scores was measured in post-testing among physicians and registered nurses in the videoconferencing group as compared with the standard teaching group ($p < 0.001$). These results suggest that videoconferencing is at least as equivalent if not better than standard CME teaching.

The following year, Rossaro's group reported results from a qualitative retrospective analysis, describing characteristics from the population of patients who received care at the Peach Tree Clinic, located in rural northern California (Rossaro *et al.*, 2008). Over the span of seven years from 2000-2007, one hundred and three patients with HCV were treated via telemedicine. Among those treated, 37% had cirrhosis and 2 were listed for liver transplant, although neither survived long enough to undergo transplantation. Sixty-four percent of patients at this clinic were treatment-naïve; treatment was recommended for 23% of these patients. Rossaro's group concluded that this descriptive analysis confirmed that there are a high proportion of patients with advanced liver disease due to HCV in rural California, many of whom may be candidates for treatment. They also suggested that consultation with specialists via telemedicine may help providers identify candidates for liver transplantation.

Around the same time period, a study from the University of New Mexico, School of Medicine in Albuquerque, was published describing the Project Extension for Community Healthcare Outcomes (ECHO) (Arora *et al.*, 2007). This telemedicine and distance-learning project aimed to link health care providers in rural clinics, the Indian Health Service, and prisons with specialists at the University of New Mexico. At the time, 32 of 33 counties in New Mexico were listed as medically underserved, and 14 counties were designated as areas with health professional shortage. Only 20% of New Mexico physicians practiced in rural or frontier areas.

Project ECHO used teleconferencing, videoconferencing, Internet-based assessment tools, online presentations, telephone, fax, and email communications to connect primary care providers with specialists, creating centers of excellence for HCV care in areas that previously had very limited options for such care. Inclusion criteria for participants in this project were Internet access, use of telephone service (including fax and speaker phone functions), and the ability to view word processing documents and presentations. Partner organizations were recruited to participate in the Project ECHO network at state-wide health care conferences and through presentations and partner contacts. Once a provider joined the network, a member of the Project ECHO team conducted an on-site, one day training session to familiarize partners with the project. Network clinicians included primary care physicians, nurse practitioners, physician assistants, and pharmacists. These clinicians were invited to spend two days at the University of New Mexico Hepatitis Clinic and to complete an orientation and training on the Project ECHO system. They were subsequently able to present their HCV cases and related questions in a weekly 2-hour telemedicine clinic in collaboration with specialists in gastroenterology, infectious disease, psychiatry, substance abuse, and pharmacology. Clinicians who participated in Project ECHO also had the opportunity to become eligible for certification in HCV treatment after managing 20 patients with HCV through one-full year of antiviral therapy.

Between 2003 and 2006, 173 clinics were initiated with 1,843 cases presented and 2,997 hours of continuing education credits issued to staff. In addition, 226 patients were treated with anti-viral therapy. The investigators proposed that the Project ECHO model could be applied to the management of many different chronic conditions and that it showed great promise to improve care to people living in medically underserved areas.

More recent data on telemedicine in HCV management was presented as an abstract at the American Association for the Study of Liver Diseases conference in 2009 entitled "*Use of telemedicine and the 'warm line' for the treatment of HCV infection in the correctional setting to reduce barriers to specialty care*" (Nachin *et al.*, 2009). In this abstract, investigators set out to identify, triage, and treat patients with HCV and estimate the prevalence of cirrhosis and end stage liver disease among inmates at the California Department of Corrections and Rehabilitation facility. To this end, the University of California, San Francisco Correctional Medicine Consultative Network held a HCV training conference in October of 2008. Primary care physicians referred patients for consultation with hepatologists via telemedicine, and a "warm line" was established to further assist primary clinicians managing HCV. This warm line was available weekdays during business hours, and responses were made within 24 hours of the request. Overall, 441 new patient consultations were performed via telemedicine between May 2008 and May 2009. The presenters concluded that use of telemedicine and the warm line offered efficient access to specialty care in this population.

In June 2011 The Project ECHO group published additional data in the New England Journal of Medicine which confirmed the utility of their model as a means to increase access to HCV treatment (Arora *et al*, 2011). In this prospective cohort study, outcomes were compared between patients who received HCV treatment at either the University of New Mexico (UNM) HCV specialty clinic (146 patients) or at one of 21 ECHO telemedicine sites located in primary care clinics in rural areas or prisons in New Mexico. There were a few baseline differences between the UNM clinic group and the ECHO telemedicine site groups. Specifically, patients treated at the ECHO sites were more likely to be male (96% of patients treated in the prison system were men). ECHO patients were also more likely to be Hispanic, and had higher mean values for weight and BMI. Despite this, there was no significant difference in sustained viral response between the two patient groups. This confirmed that HCV treatment can be delivered effectively via telemedicine in non-specialty care facilities that would otherwise have no means for delivering such care.

In summary, telemedicine has been shown to be a useful medium for communication between specialists, primary providers, and patients with HCV infection in rural areas and correctional facilities. The use and study of telemedicine in the HCV population is focused on providing guidance and training of primary care providers by hepatologists, in order to encourage them to provide anti-viral therapies to patients in those settings where hepatologists are unavailable. Whether telemedicine improves outcomes compared to standard of care in patients with HCV undergoing treatment and whether telemedicine reduces health care costs is speculative at this time.

5. Conclusion

Chronic gastrointestinal diseases are associated with significant morbidity and cost in the United States and throughout the world. Because of chronic nature of these diseases, the need for ongoing monitoring of flares of disease and the need for medications to control symptoms and prevent relapses, outcomes can be suboptimal. Telemedicine systems offer a modern, alternative monitoring/treatment method that can improve clinical outcomes, reduce time to initiation of treatment, increase patient access to treatment, improve patient and provider education, and reduce health care costs. The common thread present in all the studies summarized in this review is that when considering the management of chronic gastrointestinal disease, telemedicine is feasible and well accepted among various patient populations, improves access to care, and increases patients' sense of empowerment. Technology will continue to advance in quality and ease of use of telemedicine systems and will likely incorporate the use of hand-held devices. This progress should result in the increased use of telemedicine as a treatment alternative or as an adjunctive component to disease management in chronic digestive diseases.

Author and Year	Disease State	Telemanagement Communication	Outcomes
Castro, 2006	Inflammatory bowel disease	Physician-to-patient	Feasible method, improved patient empowerment
Cross, 2006	Inflammatory bowel disease	Physician-to-patient	Feasible method, excellent patient acceptance of technology
Cross, 2007	Inflammatory bowel disease	Physician-to-patient	Feasible method, excellent patient acceptance, improved disease activity, quality of life and patient knowledge
Cross, 2009	Ulcerative colitis	Physician-to-patient	Feasible method, excellent patient acceptance of technology
Cross, 2011	Ulcerative colitis	Physician-to-patient	High attrition rate in telemanagement arm, improved patient quality of life compared to best available care control group
Elkjaer, 2010	Ulcerative colitis	Physician-to-patient	Feasible method, excellent patient acceptance of technology
Elkjaer, 2010	Ulcerative colitis	Physician-to-patient	Improved medication adherence, quality of life, and patient knowledge; shorter flares; less clinic visits; more electronic communication in web group

Author and Year	Disease State	Telemanagement Communication	Outcomes
Enck, 2006	Irritable bowel syndrome	Physician-to-patient	Internet-based questionnaire administration is feasible
Krier, 2010	Inflammatory bowel disease	Physician-to-patient	Patient satisfaction comparable to face-to-face interaction, similar interaction times between physician and patient
Ljótsson, 2010	Irritable bowel syndrome	Physician-to-patient	Significant improvement in symptoms and quality of life in treatment group compared to control group
Rossaro, 2003	Hepatitis C	Physician-to-physician and patient	High acceptance of method among patients and local providers
Rossaro, 2007	Hepatitis C	Physician-to-physician	Improvement in hepatitis C knowledge among local providers
Arora, 2011	Hepatitis C	Physician-to-physician	Equal sustained virologic response rate in telemedicine group compared to tertiary referral center

Table 1. Summary table of key gastrointestinal telemanagement studies and outcomes

6. Acknowledgement

T32 DK067872 Research Training in Gastroenterology.

7. References

Arora S, Thornton K, Murata G, Deming P, Kalishman S, Dion D, Parish B, Burke T, Pak W, Dunkelberg J, Kistin M, Brown J, Jenkusky S, Komaromy M, & Quals C (2011). Outcomes of Treatment for Hepatitis C Virus Infection by Primary Care Providers. New England Journal of Medicine. June 2011; [doi:10.1056/NEJMoa1009370]Castro HK, Cross RK, & Finkelstein J (2006). Using a Home Automated Telemanagement (HAT) system: experiences and perceptions of patients with inflammatory bowel disease. Proceedings of *American Medical Informatics Association Annual Symposium.* 2006:872.

Crohn's and Colitis Foundation of America. http://www.ccfa.org. 2010

Cross RK, Arora M, & Finkelstein J (2006). Acceptance of telemanagement is high in patients with inflammatory bowel disease. *Journal of Clinical Gastroenterology.* March 2006; 40(3):200-8.

Cross RK, Finkelstein J (2007). Feasibility and acceptance of a home telemanagement system in patients with inflammatory bowel disease: a 6-month pilot study. *Digestive Diseases and Sciences.* February 2007; 52(2):357-64.

Cross RK, Cheevers N, & Finkelstein J. (2009) Home telemanagement for patients with ulcerative colitis (UC HAT). *Digestive Diseases and Sciences.* November 2009; 54(11):2463-72.

Cross RK, Cheevers, N, Rustgi, A, Langenberg, P, & Finkelstein J (2011). A Randomized, Controlled Trial of Home Telemanagement in Patients with Ulcerative Colitis (UC

HAT). *Proceedings of American Gastroenterological Association Digestive Diseases Week*, Chicago. May 2011.

Elkjaer, M, Burisch, J, Avnstrom, S, Lynge, E, & Munkholm, P. Development of a Web-based concept for patients with ulcerative colitis and 5-aminosalicylic acid treatment. *European Journal of Gastroenterology and Hepatology*. 2010; 22(6):695-704

Elkjaer M, Shuhaibar M, Burisch J, Bailey Y, Scherfig H, Laugesen B, Avnstrøm S, Langholz E, O'Morain C, Lynge E, & Munkholm P (2010). E-health empowers patients with ulcerative colitis: a randomised controlled trial of the web-guided 'Constant-care' approach. *Gut*. December 2010; 59(12):1652-61

Enck P, Kowalski A, Martens U, & Klosterhalfen S. Internet-based assessment of bowel symptoms and quality of life (2001). *European Journal of Gastroenterology and Hepatology*. December 2006; 18(12):1263-9.

Kane, S, Huo, D, Aikens, J, & Hanauer, S. Medication nonadherence and the outcomes of patients with quiescent ulcerative colitis. *American Journal of Medicine*. 2003; 114(1):39-43

Krier M, Kaltenbach T, McQuaid K, & Soetikno R. (2010) Broadening the Access to Specialized IBD Care Using a Consumer Grade Affordable Telemedicine System. *Proceedings of American Gastroenterological Association Digestive Diseases Week*. New Orleans, May 2010.

Lau T, Fehmi S, & Sifuentes D (2003). Application of telemedicine in the management of chronic hepatitis C in Texas prisons. *Proceedings of American Gastroenterological Association Digestive Diseases Week*, Orlando, April 2003.

Ljótsson B, Falk L, Vesterlund AW, Hedman E, Lindfors P, Rück C, Hursti T, Andréewitch S, Jansson L, Lindefors N, &Andersson G (2010). Internet-delivered exposure and mindfulness based therapy for irritable bowel syndrome--a randomized controlled trial. *Behavioral Research and Therapy*. June 2010; 48(6):531-9.

Muth ER & Switzer FS. Internet-based assessment of bowel symptoms and quality of life. *European Journal of Gastroenterology and Hepatology*. June 2008; 20(6):503-5.

Nachin P, Kerbleski M, Gaglioti A, Mahoney M, Protell R, Kohler L, & Imperial J. (2009) Use of telemedicine and the 'warm line' for the treatment of hepatitis C infection in the correctional setting to reduce barriers to specialty care. *Proceedings of American Association for the Study of Liver Diseases*, San Francisco, November 2009.

Rafuse J. (1994). University of Alberta program links northern hepatitis patients with southern consultants. *Canadian Medical Association Journal*. September 1994; 151(5):654-5.

Rossaro L, Tran T, Cole S, & Nesbitt T. (2003). Telemedicine: Improving Access to Care of Hepatitis C - Guest Editorial. *Practical Gastroenterology*. April 2003; (27):17-22.

Rossaro L, Tran T, & Ransibrahmanakhul K. (2007). Hepatitis C Videoconferencing : The Impact on Continuing Medical Education for Rural Healthcare Providers. *Telemedicine and e-Health*. 2007, 13 (3): 269-277.

Rossaro L, Aoki C, & Yuk J. (2008) The evaluation of patients with hepatitis C living in rural California via telemedicine. *Telemedicine and e-Health*. December 2008;14(10):1127-9.

Sewitch MJ, Abrahamowicz, M, Barkun, A, Bitton, A, Wild, GE, Cohen, A, & Dobkin, PL. Patient nonadherence to medication in inflammatory bowel disease. *American Journal of Gastroenterology*. 2003; 98(7):1535-44.

17

Teledermatology: Outcomes and Economic Considerations

Akhilesh S. Pathipati and April W. Armstrong
Department of Dermatology, University of California, Davis
United States of America

1. Introduction

Teledermatology is defined as the provision of dermatologic care through the use of communications technology (Goldyne & Armstrong, 2010). It offers many benefits that include increased access to dermatologic services and potential reduction in costs associated with care. Teledermatology is traditionally categorized into two different models based on the technology that is employed: store-and-forward (S&F) teledermatology, and live, interactive (LI) teledermatology (Goldyne & Armstrong, 2010). While hybrid models (a combination of S&F and LI technology) are practiced at selected institutions, this chapter focuses primarily on S&F and LI models. We will present operational flows of these two technology-enabled modalities, common outcomes measures used for evaluation of teledermatology quality metrics, and economic analyses.

At the end of the chapter (in section 5), we will consider a novel, technology-independent framework for categorizing teledermatology models as well. This system relies on classification of teledermatology based on healthcare delivery models, and serves as an alternative way to organize and evaluate the provision of teledermatologic care.

2. Store-and-forward teledermatology

Store-and-forward teledermatology is an asynchronous means for providing dermatologic care, as it relies on the *asynchronous* transmission of static digital images, patient histories, and specialist recommendations rather than real-time interaction between the specialist and the patient (Goldyne & Armstrong, 2010).

In the S&F model, a medical staff personnel at the referral site typically takes images of the relevant skin condition and obtains medical history. This information is then sent to a dermatologist via a secure internet connection. The dermatologist evaluates the patient's condition asynchronously and transmits the recommendations back to the primary care provider at the referral site (Pak et al., 2009).

2.1 Outcomes measures of store-and-forward teledermatology

Teledermatology studies have assessed numerous outcomes measures, including learning effects, length of consultation, and technical aspects (Eminovic et al., 2007). We will focus this discussion on four extensively used outcomes measures: diagnostic accuracy, diagnostic reliability, clinical outcomes, and satisfaction.

2.1.1 Diagnostic accuracy of store-and-forward teledermatology

Diagnostic accuracy refers to whether or not a diagnosis is correct, based on comparison to a gold standard reference test. While histopathological review or other laboratory tests are often used as the gold standard for diagnosis, results of these types of gold standards are not always available in clinical practice in dermatology. Furthermore, it is difficult to generate cumulative data regarding accuracy, because different studies use different methodologies and standards.

Several studies have found diagnostic accuracy of S&F teledermatology to be comparable to in-person consultations (Barnard & Goldyne 2000; High et al., 2000; Krupinski et al., 1999; Oakley et al., 1997; Whited et al., 1999). Other studies have found that in-person consultation provides a significantly greater diagnostic accuracy than S&F teledermatology (Warshaw et al. 2009a; Warshaw et al. 2009b). One study found that S&F teledermatology had a significantly greater diagnostic accuracy than in-person consultation (Lozzi et al., 2007).

Different findings on diagnostic accuracy may be attributable to several factors. First, the "gold standard" used among the studies differ from in-person evaluations to pathologic evaluation. Second, patient populations and types of skin lesions differ among the various practices that were examined. Future studies can focus on tools or interventions to increase diagnostic accuracy of S&F teledermatology, such as routine incorporation of dermoscopy (Warshaw et al., 2010a).

2.1.2 Diagnostic reliability of store-and-forward teledermatology

Diagnostic reliability is a measure of concurrence in diagnosis. It may refer to intraobserver reliability (whether one examiner makes the same diagnosis in two different examinations), or interobserver reliability (whether two different examiners make the same diagnosis). These measures of reliability may evaluate either complete agreement, which refers to comparison of the most likely diagnosis, or partial agreement, which accounts for differential diagnoses.

Studies of intraobserver reliability between S&F teledermatology and in-person consultation found that agreement ranges between 31-88% for complete diagnostic agreement, and between 50-95% for partial diagnostic agreement (Table 1).

Reference	Complete Diagnostic Agreement	Partial Diagnostic Agreement
(Romero et al., 2010)	.85	.92
(Tan et al., 2010)	.74	.88
(Heffner et al., 2009)	.82	-
(Ebner et al., 2008)	.74	.90
(Pak et al., 2003)	.70	.91
(Lim et al., 2001)	.88	.95
(Taylor et al., 2001)	.31-.64	.50-.70
(Krupinski et al., 1999)	-	.76-.90

Table 1. Intraobserver Reliability for S&F Teledermatology and Conventional Care

Studies have found that interobserver reliability ranges between 41-92% for complete diagnostic agreement and between 51-100% for partial diagnostic agreement (Table 2). A review of studies between 1997 and 2005 revealed that the aggregate complete diagnostic agreement was 60%, and partial diagnostic agreement was 80% (Romero et al., 2008).

Reference	Complete Diagnostic Agreement	Partial Diagnostic Agreement
(Tan et al., 2010)	.75-.82	.83-.89
(Heffner et al., 2009)	.69	-
(Silva et al., 2009)	.87-.92	.96-1.0
(Edison et al., 2008)	.73	-
(Ebner et al., 2008)	.71-.76	.90-.97
(Bowns et al., 2006)	.55	-
(Oakley et al., 2006)	.53	.64
(Tucker & Lewis, 2005)	.56	.68
(Baba et al., 2005)	.75	-
(Mahendran et al., 2005)	.44-.48	.64-.65
(Du Moulin et al., 2003)	.54	.63
(Eminovic et al., 2003)	.41	.51
(Lim et al., 2001)	.73-.85	.83-.89
(Taylor et al., 2001)	.44-.51	.57-.61
(High et al., 2000)	.64-.77	.81-.89
(Whited et al., 1999)	.41-.55	.79-.95
(Lyon & Harrison, 1997)	.89	-
(Zelickson & Homan, 1997)	.88	-
(Kvedar et al., 1997)	.61-.64	.67-.70

Table 2. Interobserver Reliability for S&F Teledermatology and Conventional Care

Based on this data on diagnostic reliability, it appears that S&F teledermatology is a functional and reasonably reliable tool for diagnosis of skin disorders.

2.1.3 Clinical outcomes for store-and-forward teledermatology

To date, two studies have evaluated clinical outcomes of S&F teledermatology compared to conventional care, and both studies found similar outcomes for each of the two treatment modalities (Krupinski et al., 2004; Pak et al., 2007). Specifically, Pak et al. conducted a randomized controlled trial with patients randomly assigned to either conventional face-to-face care or teledermatology. Another dermatologist, blinded to the randomization, evaluated the clinical outcomes between baseline data and after four months (Table 3). The results suggest that teledermatology and conventional care result in similar outcomes (Pak et al., 2007).

		Clinical Course Rating		
		Improved	No change	Worse
Assigned Group	Teledermatology	64%	33%	4%
	Conventional Care	65%	32%	3%

Table 3. Reported Clinical Outcomes from Pak et al.

We may also consider intermediate clinical outcomes, such as (1) time-to-intervention and (2) preventable clinic visits. Time-to-intervention is usually defined as the wait time prior to being seen by a specialist after a referral has been placed. Preventable clinic visits refers to the percentage of dermatology clinic visits that could be avoided through use of teledermatology.

The literature suggests that the use of S&F teledermatology may considerably reduce time-to-intervention. Researchers in Spain found that surgical patients managed through S&F teledermatology had a mean waiting interval 34.47 days shorter than those patients managed through conventional care (Ferrandiz et al., 2007). A similar study found that patients at primary care centers managed through teledermatology waited on average 76.31 days less than those with conventional referrals (Moreno-Ramirez et al., 2007). A study of patients at the Durham VA Medical Center found that those that received a S&F teledermatology consultation were seen on average 86 days sooner than those in the conventional system (Whited et al., 2002).

The reduced time-to-intervention may be partially due to the fact that teledermatology can help prevent unnecessary clinic visits. Indeed, studies have found that S&F teledermatology could prevent 13-58% of dermatology clinic visits (Whited, 2010).

2.1.4 Satisfaction with store-and-forward teledermatology

Satisfaction assessments may be subdivided into three categories: patient satisfaction, referring provider satisfaction, and specialist satisfaction. Studies suggest that patients were generally satisfied with receiving care through S&F teledermatology, and typically had no preference between teledermatology and usual care (Warshaw et al., 2010b). One study found that 76% of patients preferred being treated through teledermatology in order to avoid the wait time associated with a face-to-face clinic visit (Bowns et al., 2006). A common patient complaint during the S&F teledermatology process was the length of time between the consultation and being informed of the results by the primary care providers (Whited, 2010).

When referring providers were asked about their satisfaction with S&F teledermatology, referring providers provided varied feedback (Bowns et al., 2006; Collins et al., 2004; Weinstock et al., 2002; Whited et al., 2004). Many referring providers report that they improved their therapeutic and diagnostic ability due to regular feedback and interactions with the dermatologist (van den Akker et al., 2001). From the referring providers' perspective, some dissatisfaction with the S&F teledermatology process stemmed from the additional time and effort required for relaying the diagnoses to patients, prescribing the medications, or performing procedures (Bowns et al., 2006; Collins et al., 2004; Kvedar et al., 1999).

Fewer studies have evaluated satisfaction of dermatologists who practice teledermatology. While most dermatologists practicing teledermatology reported increased satisfaction (Whited, 2010), many report reduced confidence in their diagnoses (Bowns et al., 2006; Pak et al., 1999; Whited et al., 2004).

2.2 Economic considerations of sstore-and-forward teledermatology

We begin discussion of the economic aspects of S&F teledermatology with a brief review of common types of economic analysis. Three commonly used methods are cost minimization analysis, cost-effectiveness analysis, and cost-benefit analysis (Davalos et al., 2009). Cost-minimization analysis is a type of cost analysis that evaluates two systems that produce equivalent outcomes. Cost-effectiveness analysis compares monetary costs (cost) in the context of outcomes (effectiveness). However, this type of analysis generally considers only one outcomes measure. In comparison, cost-benefit analysis considers multiple economic costs as well as varied benefits within a system, and it generally includes multiple outcomes measures. Cost-benefit analyses are generally considered the most comprehensive type of economic analyses. Further information regarding economic evaluation metrics may be found in Davalos et al. (Davalos et al., 2009).

Literature shows that S&F teledermatology is generally economically viable (Table 3). While studies differed in their economic perspective and modality of S&F teledermatology delivery (e.g. triage, consultation, versus provision of care), analyses have generally established that S&F teledermatology offers a cost-effective means of providing dermatologic care especially for those living in geographically isolated communities or medically underserved communities (Pak et al., 2009; Whited et al., 2003). For example, in a cost-minimization analysis that adopted the perspective of the U.S. Department of Defense, Pak et al. concluded that the use of teleconsultations through S&F technology reduced overall costs compared to conventional care (Pak et al., 2009).

Similarly, Whited et al. performed a cost analysis of a consultative model using S&F technology from the perspective of the U.S. Department of Veterans Affairs (Whited et al., 2003). The authors found that teleconsultations are $15 more costly per patient compared to face-to-face consultation. In this study, effectiveness was defined as time-to-specialist evaluation. They found that having teledermatology consultations resulted in shorter time-to-specialist evaluation and was overall more cost-effective. Further analyses showed that, from a *societal* perspective, S&F teleconsultations would be even less costly after accounting for patients' travel time and productivity lost through face-to-face care (Whited et al., 2003).

When S&F teledermatology was used as a primary method for triaging cases appropriate face-to-face encounters, researchers found that this was an economically viable means for prioritizing patients requiring dermatologic care (Ferrandiz et al., 2008; Moreno-Ramirez et al., 2009). By comparing S&F teledermatology and conventional referrals to a skin cancer clinic in Spain, Moreno-Ramirez et al. conducted a cost-identification and cost-effectiveness analysis from a societal perspective (Moreno-Ramirez et al., 2009). The investigators assessed costs associated with travel, lost-productivity, and healthcare delivery. Effectiveness was defined as the wait-time to in-person consultation after the referral. The authors found that teledermatology triage was more cost-effective; specifically, teledermatology yielded cost-savings of €49.59 per patient compared with conventional face-to-face care (Moreno-Ramirez et al., 2009). These findings were corroborated by another cost-effectiveness study in Spain, where the investigators found that the use of teledermatology saved €122.02 compared to conventional care (Ferrandiz et al., 2008).

Reference	Type of Analysis	Teleconsultation	Conventional	Perspective
Provision of Care				
(Pak et al., 2009)	Cost-minimization	$340 / patient	$372 / patient	Department of Defense
(Whited et al., 2003)	Cost / Cost-effectiveness	$36.40 / patient	$21.40 / patient	Department of Veterans Affairs
Triage				
(Moreno-Ramirez et al., 2009)	Cost-identification / Cost-effectiveness	€79.78 / patient	€129.37 / patient	Societal
(Ferrandiz et al., 2008)	Cost / Cost-effectiveness	€156.40 / patient	€278.42 / patient	Societal
$ - US dollars; € - euros				

Table 4. Economic Analyses of Store-and-Forward Teledermatology

3. Live, Interactive Teledermatology

Live, interactive teledermatology involves synchronous interaction between the specialist and patient (Goldyne & Armstrong, 2010). Via videoconferencing or web-conferencing, the specialist obtains a clinical history, examines the patient in real-time, and communicates recommendations to the patient and the primary care provider (Wootton et al., 2000).

3.1 Outcomes measures of Live, Interactive Teledermatology

We will consider the same outcomes measures for LI teledermatology as we did for S&F teledermatology: diagnostic accuracy, diagnostic reliability, clinical outcomes, and satisfaction.

3.1.1 Diagnostic accuracy of LI Teledermatology

Studies comparing diagnostic accuracy of LI teledermatology to pathologic diagnosis are not currently available. Studies comparing diagnoses between LI teledermatology and in-person consultation generally show diagnostic agreement, and will be discussed further under diagnostic reliability.

3.1.2 Diagnostic reliability of Live, Interactive Teledermatology

Studies of intraobserver reliability between LI teledermatology and in-person consultation show complete diagnostic agreement in 59-75% of cases, and partial agreement in 76-87% of cases (Table 5).

Reference	Complete Diagnostic Agreement	Partial Diagnostic Agreement
(Loane et al., 1998b)	.71	.87
(Gilmour et al., 1998)	.59	.76
(Oakley et al., 1997)	.75	.82

Table 5. Intraobserver Reliability for LI Teledermatology

Interobserver reliability between LI teledermatology and in-person consultation ranges from 54-80% for complete diagnostic agreement, and 79-99% for partial agreement (Table 6). A review of aggregate data indicates that complete diagnostic agreement is 70%, while partial diagnostic agreement is 84% (Romero et al., 2008).

Reference	Complete Diagnostic Agreement	Partial Diagnostic Agreement
(Nordal et al., 2001)	.72	.86
(Phillips et al., 1998)	.59	-
(Loane et al., 1998b)	.60	.76
(Lowitt et al., 1998)	.80	-
(Gilmour et al., 1998)	.54	.80
(Lesher et al., 1998)	.78	.99
(Phillips et al., 1997)	.77	-

Table 6. Interobserver Reliability for LI Teledermatology

3.1.3 Clinical outcomes for LI Teledermatology

One study evaluated clinical outcomes for LI teledermatology compared to conventional care. In a retrospective analysis of patients who had two or more teledermatology consultations, Marcin et al. found that diagnosis, treatment, and patient improvement data for the teledermatology patients were consistent with existing literature regarding conventional care (Marcin et al., 2005).

Intermediate outcomes measures include (1) preventable clinic visits and (2) time for completion of consultation. Similar to the S&F modality, LI teledermatology can prevent unnecessary clinic visits. Studies found that 44.4-82% of clinic visits could be avoided through the use of LI teledermatology (Whited, 2010).

LI teledermatology can decrease total time necessary to complete a consultation visit from the patient's perspective. For example, researchers in New Zealand found that, compared to a clinic visit, the use of LI teledermatology saved patients an average of 3.45 hours of time, primarily due to reduced traveling time (Oakley et al., 2000). However, LI teledermatology does not necessarily reduce consult time for the dermatologist (Loane et al., 1999, 2001b; Oakley et al., 2000).

3.1.4 Satisfaction with Live, Interactive Teledermatology

As stated previously, satisfaction in teledermatology is categorized into patient satisfaction, referring provider satisfaction, and dermatologist satisfaction. Patients reported that they were equally satisfied with LI teledermatology and conventional care and had no strong preference for one modality over another (Whited, 2010). Some patients reported initial discomfort due to the presence of camera (Gilmour et al., 1998; Loane et al., 1998a).

Relatively few studies evaluated referring provider satisfaction in LI teledermatology. While there was some dissatisfaction associated with technical difficulties, most referring providers report being satisfied with the LI teledermatology (Gilmour et al., 1998; Jones et al., 1996).

Similar to dermatologists who practice S&F teledermatology, dermatologists who practice LI teledermatology report being satisfied with practicing LI teledermatology. However, when compared to in-person consultation, dermatologists expressed lower confidence in their diagnoses (Artiles Sanchez et al., 2004; Lowitt et al., 1998).

3.2 Economic considerations of Live, Interactive Teledermatology

Economic analyses of LI teledermatology yielded mixed conclusions regarding its economic sustainability. While some studies have shown LI teledermatology to be cost-effective, others suggested that it may be more costly than conventional care. In a cost-minimization analysis from a societal perspective, authors from New Zealand found that teledermatology consultations using LI technology appeared less costly than that of face-to-face care, especially when patients have longer travel distances (Loane et al., 2001b). In another cost-minimization study of LI teledermatology in the U.S., investigators found that consultative teledermatology using LI technology also appears to be less costly than face-to-face care from a provider perspective (Armstrong et al., 2007).

In a cost-benefit analysis from the societal perspective, Wootton et al. found that a LI teleconsultation system in the United Kingdom was more costly than face-to-face care. Sensitivity analyses showed that LI teledermatology consultations could be a less costly alternative if patients travelled longer distances for in-person consultations and incurred greater lost-productivity costs (Wootton et al., 2000).

Reference	Type of Analysis	Teleconsultation	Conventional	Perspective
(Dekio et al., 2010)	Cost-effectiveness	¥26,040 / week	¥60,500 / week	Societal
(Armstrong et al., 2007)	Cost-minimization	$274 / hour	$346 / hour	Healthcare provider
(Loane et al., 2001b)	Cost-minimization	NZ$279.23 / patient	NZ$283.79 / patient	Societal
(Loane et al., 2001a)	Cost-benefit	£146.48 / patient	£47.13 / patient	Urban Societal
(Loane et al., 2001a)	Cost-benefit	£180.22 / patient	£48.77 / patient	Rural Societal
(Wootton et al., 2000)	Cost-benefit	£132.10 / patient	£48.73 / patient	Societal
(Lamminen et al., 2000)	Cost	FM 18,627 (total cost)	FM 18,034 (total cost)	Societal
(Bergmo, 2000)	Cost-minimization	NKr 470,780 (total cost)	NKr 1,635,075 (total cost)	Healthcare provider
(Chan et al., 2000)	Cost / Cost-effectiveness	HK$57.7 / patient	HK$322.8 / patient	Healthcare provider
(Burgiss et al., 1997)	Cost	$141 / patient	$294 / patient	Societal
¥ - yen; € - euros; $ - US dollars; NZ$ - New Zealand dollars; £ - pounds; FM – Finnish marks; NKr – Norwegian kroners; HK$ - Hong Kong dollars				

Table 7. Economic Analyses of Live, Interactive Teledermatology

4. Comparison of store-and-forward and Live, Interactive Teledermatology

Approximately 42% of the United States population lives in medically underserved areas (Suneja et al., 2001). Both S&F and LI teledermatology can increase access to specialty care especially for populations living in rural or medically underserved areas (Hailey, 2005; Kailasam et al., 2010; Pak et al., 2007; Vallejos et al., 2009).

S&F and LI teledermatology present distinct advantages. S&F teledermatology appears to be very cost-effective. Specifically, compared to LI teledermatology, S&F teledermatology requires less equipment or technology costs (Pak, 2008; Watson, 2009). The requirements for administrative support and overhead also appear to be less for S&F teledermatology. Finally, the asynchronous nature of S&F modality affords greater scheduling flexibility for patients and dermatologists since coordinated appointments with specialists are not required (Finch et al., 2007; Watson, 2009). LI teledermatology, on the other hand, more closely mirrors a conventional face-to-face consultation because the specialist can interact with patients and a referring provider in real-time.

S&F and LI teledermatology have their respective disadvantages as well. In S&F teledermatology, because the ability of the dermatologist to diagnose and provide useful recommendations depends solely on the quality of images and clinical history, suboptimal images or incomplete clinical history can be frustrating for the dermatologist. Furthermore, S&F teledermatology does not allow the development of a patient-dermatologist relationship compared to LI teledermatology (Grenier et al., 2009; Onor & Misan, 2005). LI teledermatology presents alternative challenges in terms of scheduling, coordination, and costs.

Given the unique benefits that each modality offers, some providers have recently started to employ a hybrid model. In the hybrid model, the clinical encounters are conducted via videoconferencing or webconferencing, and the dermatologist reviews static digital images that were acquired by a digital camera prior to the encounter and sent to them during the encounter. Current research efforts are investigating the relative effectiveness of such hybrid systems (Baba et al., 2005; Romero et al., 2010). For example, Baba et al. found that a hybrid modality increased diagnostic accuracy by 7-9%, compared to S&F teledermatology alone (Baba et al., 2005).

5. Novel classification teledermatology based on healthcare delivery models

To date, teledermatology has been categorized by the technology it uses--S&F and LI technology. An alternative model to frame teledermatology is based on the type of healthcare delivery. Specifically, independent of the type of technology employed, we can arrange teledermatology delivery into (1) triage, (2) consultative, and (3) direct-care models. This technology-independent, healthcare delivery-based framework is accessible to policy makers and other stakeholders involved in health policy.

5.1 Triage model

In the triage model, all dermatology referrals are first seen through teledermatology. A specialist reviews the cases rapidly with the goal of prioritizing which patients are suitable for in-person evaluation. The triage model prioritizes patients based on the severity and urgency of their skin condition. This modality has been primarily practiced in Europe in prioritization patients with cutaneous malignancies (Ferrandiz et al., 2007; Moreno-Ramirez et al., 2007).

5.2 Consultative model

In the consultative model, the referring providers decide which dermatology referrals are appropriate for teledermatology evaluation. From the dermatologist's perspective, the primary goal of the consultative model is to provide detailed and useful recommendations to the primary care provider. In this healthcare delivery model, the dermatologist reviews the cases via either S&F or LI technology and provides detailed recommendations to the primary care provider. The primary care provider assumes responsibility for communicating with the patient and carrying out the recommendation plans. The consultative model is currently the most common model in the United States (Goldyne & Armstrong, 2010).

5.3 Direct-care model

In the direct-care model, the dermatologist assumes the responsibility of communicating and treating the patient. This model differs significantly from the triage or consultative

model in that the dermatologist is responsible for caring for the patient. The provision of direct care includes evaluation, communicating the treatment plan to the patient, writing prescriptions, carrying out laboratory evaluations, and monitoring disease progression.
The direct-care model has generally been practiced using S&F technology and in research settings (Chambers et al., 2010; Parsi et al., 2010; Watson et al., 2010).

6. Conclusion

As healthcare delivery becomes more patient-centered and distance-independent (Hibbard, 2004; Hogarth et al., 2010; Robinson et al., 2011), proper application of teledermatology offers a versatile means of providing high quality care to patients in their own communities. Teledermatology can be used in various healthcare delivery modalities, including triage, consultation, and direct care.
In addition to gathering the support of healthcare workers and patients for these newer models of healthcare delivery, those who work at the forefront of telemedicine need to also advocate for policy changes and technological innovations to continually improve the quality and experience of telemedicine. It is likely that the cost of technology will decline as the reliability and user-interface of technology continually improve. In this healthcare environment, innovations in teledermatology serve as examples for emerging paradigms in healthcare delivery.

7. References

Armstrong AW, Dorer DJ, Lugn NE, and Kvedar JC. 2007. Economic evaluation of interactive teledermatology compared with conventional care. Telemed J E Health 13(2):91-99.

Artiles Sanchez J, Suarez-Hernandez J, Serrano P, Vazquez C, Duque B, and Cuevas C. 2004. Evaluación cualitativa en teledermatología: Resultados del proyecto piloto en telemedicina 2000. Actas Dermosifiliogr 95(5):289-294.

Baba M, Seckin D, and Kapdagli S. 2005. A comparison of teledermatology using store-and-forward methodology alone, and in combination with Web camera videoconferencing. J Telemed Telecare 11(7):354-360.

Barnard CM, and Goldyne ME. 2000. Evaluation of an asynchronous teleconsultation system for diagnosis of skin cancer and other skin diseases. Telemed J E Health 6(4):379-384.

Bergmo TS. 2000. A cost-minimization analysis of a realtime teledermatology service in northern Norway. J Telemed Telecare 6(5):273-277.

Bowns IR, Collins K, Walters SJ, and McDonagh AJ. 2006. Telemedicine in dermatology: a randomised controlled trial. Health Technol Assess 10(43):iii-iv, ix-xi, 1-39.

Burgiss SG, Julius CE, Watson HW, Haynes BK, Buonocore E, and Smith GT. 1997. Telemedicine for dermatology care in rural patients. Telemed J 3(3):227-233.

Chambers, CJ, Parsi, K, Schupp, C, and Armstrong, AW (2010). Patient-Centered Online Healthcare Delivery Model for Psoriasis: A Randomized Controlled Equivalency Trial. Manuscript submitted for publication, University of California, Davis School of Medicine, Department of Dermatology, Sacramento, CA.

Chan HH, Woo J, Chan WM, and Hjelm M. 2000. Teledermatology in Hong Kong: a cost-effective method to provide service to the elderly patients living in institutions. Int J Dermatol 39(10):774-778.

Collins K, Bowns I, and Walters S. 2004. General practitioners' perceptions of asynchronous telemedicine in a randomized controlled trial of teledermatology. J Telemed Telecare 10(2):94-98.

Davalos ME, French MT, Burdick AE, and Simmons SC. 2009. Economic evaluation of telemedicine: review of the literature and research guidelines for benefit-cost analysis. Telemed J E Health 15(10):933-948.

Dekio I, Hanada E, Chinuki Y, Akaki T, Kitani M, Shiraishi Y, Kaneko S, Furumura M, and Morita E. 2010. Usefulness and economic evaluation of ADSL-based live interactive teledermatology in areas with shortage of dermatologists. Int J Dermatol 49(11):1272-1275.

Du Moulin MF, Bullens-Goessens YI, Henquet CJ, Brunenberg DE, de Bruyn-Geraerds DP, Winkens RA, Dirksen CD, Vierhout WP, and Neumann HA. 2003. The reliability of diagnosis using store-and-forward teledermatology. J Telemed Telecare 9(5):249-252.

Ebner C, Wurm EM, Binder B, Kittler H, Lozzi GP, Massone C, Gabler G, Hofmann-Wellenhof R, and Soyer HP. 2008. Mobile teledermatology: a feasibility study of 58 subjects using mobile phones. J Telemed Telecare 14(1):2-7.

Edison KE, Ward DS, Dyer JA, Lane W, Chance L, and Hicks LL. 2008. Diagnosis, diagnostic confidence, and management concordance in live-interactive and store-and-forward teledermatology compared to in-person examination. Telemed J E Health 14(9):889-895.

Eminovic N, de Keizer NF, Bindels PJ, and Hasman A. 2007. Maturity of teledermatology evaluation research: a systematic literature review. Br J Dermatol 156(3):412-419.

Eminovic N, Witkamp L, Ravelli AC, Bos JD, van den Akker TW, Bousema MT, Henquet CJ, Koopman RJ, Zeegelaar JE, and Wyatt JC. 2003. Potential effect of patient-assisted teledermatology on outpatient referral rates. J Telemed Telecare 9(6):321-327.

Ferrandiz L, Moreno-Ramirez D, Nieto-Garcia A, Carrasco R, Moreno-Alvarez P, Galdeano R, Bidegain E, Rios-Martin JJ, and Camacho FM. 2007. Teledermatology-based presurgical management for nonmelanoma skin cancer: a pilot study. Dermatol Surg 33(9):1092-1098.

Ferrandiz L, Moreno-Ramirez D, Ruiz-de-Casas A, Nieto-Garcia A, Moreno-Alvarez P, Galdeano R, and Camacho FM. 2008. [An economic analysis of presurgical teledermatology in patients with nonmelanoma skin cancer]. Actas Dermosifiliogr 99(10):795-802.

Finch TL, Mair FS, and May CR. 2007. Teledermatology in the UK: lessons in service innovation. Br J Dermatol 156(3):521-527.

Gilmour E, Campbell SM, Loane MA, Esmail A, Griffiths CE, Roland MO, Parry EJ, Corbett RO, Eedy D, Gore HE et al. . 1998. Comparison of teleconsultations and face-to-face consultations: preliminary results of a United Kingdom multicentre teledermatology study. Br J Dermatol 139(1):81-87.

Goldyne M, and Armstrong AW. 2010. Teledermatology Practice Guide. California Telemedicine and eHealth Center.
Grenier N, Bercovitch L, and Long TP. 2009. Cyberdermatoethics II: a case-based approach to teledermatology ethics. Clin Dermatol 27(4):367-371.
Hailey D. 2005. Technology and managed care: is telemedicine the right tool for rural communities? J Postgrad Med 51(4):275-278.
Heffner VA, Lyon VB, Brousseau DC, Holland KE, and Yen K. 2009. Store-and-forward teledermatology versus in-person visits: a comparison in pediatric teledermatology clinic. J Am Acad Dermatol 60(6):956-961.
Hibbard JH. 2004. Moving toward a more patient-centered health care delivery system. Health Aff (Millwood) Suppl Web Exclusives:VAR133-135.
High WA, Houston MS, Calobrisi SD, Drage LA, and McEvoy MT. 2000. Assessment of the accuracy of low-cost store-and-forward teledermatology consultation. J Am Acad Dermatol 42(5 Pt 1):776-783.
Hogarth M, Hajopoulos K, Young M, Cowles N, Churin J, Hornthal B, and Esserman L. 2010. The Communication and Care Plan: a novel approach to patient-centered clinical information systems. J Biomed Inform 43(5 Suppl):S6-8.
Jones DH, Crichton C, Macdonald A, Potts S, Sime D, Toms J, and McKinlay J. 1996. Teledermatology in the Highlands of Scotland. J Telemed Telecare 2 Suppl 1:7-9.
Kailasam S, Kumar S, and Dharanipragada J. 2010. Arogyasree: an enhanced grid-based approach to mobile telemedicine. Int J Telemed Appl 2010:536237.
Krupinski EA, Engstrom M, Barker G, Levine N, and Weinstein RS. 2004. The challenges of following patients and assessing outcomes in teledermatology. J Telemed Telecare 10(1):21-24.
Krupinski EA, LeSueur B, Ellsworth L, Levine N, Hansen R, Silvis N, Sarantopoulos P, Hite P, Wurzel J, Weinstein RS et al. . 1999. Diagnostic accuracy and image quality using a digital camera for teledermatology. Telemed J 5(3):257-263.
Kvedar JC, Edwards RA, Menn ER, Mofid M, Gonzalez E, Dover J, and Parrish JA. 1997. The substitution of digital images for dermatologic physical examination. Arch Dermatol 133(2):161-167.
Kvedar JC, Menn ER, Baradagunta S, Smulders-Meyer O, and Gonzalez E. 1999. Teledermatology in a capitated delivery system using distributed information architecture: design and development. Telemed J 5(4):357-366.
Lamminen H, Tuomi ML, Lamminen J, and Uusitalo H. 2000. A feasibility study of realtime teledermatology in Finland. J Telemed Telecare 6(2):102-107.
Lesher JL, Jr., Davis LS, Gourdin FW, English D, and Thompson WO. 1998. Telemedicine evaluation of cutaneous diseases: a blinded comparative study. J Am Acad Dermatol 38(1):27-31.
Lim AC, Egerton IB, See A, and Shumack SP. 2001. Accuracy and reliability of store-and-forward teledermatology: preliminary results from the St George Teledermatology Project. Australas J Dermatol 42(4):247-251.
Loane MA, Bloomer SE, Corbett R, Eedy DJ, Evans C, Hicks N, Jacklin P, Lotery HE, Mathews C, Paisley J et al. . 2001a. A randomized controlled trial assessing the

health economics of realtime teledermatology compared with conventional care: an urban versus rural perspective. J Telemed Telecare 7(2):108-118.

Loane MA, Bloomer SE, Corbett R, Eedy DJ, Gore HE, Hicks N, Mathews C, Paisley J, Steele K, and Wootton R. 1999. Patient cost-benefit analysis of teledermatology measured in a randomized control trial. J Telemed Telecare 5 Suppl 1:S1-3.

Loane MA, Bloomer SE, Corbett R, Eedy DJ, Gore HE, Mathews C, Steele K, and Wootton R. 1998a. Patient satisfaction with realtime teledermatology in Northern Ireland. J Telemed Telecare 4(1):36-40.

Loane MA, Corbett R, Bloomer SE, Eedy DJ, Gore HE, Mathews C, Steele K, and Wootton R. 1998b. Diagnostic accuracy and clinical management by realtime teledermatology. Results from the Northern Ireland arms of the UK Multicentre Teledermatology Trial. J Telemed Telecare 4(2):95-100.

Loane MA, Oakley A, Rademaker M, Bradford N, Fleischl P, Kerr P, and Wootton R. 2001b. A cost-minimization analysis of the societal costs of realtime teledermatology compared with conventional care: results from a randomized controlled trial in New Zealand. J Telemed Telecare 7(4):233-238.

Lowitt MH, Kessler, II, Kauffman CL, Hooper FJ, Siegel E, and Burnett JW. 1998. Teledermatology and in-person examinations: a comparison of patient and physician perceptions and diagnostic agreement. Arch Dermatol 134(4):471-476.

Lozzi GP, Soyer HP, Massone C, Micantonio T, Kraenke B, Fargnoli MC, Fink-Puches R, Binder B, Di Stefani A, Hofmann-Wellenhof R et al. . 2007. The additive value of second opinion teleconsulting in the management of patients with challenging inflammatory, neoplastic skin diseases: a best practice model in dermatology? J Eur Acad Dermatol Venereol 21(1):30-34.

Lyon CC, and Harrison PV. 1997. A portable digital imaging system in dermatology: diagnostic and educational applications. J Telemed Telecare 3 Suppl 1:81-83.

Mahendran R, Goodfield MJ, and Sheehan-Dare RA. 2005. An evaluation of the role of a store-and-forward teledermatology system in skin cancer diagnosis and management. Clin Exp Dermatol 30(3):209-214.

Marcin JP, Nesbitt TS, Cole SL, Knuttel RM, Hilty DM, Prescott PT, and Daschbach MM. 2005. Changes in diagnosis, treatment, and clinical improvement among patients receiving telemedicine consultations. Telemed J E Health 11(1):36-43.

Moreno-Ramirez D, Ferrandiz L, Nieto-Garcia A, Carrasco R, Moreno-Alvarez P, Galdeano R, Bidegain E, Rios-Martin JJ, and Camacho FM. 2007. Store-and-forward teledermatology in skin cancer triage: experience and evaluation of 2009 teleconsultations. Arch Dermatol 143(4):479-484.

Moreno-Ramirez D, Ferrandiz L, Ruiz-de-Casas A, Nieto-Garcia A, Moreno-Alvarez P, Galdeano R, and Camacho FM. 2009. Economic evaluation of a store-and-forward teledermatology system for skin cancer patients. J Telemed Telecare 15(1):40-45.

Nordal EJ, Moseng D, Kvammen B, and Lochen ML. 2001. A comparative study of teleconsultations versus face-to-face consultations. J Telemed Telecare 7(5):257-265.

Oakley AM, Astwood DR, Loane M, Duffill MB, Rademaker M, and Wootton R. 1997. Diagnostic accuracy of teledermatology: results of a preliminary study in New Zealand. N Z Med J 110(1038):51-53.

Oakley AM, Kerr P, Duffill M, Rademaker M, Fleischl P, Bradford N, and Mills C. 2000. Patient cost-benefits of realtime teledermatology--a comparison of data from Northern Ireland and New Zealand. J Telemed Telecare 6(2):97-101.

Oakley AM, Reeves F, Bennett J, Holmes SH, and Wickham H. 2006. Diagnostic value of written referral and/or images for skin lesions. J Telemed Telecare 12(3):151-158.

Onor ML, and Misan S. 2005. The clinical interview and the doctor-patient relationship in telemedicine. Telemed J E Health 11(1):102-105.

Pak H. 2008. Teledermatology: A User's Guide. New York: Cambridge University Press.

Pak H, Triplett CA, Lindquist JH, Grambow SC, and Whited JD. 2007. Store-and-forward teledermatology results in similar clinical outcomes to conventional clinic-based care. J Telemed Telecare 13(1):26-30.

Pak HS, Datta SK, Triplett CA, Lindquist JH, Grambow SC, and Whited JD. 2009. Cost minimization analysis of a store-and-forward teledermatology consult system. Telemed J E Health 15(2):160-165.

Pak HS, Harden D, Cruess D, Welch ML, and Poropatich R. 2003. Teledermatology: an intraobserver diagnostic correlation study, part I. Cutis 71(5):399-403.

Pak HS, Welch M, and Poropatich R. 1999. Web-based teledermatology consult system: preliminary results from the first 100 cases. Stud Health Technol Inform 64:179-184.

Parsi, K, Chambers, CJ, and Armstrong, AW (2010). Cost-Effectiveness Analysis of a Patient-Centered Online Care Model for Management of Psoriasis. Accepted for publication by the Journal of the American Academy of Dermatology.

Phillips CM, Burke WA, Allen MH, Stone D, and Wilson JL. 1998. Reliability of telemedicine in evaluating skin tumors. Telemed J 4(1):5-9.

Phillips CM, Burke WA, Shechter A, Stone D, Balch D, and Gustke S. 1997. Reliability of dermatology teleconsultations with the use of teleconferencing technology. J Am Acad Dermatol 37(3 Pt 1):398-402.

Robinson JD, Turner JW, Levine B, and Tian Y. 2011. Expanding the walls of the health care encounter: support and outcomes for patients online. Health Commun 26(2):125-134.

Romero G, Cortina P, and Vera E. 2008. [Telemedicine and teledermatology (II): current state of research on dermatology teleconsultations]. Actas Dermosifiliogr 99(8):586-597.

Romero G, Sanchez P, Garcia M, Cortina P, Vera E, and Garrido JA. 2010. Randomized controlled trial comparing store-and-forward teledermatology alone and in combination with web-camera videoconferencing. Clin Exp Dermatol 35(3):311-317.

Silva CS, Souza MB, Duque IA, de Medeiros LM, Melo NR, Araujo Cde A, and Criado PR. 2009. [Teledermatology: diagnostic correlation in a primary care service]. An Bras Dermatol 84(5):489-493.

Suneja T, Smith ED, Chen GJ, Zipperstein KJ, Fleischer AB, Jr., and Feldman SR. 2001. Waiting times to see a dermatologist are perceived as too long by dermatologists: implications for the dermatology workforce. Arch Dermatol 137(10):1303-1307.

Tan E, Yung A, Jameson M, Oakley A, and Rademaker M. 2010. Successful triage of patients referred to a skin lesion clinic using teledermoscopy (IMAGE IT trial). Br J Dermatol 162(4):803-811.

Taylor P, Goldsmith P, Murray K, Harris D, and Barkley A. 2001. Evaluating a telemedicine system to assist in the management of dermatology referrals. Br J Dermatol 144(2):328-333.

Tucker WF, and Lewis FM. 2005. Digital imaging: a diagnostic screening tool? Int J Dermatol 44(6):479-481.

Vallejos QM, Quandt SA, Feldman SR, Fleischer AB, Jr., Brooks T, Cabral G, Heck J, Schulz MR, Verma A, Whalley LE et al. 2009. Teledermatology consultations provide specialty care for farmworkers in rural clinics. J Rural Health 25(2):198-202.

van den Akker TW, Reker CH, Knol A, Post J, Wilbrink J, and van der Veen JP. 2001. Teledermatology as a tool for communication between general practitioners and dermatologists. J Telemed Telecare 7(4):193-198.

Warshaw EM, Gravely AA, and Nelson DB. 2010a. Accuracy of teledermatology/teledermoscopy and clinic-based dermatology for specific categories of skin neoplasms. J Am Acad Dermatol 63(2):348-352.

Warshaw EM, Hillman YJ, Greer NL, Hagel EM, Macdonald R, Rutks IR, and Wilt TJ. 2010b. Teledermatology for diagnosis and management of skin conditions: A systematic review. J Am Acad Dermatol.

Warshaw EM, Lederle FA, Grill JP, Gravely AA, Bangerter AK, Fortier LA, Bohjanen KA, Chen K, Lee PK, Rabinovitz HS et al. . 2009a. Accuracy of teledermatology for nonpigmented neoplasms. J Am Acad Dermatol 60(4):579-588.

Warshaw EM, Lederle FA, Grill JP, Gravely AA, Bangerter AK, Fortier LA, Bohjanen KA, Chen K, Lee PK, Rabinovitz HS et al. . 2009b. Accuracy of teledermatology for pigmented neoplasms. J Am Acad Dermatol 61(5):753-765.

Watson A, Pena, V., Kvedar, J.. 2009. Teledermatology. eMedicine.

Watson AJ, Bergman H, Williams CM, and Kvedar JC. 2010. A randomized trial to evaluate the efficacy of online follow-up visits in the management of acne. Arch Dermatol 146(4):406-411.

Weinstock MA, Nguyen FQ, and Risica PM. 2002. Patient and referring provider satisfaction with teledermatology. J Am Acad Dermatol 47(1):68-72.

Whited JD. 2010. Summary of the Status of Teledermatology Research. Teledermatology Special Interest Group - American Telemedicine Association.

Whited JD, Datta S, Hall RP, Foy ME, Marbrey LE, Grambow SC, Dudley TK, Simel DL, and Oddone EZ. 2003. An economic analysis of a store and forward teledermatology consult system. Telemed J E Health 9(4):351-360.

Whited JD, Hall RP, Foy ME, Marbrey LE, Grambow SC, Dudley TK, Datta S, Simel DL, and Oddone EZ. 2002. Teledermatology's impact on time to intervention among referrals to a dermatology consult service. Telemed J E Health 8(3):313-321.

Whited JD, Hall RP, Foy ME, Marbrey LE, Grambow SC, Dudley TK, Datta SK, Simel DL, and Oddone EZ. 2004. Patient and clinician satisfaction with a store-and-forward teledermatology consult system. Telemed J E Health 10(4):422-431.

Whited JD, Hall RP, Simel DL, Foy ME, Stechuchak KM, Drugge RJ, Grichnik JM, Myers SA, and Horner RD. 1999. Reliability and accuracy of dermatologists' clinic-based and digital image consultations. J Am Acad Dermatol 41(5 Pt 1):693-702.

Wootton R, Bloomer SE, Corbett R, Eedy DJ, Hicks N, Lotery HE, Mathews C, Paisley J, Steele K, and Loane MA. 2000. Multicentre randomised control trial comparing real time teledermatology with conventional outpatient dermatological care: societal cost-benefit analysis. BMJ 320(7244):1252-1256.

Zelickson BD, and Homan L. 1997. Teledermatology in the nursing home. Arch Dermatol 133(2):171-174.

18

Screening for Retinopathy of Prematurity

Claire Hartnett and Michael O'Keefe
Children's University Hospital, Temple Street, Dublin 1
Ireland

1. Introduction

All ophthalmologists and neonatologists are aware that the condition of retinopathy of prematurity is potentially blinding to the premature infant. However it is also one of the few causes of childhood visual disability which is largely preventable. Many extremely preterm infants will develop some degree of retinopathy of prematurity although in the majority this never progresses beyond the level of mild disease which resolves spontaneously without treatment. A small proportion of premature infants develop potentially severe retinopathy which can be detected through retinal screening. If untreated, severe disease can result in serious vision impairment and consequently all babies at risk of sight-threatening retinopathy of prematurity should be screened.

2. The aim and importance of screening for retinopathy of prematurity

Retinopathy of prematurity is a proliferative disease of the retinal vasculature and is a potentially blinding disorder of premature infants (Hunter et al. 1992, Gibson et al. 1990). The condition is characterized by proliferation of abnormal fibrovascular tissue at the border of vascularised and non-vascularised retina (Flyn et al. 1977). Timely and accurate screening of this condition is of utmost importance because of the short window of opportunity during which treatment is effective. The 1984 Classification of Retinopathy of Prematurity (An International Classification of Prematurity, 1984) and the 1988 Cryotherapy for Retinopathy of Prematurity (CRYO-ROP) Study (Cryotherapy for retinopathy of prematurity cooperative group. 1988) both confirmed the success of treatment for retinopathy of prematurity and made screening mandatory. Screening has subsequently improved the visual prognosis of this condition. Improved survival of premature infants of gestational age less than 25 weeks gestation and very low birth weight has resulted in an increased incidence of retinopathy of prematurity and an increase in blindness. These factors have significantly increased the importance of screening. Treatment is effective in altering the course of the disease and can prevent blindness. This means that screening infants is the fundamental first step. The Early Treatment for Retinopathy of Prematurity (ETROP) study also confirmed the importance of screening. National based screening guidelines have been based on the varied incidence of disease between countries (Early Treatment of Retinopathy of Prematurity Cooperative Group. 2003). Many developed countries have adopted guidelines and screening criteria based on weight and gestational age and these are modified according to population based studies on the incidence of retinopathy of prematurity. There is a varied incidence of the condition in developed countries compared to developing countries (Gilbert et al. 1997).The incidence of retinopathy of prematurity is much higher in developing countries and there is a greater prevalence of the disease in heavier and older premature infants (Phan et al. 2003).

3. Indications for screening

Various guidelines for screening of retinopathy of prematurity exist. All guidelines for screening are evidence-based.

3.1 Screening criteria

The American Academy of Ophthalmology, the American Academy of Paediatrics and the American Association of Paediatric Ophthalmology and Strabismus have recommended screening infants with birth weights under 1500g or gestational age of 30 weeks or less and selected infants with a birth weight between 1500 and 2000g or a gestational age greater than 30 weeks with an unstable clinical course who are considered at high risk by their paediatrician or neonatologist (2006). In 2007, after an extensive review of the literature, updated United Kingdom national guidelines recommended retinopathy of prematurity screening for babies of birth weight less than 1501g and / or gestational age less than 32 weeks (up to 31 weeks and six days)(Royal College of Paediatrics & Child Health & Royal College of Ophthalmologists. 2007).

3.2 Screening protocol

The American guidelines on screening recommend that in babies born up to 27 weeks the first retinopathy of prematurity screen should be performed at 31 weeks post menstrual age. Those born at 28 weeks gestation or older are screened at 4 weeks after birth. The United Kingdom guidelines recommend that babies born before 27 weeks (up to 26 weeks and 6 days) the first retinopathy of prematurity screen should be performed at 30 to 31 weeks postmenstrual age. Those born at 27 to 31 weeks and 6 days gestational age should have their first screen between four to five weeks after birth. It is recommended that repeat examinations should take place every two weeks thereafter. However repeat examinations should take place weekly when the vessels end in zone 1 or posterior zone 2, there is plus or pre plus disease or there is any stage 3 disease in any zone. Of particular importance is the retinopathy of prematurity examination at about 34 weeks post menstrual age as this is the age at which the risk of severe disease is considered greatest. In countries where resources and personnel for screening are scarce, the 34 week screen may be the only examination to take place and is also labelled as the one stop examination. Although screening for retinopathy in premature babies should follow the above protocol, it is acknowledged that there may be clinical or organisational circumstances which prevent this. Where a decision is made not to screen a baby, the reason for doing so should be clearly stated in the baby's medical record and the examination should be rescheduled within one week of the intended examination.

3.3 Threshold disease

The presence of threshold disease signals the need for treatment. Threshold disease is defined by the Cryotherapy for Retinopathy of Prematurity (CRYO-ROP) Study as at least five continuous or eight cumulative clock hours of Stage 3 retinopathy of prematurity in zone I or II with plus disease. There are other definitions of threshold disease in use, for example, the broader United Kingdom guidelines which in addition to the above also include five continuous clock hours or eight cumulative clock hours of stage 3 retinopathy of prematurity in zone III with plus disease. The Supplemental Therapeutic Oxygen for Prethreshold Retinopathy of Prematurity (STOP-ROP) study had different criteria for zones I and II threshold retinopathy of prematurity; for zone II disease it used the same definition as the CRYO-ROP study, but in zone I, it defined as 'threshold' any stage of retinopathy of prematurity with plus disease, or stage 3 retinopathy of prematurity with or without plus disease.

3.4 Prethreshold disease

The ETROP study however highlighted the importance of the recognition of prethreshold disease and the need for earlier treatment in some babies. This study emphasises the importance of pre plus disease and aggressive zone I and zone II retinopathy of prematurity.
Infants screened prior to 30 weeks gestation have hazy corneas and fundoscopy is more difficult. This makes screening prior to 30 weeks difficult and attempting laser treatment is almost impossible. The early onset of threshold disease has been referred to as "rush disease" by some ophthalmologists. It has been reported at 31 to 32 weeks gestational age (Subhani et al. 2001). As a result, the United Kingdom guidelines for screening recommend that the more premature infants should undergo the first screening examination at 30 to 31 weeks post menstrual age.

Early Treatment of Retinopathy of Prematurity (ETROP) Classification:

Type 1 ROP should be treated:
Zone I any stage of ROP with plus disease
Zone I Stage 3 ROP with or without plus disease
Zone II Stage 2 or 3 ROP with plus disease

Type 2 should be observed, and only undergo treatment if it progresses to type I or threshold disease:
Zone II Stage 1 or 2 ROP without plus disease
Zone II Stage 3 ROP without plus disease

Fig. 1. Classification of treatment guidelines from the Early Treatment of Retinopathy of Prematurity (ETROP) Study.

3.5 Termination of screening

Screening for retinopathy of prematurity should continue in accordance with the guidelines until there is no risk of sight threatening disease. The advice in the UK is to continue screening until retinal vascularisation has extended into zone 3 or at 37 weeks in infants in whom no retinopathy of prematurity has developed. In infants who have developed retinopathy of prematurity, screening may cease once regression has been seen on two consecutive examinations. The American guidelines advise ceasing screening when zone 3 or the entire retina is vascularised, the infant is 45 weeks post menstrual age or the retinopathy of prematurity has regressed.

Screening for retinopathy of prematurity must be safe, cost effective and target those most at risk. Effective screening eliminates unnecessary examinations and reduces wastage of resources and personnel. Retinopathy of prematurity screening requires experience and skill. The ability to recognise severe disease is crucial. All neonatal units should have an agreed policy on screening. Screening includes input from the ophthalmologist, neonatologist and neonatal nurses. Of great importance is the involvement of the neonatal nurses. They play an invaluable role in ensuring infants are included in the screening process at the correct gestational age. They ensure that the pupils are dilated prior to the eye examination and also assist at examinations. The neonatal nurses also play a key role in liaising with both the ophthalmologist and the neonatologist. Screenings should not be delayed or missed as this can result in a poorer visual outcome.

4. The technique of the screening process

The screening examinations are usually performed in the neonatal unit with the infant in the incubator and the trained neonatal staff present. The examination requires a well-dilated pupil so that the peripheral retina can be fully visualised. Mydriatic eye drops should be instilled approximately 60 minutes and 30 minutes prior to the examination. A combination of eye drops is preferable to using one single agent. Various combinations of dilating drop regimes exist. Popular combinations include 0.5% cyclopentolate and 2.5% phenylephrine or 0.5% tropicamide and 2.5% phenylephrine. Most, if not all examinations require a sterile lid speculum. An indenting device may be required in some cases to gently rotate or manipulate the globe.

An indirect ophthalmoscope and a hand held 28 or 30 dioptre convex lens are necessary to perform the retinal examination. The classification scheme for retinopathy of prematurity divides the retina into zones and 12 clock hours and in addition documents the presence or absence of plus or pre plus disease. The examiner should therefore be very familiar with a visual representation of the zones of the retina.

The examiner should first visualise the posterior pole looking for retinopathy of prematurity and in particular note the presence or absence of plus disease. The posterior pole must be scrutinised for flat retinopathy of prematurity and importantly the examiner should be aware that advanced disease in this region may not form a ridge. Failure to recognise this may lead to a delay in treatment and a poorer visual outcome. The nasal and temporal retinal peripheries must then be visualised.

4.1 Classification of retinopathy of prematurity: zone of retinal involvement

An important component of the classification of ROP is the zone in which the disease occurs. Zone 1 is a circular area, the radius of which is twice the distance from the optic disc to the fovea (Fig 2). Zone 11 extends concentrically from the edge of zone 1 and its radius extends from the centre of the optic disc to the nasal ora serrata and extends to the equator on the temporal side. Zone 111 consists of the residual temporal crescent of retina (Fig 2).

4.2 Classification of retinopathy of prematurity: the stage of the disease

The second component of the classification system is the stage of the disease. Stage 1 retinopathy of prematurity is a thin, flat tortuous, grey-white line that runs approximately parallel with the ora serrata and divides the vascular from the avascular retina (Fig 3).

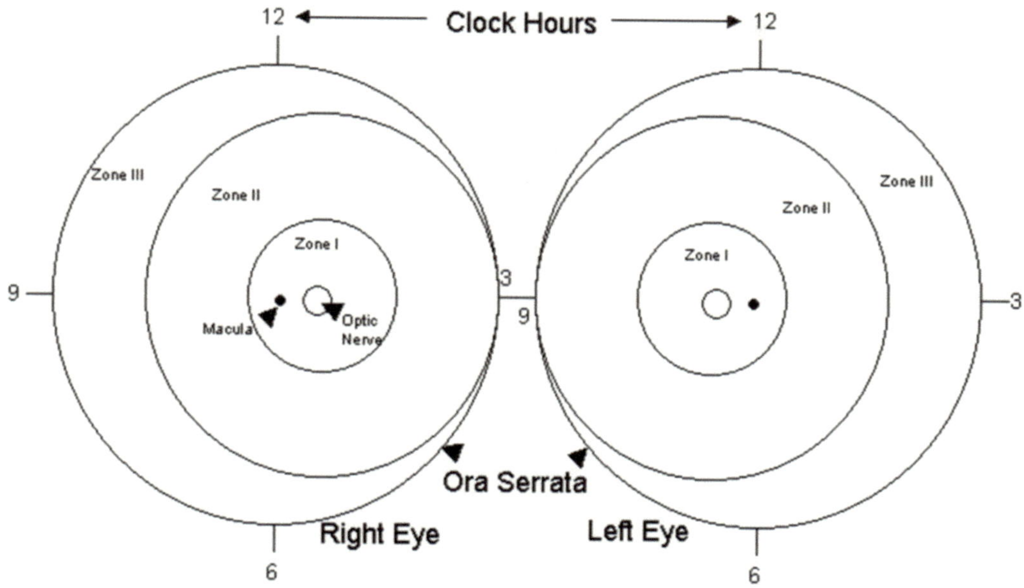

Fig. 2. Zones of the retina and clock hours.

Stage 2 retinopathy of prematurity arises in the region of the line and has height and width and extends above the plane of the retina (Fig 4). Stage 3 signifies extra retinal neovascularisation (Fig 5). The fibrovascular proliferation extends from the ridge into the vitreous, continuous with the posterior aspect of the ridge, causing a ragged appearance as the proliferation becomes more extensive. Stage 4a indicates extra foveal retinal detachment (Fig 6). Stage 4b indicates macular detachment (Fig 7). The detachment is generally concave and circumferentially orientated. In progressive cases the fibrous tissue continues to contract and the detachment increases in height and extends posteriorly and anteriorly. Stage 5 (Fig 8) is present when there is a total retinal detachment and it can be an open or closed funnel shape.

4.3 Plus and pre-plus disease

The third diagnostic feature is the presence or absence of plus disease which is diagnosed by the presence or absence of vessel dilatation and tortuosity (Fig 9), increasing preretinal and vitreous haemorrhage, vitreous haze and failure of the pupil to dilate. Plus disease signifies a tendency to progression. Pre-plus disease is characterized by abnormal dilatation and tortuosity that is insufficient to be designated as plus disease (Fig 10).

4.4 Stress-reduction techniques

The retinopathy of prematurity screening examination process can be distressing for the infant. Distress can be caused by handling the infant in the incubator, inserting the eyelid speculum and use of an indenter to rotate, manipulate or indent the globe. Examinations which extend to more than 2 minutes long are not well tolerated by the infant. There is conflicting evidence as to the physiological changes which occur secondary to the distressing examination. A report by Laws et al. (1996) showed an increase in heart rate of seven beats per minute and a 3% drop in oxygen saturation after the examination. However,

Slevin et al. (1997) reported no significant change in heart rate or oxygen saturation but noted that infants expressed distress by their crying patterns and body and limb movements. It was recommended that infants undergoing a screening examination should be placed on a soft padded surface with boundaries that maintained them in a flexed position but allowed for unrestricted movement of the body and limbs. This method of handling may reduce the distress experienced by the infant during the examination process. Other comfort care techniques including administering sucrose solution, nesting, swaddling and/or the use of a pacifier during the screening examination may also be considered. Ophthalmological notes should be made after each screening examination, detailing zone, stage, and extent in terms of clock hours of any retinopathy of prematurity and the presence of any plus or pre-plus disease. These notes should include a recommendation for the timing of the next examination (if any) and be kept with the baby's medical record.

4.5 Indirect ophthalmoscopy and retcam digital imaging

Indirect ophthalmoscopy is recognised as the gold standard for retinopathy of prematurity screening. However screening for retinopathy of prematurity with digital imaging has been proposed as a potential alternative. The RetCam 120 (Massie Research Laboratory Inc., Dublin, California) is a digital retinal camera used frequently in paediatric ophthalmology. It is becoming more important for the photo-documentation of retinal conditions in infants with retinopathy of prematurity and retinal haemorrhages associated with "shaken baby syndrome". The hand-held camera is placed gently on the cornea interfaced with ophthalmic lubricant. It produces excellent reproducible images and its advantage over conventional indirect ophthalmoscopy is that of data and image recording and also its ease of use. It is also a very gentle examination in comparison to sclera indentation. However Adams et al. (2004) reported a case of retinal haemorrhaging after RetCam 120 use, highlighting the fragility of the infant retinal vascular system. The RetCam can detect disease up to anterior zone 11 which accounts for over 90% of retinopathy of prematurity requiring treatment. Despite this, the suitability of the RetCam for screening for retinopathy of prematurity, its sensitivity and specificity for detecting the various stages of the disease remains underdetermined but is gaining more and more acceptance. Yen et al. (2002) concluded that RetCam images had insufficient sensitivity to replace the indirect ophthalmoscope. In contrast, Ells et al. (2003) reported that over the course of a longitudinal series of examinations that digital photography can identify eyes at risk for progression to severe retinopathy of prematurity which would require treatment. Based on a pilot study they reported excellent specificity and sensitivity for remote detection of severe retinopathy of prematurity using the digitised images which were examined remotely by an experienced reader. Wu et al. (2006) compared screening and management results recommended by both indirect ophthalmoscopy and RetCam users and concluded that digital photography had a sensitivity of 100% and a specificity of 97.5%. In 43 infants they noted that screening and management of retinopathy of prematurity using RetCam imaging did not fail to detect pre-threshold or threshold disease when images could be obtained. However it was noted that indirect ophthalmological examinations were required in 20% of cases due to poor image quality or overestimation of retinopathy of prematurity. RetCam digital screening has been used with great success in some countries such as Germany.

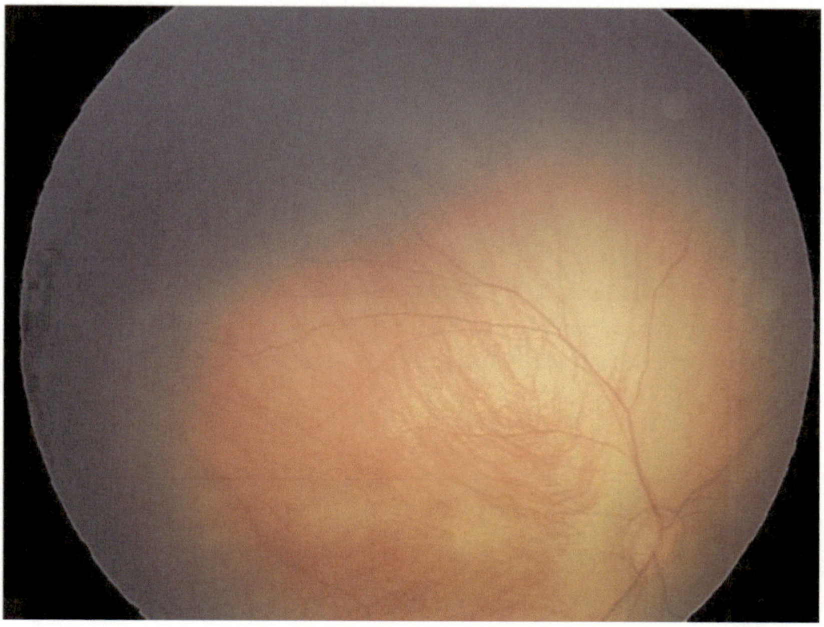

Fig. 3. Stage 1 retinopathy of prematurity. Demarcation line: This is a definite structure that separates the avascular from the vascular retina.

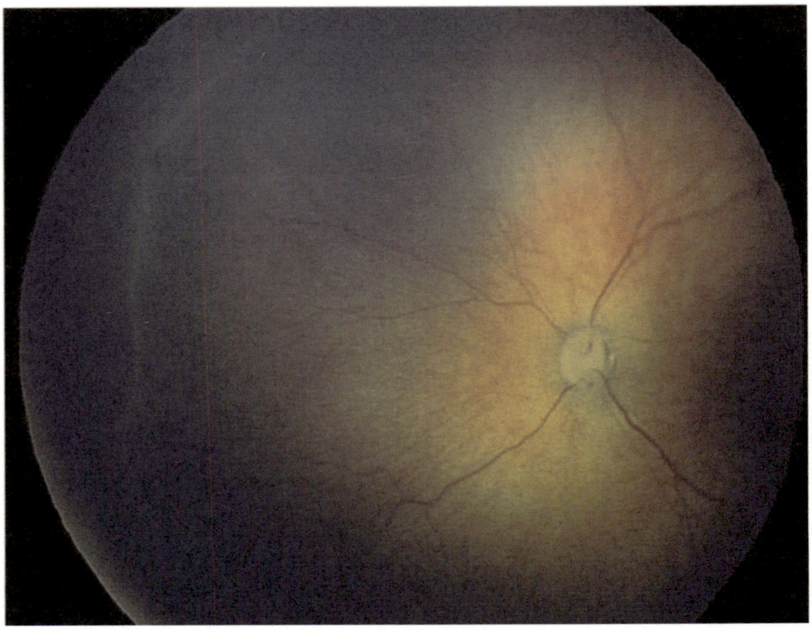

Fig. 4. Stage 2 Retinopathy of Prematurity. The Ridge: This is the hallmark of the stage 2 disease. It arises from the demarcation line and has length and width. It extends above the plane of the retina.

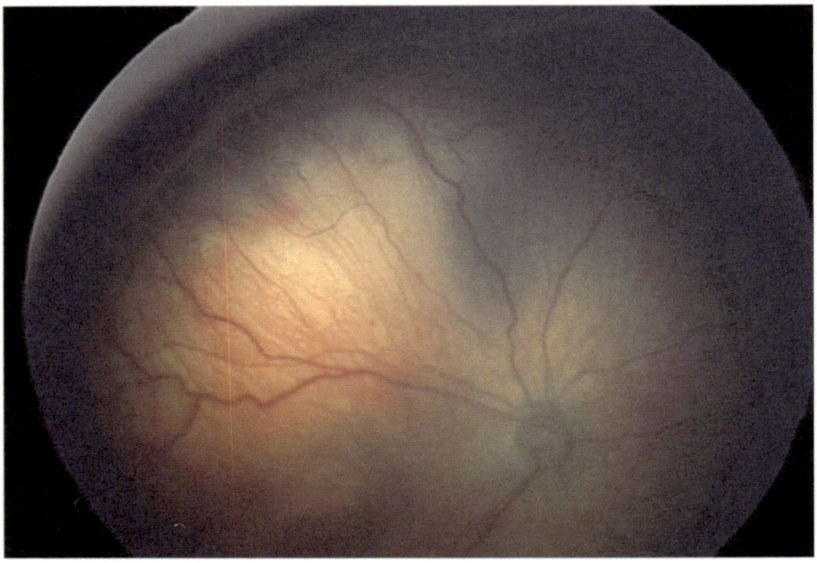

Fig. 5. Stage 3 retinopathy of prematurity. Extra retinal fibrovascular proliferation: Extends from the ridge into the vitreous. It can be divided into mild, moderate and severe depending on vitreous involvement.

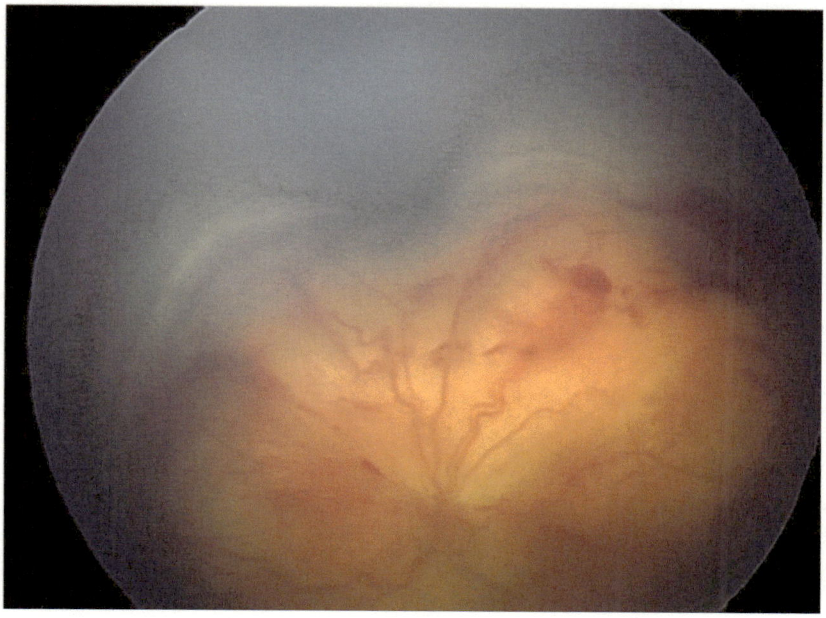

Fig. 6. Stage 4a retinopathy of prematurity: Extra-foveal partial retinal detachment.

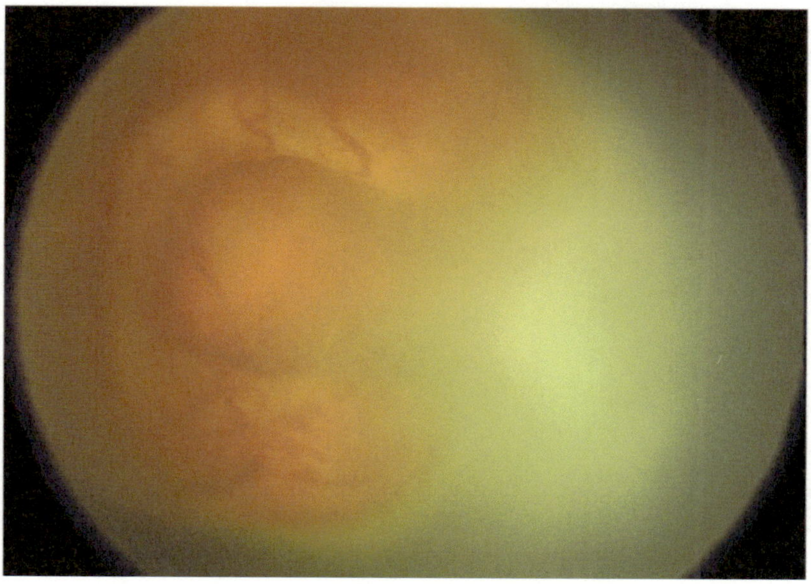

Fig. 7. Stage 4b retinopathy of prematurity: Foveal partial retinal detachment.

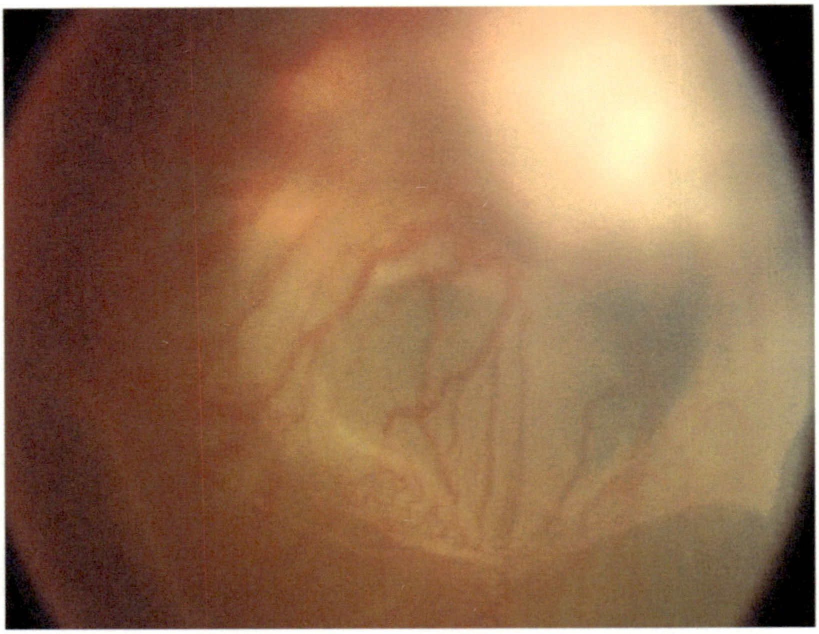

Fig. 8. Stage 5 Retinopathy of prematurity: Total retinal detachment. These detachments are generally tractional and may occasionally be exudative. They are usually funnel shaped.

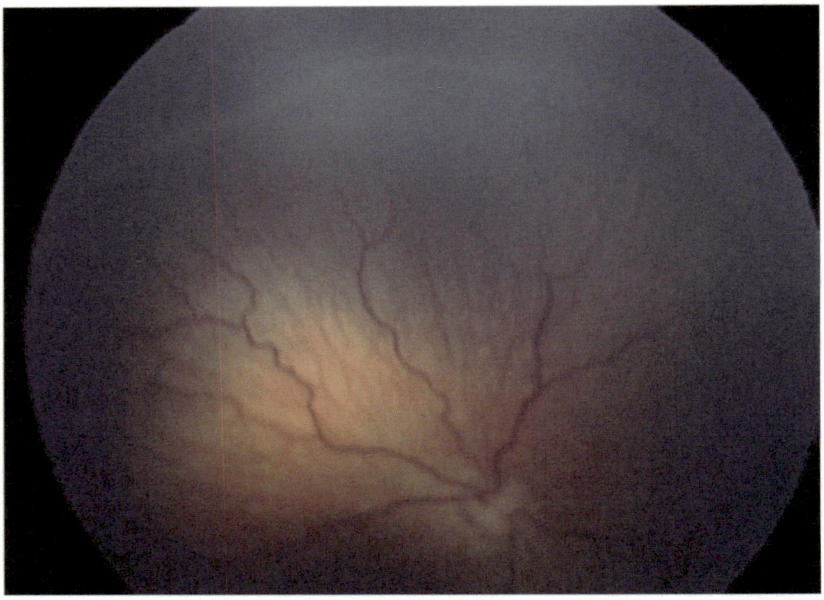

Fig. 9. Plus disease: These are additional signs indicating the severity of active retinopathy of prematurity disease. 1. Venous dilation, anterior tortuosity of posterior pole vessels. 2. Iris vascular engorgement. 3. Pupil rigidity. 4. Vitreous haze.

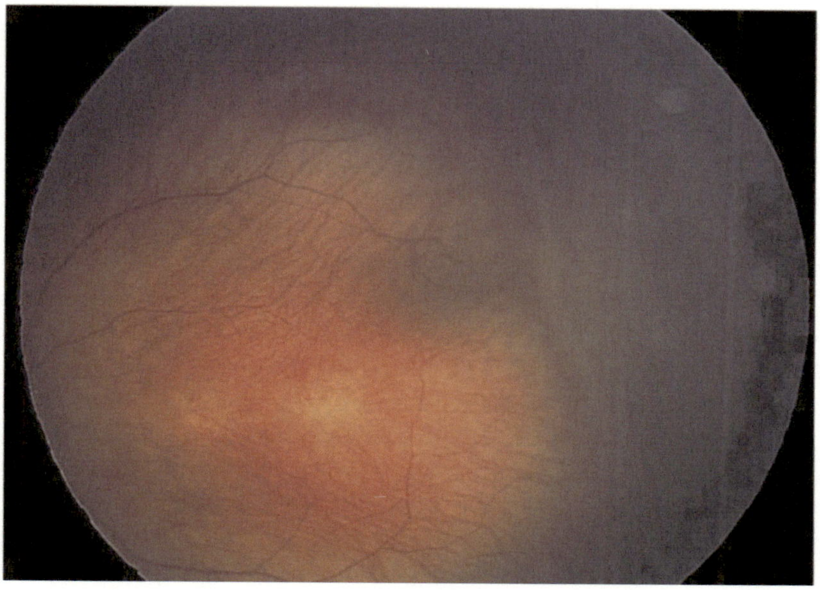

Fig. 10. Pre-plus disease: This is defined as vascular abnormality of the posterior pole but insufficient to form a diagnosis of plus disease but demonstrates more arterial tortuosity and more venous dilation than normal.

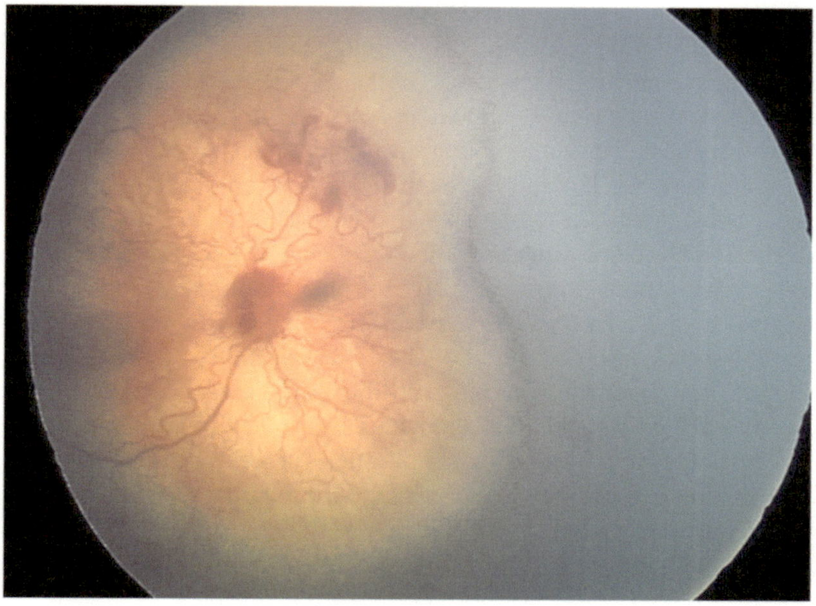

Fig. 11. Aggressive posterior retinopathy of prematurity. This is a rapidly progressive form of retinopathy of prematurity. It can progress to stage 5 retinopathy of prematurity. It has a posterior location with prominence of plus disease. It is observed in zone I or posterior zone II.

5. Future advances in screening

The advent of the telemedicine approach to screening in retinopathy of prematurity raises some important issues. With increasing survivals and expectations for premature infants this is a growing area in terms of litigation. Many ophthalmologists no longer screen for this condition and specialist expertise in retinopathy of prematurity staging is frequently not available in the peripheral hospitals. The reading of digital images by a remote expert could potentially improve the accessibility, quality and cost of retinopathy of prematurity management (Richter et al. 2009). There is the potential for trained neonatal nurses to carry out retinopathy of prematurity screening examinations safely and effectively with the RetCam. This could dramatically reduce the number of indirect ophthalmoscopy examinations needed to be carried out. As a result there would be the potential to maximise effective screening whilst minimising valuable personnel resource time. Diagnostic accuracy and reliability of remote imaging interpretation by experts would have to be assured. Lorenz et al. (2009) reported the success with using wide field digital imaging (RetCam 120) based telemedicine over a six year period where 1,222 infants were screened. They concluded that all treatment requiring retinopathy of prematurity was detected in time with sensitivity for detecting suspected treatment-requiring retinopathy of prematurity at 100% and a positive predictive value for treatment-requiring retinopathy of prematurity 82.4%. This study is a very positive endorsement for the potential future of telemedicine in retinopathy of prematurity screening. The RetCam is expensive however and may not be cost-effective in those centres where a limited number of infants require screening.

6. Conclusion

Screening for retinopathy of prematurity in a timely manner remains the most important initial step in the detection and management of the condition. This is of great importance as it is acknowledged that earlier treatment of the condition results in improved visual outcomes and prognosis. It is becoming increasingly recognized that retinopathy of prematurity is a disease for life and there are significant long-term sequelae. All neonatal units caring for babies at risk of retinopathy of prematurity should have a written protocol in relation to screening. During the screening examination techniques such as nesting the baby will reduce the infants stress and pain and this should be encouraged. Training of ophthalmologists in the technique of screening for retinopathy of prematurity and the recognition of the disease should not be overlooked so that a larger pool of ophthalmologists can perform screening in the peripheral hospitals. Whilst indirect ophthalmoscopy is the gold standard examination device, RetCam digital image systems are becoming increasingly important. The application of telemedicine to retinopathy of prematurity screening is encouraging and positive and in larger neonatal units telemedicine may almost certainly play a much bigger role in the future.

7. References

Hunter DG, Mukai S. (1992). Retinopathy of prematurity: pathogenesis, diagnosis andtreatment. *Int Ophthalmol Clin* 1992;32:163-84.

Gibson DL, Sheps SB,Uh SH, Schechter MT, McCormick AQ.(1990). Retinopathy of prematurity- induced blindness: birth weight-specific survival and the new epidemic. *Paediatrics* 1990;86:405-12.

Flyn JT, O' Grady GE, Herrera J, Kushner BJ, Cantolino S, Milam W. (1977). Retrolental fibroplasias: clinical observations. *Arch Ophthalmol* 1977;95:217-23.

An international classification of retinopathy of prematurity. (1984). *Paediatrics*1984;74(1):127-33.

Multicenter trial of cryotherapy for retinopathy of prematurity. Preliminary results. Cryotherapy for retinopathy of prematurity cooperative group. (1988). *Arch Ophthalmol.* 1988;106(4):471–479.

Early treatment for retinopathy of prematurity cooperative group. (2003). Revised indications for the treatment of retinopathy of prematurity: results of the early treatment for retinopathy of prematurity randomized trial. *Arch Ophthalmol.* 2003;121(12):1684–1694.

Gilbert C, Rahi J, Eckstein M, O'Sullivan J, Foster A. (1997).Retinopathy of prematurity in middle-income countries. *Lancet.* 1997;350(9070):12–14.

Phan MH, Nguyen PN, Reynolds JD.(2003). Incidence and severity of retinopathy of prematurity in Vietnam, a developing middle-income country. *J Pediatr Ophthalmol Strabismus.* 2003;40(4):208–212.

Screening examination of premature infants for retinopathy of prematurity.(2006).Section on Ophthalmology, American Academy of Pediatrics, American Academy of Ophthalmology American Association for Pediatric Ophthalmology and Strabismus. *Pediatrics.* 2006;117:572–576.

UK Retinopathy of Prematurity Guideline . Royal College of Paediatrics & Child Health & Royal College of Opthalmologists. 2007.

Subhani M, Combs A, Weber P, Gerontis C, DeCristofaro JD. (2011). Screening guidelines for retinopathy of prematurity: the need for revision in extremely low birth weight infants. *Pediatrics.* 2001;107(4):656–659.

Laws DE, Morton C, Weindling M, Clark D. (1996). Systemic effects of screening for retinopathy of prematurity. *Br J Ophthalmol.* 1996;80(5):425–428.

Slevin M, Murphy JF, Daly L, O'Keefe M.(1997). Retinopathy of prematurity screening, stress related responses, the role of nesting. *Br J Ophthalmol.* 1997;81(9):762–764.

Adams GW, Clark BJ, Fang S, Hill S.(2004). Retinal haemorrhages in an infant following RetCam screening for retinopathy of prematurity. *Eye.* 2004;18:652-653.

Yen KG, Hess D, Burke B, Johnson RA, Feuer WJ, Flynn JT. (2002). Telephotoscreening to detect retinopathy of prematurity: preliminary study of the optimum time to employ digital fundus camera imaging to detect ROP. *J AAPOS.* 2002;6(2):64–70.

Ells AL, Holmes JM, Astle WF, Williams G, Leske DA, Fielden M, et al. (2003).Telemedicine approach to screening for severe retinopathy of prematurity: a pilot study. *Ophthalmology.* 2003;110(11):2113–2117.

Wu C, Petersen RA, VanderVeen DK. (2006). RetCam imaging for retinopathy of prematurity screening. *J APPOS.* 2006 ;10(2):107-11.

Richter GM, Williams SL, Sarren J, Flynn JT, Chiang MF. (2009). Telemedicine for retinopathy of prematurity diagnosis: evaluation and challenges. *Surv Ophthalmol.*2009;54(6):67-85.

Lorenz B, Spasovska K, Elflein H,Schneider N. (2009). Wide-field digital imaging based telemedicine for screening for acute retinopathy of prematurity (ROP). Six-year results of a multicentre field study. *Graefes Arch Clin Exp Ophthalmol.* 2009;247(9):1251-62.

19

Teleophthalmology

Manoj Kulshrestha[1], Simon P Kelly[2] and Usman Mahmood[1]
[1]Aberystwyth Eye Centre/Hywel Dda Local Health Board
[2]Royal Bolton Hospital
United Kingdom

1.Introduction

In the recent years there has been significant growth in Information Technology. The internet has also transformed clinical care. IT interventions and consultations are being introduced rapidly and on a large scale across health care. These telemedicine consultations can be divided into two categories: 'synchronous telemedicine' utilizes telecommunications for real time interactions between participants (e.g. video conferencing), and 'store-and-forward' telemedicine which involves the capture of patient data for subsequent interpretation by a remote expert.

In image-oriented specialties such as ophthalmology, radiology, cardiology, and dermatology, diagnostic decisions are often based on review of photographic/imaging studies and which are often captured by technicians. Therefore, remote diagnosis using store-and-forward telemedicine may be a promising strategy for improving the delivery and accessibility of care in image-oriented fields.

Randomised controlled trial evaluation of such service innovations on service provision would be ideal, but are rarely possible. A recent such report by Chiang MF et al., 2010 favourably compared telemedicine examination in retinopathy of prematurity infants against direct examination. A service evaluation by Stoves J et al., 2010 showed e-consultation with hospital nephrologists promotes effective management of patients with mild-to-moderate chronic kidney disease in primary care in the National Health Service (NHS). In areas where accessibility to clinical care is problematic such as in parts of Canada, Australia, India and Wales, there are major challenges to healthcare. Advances in videoconferencing technologies have had a positive impact in telemedicine care in such rural regions. We have worked in ophthalmology in rural Wales, where district general hospitals and community hospitals have excellent telemedicine links. This chapter provides case studies from telemedicine in ophthalmology based on our experience and that of others elsewhere.

Rurality has its own unique problems for healthcare, patients, medical and nursing staff. All usually have longer distances to travel compared to urban areas. There are increased fuel and transport costs and often poor transport infrastructure. However such rural areas in Wales (Figure 1) may have a high concentration of elderly people with sight problems.

The learning goal of this chapter is better understanding of novel technology for ophthalmic disease management deployed in the digital heath environment. This is a topic of considerable significance in retinal care given the explosion of relevant clinical imaging technology and the huge burden of certain retinal disease (age-related macular degeneration, retinal vein occlusion and diabetic retinopathy) and which are set to expand even more.

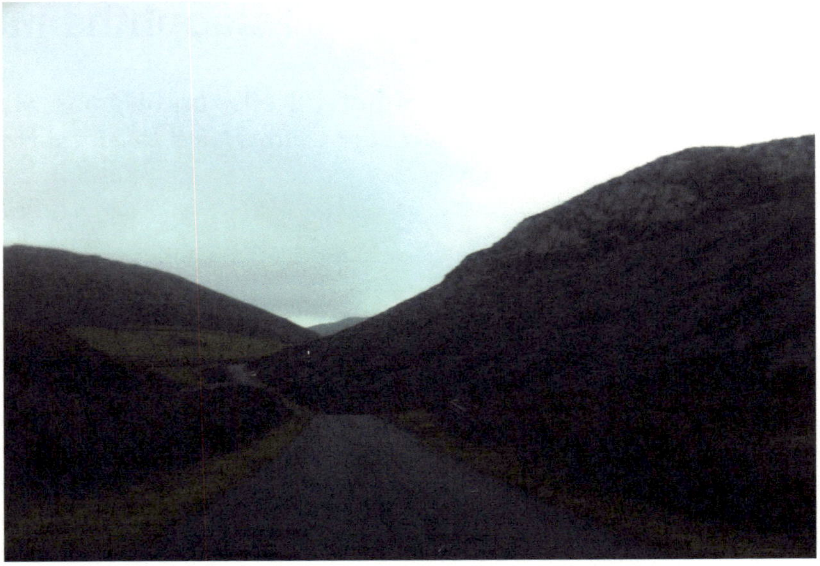

Fig. 1. Sparsely populated rural environment in Wales.

Smarter ways of working, using new technology, are required to cope with this clinical need and organisational burden. The need includes better use of IT infrastructure; innovation in primary to secondary care referral management and enhanced productivity in secondary care. Some **clinical IT/imaging driven solutions** to such challenges will be explored.

Teleophthalmology may be considered a division of telemedicine and is technological method by which medical expertise from an ophthalmologist is provided electronically to another clinical location, sometimes in rural or remote areas. Teleophthalmology includes enabling the ophthalmologist to interact with patients at a remote location through video conferencing, share data, and diagnose the patient with the help of local non ophthalmologist doctor or nurse or other practitioner who uses ophthalmic diagnostic equipment to digitally transfer images.

Telemedicine in general is an area which brings collaboration between secondary and primary care, enabling secure transmission of information and in particular for ophthalmology, transfer of digital clinical images. Ophthalmology relies greatly on clinical visual information. Dermatology is another specialty with similar matters. The pilot project of teledermatology in Bristol described in the Practical Commissioning Magazine (2009) found that referrals fell by about 62% in a single practice, providing patients with a faster, closer service. Safety and cost effectiveness of any telemedicine specialty needs further assessment. The provision of a safe, reliable and fast telemedicine ophthalmic service to the public may have merit in rural areas.

Currently there are only 2.3 ophthalmologists per 100,000 population in the UK. This is fewer, pro rata, than in any other European Union nation (European Union of Medical Specialties www.uems.net). Together with a high level of undetected, yet treatable visual morbidity and an increasing elderly population, improvements in primary eye care are needed. Telemedicine in ophthalmology, or teleophthalmology, offers some merit in responding to these pressures in the digital era in both developed and emerging economies with sparse ophthalmic manpower and in any economy where distance to the ophthalmologist is a problem. The latter is especially relevant in rural and remote areas.

2. Digital retinal fundus photography imaging

Modern fundus cameras (such as the Topcon non-mydratic camera shown in Figure 2) have high resolution and an ability to alter contrast and colour thereby allowing for such manipulation of images that at times might not be possible even with direct view. Such cameras are presently employed for diabetic retinopathy (DR) screening in the community. All diabetic patients in the UK are now able to have regular screening for sight threatening diabetic retinopathy and such screening significantly reduces visual morbidity. High resolution fundus photographs are taken and linked via servers to trained primary retinal screeners who grade the image by retinopathy severity status and arrange referral if needed. Such diabetic patients often may not need to travel to the hospital. Secondary or tertiary screeners can also undertake remote digital imaging screening.
(www.diabetes.org.uk/About_us/Our_Views/Position_statements/retinal_screening)

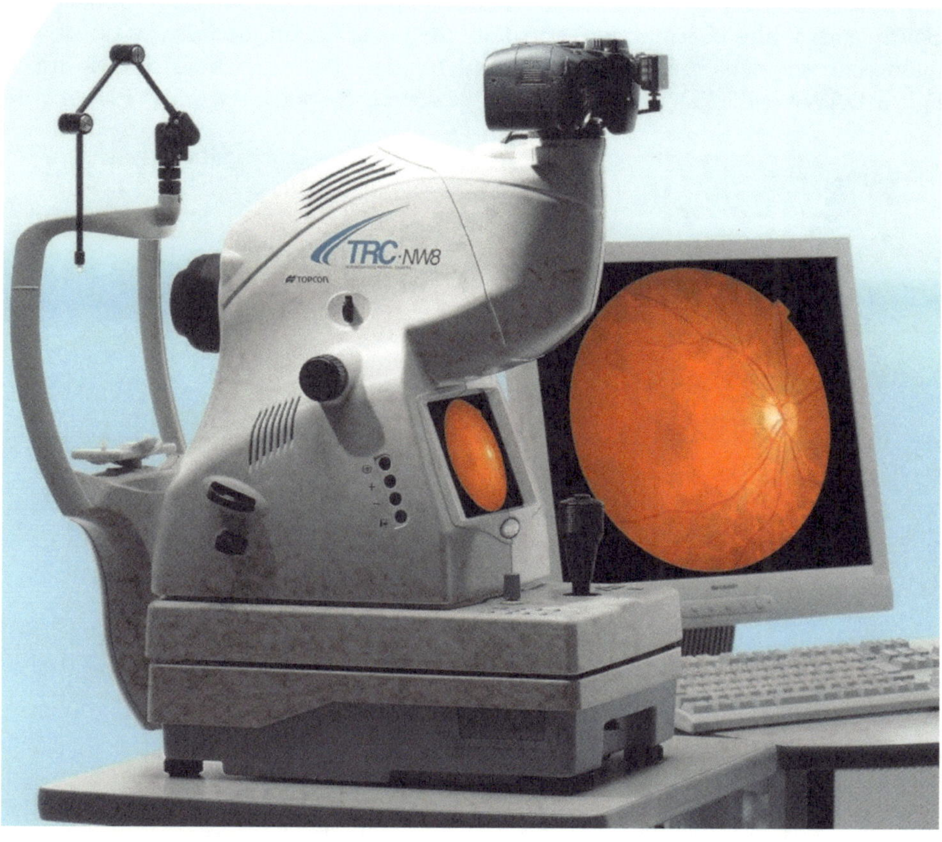

Fig. 2. Digital fundus camera. (Topcon)

The Central Ophthalmology Receiving Unit in NHS Fife, Scotland reported the benefits of improving use of existing resources to bridge the gap between primary and secondary ophthalmic care (Cameron JR et al., 2009). Hansen C et al., 2008 have described a similar government funded scheme in Alberta and in the Northwest Territories of Canada (www.teleophthalmology.com) which allows remote rural optometrists to transmit fundus photographs to retinal specialists in the regional centre.

In countries where such an infrastructure does not currently exist, Universal Service Funds (USFs) could be utilised for this purpose. These are internationally available funds that accompany government tax breaks (Nakajima L ,2010). USF promotes the development of telecommunication services in un-served and under-served areas throughout the length and breadth of a country. They help to bring the digital image transfer to a rural population and increase the level of connectivity significantly in the rural areas through effective and fair utilization of the fund. They help towards significant advances towards enhancement of e-services, both in rural as well as urban areas of the country.

2.1 Diabetic retinopathy screening service for Wales

In Wales all diabetic patients undergo annual screening for retinopathy in local community hospitals or GP surgeries depending on the rural location. Digital fundus imaging is carried out with dilation of the patients' pupils. The photographs are saved onto laptops with strict security access codes. Images are stored in data centres in North Wales, (Carnaervon), Mid and South West Wales (Carmarthen) and Trefforest near Cardiff at Fairway Court which is the main centre to which all images are sent for data backup. These centres are linked through a $DAWN_2METRO$ VPN (Figure 3). A virtual private network (VPN) is a secure

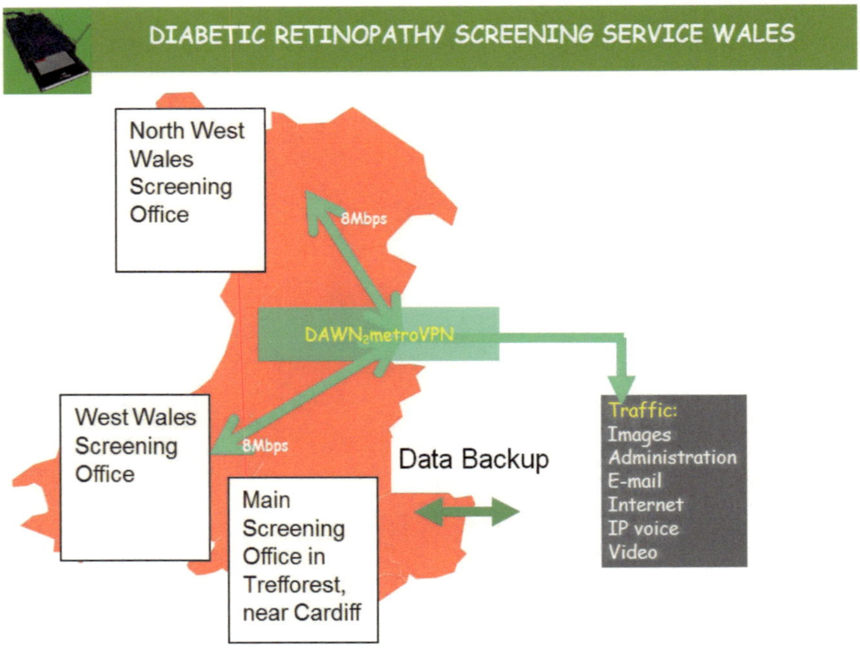

Fig. 3. Overview of IT Links between 3 Sites in Wales for Diabetic Retinopathy Screening Service for Wales using $DAWN_2$metroVPN

authentication to a network enabling a gateway for all computers at all sites to be connected. Tele-ophthalmology is enabled as all computers are on the same network. Graders at Trefforest carry out primary and secondary retinal screening across this VPN.

2.2 Teleophthalmology for paediatric retinal disorders

Retinopathy of prematurity (ROP) is a leading cause of irreversible visual impairment in childhood. Timely treatment usually prevents blindness. Provision of objective documented clinical images is critical in ROP care. Digital retinal image capture is used for screening of premature or low birth weight babies for retinopathy of prematurity. Images are captured with a digital retinal camera, most often the Retcam instrument (Fig 4). Furthermore such images can be captured by non-ophthalmic staff in the neonatal intensive care unit. Validation studies of telemedicine for ROP diagnosis have demonstrated that its accuracy, intergrader reliability, and intra-grader reliability are high and are comparable to or better than that of other widely accepted diagnostic tests (Victor G et al., 2009).

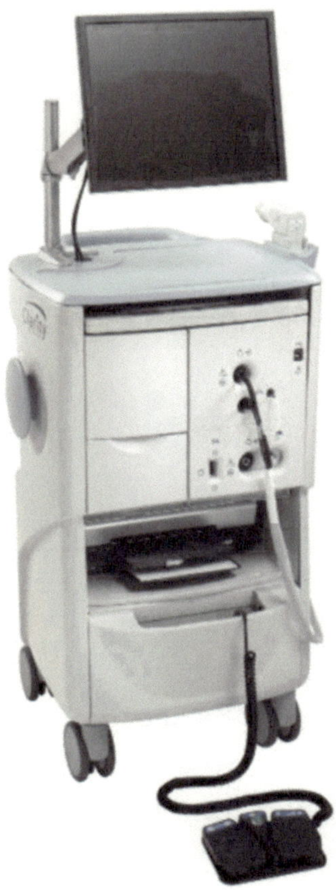

Fig. 4. Retcam instrument (Clarity Medical Systems) for retinopathy of prematurity screening

Skilled ROP screeners may grade neonatal retinal images in a central location that can be remote from the neonatal unit. Where a shortage of ophthalmologists capable of undertaking or providing ROP screening exists, this mode of teleophthalmology is a solution to maintaining a credible and efficient screening service. Other urgent paediatric ophthalmic pathology, such as retinoblastoma, can also be imaged via the Retcam. Fundus images of retinae of suspected non-accidental injury (shaken babies) for diagnostic and medico legal purposes can also be taken via a Retcam and the images subsequently transferred for expert opinion.

Advantages of the Retcam include its portability and manoeuvrability to the bedside in constrained areas such as on the Neonatal Intensive Unit. It can be transported between hospitals and clinics, and allows transfer of retinal images to any networked system. It allows timely remote evaluation of patient images and provides advanced image analysis and comparison capability of previous images with review software.

3. Urgent eye care and teleophthalmology

Anterior segment cameras (Figure 5) can be used in Accident and Emergency settings by nurses and ophthalmologists. Images from such instruments are similarly uploaded via a central server. The ophthalmologist in a central location is then able to make decisions on the urgency of an ophthalmic opinion, suggest treatment online that can be accessed by the remote practitioner after a specified time (very similar to PACS reporting of radiology images) or arrange a referral. This allows rural populations to benefit from an emergency ophthalmic service.

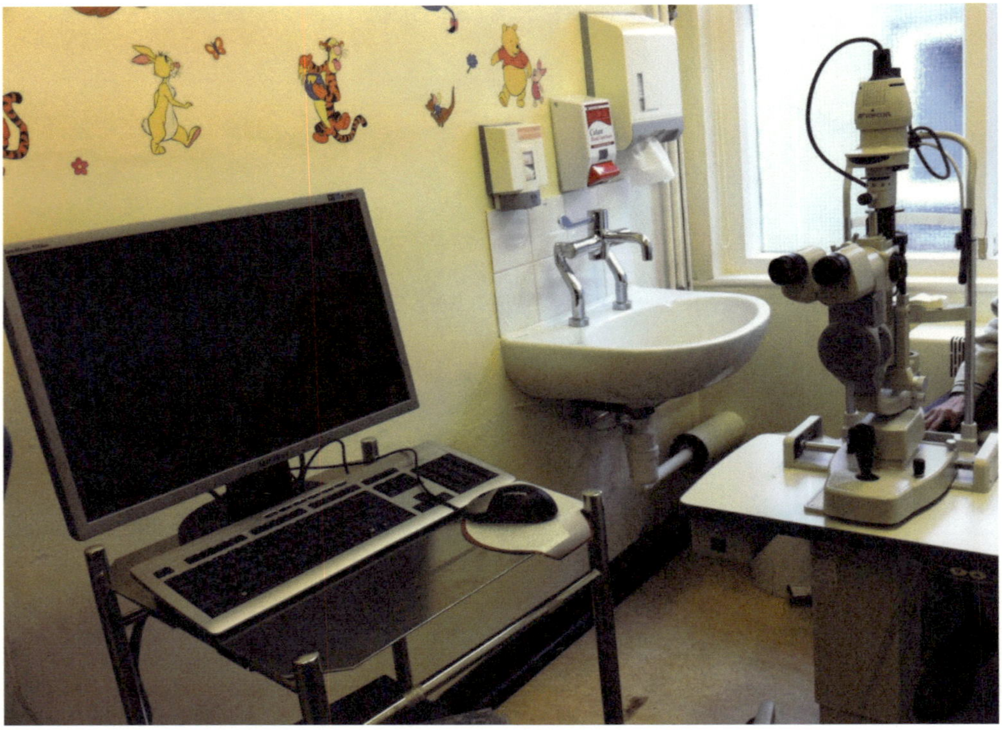

Fig. 5. Anterior segment digital camera in peripheral clinic in Wales.

Ophthalmologic accidents and emergencies,) are an important public health matter and component of hospital workload. (Bhopal RS (1993). The most prevalent such problems are corneal foreign bodies, corneal abrasions and conjunctivitis (Girard B et al., 2002). In rural areas, such patients are usually seen by general practitioners, who often lack expertise or the equipment for the management of eye emergencies.

3.1 The Welsh experience of teleophthalmology for urgent eye care

We piloted a teleophthalmology service in rural Wales, as described by Kulshrestha MK et al., 2010. Tywyn Hospital is located in a rural setting in Gwynedd, Snowdonia, North Wales (Figure 6). Ophthalmic medical staff are based at Bronglais District General Hospital, Aberystwyth, which lies in the neighbouring county of Ceredigion. Management of ophthalmic services is controlled from Carmarthen, in South Wales. There is poor provision of public transport between Tywyn and Aberystwyth which is one hour away by car. The road journey from Carmarthen to Tywyn is three and a half hours. The region therefore extends over a wide area of North and West Wales.

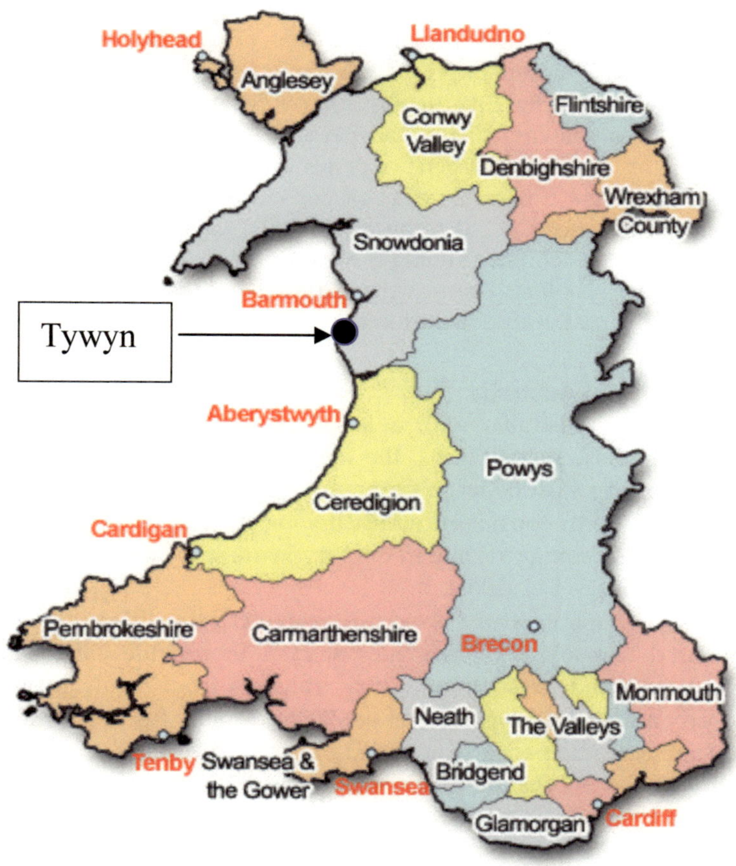

Fig. 6. Map of Wales and Counties, showing location of Tywyn, in South Gwynedd (Snowdonia)

More than 80% of the population live in rural areas and there are 1.88 ophthalmologists per 100,000 population, with narrow roads and poor transport links. This is lower than the UK average figure of 2.3 ophthalmologists per 100,000 population.

This teleophthalmology service involved nurses, IT professionals and managers from the Betsi Cadwaladr Local Health Board (Gwynedd, Snowdonia) and ophthalmologists from the neighbouring Hywel Dda Health Board (Carmarthenshire, Ceredigion and Pembrokeshire), illustrating partnership by working across these two different Health Boards.

All ophthalmic emergencies from South Gwynedd are assessed by nurses in Tywyn Accident and Emergency Department. Any patients who require a consultant ophthalmologist's opinion need referral to Bronglais Accident and Emergency for specialist referral.One hundred and twenty four eye emergencies were seen in Tywyn Accident and Emergency Department in 2008. Consultant Ophthalmologist clinics are held once every two weeks. Some emergencies are seen in the eye clinic, but if these urgent cases occur/present at other times and require a ophthalmic opinion, transfer to Aberystwyth by ambulance is required. A teleophthalmology service has now been developed between the peripheral unit in Tywyn and the central unit at Bronglais Hospital, so eye emergency patients seen by the nurses on duty in Tywyn can be better treated. Ophthalmic signs are visualised by transmission of images from a Topcon SL D7 Slit Lamp camera (Fig 5) in the peripheral clinic through a Polycom or NEC Videoconferencing Unit (Figure 8) to the central Bronglais Hospital, Aberystwyth. Live or real time video tele-consultations with patients and staff can be held to initiate immediate management, treatment and advice.

Fenton et al found in an audit of emergencies presenting to a city centre eye department in Dublin that 60 - 70% of these referrals did not constitute accidents or urgent conditions needing urgent specialist attention . (Fenton et al., 2001) Given this scenario, an internet-based system for eye care (teleophthalmology) would help to avoid unnecessary transfer of patients with non-urgent problems by emergency ambulance or helicopter, saving transport costs and time, as well as road traffic pollution in rural areas.

3.2 Tele-ophthalmology in Australia

In the state of Western Australia, with a land area ten times larger than UK, most ophthalmologists are based in Perth, the major city of this region. Models of teleophthalmology services exist between Carnarvon in North West Australia, where clinics are run by nurses and Perth consultant ophthalmologists (Figure 7). Patients detected to have an urgent sight threatening problem in Carnarvon are sent by helicopter for emergency treatment in Perth (Kumar S et al., 2006).

Access to emergency treatment in rural areas can often mean the difference between life and death. Internet-based technologies have the potential to provide earlier diagnosis and intervention, save lives and avoid unnecessary transfers from rural hospital emergency departments to urban hospitals (Kumar S et al., 2006) Benefits for rural healthcare staff in skills acquisition and education are also evident.

There is a real need for ophthalmic emergency services in rural regional hospitals. An internet service may be the most efficient way to triage these emergencies. A decline (15%) in the number of eye related cases in Carnarvon, Australia may be related to a number of people presenting themselves directly for the teleconsultation service.

While acknowledging that the time comparisons need to be more appropriate by comparing 'like-for-like', at Carnaervon, the average time of an internet consultation was 30 min against a 2-h and 45-min turnaround time for an emergency department evaluation (Ellis et al.,

2001). A variety of emergency complaints were managed effectively using relatively low-cost internet-based telemedicine technology, thereby eliminating the need for transportation of the distant patient to the city-centre emergency department.

Specialist diagnostics is readily available and a better assessment of patient's evacuation urgency is made using the internet service. Other benefits included earlier diagnosis and intervention, a shorter stay in hospital (if hospitalisation is deemed necessary) and avoided traveling for the patient.

While conventional, face-to-face consultation with a specialist doctor is beneficial; availability, access and costs are often barriers in remote regions. Internet services offer a substitution for conventionally provided emergency services in rural and remote regions. Furthermore, urban specialists are usually satisfied with such arrangement as it may enhance potential income, skill and practice, without disrupting conventional consultations at central hospital facilities.

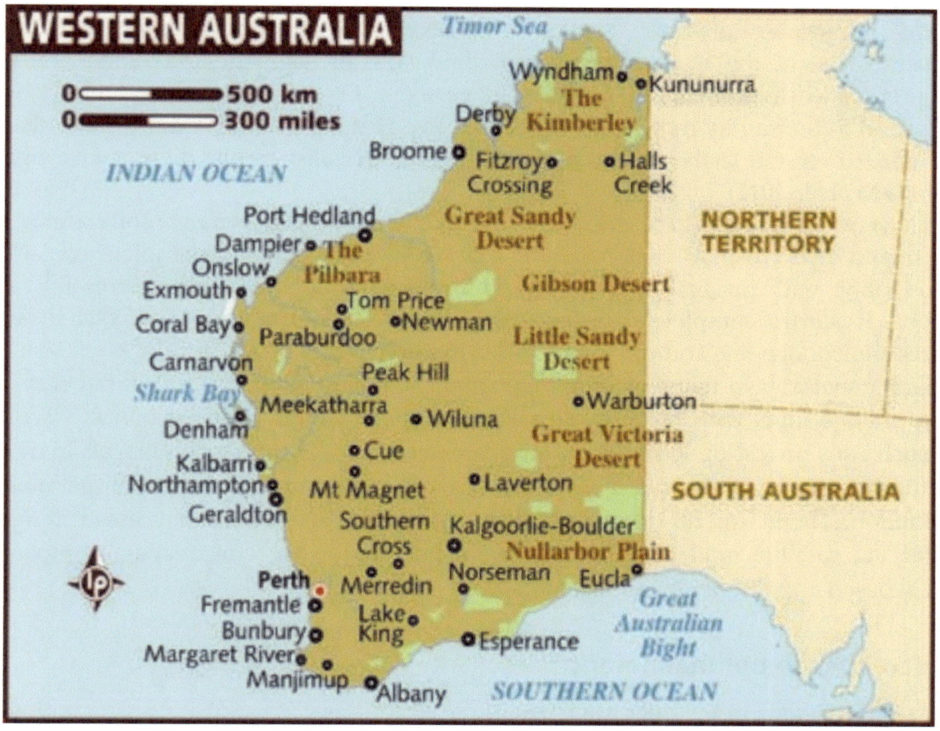

Fig. 7. Map of Western Australia showing Carnarvon to the NorthWest where Nurses have Teleophthalmology equipment and Perth on the South West Coast where Consultant Ophthalmologists can obtain photographic or live video images

The cost of an established tele-ophthalmology service has been compared with the cost of three other existing eye-care service delivery options by Kanagasingam and Yogesan K, 2006. During a 12-month study period, 118 persons took part in the tele-ophthalmology consultations between a rural clinic located approximately 900 km from the Lions Eye Institute in Perth. The variable costs of tele-ophthalmology were \$166.89 (AUD) per patient, and the alternatives cost \$445.96, \$271.48 and \$665.44 per patient. Tele-ophthalmology incurred a set-up cost of \$13,340. The threshold at which tele-ophthalmology became cheaper than any of the alternative options occurred at a total workload of 128 patients. Tele-ophthalmology therefore offered a viable alternative to conventional eye-care service in rural and remote areas.

3.3 Experience in India with teleophthalmology

Eighty percent of India's population lives in rural areas (Gullapi N, 2000). However, seventy percent of the healthcare resources are in urban areas. There is one ophthalmologist per 100,000 population, 70% of whom practice in urban area.

Teleophthalmology reduced the need to travel and holds potential for improved quality, access and affordability of healthcare. There can be at least 50 community centres attached to one tertiary hospital centre (http://www.laico.org/v2020res ource/files/teleophthalmolo g_in_india.PDF). In these 'Vision Centres' there are mid level ophthalmic personnel (MLOP), who are similar to trained Ophthalmic Nurse Practitioners (htt p://www.lai co.org/v2020reso urc e/f il es/m lopICO.pdf). They are trained to take anterior segment and retinal images and perform intraocular pressure checks. They communicate online with a consultant ophthalmologist at the main hospital providing anterior segment and retinal images as appropriate and discuss clinical details of the patient. Of 91698 patients examined by this means from 5 community centres at the Aravind Eye Hospital, Tamil Nadu, South India, only 12.5% needed referral to the main centre for surgery, specialist consultation or investigations (Khurana M et al., 2011).

Eyestalk (www.aravind.org/telemedicine/eyestalkhome.htm) is dynamic software in use at the Aravind Eye Hospital that makes it safe and simple to send complete consultation records along with images from slit lamps to specialists at main eye centres for second opinions. It allows complete confidentiality of patient information. This system simply requires a telephone line and computer with a modem to function.

The Sankaranethralaya teleophthalmology network as described by Thulasi Bai et al., 2007 utilizes mobile units with teleophthalmology equipment with satellite connectivity. There are 6 such vans providing local ophthalmic care in community outreach villages. In over 800 community camps over 15,000 patients have benefited from a teleophthalmological consultation. There was no degrading effect on compressed or uncompressed images on transfer via satellite, and consultations were extremely cost effectiveness compared to hospital based appointments.

4. Video links in ophthalmology

Live or synchronous video links are currently used in Wales, Australia, Canada and remote parts of the USA to allow patients in remote or inaccessible areas to be examined in emergency settings by an ophthalmologist (Figure 8). Before the advent of teleophthalmology either treatment was delayed or patients needed to be evacuated to a central hospital. Video links allow live anterior ocular segment examination and also a direct communication with the patient. Fundus cameras and optical coherence tomograpahy (OCT) imaging can also be employed for retinal examination.

The zoom control function allows accurate assessment of ocular motility, allowing assessment of trauma/falls and accident cases where there has been orbital injury. In case of suspected orbital fracture the nurse practitioner or doctor can be instructed to check the infra-orbital nerve sensation and a management plan/treatment can be given over the video-link by the ophthalmologist without the need for the patient to travel to the main centre. Orbital radiological imaging is also undertaken taken locally and are available for viewing by the radiologist through the PACS system.

The Sony or Canon pan/tilt/zoom video cameras used with many of the desktop videoconferencing systems can also be used for acquiring diagnostic still images, as well as video clips during the ocular motility assessment. These cameras generally have at least 470 horizontal lines of resolution, which is equivalent to a digital still image resolution of 640 x 480 pixels.

Most of these cameras have either a composite or S-video signal output to allow the video signal from the camera to be transferred to any standard PC video capture card. Thus, both still image captures of the ocular alignment in primary gaze can be obtained. The PC video capture card is purchased separately and should be TWAIN compliant. Flashbus, Pinnacle, AVI, Matrox video capture cards are some of the popular video capture cards used in many of the telemedicine systems. The video capture card chosen should support JPEG, TIFF, MPEG, and AVI file formats. Cards that support MJPEG or MPEG-2 compression formats would be ideal, because they provide higher image quality. Some healthcare organisations such as NHS Trusts, however do not support storage of clinical data on video cards and only support clinical data storage on the networked central server.

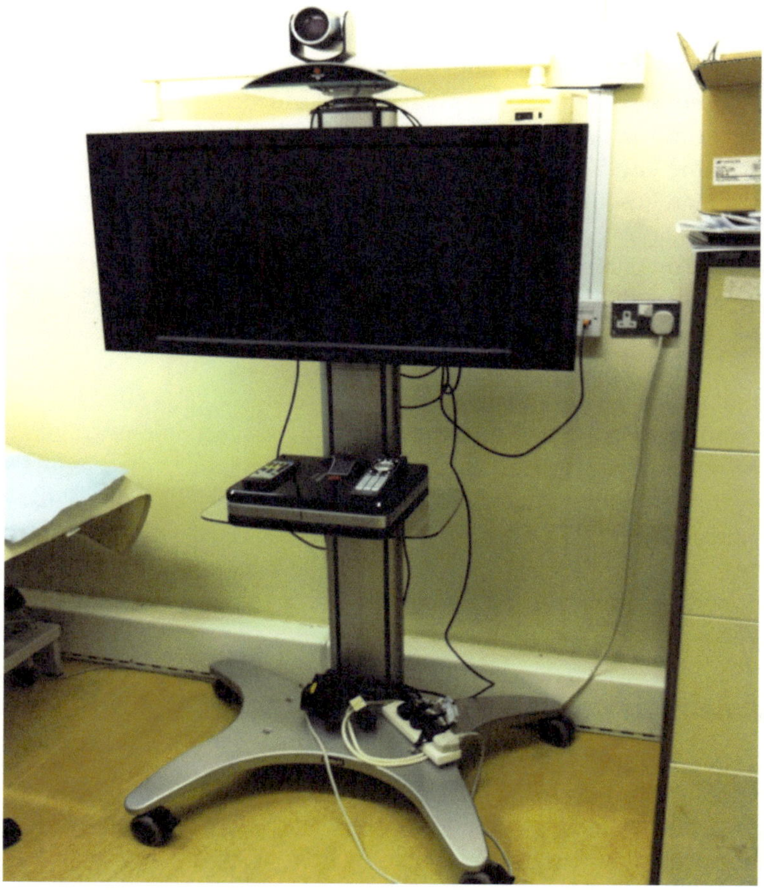

Fig. 8. Videoconferencing instrument at Tywyn Hospital

Pre-recorded video files can be used by optometrists and nurse practitioners. Video files record anterior segment, retinal or fluorescein imaging and these are uploaded via a central server and examined and reported by an ophthalmologist. The ophthalmologist may be able to access the video AVI file from the central server at any location within the region providing the community hospital has teleophthalmology equipment which is linked to the main server.

4.1 Clinical advantages include

- Increase productivity of healthcare professionals
- Strengthen referral patterns
- Effectively educate hospital staff, clinicians and the community
- Extend patient care and expertise to remote areas
- Improve patient care

4.2 Non-clinical and administrative advantages include

- More effective planning and administrative meetings with point-and-click sharing of content
- Remote connection for executive and business meetings avoids unnecessary travel and expenses. In rural healthcare settings staff attending business meetings from different areas, often involves a large amount of travelling to a central location for managers and clinicians based at community hospitals. Use of videoconferencing has helped teams to make maximum use of the time available in the day, with minimum disruption to the general working day. This has dramatically reduced travelling times for staff in Wales
- Support Human Resources, which may be located far away from the main hospital, eye clinic. At community hospitals workforce issues may arise on a daily basis and Human Resource departments may be anything from 2-4 hours away by car in Wales. Use of videoconferencing to members of the human resources department has helped to resolve emergency staffing issues

4.3 Educational advantages include

- **Attend Continuing Medical Education events** by videoconference. Community nurses have attended teaching sessions at the main hospital via live videoconferencing and live power point presentations, thereby enhancing their knowledge and skills.
- **Conduct video grand rounds** sharing PC content, live patient encounters, or recorded procedures
- **Video connect to nursing schools** for up to date training and medical information
- **Conduct administrative training and medical education** using live or streaming video

5. Optical coherence tomography (OCT) and retinal imaging

Optical coherence tomography (OCT) imaging (Huang D et al.,1991) is a relatively new, non-invasive, tool in clinical imaging. In ophthalmic clinical practice OCT allows real time imaging of the layers of the retina. OCT allows much better diagnosis of retinal conditions than conventional ophthalmoscopy and or retinal photography. Importantly, many retinal conditions can be diagnosed rapidly using OCT scanning, where undertaken, and in our opinion referral triage be improved upon. In 'virtual macular clinics' review of OCT images, combined with fundus photographs for review of patients with macular degeneration is now being used. Fluorescein angiogram images can also be correlated in these virtual clinics, with OCT and other retinal images.

5.1 Teleophthalmology and age-related macular degeneration (AMD)

Age-related macular degeneration (AMD) is the leading cause of blindness in developed economies. Neovascular or wet-AMD accounts for more than half of all cases of registered sight and severe sight impairment (Bruce C et al., 2010) and approximately 26,000 new cases of wet-AMD develop every year in the UK (Owen et al., 2003). There have been major recent advances in the treatment of wet-AMD with the use of biological agents and in particular with vascular endothelial growth factor (VEGF) inhibitor medications - frequently termed 'anti-VEGF agents'- following publication of key trial results, (Gragoudas et al., 2004, Rosenfeld et al., 2006 Brown DM et al., 2006). These studies showed that wet-AMD patients treated with monthly intravitreal injections of anti VEGF agents had a greatly reduced risk of visual loss compared to no treatment or other existing treatments. Wet-AMD patient care requires regular injections of such anti-VEGF medication whenever visual acuity drops or the retina is found to thicken on monthly OCT scanning. This is thus an area of both high volume, frequent, time sensitive care. Delay in access to treatment for wet AMD patients was found to be a major problem in a recent review of NHS patient safety data across England and Wales (Kelly and Barua, 2011). Pressures on AMD services are mounting as the numbers of such patients enlarge. For example in West Wales, Aberystwyth, in February 2010, 51 patients were undergoing such treatment. This increased to over 200 such patients by February 2011. Nurses in the clinic have been trained to undertake OCT imaging, facilitating timely review of patients' results by the consultant ophthalmologist to determine whether a further VEGF inhibitor injection is indicated.

The use of nurses and assistant nurse practitioners (Figure 9) to capture OCT images has allowed our AMD service to develop. Feed back from patients is positive. Nurses have been involved with formulating an electronic record incorporating the OCT scans for individual patients and in setting up a local community hospital service using telemedicine facilities. There has been improvement in the quality of life for the elderly patients in our community as a result of maintaining eyesight. Poor vision is associated with depression, suicide, falls and fractures.

5.2 Virtual clinics in macular disorders

Virtual macular clinics have been organised in centres to cope with increasing demand of retinal disease and to free up capacity issues within the hospital service. Such innovation may allow patients to be managed with the click of a mouse. The multidisciplinary team undertakes clinical history review and carries out digital fundus photography and optical coherence tomography imaging. These clinical images together with an electronic -or paper based- clinical record are reviewed by a consultant ophthalmologist either in the eye clinic or possibly at another location. Such clinics are becoming established at facilities for wet AMD patient care such as Sheffield, Cheltenham and Gloucester and West Wales.

Ophthalmology medical staff may not need to examine every patient, provided they are still involved in the decision making process at vital points in the patient pathway. Face-to-face patient contact can be undertaken by suitably skilled nursing and optometry staff. Consideration can also be given to electronic transfer of ophthalmic images from the community for review at the hospital. This can be problematic, due to IT issues, but is

possible. This type of digital image transfer is currently under investigation at community hospitals in West Wales using videoconferencing equipment.
In the North West of England we are piloting use of the PACS system, (mostly used for radiology at this time), for OCT and fundus images, with transfer of such images to ophthalmologists in other locations, clinics and hospitals for consultation or review. The iPhone and iPad have an application into which OCT images may be downloaded for viewing at remote locations (Figure 10)

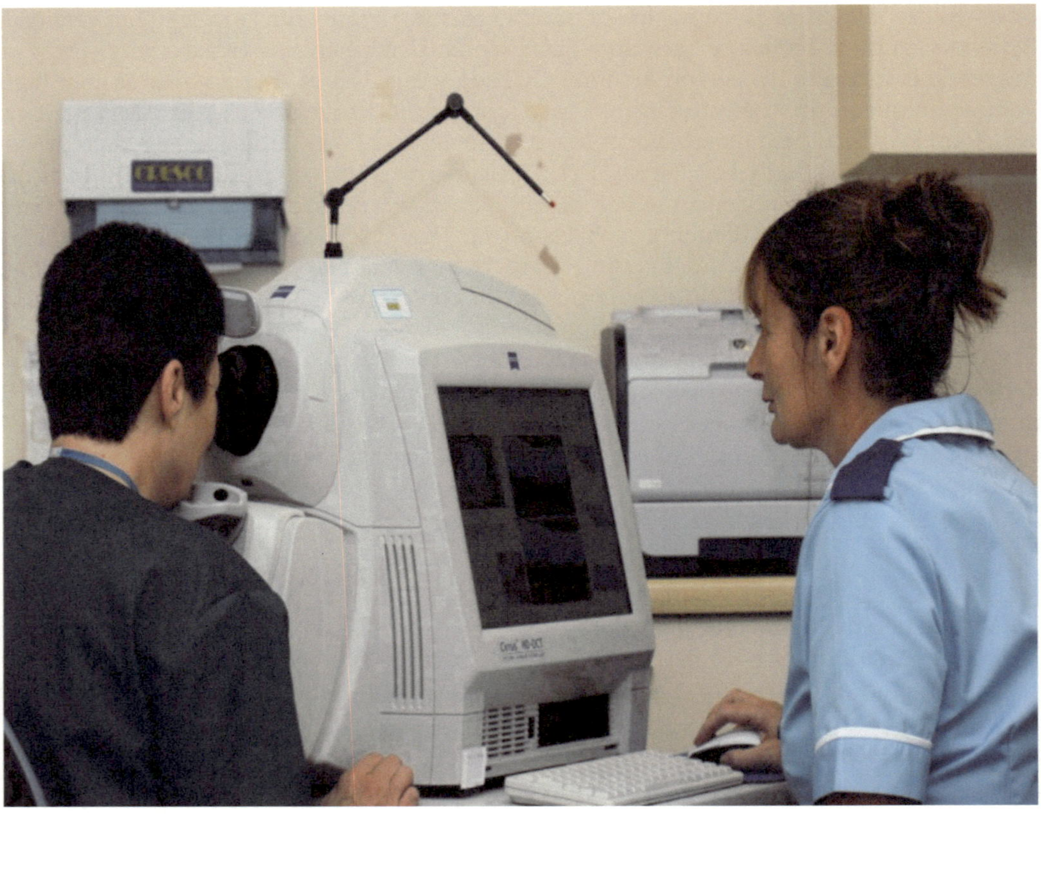

Fig. 9. Nurse undertaking optical coherence tomography examination

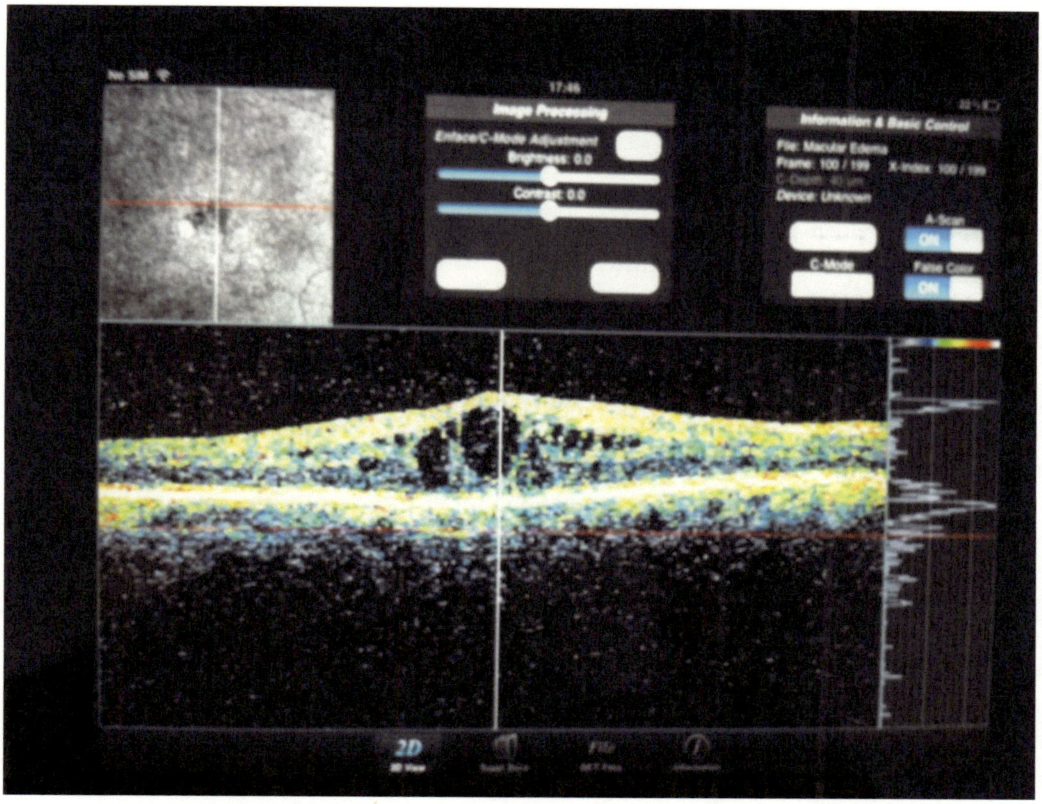

Fig. 10. OCT Scan showing abnormal macular fluid accumulation and which has been wirelessly downloaded to an Apple iPAD through an app downloaded from iTUNES

Large size clinical image transfer in the NHS requires N3 connectivity. Image exchange portal (IEP) services are being commissioned by NHS at present. Such facilities may be an additional tool for ophthalmology image transfer. Comprehensive ophthalmic image data management systems such as EyeRoute Synergy (Topcon Medical Systems) and Forum (Carl Zeiss Instruments) are available to assist such teleophthalmology endeavours. Interoperability with electronic medical records leads to enhanced productivity in busy ophthalmic clinics and across clinical boundaries.

It is likely that such systems will be more integrated into more ophthalmology clinics and thus facilitating development of virtual clinics and the introduction of wireless technology instruments into clinical care.

Some optometrists are now using NHSmail and which enables secure electronic transmission of patient information. NHSmail accounts are available to optometrists in Scotland and England. As such connectivity to NHSmail to community optometrists is available, publicity within the optometry profession to encourage uptake is now required. Use of NHSmail has successfully allowed collaboration between consultant ophthalmologists and community optometrists in Bolton in a pilot clinical study, allowing the rapid access of patients into treatment for AMD and other retinal disorders when required. However, if large file sizes are being transmitted N3 connections are required. N3 connectivity provides a centrally funded, resilient network connection for every NHS site in

England. Placement of virtual clinics in the correct place in the patient pathway is critical for success

Multiple OCT units have been successfully integrated in Australia through the beta release ofV5.2 software for the Zeiss Cirrus OCT instrument. This enables the sharing of OCT raw data between multiple Cirrus units via FORUM 2.6 software. (Person communication C Hawke, Zeiss Australia). Depending on internet connection speed this could also be performed between multiple sites. This could either be running live or possibly by synchronisation via scheduled transfer of data, perhaps overnight. There are also future developments underway by Zeiss not only for OCT data synchronisation but all ophthalmic data synchronisation. Such a setup may perhaps better facilitate integration of ophthalmic image data files between diverse departments, such as rural community clinics and the central departments. Such innovation may facilitate the better development of virtual clinics.

Similarly EyeRoute Synergy Ophthalmic Data Management System from Topcon integrates images and reports from many instrument manufacturers into a single, secure, digital environment. With the ability to view, compare, annotate and transmit patient images, EyeRoute Synergy provides for fluent workflow efficiency. The web based system allows for rapid access to patient information, anytime, from virtually anywhere, including workstations and remote computers. As this system can store, manage and share data and images from many medical devices and can facilitate better sharing of information between colleagues in real time through a secure Synergy Community Portal. It has been used in remote diabetic retinopathy screening in the USA.

6. Glaucoma and optic disc imaging

Glaucoma is a common condition and a potentially blinding eye disorder for which effective treatment (usually with eye drop medications) exists and guidance from NICE is present. http://guidance.nice.org.uk/CG85

Delay in NHS glaucoma patient follow up appointment provision emerged from a review by the National Patient Safety Agency (NPSA). A NPSA alert followed in 2009 seeking to improve patient safety in this area of high volume care.

http://www.nrls.npsa.nhs.uk/resources/type/alerts/?entryid45=61908

Optic disc OCT imaging is useful in glaucoma and can record progression of nerve fibre layer thinning. The findings obtained with OCT can be used in conjunction with visual field tracings, also recorded digitally and thus available remotely. The glaucoma service in West Wales is presently being modified to increase the role of the community diagnostic and treatment centres with glaucoma teams who record the visual fields, the intraocular pressures and optic disc OCT image and digital photograph. The glaucoma specialist can make decisions on the need for referral or indeed the need for the patients to be seen in the hospital or not , based on assessment of images of visual fields, optic discs, optic disc OCT and an updated patient electronic record.

Once glaucoma or ocular hypertension is diagnosed and treatment initiated, some patients can be managed via virtual glaucoma clinics. There are models which have been developed for Virtual Glaucoma clinics in South Wales, (Llandeilo and Swansea), with Diagnostic Centres control stations, where decisions are made through telemedicine by a consultant

ophthalmologist with a specialist interest in glaucoma at the main University Hospital. Though futuristic, there are plans underway to role these clinics out throughout urban and rural Wales using the community hospitals as diagnostic and treatment centres. Training is in place in the Carmarthenshire Glaucoma Referral Refinement Scheme to ensure nurses and community optometrists have the skills to take part in these glaucoma teams, as described by Devrajan et al., 2011.
Tele-glaucoma clinics have been piloted in Finland. Tuulonen compared patients seen in community telemedicine clinics in Finland and those seen in the hospital. (Tuulonen A et al., 1999). Both patient groups were equally satisfied with the ophthalmic service. Nearly all patients in the telemedicine group (96%) wanted to have their next visit in their own healthcare centre instead of the university eye clinic. The most important reasons were reduction in travelling (97%), costs (92%), and time (92%). The costs of the telemedicine and conventional care visits were equal, but decreased travelling with telemedicine option saved $55 per visit. With greater emphasis on team leadership, introduction of these clinics to rural areas will help cope with the increased demands of seeing an ever increasing number of follow up patients on time.

7. Conclusions

Telemedicine is well suited to ophthalmology patient care. The term teleophthalmology provides a framework for such innovation. Teleophthalmology also offers benefits to the organisation of patient care and enhances the skills of local first level eye care practitioners, such as community optometrists and ophthalmic nurses. Teleophthalmology has merit both in urban and rural settings. Better integration of teleophthalmology with local services is improving emergency eye care, diabetic eye screening and virtual macular and glaucoma clinics. Teleophthalmology helps reduce costs while maximising productivity, and reduces patient travel or transfer. It is not intended that teleophthalmology consultations would replace face to face ophthalmic consultations and clinical examination. Rather electronic referral of ophthalmic images, rather than of patients, is a useful and rapid tool to assist, prioritise and refine referral of many ophthalmic patients, especially retinal patients in the digital age. This is the case in our experience in Wales. (Kulshrestha et al 2010)
There are many advantages of this exciting technology in revolutionising the way care is provided given an expanding numbers of ophthalmic patients. Furthermore there are increasing applications for emergency and out of hours care; management and administrative meetings; CPD and educational training. These advantages are particularly relevant in rural areas, with patients who may otherwise have to travel long distances to access ophthalmic care. Importantly the introduction of virtual clinics allows greater team working between primary and secondary care and may thus help to solve some of the problems of slippage and delay in hard pressed retinal and glaucoma patient care.
Although there is strong evidence that teleophthalmology is particularly useful in the treatment of retinal disease, 93% of published projects in a recent review concern 'store and forward' applications rather than transfer of real time images schemes Over 90% of projects in that review had a positive view on teleophthalmology services, indicating its role as a reliable method of eye care delivery.

http://www.intechopen.com/source/pdfs/14329/InTechAdvances_in_teleophthalmology_summarising_published_papers_on_teleophthalmology_projects.pdf
The use of modern wireless technologies in mobile and hand held devices -such as smart phones (eg Apple iPhone) and tablets (eg Apple iPad), - together with the potential wider use of PACS to allow image transfer is likely expand the options and usage of teleophthalmology solutions in the future.

8. Acknowledgements

We thank Dr Alan Axford, Medical Director, Bronglais Hospital, Aberystwyth for his guidance and direction in formulating ophthalmic telemedicine projects and Delyth Lewis, Telemedicine Project Manager, Bronglais Hospital for her support. Professor David Owen, Professor Emeritus, University Hospital Cardiff, provided slides on diabetic retinopathy screening. David O'Sullivan, Optometrist, South Wales and Mr Michael Austin, Consultant Ophthalmologist, Singleton Hospital Swansea provided information on virtual glaucoma Clinics. Cameron Hawke Zeiss Australia provided information on the future of the Zeiss FORUM system.

9. References

Bhopal RS, Parkin DW, Gillie RF, Han KH. (1993) Pattern of ophthalmological accidents and emergencies presenting to hospitals. *J Epidemiol Commun Health*, 47: 382–387.

Brown DM, Kaiser PK, Michels M, Soubrane G, Heier JS, Kim RY, *et al.*, (2006) the ANCHOR Study Group. Ranibizumab versus verteporfin for neovascular age-related macular degeneration. *N Engl J Med* 355: 1432–1444

Bunce C, W Xing W and Wormald R. (2010) Causes of blind and partial sight certifications in England and Wales: April 2007–March 2008. *Eye.* 24: 1692–1699

Cameron JR, Ahmed S, Curry P, Forrest G, Sanders R. (2009) Impact of direct electronic optometric referral with ocular imaging to a hospital eye service. *Eye*. 23:1134-40.

Chiang MF, Wang L, Kim D, Scott K, Richter G, Kane S, Flynn J, Starren J. (2010) Diagnostic performance of a telemedicine system for ophthalmology: advantages in accuracy and speed compared to standard care. *AMIA Annu Symp Proc.* Nov 13;2010:111-5.

Devarajan N, G S Williams, M Hopes, D O'Sullivan and D Jones (2011)The Carmarthenshire Glaucoma Referral Refinement Scheme, a safe and efficient screening service43-49 *Eye* 25:1

Ellis DG, Mayrose J, Jehle DV, et al. (2011)A telemedicine model for emergency care in a short-term correctional facility. *Telemed J E Health.* 7(2):87-92.

European Union of Medical Specialities. www.uems.net

Fenton S, Jackson E, Fenton M. (2001)An audit of the ophthalmic division of the accident and emergency department of the Royal Victoria Eye and Ear Hospital Dublin. *Ir Med J* 2001: 94 (9): 265-6.

Girard B, Bourcier F, Agdabede I, Laroche L (2002) Activity and epidemiology in an ophthalmological emergency centre. *J de France d'Ophthalmol* 25:701-711

Gragoudas ES, Adamis AP, Cunningham ET Jr, Feinsod M, Guyer DR, (2004)for the VEGF Inhibition Study in Ocular Neovascularization Clinical Trial Group. Pegaptanib for neovascular age-related macular degeneration. *N Engl J Med*. 351:2805-2816.

Gullapalli N, Rao (2000) Ophthalmology in India *Arch Ophthalmol*, 118:1431-1432
Hanson C, Tennant MT, Rudnisky CJ. (2008) Optometric referrals to retina specialists; evaluation and triage via teleophthalmology. *Telemedicine and Journal e-Health.*14:441-5.
http://www.aravind.org/telemedicine/eyestalkhome.htm
http://www.diabetes.org.uk/About_us/Our_Views/Position_statements/retinal_screening
http://guidance.nice.org.uk/CG85
http://www.image-exchange.co.uk/index.php
http://www.intechopen.com/source/pdfs/14329/InTechAdvances_in_teleophthalmology_summarising_published_papers_on_teleophthalmology_projects.pdf
http://www.nrls.npsa.nhs.uk/resources/type/alerts/?entryid45=61908
http://www.teleophthalmology.com
Huang D, Swanson EA, Lin CP, et al. (1991) Optical coherence tomography. *Science 254:1178–81.*
Kanagasingam and Yogesan K (2006) Remote ophthalmology services: cost comparison of telemedicine and alternative service delivery options. J *Telemed Telecare*,12:19-22
Kelly SP and A Barua A. (2011) A review of safety incidents in England and Wales for vascular endothelial growth factor inhibitor medications. *Eye* advance online publication, April 29, 2011.
http://www.nature.com/eye/journal/vaop/ncurrent/full/eye201189a.html
Kulshrestha MK, Williams C, Lewis D, Axford A (2010) A pilot trial of tele-ophthalmology services in north Wales. *J Telemed Telecare,* 16: 196-197
Kumar S, Yogesan K, Hudson B, Tay-Kearney M-L and Constable IJ(2006) Emergency eye care in rural Australia: role of internet *Eye,* 20, 1342–1344.
Khurana M, Ramakrishnan R, Kader MA (2011) Teleophthalmology aided vision centres in rural south India:Role and utilisation of services *ARVO Abstract* Fort Lauderdale 4 May 2011
Nakajima I. (2010)Worldwide trends in universal service funds and telemedicine. *Journal of Medical Systems*, 34; 1105-10.
Owen, C.G., Fletcher, A.E., Donoghue, M., Rudnicka, A.R. (2003) How big is the burden of visual loss caused by age related macular degeneration in the United Kingdom? *B J Ophthalmol* 87: 312-317.
Practical Commissioning Magazine (2009) How Telemedicine Can Cut Referrals,29.
Richter GM, Williams SL, Starren J, Flynn JT, Chiang MF. (2009)Telemedicine for retinopathy of prematurity diagnosis: evaluation and challenges. *Survey of Ophthalmology* Nov-Dec;54(6):671-85.
Rosenfeld PJ, Brown DM, Heier JS, Boyer DS, Kaiser PK, Chung CY, *et al.*, the MARINA Study Group.(2006)Ranibizumab for neovascular age-related macular degeneration. *N Engl J Med* 355: 1419–1431
Stoves J, Connolly J, Cheung CK, Grange A, Rhodes P, O'Donoghue D, Wright J (2010) Electronic consultation as an alternative to hospital referral for patients with chronic kidney disease: a novel application for networked electronic health records to improve the accessibility and efficiency of healthcare. *Qual Saf Health Care.* Oct;19(5)
Thulasi Bai, V. Murali, R. Kim, S.K. Srivatsa (2007) Tele-Ophthalmology Based Rural Eye Care in India *Telemedicine and e-Health.*, 13(3): 313-321.

Tuulonen A, Ohinmaa T, Alanko HI, Hyytinen P, Juutinen A, Toppinen E (1999) The application of teleophthalmology in examining patients with glaucoma: a pilot study. J Glaucoma., 8(6):367-73.

20

Telemedical Solutions - Practical Approach in Bulgaria

Polina Mihova
New Bulgarian University
Bulgaria

1. Introduction

The electronic communication network is an umbrella term, which generally is associated with computer and communication through modern information and communication technologies. These structures allow the workflow of data at different time and from different locations, using an e-mail address lists, electronic forums, online conferences, etc. The exchange of information over the Internet is a standard procedure, the main component of network communications and technological achievements, but this approach in the field of medicine and healthcare actually changes patients' lives!

Life in a network allows us to create virtual communities of various specialized organizations and entities working together on specific issues through the exchange of information. In essence, the Internet is a democratic, social and non-discriminatory information and technological environment, the ideal instrument for achieving common objectives which provide unpredictable opportunities for individual systems and experts.

Users of the World Wide Web in all its aspects and forms get more data, information, evidence, knowledge and experience through:

exchange of information substrates implementing technology tools and services to assist the communication process new automated methods of information processing conglomerates and statistical evaluation of any information products change in qualification - both for training and skills in technology assisted work.

By definition, telemedicine is a branch of medicine based on telecommunication and information technologies to ensure medical services and work as their main goal is quality care for all patients regardless of their location and social position.

Today the main priorities of medicine are: in economic terms - the financing of medical science and development of medical work to achieve higher efficiency; at international level - to what extent the poor and developing countries imitate the patterns of rich countries with expensive technologies and how to standardize and make consistent the information activities; in research plan - new technologies and sciences which serve medicine, how, in what dose, and appropriate application.

eHealth is strongly dependent on economic policy, infrastructure investment patterns and changes in health care facilities that provide opportunities to implement advanced technological solutions. Other fundamental factors are the pricing policy and legal framework and organization of this new kind of payments and services. There are no regulations and standards for the exchange of information and transfer of personal data processing and storage. The staff is not well trained in terms of computer skills, which means investments in education and changes in the curricula of medical colleges and universities.

Business models and management approaches should first seek benefits for patient satisfaction by providing healthcare services through easier access. Professional communities must also be motivated by promotion and presentation of the advantages and benefits about:

- methods for data presentation;
- methods of access;
- methods for data integration;
- network services.

Notwithstanding increasingly aware of the role of IT in healthcare and global experience with proven benefits of eHealth, its introduction is associated with number of obstacles to overcome:

- Difficulty in converting these data - the necessity to integrate and digitize
- Standardization of medical records – personal information is stored from the patients, and on the other hand – locally, in the hospital. When all the participants are connected in the process of health care we will have continuous updates and a single database. Overall, this is a problem in any kind of systems, not just for medical ones.
- Confidentiality - in healthcare, this parameter refers both to the information stored on paper and data in electronic format
- Hardware limitations - the effective practice of an EHR system requires the presence of sufficient number of computers - desktops and notebooks in a hospital
- Inertia - Most large organizations have opposed the changes. The shocking transition to a new system in each institution should be made by the governing bodies. According to studies, introduction of the EHR system comes within the so-called 80/20 rule, i.e. - 80% of the work involves issues of managing change and only 20% work - technical issues

The standard medical practice, as such, exists from the Hippocrates times - face to face contact with a suffering patient, personal experience to suggest accurate treatment and legitimacy to the laws in Bulgaria are just some of the advantages and established standards of practice. On the other hand, paper documentation that is still the practice in our healthcare system, the possibility of intentional or accidental error, lack of sufficient practical experience in a particular case, present just some of the factors that describe the current status of our system as old-fashioned, unsatisfactory and risky for the health of the patient.

However, telemedicine is facing many other problems that lead to fear and reluctance from consumption of new working models. It requires modern standards of employment, security for the patient by several expert opinions, prevention and minimization of possibility of errors in the final diagnosis, the provision of care 7 days a week, 24 hours a day. Of course, the difficulties and obstacles in this scheme of work, which are related to the willingness of medical experts, placed in a competitive regime, the lack of ethical and legal frameworks that limit abuses and skills required to work with information technology are only a few of the barriers to implement that service.

In this chapter the standard medical practice will be discussed contrasting it with telemedical solutions and benefits based on deep investigation and SWOT analysis. The term telemedicine will be presented with 60 different definitions and comments, in combination with a basic set of workstations for telemedical consultations. For the purposes of the investigation an inquiry model is realized, evaluating telemedical systems with 61 basic questions.

Tasks that we have pointed out in this chapter are to offer a short historical overview of telemedicine in Bulgaria, to demonstrate juxtapositions between different specialized terms as telemedicine, telemetry and telematics; to present one Bulgarian solution for telemedical services, to discuss the pros and cons from three different points of view - patients, doctors and hospital managers.

2. Investigation of telemedicine – SWOT analysis, confrontations, definitions

Health is the foundation of human life and therefore it must be supported by effective policies and actions in the country members of the European Community and worldwide. Article 152 of the EC Treaty requires "the development and implementation of all policies and actions to ensure a high level of protection of human health."

From January 1, 2007 provisions of EU regulations governing matters of social and health insurance are directly applicable in Bulgaria - in the context of the right of free movement of people within United Europe.

Bulgarian citizens who have continuous health insurance rights under Bulgarian law, if necessary, may use medical assistance in countries of the European Community.

eHealth challenges include developing common standards and interoperability of health products, systems and services at European level.

Given the recent accession of Bulgaria to the EU, it is an appropriate and timely investment in the development of eHealth in the country.

According to the National Health Development Strategy 2008-2013 [50] the following are outlined as key priorities:

- Providing health services on-line;
- Implementation of electronic health cards.
- Implementation of personal electronic health records.
- Implementation of integrated software applications for processing and sharing information in real time, including: electronic directions, recipes, expert findings, laboratory and diagnostic data, etc.
- Development of complex integration models, working with external applications and systems.
- Creation of hospital information systems for electronic medical records.
- Construction of required infrastructure for normal functioning of healthcare system - networks that connect devices, and other devices.
- Construction of appropriate infrastructure for the deployment of telemedical applications.

eHealth, by definition, is a rapidly developing field where medical informatics, public health, supply of healthcare services and modern information and communication technologies interact. It features technology development for improvement of health services at local, regional and global levels.

The European Commission published in April the results of an Europe-wide survey on electronic services in healthcare (eHealth), which found that 87% of GPs use a computer, 48% have a broadband connection. Doctors in Europe store and send data electronically to patients, such as laboratory results.

According to the submitted study entitled "Evaluation of ICT use among General Practitioners in Europe" eHealth applications play a growing role in medical practice.

Advantages	Weaknesses
Needs of patients	respect, uncertainty and even fear of the unknown, arising from outdated entity, where medical informatics has no fixed place
access to care	lack of highly qualified specialists in the field of communication services
immediate assistance from specialist	lack of professional culture and teamwork with experts from other fields
24-hour coverage by a doctor for all hospitals	interactivity is achieved through a terminological language - communication strategies
Needs of specialists	
opportunity to communicate with all specialists in fields/community	
earlier medical intervention	
reduction illness time	
saves lives	
improved methods and treatment regimens	
medical advice and constant support at any time,	
at any place, any condition	
part of the digitalization of society and health care	
reform that reduces health inequalities	
construction of a modern technological infrastructure and information systems	
change of quality of medical work and training of experts in the most accessible way	
interactivity and good practices	
Opportunities	**Impendences**
improved access to the needy of health care qualitative improvement and effectiveness of diagnostic and therapeutic activity	lack of sufficient entrepreneurial spirit and motivation among professionals
benefits and satisfaction of patients and medical professionals	not popular business models of behavior and application of these services
Information Management	political management methods from the recent past, marked by different political motives
different communities - professional and patients	legislation
modernization of health policy	lack of regulations and pricing

Table 1. SWOT analysis of the Telemedicine as a new type of practice [48]

Standard medical practice		Telemedicine	
For	Against	For	Against
tradition of medical practice – changing with the generations		simultaneous operation of several organizations	costs for equipment
tested in time – fixed and accepted as routine practice		simplified and standardized process	knowledge of electronic standards and requirements
paper does not require any technology	risk of information loss	improved health services	new public nature of the profession
face-to-face contact	expenditure of financial and time resources to remote patients and their families	provision of care anytime, anywhere and by anyone	problems with persuasiveness and reliability
subjective – the record is done by one author	possible errors or omission	transfer of various data formats	Perceptions of staff to work with the new system
Law legitimacy	opportunity for abuse and manipulation of information	various forms of diagnostic techniques	competency requirements for more than narrow specialization
written responsibility, verified with personal signature	delay in time	consultation with multiple specialists together	competitive moment
results of communication with patients	poor results of aging assets	Provision of care 24 hours at home	ongoing commitment
		education from a distance in real time	Pricing - Who decides?
		human interaction - PC	PC equipment
		objectivity of opinions	ethical issues
		reduce professional isolation	Lack of political will to implement
		increased confidence by specialist	Institutional will
		providing the best experts in the field	prudence
		new working standards, fast and efficient, information transfer Real teamwork	lack of legal framework

Table 2. Standard medical practice vs telemedicine [48]

Basic applications of telemedicine in Bulgaria today are:

- Clinical telemedicine
- Military (and other specialized types of specializations) telemedicine
- Other health care information systems with various functions

- Remote training and retraining of experts and creation of new health concerns, consumer standards and mass cultural practices of users of these services, activities and expertise resident in the complex dynamics between health and disease.

Telemedical practice can be divided as follows:

1. technical devices for recording and transfer of data to the required distance
2. technologies, asisting medical decisions
3. experts to interpret the specialized information
4. agreement for real-time management of patient from a distance

The need for specialized information stems from the scope of work and medical practice relating to:

Key objectives of information systems in medicine are:

- projection and automation of entire information process to achieve the minimum possible risk of error
- improve and accelerate the selection of management decisions, planning and forecasting
- regulate information exchange in vertical and horizontal direction
- relief staff in its routine activities
- modification in the exchanging system with the environment - in this respect, telemedicine and computer networks are a genuine revolution in the filling and retransmission of data gathering and any kind of multimedia.

Key tasks that computer systems in medicine pursue:

- Unambiguous classification of information and processing of international standards that ensure objectivity, comparability and adaptation in operation modes and their possible use by other experts and classifiers - resources, statistics, diagnostics, certificate, health insurance, research and training
- Standardization of methods for retrieval of medical information and its carriers by type (computer file - Electronic Medical Record)
- Automation of processes input from various devices, technical and technological facilities and equipment (clinical and paraclinical)
- Coding and total control of information through design of menus, dialog with a PC, which guarantees the same standards
- Creation of databases for objects of local IP connections to other databases, with access to software, designed for different users

Telemedicine - method for remote consultations, personalized medicine by distance. Thus conceptual correlation value of the selected title in the enrichment of already developed or in designing new CIS adds additional feature that allows medical practice without physical contact, working from multiple different locations and at different time, repeatability and verifiability of decision processes and management choices of the source.

Telemedical functions aim to change the characteristics of medical work, which allow practice under evidence-based medicine, often described as a scientifically based medicine.

Defining the term telemedicine

Telemedical essence is a basic and fundamental type of service, a version of eHealth.

The variety of technological solutions in eHealth applications correspond to the following aspects:

- Tele-medicine / Tele-health
- Web Health Services
- I-medicine / I-health

- Cyber-medicine / Cyber-health
- Medicine online
- High-tech medicine
- Website and Portal

Telebridge in medicine and health [68]

1. Type of information (History of disease, video, X-rays, microscopic samples, data from literary analysis, etc.)
2. Transmitting medium (telephone line, satellite);Telemedicine is the main application area, where the following components are present:

1. Technology (measuring instruments, monitoring systems, channels of contact and communication video, workstations, databases, expert systems, etc.).
2. Medical education (distance education, computer workstation, and international inter-university educational programs)
3. Medical science
4. Library databases and knowledge systems
5. Social Medicine
6. Clinical Medicine
7. Health Policy
8. Management, law and of administration
9. Medical specific areas of knowledge (space biomedicine and ecomedicine, disaster, military telemedicine, etc.).
10. Interdisciplinary areas and activities, related to theoretical and applied aspects of human health.

The origin of the term telemedicine is a formation of two parts: "tele" in this phrase originates from the term "telematics" and added to the medical interpretation as a kind of modern medical science, practiced by means of telematics.

In it's contemporary sense, the actual concept of telemedicine exists since 1924. It appeared in the U.S. in Radio News article, the cover painted with a doctor who examines the patient and sends his results on the radio and the new chain scheme "Doctor on the radio. The first demonstration was made in 1951 at the World Fair in New York and in 1955 Dr. Albert Dzhutras began teleradiology practice in Montreal. In 1959 for the first time were transmitted diagnostic results between United States and Canada by coaxial cable.

Also, Cecil Whitson from the Institute of Psychiatry in Nebraska began the first courses in teleeducation and telepsichiatry. In Bulgaria, the theme is related to the development of aviation medicine and its basic methodology - aviation biotelemetry into a new mode - space medicine.

The term telemedicine was introduced into medical literature in 1974 by RGMark (Telemedicine system: the missing link between homes and hospital Mod.Nurs.Home-1974, N 32 (2). In the MEDLINE database there are previously published works which concerned the concepts of its place, role and possible development, without mentioning the term itself.

According to the Telemedicine Glossary [66]: "Telematics is the use of information and telecommunication technologies and services, usually in individual combinations to meet the specialized medical and consumer health needs and problems.

Telemedicine can be defined as a "system to expand and enhance the capabilities of medicine through electromagnetic field (EMF), suggesting a variety of information and management functions [67]."

For many, a commonly accepted definition is hard to designate, but there are several clear principles that are enshrined in the integrated multiple components of medical practice:
"The use of electronic information and communication technologies to deliver and maintain healthcare services, when distance separates the participants." [30] These technologies have applications in providing any care for the sick, education, research, administration and health care, overcoming distance and isolation [2]. Probably the most comprehensive is "Telemedicine covers everything from health, education, information and administrative services that can be transmitted at a distance via telecommunication technology." [40] "Telemedicine is a logical development of the first medical consultation by telephone, made at the beginning of XX century ". [41] Indeed, from a technical standpoint, it performs rational development and integration of informatics in medical practice.
"Telemedicine is the use of telecommunication technologies as a medium for delivery of medical services - diagnosis and patient care in locations that are remote from the supplier." This concept covers everything from the use of standard telephone service to high speed digital signals between computers, optics, satellites and other peripheral devices and software.
Another definition, that focuses more on the tools that telemedicine provides: "Telemedicine is based on the use of electronic communication and information technologies to provide or support clinical care from any distance." [1]
"Remote alternative medical practice - via telecommunications and video technologies, used for education, transmission of medical or other specialized data and its subsequent processing." [70]
According to the American Telemedicine Association: "The subject of telemedicine is transmission of medical information between remote points, where there are patients, doctors or other health care providers. It involves use of telecommunications to link diagnosis, treatment, advice and continuous training. [79]
In the next few specific definitions, the term is interpreted from a technical rather than a medical perspective, focusing on the means of transmission of information and methods of transmission:
"Telemedicine is the rapid provision of medical knowledge at a distance using telecommunications and information technologies, regardless patients location and the necessary information about his case. [18]
Section of medicine that deals with the remote control of the pilots health , astronauts, and then about a decade afterwards has become very famous and popular as telemedicine. [30]
"Telemedicine is one of the applied fields of medical science with systemic nature, which supposes combination of medical apparatus with telecommunications network equipment, software and specialists from several areas. [29]
“Unique variety of system applications of telecommunication technologies for medical purposes.” [115]
"It is a combination of medical and technological systems implemented on the basis of computing and telecommunications, medical consultation, diagnosis and choice of therapeutic effects from distance and control of medical resources." [116]
"It is a system for delivery access to modern medical resources, a conglomerate of funds and complexes for potential realization of modern information and telecommunication technologies in medicine and healthcare, in harmony with the respective financial and legal certainty.” [34]

"The tasks of research and development in the field of telemedicine are expressed in association between information and communication technology in a way that will provide services in health medicine and ability to systematically use the medical resources that are outside the local organization." [117]

A definition, which essentially illustrates this development, was published in 1990 in a paper in «Clinical Informatics in Medicine, Pathology and pediatricians»: "Telemedicine is the introduction of built-in Medical Information Systems (MIS) - new technological tools for data processing, now united as an entire technology systems for communication to create, distribute and store information products (data or knowledge) with minimal loss in order to carry out remedial and diagnostic activities, training and administration of patients in need in the right time and place. [18]

At http://ritmru.chat.ru/ [82], one of many sites, dedicated to the development of telemedicine in Russia, are published about 15 interpretive definitions of telemedicine from the most popular Russian authors.

"It is unity of telecommunications and information technologies for medical or health purposes. This must be done cost effectively by stimulating growth and usability of medical resources, which could be attainable through deployment of intellectual resources to establish information management systems." [118]

"The scope of telemedicine is to transmit medical information between distant points where patients, physicians and other providers of medical care and services are situated between medical establishment purposes: diagnosis, treatment, advice and continuous training." [1]

"Telemedicine is a system of agents, complexes and methods that realize the potential of modern information and telecommunication technologies in medicine and healthcare, in harmony with legal regulations, licensing rights and standards of work, corresponding to financial security." [66]

Distance is also cited as a major digitalization of medical services and activities and their intended transmission when it is necessary. This capability is achieved thanks to the unique connection principles of all participants in the therapeutic-diagnostic process.

To enrich the functional range of conversion, the process of medical and paramedical information would be used not only for treatment but also for training, organization, management, and control and business functions.

"Telemedicine is a system for accomplishment of remote medical expertise in any circumstances. It incorporates three main components: the domestic (and other non-clinical) registrations and care (the use of various types and quality biosensors) and centers for collection and analysis of received information, which work together." [73]

"It is not a tool that you buy to examine patients. It is important to remember that its impact is much greater than what we've seen when it introduces a new method and methodology in our work. This is the result of complex interaction of advanced technologies and human factors that would inevitably lead to social changes. The success of these changes and their usefulness is dependent on many different people - consumers and experts who work together. " [10]

This is the place to quote the original definition of Medical Informatics, Edward Shortliffe:

"Medical informatics is the study of rational ways for interpreting the patient's condition and its treatment approaches, which we define and develop over time; an examination of how medical knowledge is formed, distributed and applied." [62]

Telemetry	Telematics	Telemedicine
Use of telecommunications for automatically indicating radio beacons or recording measurements at a distance from the measuring apparatus. [107] Scientific method for measuring, registration and transport of medical data through communication tools. Transmission of data (i.e. registered and measured variables) - they can be measured and recorded manually and automatically	Refers to industry related to computers, interconnected via telecommunication devices and systems. This includes dial-up services to the Internet [108] Scientific method for data and / or information with selected communication tools. *Transmission of data and information with selected ICT*	Method for providing medical services, where distance is a critical factor. These services are performed by medical professionals, using information and communication technologies (ICT) for obtaining information needed for diagnosis, treatment and prevention. [95] Scientific specialty, which aims to realize the transportation of medical and health data and information through ICT between unlimited number of experts in real and / or another selected time/ experts. Automated or automatic transmission of data and information through ICT.
Scientific method, associated technology of automatic recording and transmission of data from a remote source to receiver. [103]	Combination of resources and services in computer science and telecommunications. [109]	Use of ICT the provision of medical care from a distance. [94]
Transmission at distance of measured values by radio or telephone coded amplitude, frequency, phase and pulse. The data are received and stored on a remote station. [92]	Technology that allows converting digital images to analog. [110]	Use of computers, Internet and other communication technologies to provide medical care to remote patients. [57]
Electronic device that carries specific data (measurements) to a remote receiver. Data are recorded electronically. [119]	Refers to the synthesis of various technologies, which generally are telecommunication technologies, computers, methods of data processing [111]	Telemedicine is not sub discipline of medical and therapeutic aids and surgical specialties. This concept includes the availability of telephone system, high-speed system for information transmitting through fibrooptics, satellites or

		combination of terrestrial and satellite communication technologies. [49]
Process of measuring quantities from a remote location, which is recorded and further processed by another one. [9]	Focal function between telecommunications and informatics (information science). [14]	Medical care at a distance - the images are transmitted, because patient and treating physician are not located at the same place. [76]
Computer-based monitoring and communication with remote objects. The term comes from the Greek tele = remote, and metron = measure. [120], [105]	Telecommunications and Informatics show the relationships between IT systems, digital data, etc. [107]	Integrated system for providing medical care using telecommunications and computer technology rather than direct contact between patient and doctor. [25]
System through which a signal is transmitted to a remote location in order to control the process, to perform specific functions and tasks. [25]	Realization of relationships between computer and information technologies. [41]	Provision of medical assistance to any point on the globe, using combination of communication technologies and medical expertise. [23]
Linkage, registered through specialized equipment using radio signals [95]	Wireless communication system designed for storage and dissemination of data. Applications: electronic systems in the industry, mobile phones, tracking vehicles and GPS systems, health and emergency assistance. [52]	Rapid provision of medical knowledge at a distance using telebridge and information technology, regardless of where the patient is located and where the information is needed. [109]
Technology, including wireless transmission of signals. The term is used to define the electronic technology, used for registration of several mechanical functions and sending process to a remote receiver.[32], [40]	Science for transmitting, receiving and storing information via telecommunication systems. [53]	Combination of medical information systems, fundamentally new means and methods of data processing technologies, integrated into a comprehensive system providing the creation, transmission and storage of information products - data and knowledge - in order to conduct therapeutic and adequate diagnostic measures, and perform the necessary

		training at the necessary time. [91]
Measurement of different electrical parameters by using feedback from a particular receptor device. In the T-level - the lowest level at which the signal stimulates the recipient and identify irritation. [35]	Integration of wireless communication technologies to create systems and monitoring devices. [54]	Method for remote assistance and exchange of specialized information on the basis of modern telecommunications technologies. [48]

Table 3. Comparison Telemetry / Telematics / Telemedicine [48]

Our definition of telemedicine is: Information network organization based on information and communication technology that connects medical experts together for medical care delivery from a distance.

Progress in the informatics science leads to personalized care and prevention of diseases, in contrast to longer treatment episodes in the status "invalid". The patient plays a major role in automated systems and telemedical networks.

In detailed steps, telemedicine can be described as a combination of:

1. Specialized monitoring, care and support for the sick through the use of systems that enable access to expert advice and information, regardless of the places where the need and source of information are located.
2. Application of electronic information and communication technologies to offer medical care and support, in the case of distance between actors.
3. Delivery of healthcare where the distance factor is prevented from applying any medical and health methods through the use of information and telecommunication technologies such as the right to exchange information concerning diagnosis, treatment, prevention of diseases and injuries, research, further training, continuing education and health care interests that are related to health and its preservation.
4. Any activity, which is a manifestation of health care (including diagnosis, consultation or advice, treatment and monitoring) that normally exhibit a professional and a patient (or two professionals, if located at the different places) and it is implemented through exchange of information and communication technologies.

The mainstream media where the telemedical system functions is the Internet. There are versions of medium - telephone, webcasts, specialized hardware for videoconferencing systems, but as a general definition from 90s, web-space is the chief mediator and underlying factors for operation of telemedical systems.

What benefits should Internet suppose?

- Accessibility of each
- Efficiency
- Low cost
- Compliance
- Possibility of transmission of any data
- Opportunity to record videocommunication
- Relatively high literacy in a Web environment

Based on the international experience and tendencies, and reflecting the above advantages, it can be concluded that for the development of e-health and telemedicine in particular, the necessary condition is an effective technology infrastructure (ICT) at each level in the health sector to ensure communication and transmission of information via the Internet.

Configuring the telemedical system

In Bulgarian medical hospitals, clinics and other private institutions have particular projects and implementations, which are not sponsored by the government. We have Leonardo Da Vinci in Pleven city, several solutions for the Military academy and few projects in medical hospitals. There are different projects in separate wards and departments, which often even are not popularized and published in the press and special journals.

The main stakeholders in Bulgarian healthcare system are the Parliament, the Ministry of Health, the NHIF and the Higher Medical Council. A number of other ministries own manage and finance their own health care facilities, including the Ministry of Defense, the Ministry of Internal Affairs and the Ministry of Transport. Private practice has expanded significantly, now including dental practices, pharmacies, physicians' surgeries, laboratories and outpatient clinics and polyclinics.

There have been advances in overall investment for the IT sector in Bulgaria as well as for IT in the healthcare system. In 2005, information and communication technology expenditure accounted for 3.77% of GDP and there were 59 personal computers (PCs) per 1000 inhabitants in 2004, compared to 47 in 2001.

Use of the Internet is also increasing. A recent survey conducted by the Alpha Research Agency found that 53% of adult Bulgarians used the Internet in 2010.

IT enjoys an ever-expanding application in outpatient care medical centres and in hospitals. Thanks to a financial donation from the World Bank, every GP now has a PC workstation and all PCs report in a digitalized format. In 2003, the Ministry of Health together with the Ministry of Finance and the NHIF countersigned the so-called "road map" setting forth the particulars of the coming incorporation of a diagnosis-related group (DRG) system within the reporting processes of hospitals. According to the "road map", and with the support of USAID and 3M Health Information Systems, a pilot project with 43 hospital beneficiaries was developed and implemented. 2004 marked the second year in which the relevant data necessary to calculate relative weights were collected. The National Centre for Health Informatics is also currently working on a project related to the introduction of uniform information standards within the health system under which in 2004–2005 all regional health care centers were updated with modern IT equipment.

The Health Card is one of the key technologies currently being developed and introduced in Bulgaria for health sector optimization, more efficient transactions between the health care institutions, more secure, flexible and transparent exchange of information, standardization of services and activities, and ensuring future interoperability with other European countries and healthcare systems. At the time of writing, there is no exact information about the dates for the launch of the system.

According to the "road map", and with the support of USAID and M Health Information Systems, a pilot project with hospital beneficiaries was developed and implemented. 2009 marked the second year in which the relevant data necessary to calculate relative weights were collected. The National Centre for Health Informatics is also currently working on a project related to the introduction of uniform information standards within the health system under which all regional health care centers were updated with modern IT equipment.

The Health Card is one of the key technologies currently being developed and introduced in Bulgaria for healthcare sector optimization, more efficient transactions between the health care institutions, more secure, flexible and transparent exchange of information, standardization of services and activities, and ensuring future interoperability within European countries and health systems. At the time of writing, there is no exact information about the dates for the launch of the system [119].

A telemedical system is basic set of workstations connected to each other, designed to bridge the knowledge in clinical medicine and scientific tasks using telemedical procedures.

The simplest system is a telemedical link between patient and nurse through a telephone line - fixed or GSM. More complex systems include video surveillance and audio connection. They consist of high standard telephone lines, digital information technology, computers, peripheral equipment, satellite connection and software security. In dissertation "Telemedical functions of Medical Information System", published at http://eprints.nbu.bg/view/subjects/MET.html are discussed in details different solutions, schemes and configurations.

It is not yet known throughout the country form of telemedical connection between two hospitals that provide continuous contact of experts, available for patients, permitting remote consultations by sending some kind of standard tests and images.

Telemedical Information System (TIS) is by definition an information system implemented to provide telemedical services and has several components (attributes):

- Hospital Information System
- Electronic Health Record
- Systems for Image Processing
- Health Information Network
- Applications for support of distance learning

The purposes of a TIS can be determined:

- Registration of selected key information in the data source
- Provide a platform for automated processing of that information
- Communication platform for its transmission
- Provision of expert support with a choice of clinical decisions
- Ensuring confidentiality during transmission of patients` personal data
- Assisting the patients in managing their own health

For the Bulgarian healthcare system, as for every other too, there are strict requirements for healthcare delivery and payment organization. Before starting the practical work for development of software we have analyzed the hospital structure, working personnel, technology infrastructure - both, PC periphery and specialized medical apparatuses, etc. We have developed special Questionnaires for each user that was expected to work with the software.

After processing the inquiry results, our working team pointed out the following tasks:

- development of software for telemedicine purposes where the user should identify every single step with a digital signature - requirement from the Ministry of Health.
- development of web portal for popularization of the project
- assurance of the required technologies:
- Laptop with camera, microphone and audio system for every General Practioner (GP) in the municipalities
- Digital stethoscope and digital ECG apparatus for distance transmission of data
- Specialized videoconference software for communication between the users

- Professional hardware for videoconference rooms

Doctors use four types of forms – „Consulted“, „Not checked“, „Consulted but with necessity for more information“ and „Returned forms with additional information“. After starting a request for consultation there are the following types of fields:

Paraclinic examinations - Identical with the paper original: blood tests, patomorphologic, urine tests, image examinations (ECG, X-ray, Echocardiography, Velotest, Holter, Scanner, Mammography and etc.)

Unlimited number of uploads are allowed – both for the consulting and giving consultations experts; also zooming of the image to the original size.

User parameters that the system registers are name, action, host, ip address, day, month, year, hour, minutes and seconds. It allows filtering of any of the above mentioned parameters, Microsoft Excel export format of the references, chronology control.

The Administrator performs a connection between users and software developers, which is realized as an e-mail box with all the standard parameters.

The system has 69 different statistics.

1. *Doctor statistics* - From date to date; Number of required consultations; Number of accomplished consultations
2. *Hospital statistics*

- From date to date; Number of required consultations; Number of accomplished consultations

3. *References with export to Microsoft Word, Microsoft Excel and with graphical visualization:*

- Number of consultations per period
  - Filtering through start and end date, level of consultation
- Number of consultations with result 'hospitalization'
  - Filtering through starting and ending date, level of consultation
- Percentage distribution according to specialists
  - Filtering through start and end date, level of consultation and specialty
- Number of consultations with second consultation
  - Filtering through start and end date, level of consultation
- Percentage distribution of correspondence between working and final diagnoses
  - Filtering through start and end date, level of consultation
- Percentage distribution of final diagnoses according to disease types
  - Filtering through start and end date, level of consultation

4. One of the most important statistics is actually the chronology of the system and control of each activity of every person

We have accomplished 150 consultations and 2000 registered activities. Our purposes are to adopt the model and to implement it in 5 municipalities at first and afterwards in every municipality on Bulgarian territory.

What types of patients is this healthcare method intended for?

1. For patients with "no time" - particularly active and financially supported to seek maximum quality of service they want to vote and to participate in making "the second / other opinions.
2. For patients with "no option" - single adults and people with a bunch of diseases who are in a physical difficulty to contact a doctor.
3. For patients with "no contact conditions" - those who can not receive direct medical services due to any unique circumstances and large contingents of people (from living in remote locations to space flights and military operations).

4. For patients like "I have the right of consultation" - prompted by the Constitution to regulate access to health care with the appropriate quality and prices should be clearly defined by the authors and be affordable for consumers.

Our software solution is implemented in 2 remote hospitals - Aeroclinic in Sofia and Municipal Hospital in the town of Svoge which is about 50 km far from the capital. According to the Personal Data Protection Law (PDPL) "processing of personal data" means any operation or set of actions that is made in respect of personal data by automatic or other means, such as collection, recording, organization, storage, adaptation or alteration, retrieval, consultation, use, disclosure by transmission, dissemination, making available, alignment or combination, blocking, erasure or destruction of data [37].

In remote consultation only initials of names, sex and age of patient are used.

The other protection method, covering the legitimacy of the diagnosis, is the electronic signature that the system requires to start working with.

Under Bulgarian law the electronic document signed with a valid digital signature is fully equivalent to the corresponding paper. The recipient of the electronic document does not need to possess a digital signature.

We have developed a representative analysis with 19 points that clearly shows the benefits form telemedicine.

Comparative analysis

In order to illustrate the merits, while outlining the challenges, facing the Bulgarian telemedicine, we will present a popular and close by construction, but far more extensive, solution - HEALTH OPTIMUM project.

This is European international project that involves 3 countries – Italy, Denmark and Spain. Italy participates with 6 neurosurgical telecounselling centers and Tele-laboratory; 1 telecounselling center and 1 tele-laboratory for Spain, and in Denmark – tele-diabetes center and tele-cardiology center.

The HEALTH OPTIMUM comprises the following services:

Tele-counselling - general hospital specialists/GP requests the opinion of the tertiary hospital specialists on a clinical case. The service can be provided according to various modalities:

- Asynchronously (secure e-mail type interaction) - the requesting professional sends the query to the tertiary hospital specialists and waits for a reply. The maximum delay in replying to a query must have been agreed beforehand between the requester and the tertiary hospital. Both the request and the counsellor answer make use of standard forms, agreed among all the actors involved in the tele-counselling. Such forms must contain all the clinical and anamnesis information needed to provide a feedback through tele-counselling. Moreover such forms must be validated through digital signature according to EU and national regulations.

1. Interactively (through videoconferencing facilities) - in this case the healthcare professionals can talk and see at each other, sharing information about the patient. This modality normally requires booking an appointment with the tertiary hospital specialist as in the case of a normal referral unless standby or emergency arrangements are in place between the requesting party and the tertiary hospital.
2. Virtual referral - general hospital specialists or exceptionally a General Practitioner carries out a virtual referral with the tertiary hospital specialist while the patient is in his/her clinic. This service normally requires booking an appointment with the tertiary hospital specialist as in the case of a normal referral unless standby or emergency

arrangements are in place between the requesting party and the tertiary hospital. Notification services

- This family of services will notify the referring medical doctor (general hospital specialist or GP) about relevant events concerning the evolution inside the tertiary hospital of the patient they have referred. Three types of events requiring notification have already been identified in a previous eTEN project (C^3 - Comprehensive Continuous Care): Notification of Admission; Notification of Transfer and Notification of Discharge (this includes death as one of the possible reasons for discharge).

Before	*After*
Transport to hospital	*Instant Consultation*
Using an expert	*Using more experts*
Paper archive	*Electronic data base + paper archives*
Losses in transmission of data and research	*Digitized archive of record with 2 seats*
More costs to the patient / relatives	*Less cost to the patient / relatives*
Multiple visits	*Number of visits*
Expenditure of time for specialist	*Only if necessary*
Healthcare in hospital	*Healthcare at home*
Isolation of experts	*Improving relations in expert community*
Charge for the hospital:	*Only if necessary*
- For professionals	*Only if necessary*
- Transport	*Only if necessary*
- Time	*Only if necessary*
- Technology	*Off with long-term returns*
Loss of time for patient	*Only if necessary*
Limited disease prevention	*Disease prevention*
Patient access to specialists at the local level	*Patient access to specialists at national level*
Need for direct contact with national specialists	*Remote specialist consultation at national level*
Limited free time	*Increase the creative work*

Table 4. Before/after implementation of telemedical software analysis [48]

Shared clinical records - a referring general hospital specialist and tertiary hospital specialists will have access to the same set of patients clinical records during a virtual referral or during the entire stay of the patient in a tertiary hospital. This allows the referring specialist not to lose touch with his/her patient.

Tele-laboratory - it allows to carry out tests which are usually executed inside a clinical laboratory practically in any place thanks to portable analysis equipment which can be checked remotely, data transmission and a PKI infrastructure which guarantee the authenticity the confidentiality and the legal value of the data transmitted. [122]

Throughout Bulgaria is not yet known form of telemedical scheme between two hospital units that provide continuous contact between the experts, available for patients and permits remote consultations by sending any kind of standard tests and imaging, as parts of the DH (disease history) treated.

TELECONSULT is organized as follows:

- Main software desktop solution, divided according to the operational level into three main parts- three different management modules that are developed according to the requirements and necessary functions for each participant in the telemedical process.
- Audio and video streaming through specialized software.
- Video communication through newly developed application with individual virtual rooms, locked and password protected meetings.

With this integral solution is performed the ability to verify whether a receiving physician presents; if the receiving system is able to process the transmitted files and whether the receiving system has approved all prior files. Each patient is identified only with age, sex and physical conditions, in order to keep the patients privacy and confidentiality.

Expert's module is designed and conformable to the specific telemedical consultation characteristics - each variant of consultation: required, consulted, not checked and with request for more information, is differentiate with its own color. The system checks every 30 seconds about newly arrived requests for consultations, and ensures sound and visual signalization to attract the expert's attention.

The operator's module is the main coordinator in the system, where the Operator manages the expeditiousness of the process of giving consultation, and in case delay of 24 hours, the system allows redirecting the form according to the available specialists. In case of few requirements for the same specific condition consultations arrive at the same moment, the system distributes through the available specialists in the corresponding specialty.

The Administrator performs functional connection between users and software developers, which is realized with system mailbox. He has the authorization to make any kind of statistics for anybody at any time.

Administrator's panel is developed in order to assure the correct performance of the processes, committing full access to every single user parameter that the system registers: name, activity, host, ip address, day, month, year, hour, minutes and seconds. The system allows filtering of any of the above mentioned parameters, Word & Excel export of the references, chronology control, and graphical representations in bars. Statistical basis is organized in 69 different sections. In order to prove the usability and benefits from telemedical investments, there are two statistics about percentage of application for a medical expert and for a hospital.

The comparative analysis is developed on the base of published and accessible documents for both projects.

The asterix indicates that the value of the first 4 parameters is doubled, because of their importance and significance to the realization of telemedical solutions. The rest: are also important, but required for any kind of software solution.

Teleconsult performs videoconsultaions through specialized software, Health optimum states that the interactive form of consulation is done through video-conferencing facilities, where the healthcare professionals can talk and see each other and thus share information about the patient.

Teleconsult doesn't have Telelaboratory, Health Optimum develops four

In Bulgarian practice still it is not familiar as a working model the HL7 standard, while Spain, Denmark and Italy investigate efforts.

DICOM is not implemented and used in Teleconsult, in contrast to Health Optimum.

IDC 10 is introduced in both system as working coding system.

By Notification services we mean services, ensuring that the experts attention would be kept and he would be able easily to asses the situation. In Teleconsult there are 4 types of consultations: Required, Consulted, Not checked and With request for more information, while in Health Optimum are performed as follows: Notification of Admission; Notification of Transfer and Notification of Discharge.

Email connection is with 2 points for both softwares, because Teleconsult has internal email system within the software solution. It doesn't perform, for example - patient-doctor connection. Health Optimum, on the other site organizes secure e-mail type interaction - the requesting professional sends the query to the tertiary hospital specialists and waits for a reply.

Exchange of files and records is well organized in Teleconsult, because it allows sending and receiving any kind and format of documents. Health Optimum experts have access to patients' clinical records in a single data repository.

PKI infrastructure in Teleconsult is represented with digital signature - requirement of Bulgarian law, the system requires authenticity of medical specialist - the private key is connected to his unique ID number, when any action is performed by him in Teleconsult. In Health Optimum data transmission and a PKI infrastructure guarantee the authenticity, confidentiality and legal value of the transmitted data.

Emergency arrangements is a parameter, that ensures fast reaction from the system itself, when there is an urgent situation. Teleconsult guarantees express actions, which include light and signal alarms. Health Optimum performs asynchronous services through secure e-mail type interaction, where the maximum delay in replying to a query must have been agreed beforehand between the requester and the tertiary hospital.

Clinical anamnesis information is presented through introduction of concrete data from the patient's record. In Health Optimum - the experts have access to the whole patient's record from a centered repository.

Multilingual interface - Teleconsult is developed into Bulgarian and English, while Health Optimum is a three different countries product

Both systems get 2 points for System verifications. Teleconsult consultation forms have obligate fields, which filled incorrect, do not allow sending the request.

Teleconsult executes 69 different references and system statistics.

Archive is well organized in Teleconsult with high level of security and RAID 5.

Level of introducement - Teleconsult is a national project within 2 hospitals, while Health Optimum is an international development.

Specialists on call use the company network with a private ADSL (or ISDN) - both software solutions ensure that parameter.

Teleconsult can perform GPRS connection, but at the current moment this feature is not specifically developed. Tele-laboratory makes use of the existing company network for

connections to elderly homes and a GPRS or similar connection with mobile POCT devices for use in home assistance.
HIS connection with the telemedical module has 4 points for Teleconsult, because actually it is pat of a HIS. Health Optimum works within a hospital institutions but it is not clearly stated that it is part of a HIS.
Teleconsult has 4 points for Open system, because it is organized easily to update and expand.
Multifunctional system. We haven`t found data about System statistics, Archive and Open system for HEALTH OPTIMUM.
The maximum result of the 23 parameters analysis is 84. HEALTH OPTIMUM is with 77% accomplishment, while Teleconsult is with 68%. The system allows unlimited number of participants, but to the current moment different legal limits and obstacles do not allow spreading.

Comparative analysis

System / Parameter	TELECONSULT	Health Opitmum
Videoconference connection *	4	2
Telelaboratory *	0	4
HL7 *	0	3
DICOM *	0	4
IDC 10	4	4
Notification services	3	4
Email connection	2	2
Exchange of files and records	3	2
PKI infrastructure	3	4
Emergency arrangements	4	2
Clinical anamnesis information	3	4
Multilingual interface	3	4
System verifications	2	2
System statistics	3	No data
Archive	3	No data
Level of introduction	National	International
ADSL connection	4	4
GPRS connection	1	2
HIS connection with the telemedicine module	4	3
Open system	4	No data
Multifunctional system	4	2
	58	65

Legend: 0 - missing; 1 - bad organization; 2 - exists; 3 - good organization; 4 - excellent organization

3. Conclusion

eHealth and its practical application options are necessary, inevitable part of electronization of society. This requires not only investing in technology, but also to think about training and qualifications of medical experts to offer it as an important and effective version of healthcare services.

The results of the surveys from three different points of view - patients, doctors and hospital managers, confirmed the usefulness of such a decision. More than 4/5 of patients find it satisfactory and do not worry about the lack of physical contact with the treating expert. Physicians reported their positive attitude about this contemporary method of work, supporting it in about 90%. Of course, our findings are based on a limited number of statistical observations.

Clearly recognized is the natural caution and even fear when introducing a new practicing method - both for the quality of provisioning methodology and technology, either for data protection and natural tendency towards tradition of natural communication, we believe that we have made the first step. There are no registered complaints and mistakes; the intake is a natural and good feedback. It is important to indicate the originality of presented telemedical system - in our country there is lack of experience, no attitudes, limited research and publications.

On these grounds we can determine Teleconsult as an example of High-tech medicine. Patients should have personal respect and a culture of their own health management - to seek and comply personal medical and health data and information. Clinical approbation and subsequent implementation show that more than 60% of consulted patients are reallocated after hospitalization for teleconsultation and in over 25% there is a positive effect on hospitalized with a result - reduce of their hospital stay. In more than 10% of cases is demonstrated complete consistency between the views of consultants.

4. Acknowledgment

The thesis, summarized in this chapter, arose in part out of years of research that has been done since I came to the Biomedical department of sciences. In the first place, I would like to express my gratitude to prof. Jivka Vinarova, PhD, DMSc for her supervision, advice, and guidance from the very early stage of this research as well as for giving me extraordinary experiences through out the work. Above all and the most needed, she provided me with unflinching encouragement and support in various ways. Also, I gratefully acknowledge chief. ass. prof. Iliq Pendzhurov, PhD for his advice, supervision, and crucial contribution, which made him the backbone of this research and so to this thesis. His involvement with originality has triggered and nourished my intellectual maturity that I will benefit from, for a long time to come.

5. References

[1] Ablaza V., Fisher J. Telemedicine and wound care management // Home Care Provid.-1998.-Vol.3,N4.-P.206-213.

[2] Adeyinka M. The teleambulance//J.Telemed.Telecare.-1996.-Vol.2,N1.-P.76-79.

[3] Aims and Scope//J.of Telemed and telecare.-1995, Vol.1, N1, p1

[4] Bashshur R.L. On the definition and Evaluation of Telemedicine// Telemed J.-1995, Vol.1, N1, p34-38
[5] Beals D., Fletcher J. Telemedicine and pediatric surgery // Semin.Pediatr.Surg.-2000.-Vol.9,N1.-P.40-47.
[6] Benger J. A review of minor injuries telemedicine // J.Telemed. Telecare.-1999.-Vol.5,N3.-P.5-13.
[7] Beolchi L., Telemedicine Glossary, 5 Edition, 2003 Working Documents, Glossary of Concepts. Technologies, Standards and Users, September 2003, European Commission, Information Society Directorate-General, Brussels
[8] Bergeron B.P. Telepresence and the practice of medicine. Look for machines to assist you, not replace you // Postgrad Med.- 1998.- Vol.103,N4.
[9] Billica R., Sargsyan A., Simmons S. Telemedicine aboard the International Space Station (ISS): an operational system and a testbed-http://www.telemed.ru
[10] Coiera E, "Guide to Medical Informatics, the Internet and Telemedicine", 1998, p.376.
[11] Darkins A., Fisk N., Garner P. et al. Point-to-point telemedicine using the ISDN // J.Telemed.Telecare.-1996.-Vol.2,N1.-P.82-83.
[12] DeBakey M. Telemedicine has now come of age// Telemedicine Journal.-1995.-Vol. I, No. 1.-P.44-52.
[13] Demartines N., Mutter D., Marescaux J., Harder F. Preliminary assessment of the value and effect of expert consultation in telemedicine // J.Am.Coll.Surg.-2000.-Vol.190,N4.-P.466-470.
[14] Demartines N., Mutter D., Vix M. et al. Assessment of telemedicine in surgical education and patient care // Ann.Surg.-2000.-Vol.231,N2.-P.282-291.
[15] Eelsalu H. Telematic application for nurses: integration and dissemination of European nursing terminology in information technology // I International Virtual Conference "High Technologies in Medicine".-Donetsk, 1999.-P.26.
[16] Field M. J. Telemedicine: a guide to assessing telecommunications in health care. Washington, DC: National Academy Pr; 1996
[17] Foster D., Werner F., Murray D., Somerset J. Telemetry instrumentation for kinesiologic studies of knee motion //Med.Res.Eng.-1980.-Vol.13,N2.-P.17-21.
[18] Guber E., Informatics in clinical medicine, pathology and pediatrics, Leningrad, Medicine, 1990
[19] Goldberg M.A. Telemedicine an overview// Telemed J.-1995, Vol.1, N1, p20-25
[20] Grigsby J, Kaehny M.M., Schlenker RE, Shaughnessy PW, Beale SK. Telemedicine: literature review and analytic framework. Denver: Center for Health Policy Research; 1993; Office of Technology Assessment, U.S. Congress. Bringing health care online. Washington, DC: US Gov Pr Office; 1995;
[21] Grundy B., Crawford P., Jones P. et al. Telemedicine in critical care: an experiment in health care delivery // JACEP.-1977.-Vol.6,N10.-P.439-444.
[22] Harr D.S., Balch D.C., McConnell M.E.Next generation telemedicine. The future is now// NC Med. J.- 1997.-Vol. 58,N6.
[23] Heneghan C., Sclafani A., Stern J., Ginsburg J. Telemedicine applications in otolaryngology // IEEE Eng.Med.Biol.Mag.-1999.-Vol.18,N4.-P.53-62.
[24] Jerant A. Home telemedicine: merging the old and new ways // Am.Fam.Physician.-1999.-Vol. 60,N4.-P.1096-1098.

[25] Jusupuva R., R. Polonnikova, "Telemedicine: new information technology in XX century ", Sankt Peterburg, 1998
[26] Kalaidjieva M., Protection of perosnal data in the process of eHealth adoption, http://www.kaminata.net/viewtopic.php?f=131&t=12920 [accessed 2011 March 22]
[27] Kayser K., Drlicek M. Accessedual telecommunication for expert consultation of intraoperative sections // Zentralbl.Pathol.-1992.-Vol.138,N6.-P.395-398.
[28] Kazakov V.N., V.G. Glymovickyy, Liah U.E., Vladzymyrskyy A, Kolodejdnyy A.V.,. Use of telemedical system in traumatology and orthopedics in «UkrMedNet» // XIII Congress of orthopedic trauma Ukraine, "Lebed",2001.p.413-416.
[29] Kazakov V.N., V.G. Glymovickyy, Vladzymyrskyy A, Telemedicine, ISBN 966-556-010-7, Donetzk, 2002
[30] Kennedy M. Technology opens new doors for trauma and care//WMJ.-1999.-Vol.98,N7.-P.12-18.
[31] Khandheria B.K. Telemedicine: An application in search of users//Mayo Clin.Proc. - 1996 - Vol.71 - P.420-421
[32] Kuvakin V.I., Telemedicine: definition, basic direction and history - http://www.telemed.ru [accessed 2010 May 12]
[33] Kuvakin V.I., Teplynskyy V.N., General design of telemedical systems. Development and technical approach // I International electronic scientific coneference "Hightech in medicine".- Donetzk, 1999.-p.33-35.
[34] Lambrecht C. Emergency physicians' roles in a clinical telemedicine network // Ann.Emerg.Med.-1997.-Vol.30,N5.-P.670-674.
[35] LaPorte R.E. Global public health and the information superhighway //BMJ.-1994.-Vol.308,N6945.-P.1651-1652.
[36] Law for digital document and digital signature
[37] Law for protection of personal data
[38] Liah U.E., Vladzymyrskyy A, Introduction in telemedicine, Series: Essays in biological and medical informatics, Donetzk, Lebed, 1999.-102 p.
[39] Lipson L, Henderson TM., State initiatives to promote telemedicine, Washington, DC: Intergovernmental Health Policy Project, George Washington University; 1995.)
[40] Mahau M., A. Allen, E-Health & Telehealth Glossary, http://www.telehealth.net/glossary.html, [accessed на 01.10.2008]
[41] Mahau M., P.Whitten, A.Allen, E-Health, Telehealth and Telemedicine, A guide to start-up, ISBN:0-7879-4420-3, Jossey-bass, 2000
[42] Marilyn J. Field, Editor; Committee on Evaluating Clinical Applications of Telemedicine, Institute of Medicine Telemedicine, A guide to assessing telecommunications in healthcare, National Academy of Science, ISBN-10: 0-309-05531-8, ISBN-13: 978-0-309-05531-4
[43] Materna B., Advances in international telemedicine and e-health around the world, ISBN 978-83-89769-22-0
[44] Meindl J., Ford A. Implantable telemetry in biomedical research // IEEE Trans.Biomed.Eng.-1984.-Vol.31,N12.-P.817-823.
[45] Meldrum S. The current status of medical telemetry//J.Med.Eng.Technol.-1980.-Vol.4,N1.-P.1.

[46] MIE 2005 The XIX International Congress of the European Federation for Medical Informatics, Vol I No 1, 2005; ISSN 1861-3179

[47] Mihova P., „Telemedical functions of Medical Information System", dissertation work for scientific degree "Philosophy doctor of NBU", scientific code 03.01.53, 2009

[48] Moore M., "Elements of Success in Telemedicine Projects", 1996

[49] National health strategy 2008 – 2013 year

[50] Nerlich M., Kretschmer R. The Impact of Telemedicine on Health Care Managment.- Amsterdam, Berlin, Oxford, Tokyo,Washington: IOS Press,1999.-281 p.

[51] NLM National Telemedicine initiative, Summaries of awards announced October 1996// US National Library of medicine – 1996 - N3-9 p.

[52] Perednia DA, Allen A., Telemedicine technology and clinical applications. JAMA. 1995; 273:483-8; Physician Payment Review Commission Annual Report to Congress, Washington, DC: PPRC; 1995

[53] Pozen M., Berezin M., Kulp R. Cost and utility considerations in implementing ambulance telemetry // Heart.Lung.-1980.-Vol.9,N5.-P.866-872.

[54] Screnci D., Hirsch E., Levy K et al. Medical outreach to Armenia by telemedicine linkage // J.Med.Syst.-1996.-Vol.20.N2.-P.67-76.

[55] Shortliffe E., L.Perreault, G. Wiederhold, Lawrence M. Fagan, Medical Informatics: Computer Applications in Health Care and Biomedicine (Health Informatics), ISBN: 0387984720

[56] Siderfin C. Low-technology telemedicine in Antarctica // J.Telemed.Telecare.-1995.-Vol.1,N1.-P.54-60.

[57] Stanberry B. The legal and ethical aspects of telemedicine. Telemedicine and malpractice// J. Telemed.Telecare.- 1998.-Vol.4, N2.-P.13-22.

[58] Telemedicine Glossary, printed by DG INFSO - B1, Version 4.2.6., February 2002

[59] Telemedicine Recourses and Services: American Telemedicine Association// The Univ. of Texas at Austin., 1994 - 4p.

[60] Telemedicine: Fad or Future? Editorial,//Lancet -1995, Vol.345, N89, p.42

[61] Telemedicine: Theory and Practice // R.Bashshur et al.-Springfield: Ch.C.Thomas Publisher Ltd., 1997.-320 p.

[62] Thrall J., Boland G. Telemedicine in practice // Semin. Nucl. Med.- 1998.- Vol. 28,N2.

[63] Tracy J., A Guide to Getting Started in Telemedicine, Telemedicine Technical Assistance Documents, , University of Missouri – School of Medicine

[64] Traubman L. The saving of Oleg. A USA-USSR medical success using packet and ham radio, facsimile, and electronic mail // Ann.NY Acad.Sci.-1992.-N670.-P.229-243.

[65] Vinarova J., M.Vukov, textbook and Glossary in telemedicine, translation of "European Telemedicine Glossary", Glossary of standards, concepts, technologies and users, edited by DG INFSO, May 2001, editor prof. Luciano Beolchi, ISBN954-535-269-8, NBU, Sofia, 2002

[66] Vinarova J., "Theoretic and applied aspects of medical and health information", dissertation work for or scientific degree "Doctor of Philosophy", scientific code 03.01.53, 2007

[67] Vinarova J., P.Mihova, St.Tonev, A.Petkov, textbook "eHealth", ISBN 13: 978-954-516-910-6, Letera, Sofia, 2009

[68] Vinarova J., P.Mihova, textbook "Medical informatics", ISBN 13: 978-954-535-515-8, NBU, Sofia 2008

[69] Vladzymyrskyy A, "Telemedical glossary", ISSN 1728-936X 2007
[70] Vladzymyrskyy A, Clinical teleconsulting (Doctors guide), ISBN 966-7968-45-6, Donetzk 2005
[71] Vladzymyrskyy A, Guie in telemedicine for General Practitioners, ISSN 1728, Donetzk 2005
[72] Vladzymyrskyy A, Liah U.E., Structure of telemedical system for consultaion form distance// Modern problems in informatics- Abstracts of IV International electronic scientific coneference, Voronej,1999.-p.136.
[73] Vladzymyrskyy A., „Evaluating telemedical effectiveness", ISBN 978-966-335-031-8, Donetzk 2007
[74] Vladzymyrskyy A., Problems in telemedical terminology // Arch.clin.exp.med.-V.10,№1.-2001.-p.108-112.
[75] Wirthlin D., Buradagunta S., Edwards R. et al. Telemedicine in vascular surgery: feasibility of digital imaging for remote management of wounds //J.Vasc.Surg.-1998.-Vol.27,N6.-P.1089-1100.
[76] Wright D.The International Telecommunication Union's report on Telemedicine and Developing Countries// J. Telemed. Telecare.- 1998.- Vol.4, Suppl. 1.
[77] Yamamoto L. Wireless teleradiology and fax using cellular phones and notebook PCs for instant access to consultants // Am.J.Emerg.Med.-1995.-Vol.13,N2.-184-187.

Webography

[78] http://www.americantelemed.org/i4a/pages/index.cfm?pageid=1 [accessed 2011 January 11]
[79] http://intra.rfbr.ru/pub/vestnik/V4_99/1_11.htm,О.С.Медведев, МГУ, И.Н.Столяров, РосНИИРОС, [accessed 2011 January 11]
[80] http://iol.spb.osi.ru/IOL1999/DB/DOC/get_thes.php3?id=338, [accessed 2011 January 11]
[81] http://ritmru.chat.ru/, [accessed 2011 January 13]
[82] www.nlm.nih.gov/pubs/cbm/telembib.html, [accessed 2011 January 14]
[83] www.sno.msmi.minsk.by/PRESS/9NOMER/telemed..html, [accessed 2011 January 11]
[84] http://www.astm.org/COMMIT/COMMITTEE/E31.htm, [accessed 2011 January 10]
[85] http://www.telemed.net.ua/, [accessed 2010November 11]
[86] www.b4uclose.com/index_files/glossaryofterms.htm, [accessed 2011 January 6]
[87] http://www.inftech.webseraccessedru/it/conference/isanditc/2000/section6/index.html, [accessed 2010 November 11]
[88] http://www.gmds2006.de/Abstracts/129.pdf , [accessed 2011 January 14]
[89] http://www.stsc.hill.af.mil/crossTalk/2001/06/bowman.html, [accessed 2011 January 14]
[90] http://www.jmir.org/2005/1/e9, [accessed 2010 November 11]
[91] casde.unl.edu/glossary/t.php, [accessed 2010 November 18]
[92] www.flowmeterdirectory.com/sensor_terminology_a.html, [accessed 2010 November 18]
[93] amsglossary.allenpress.com/glossary/browse, [accessed 2010 November 18]
[94] www.sciencelobby.com/dictionary/t.html, [accessed 2010 November 18]
[95] www.w4kwh.org/radio/satellite.html, [accessed 2010 November 18]

[96] www.nps.gov/archive/yell/yellowstoneindepth/episode4glossary.htm, [accessed 2010 November 18]
[97] www.suite101.com/lesson.cfm/17337/573/2, [accessed 2010 November 18]
[98] en.wikipedia.org/wiki/Telemetry, [accessed 2010 November 18]
[99] en.wiktionary.org/wiki/telemetry, [accessed 2010 November 18]
[100] www.thesaudi.net/vsat/vsat-glossary.htm, [посетен 2008 Ноември 18]
[101] www.angelfire.com/anime3/internet/communications.htm, [accessed 2010 November 18]
[102] www.unesco.org/education/educprog/lwf/doc/portfolio/definitions.htm, [accessed 2010 November 18]
[103] www.equivalence.com/labor/lab_vf_glo_e.shtml, [accessed 2008 November 18]
[104] www.quantum3.co.za/CI%20Glossary.htm, [посетен 2008 November 18]
[105] www2.plymouth.ac.uk/distancelearning/course/glossary.doc, [accessed 2008 November 18]
[106] www.asklepios-future-hospital.com/english/glossary.asp, [accessed 2010 November 18]
[107] www.highland.gov.uk/yourenvironment/planning/developmentplans/localplans/glossary.htm, [accessed 2010November 18]
[108] www.libanphone.com/gsm-glossary-of-terms.htm, [accessed 2010 November 18]
[109] en.wiktionary.org/wiki/telematics, [accessed 2010 November 18]
[110] www.accesswireless.org/general/glossary.cfm, [accessed 2010 November 18]
[111] http://www.healthoptimum.info/archive/index.jsp.12.html, [accessed 2011 January 09]
[112] www.nas.nasa.gov/About/Education/Racecar/glossary.html, [accessed 2008 May 8]
[113] www.wbopdc.govt.nz/Projects/OmokoroaCommunityWastewaterProject/Learningthelingo.htm [accessed 2008 November 18]
[114] http://medical.nema.org/, [accessed 2011 January 25]
[115] http://videoconferencing.hit.bg/str_6.html, [accessed 2011 January 17]
[116] http://tele.med.ru/u15.htm [accessed 2011 January 11]
[117] http://www.who.int/en/ [accessed 2011 January 11]
[118] www.euro.who.int/__data/assets/pdf_file/0006/80592/E90023.pdf [accessed 2011 March 23]

21

Practical Results of Telemedicine System Between Antarctic Station and Japan

Giichiro Ohno
National Institute of Polar Research, Tokyo
Department of Surgery, Tokatsu Hospital, Chiba
Japan

1. Introduction

It is as sure as ice is ice that being a medical doctor is a rewarding job. A good surgeon starts and ends the day to save many precious lives in the operating room with the most powerful team. Though he is satisfied with his role, the doctor notices one day that he does not know whether it is raining or sunny outside, or even what the season is now. At that time, it creeps into his heart that he wants to work by himself with a daily awareness of nature in every respect, for instance as a doctor in Antarctica.
He tries working in Antarctica to find unexpected extreme medicine waiting for him.

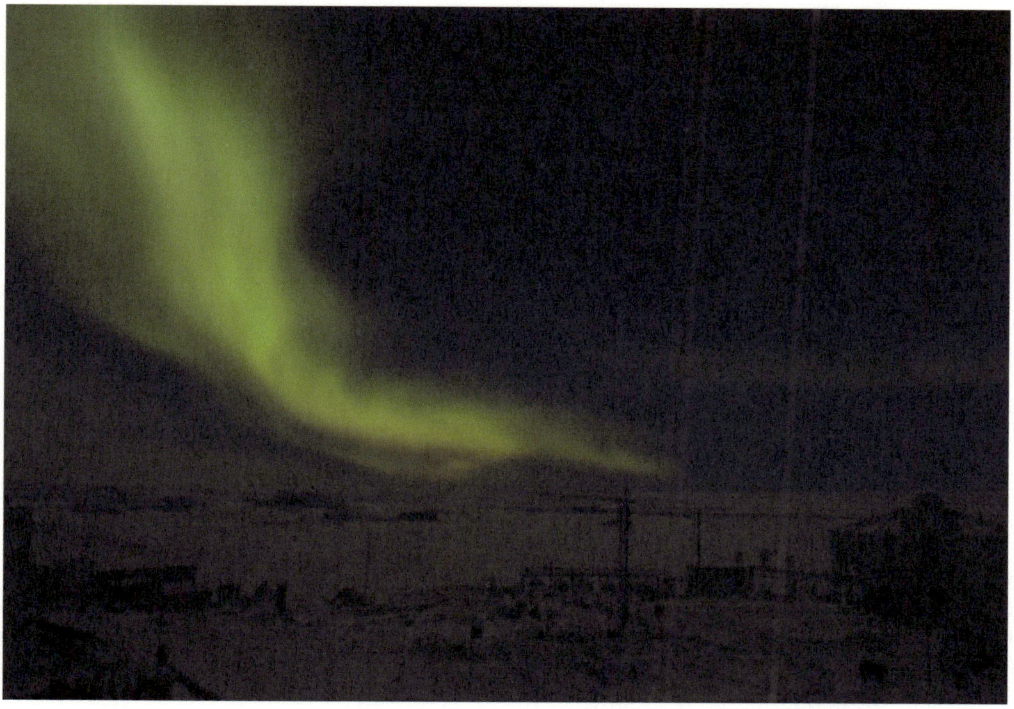

Photo by Toyama Y.

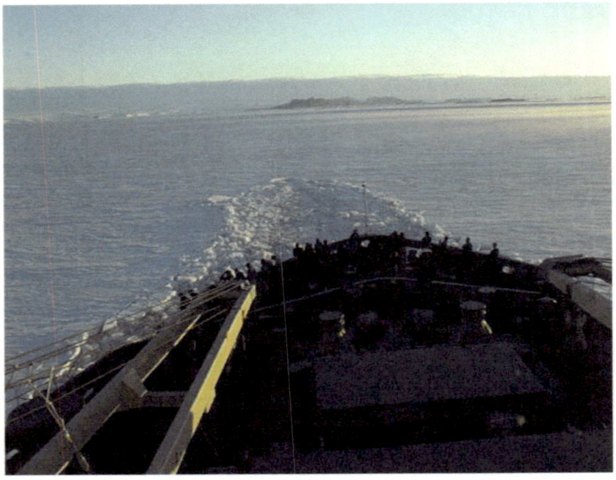

2. Antarctic research tells us about tomorrow's earth and space

The Japanese Antarctic Research Expedition (JARE) has had a continued presence in Antarctica, and has continued the survey with winter-over operation since 1956 at Syowa station (S69°,E39°)

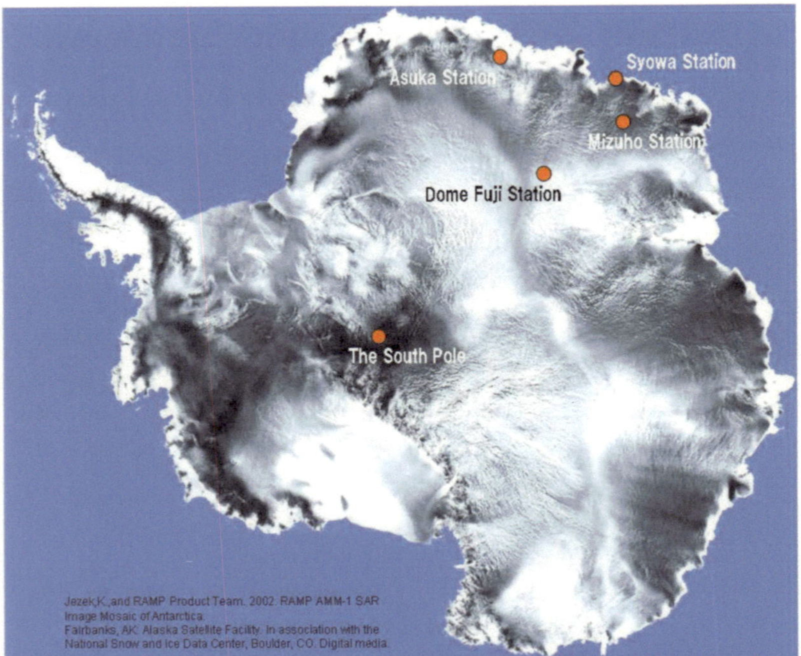

At the dawning of the expedition, it was a life-risking enterprise for its own sake to spend a winter in such an unapproachable and potentially hostile environment. After setting up the station and refining operational methods, energetic researches were made to clarify the last unexplored area including the mysterious aurora, many unique forms of life, climatic conditions and meteorology, the nature of the huge ice cap covering the continent 2000m in thickness and the continent itself concealed beneath. These riddles continue to attract many researchers to this day. Recently Antarctica has been noticed afresh. The location, isolated and far from civilized society makes Antarctica the most sensitive monitor of climate change and its cooling system is the key of the earth warming. The Ozone layer shows Antarctica as a forerunner of world environmental disruption. It becomes clear that the Aurora influenced by solar wind and Antarctic meteorites teach us about solar system and earth. The Antarctic continent has a large part to play in understanding plate tectonics. Antarctic research expeditions have been going on for a half century history and will continue.

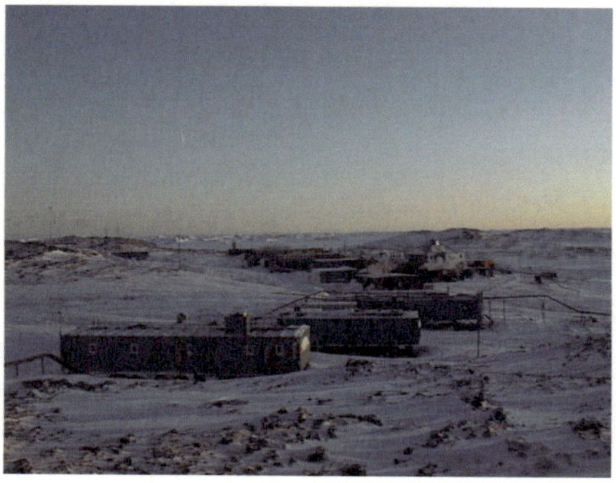

Syowa Station

3. Complete isolation in icebound Antarctica

It is a particular luxury to appreciate extreme nature through the window from a warm comfortable room. The Japanese Antarctic station has been repaired every year and updated with the latest technology so that participants are able to stay not only without the dangers of the past but also with a comforts of home. But once they step out of the door, the ferocity of nature is still there, yet many outdoor operations and field investigations are managed. It is even impossible to go the next building just in the station area without a degree of danger. The sole victim of Japanese expedition over the years, was lost when he attempted to go the doghouse from main building within the base area.

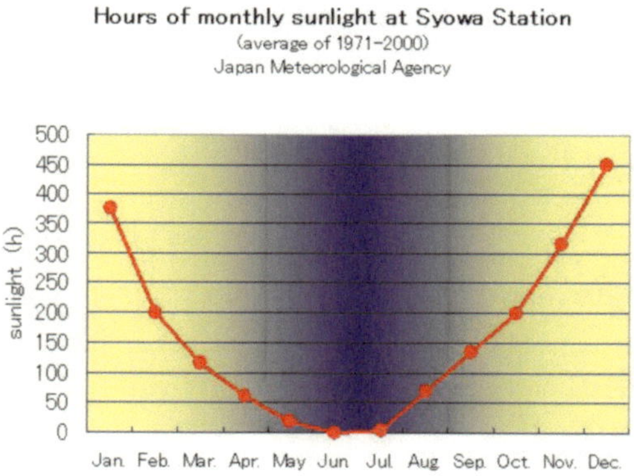

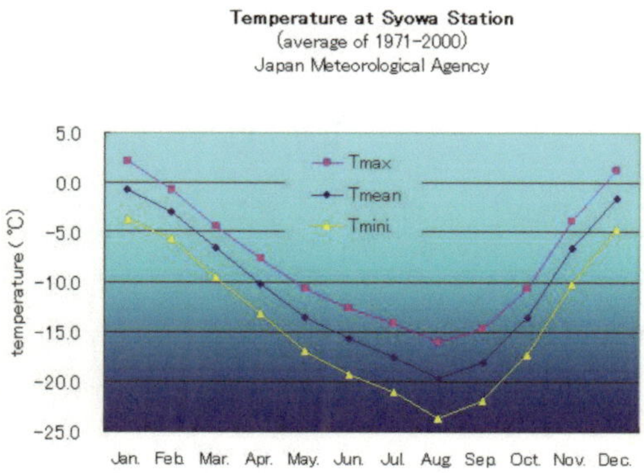

Syowa station is a coastal one and the temperature is -5°C in summer and -40°C in winter. The Antarctic continent is covered by a thick ice sheet that has an average thickness of over two thousand meters. The temperature becomes drastically lower inland on the ice sheet. Dome Fuji, one of Japanese Antarctic bases is S 77°, E39°, and 3810 meters above sea level. The temperature is -20°C in summer and -80°C in winter.

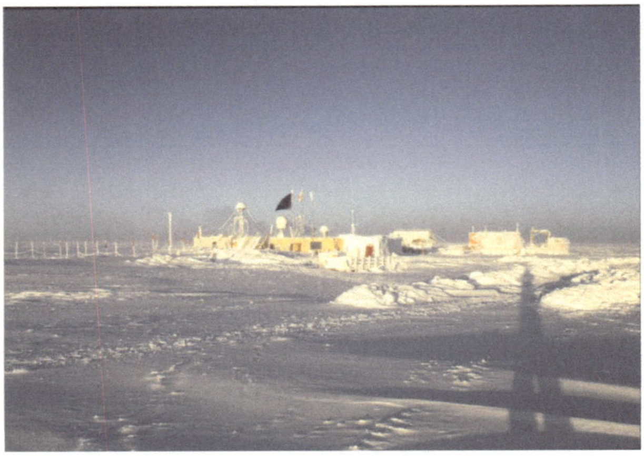

Dome Fuji Base

Day length and Sunlight change is also one particular characteristic in the polar region. At Syowa station on the edge of the Antarctic circle at S69°degrees, there is night with the midnight sun for one and half months then the sunlight shortens 5 hours every month to the polar night with no daylight. Loss of day light and night causes problems with circadian rhythms leading to insomnia, EEG changes, and autonomic nervous system dysfunction with ECG abnormalities. Excessive change of sunlight hours can also cause emotional instability.

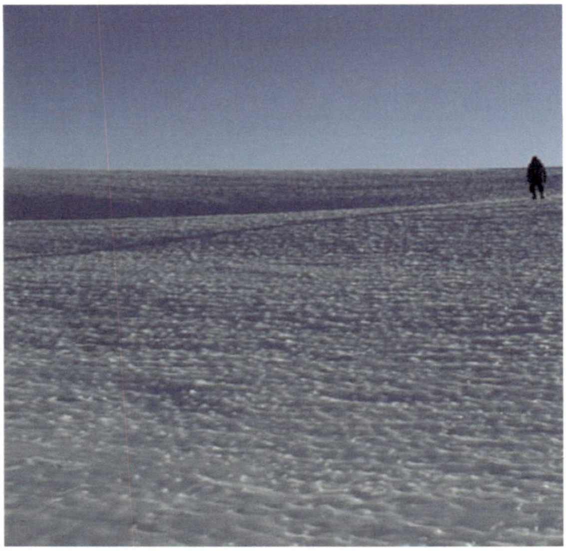

Wintering teams continue nevertheless to grapple with many field operations including high altitude work, diving in the sea and so on.

Each field operation needs several weeks to a few months away from the station with snow tractors and snow mobiles for locomotion and living space. There are crackles on the sea ice as crevasses on the ice sheet wide enough to swallow the mobiles. There are hypobaric effect at high altitude, strong ultraviolet ray under ozone hole, large marine animals can harm divers and so on the risks to health and wellbeing are great. The cold increases with wind chill effects and it is said someone who is immobile with injuries, can only survive for up to an hour or two, though it may take a few days to rescue from station and even this is impossible in stormy weather.

It is impossible not to be exposed to wild nature in any field operations.

The station is 15000km distance from Japan. The only means of access is an icebreaker ship which plies between Tokyo and the station once every Austral summer. The ship takes in new winter-over team with the whole commodity to survive for one year and brings the previous team back to Japan. Once the ship leaves, there is no regular transport to the station and in winter it is completely impossible to approach because of huge sheets of oceanic ice and polar darkness.

There are about thirty stations altogether engaged in wintering but none of them is close enough to Syowa station to permit mutual help for each other in an emergency. It may be said that there is no evacuation to or rescue from outside possibly during winter months.

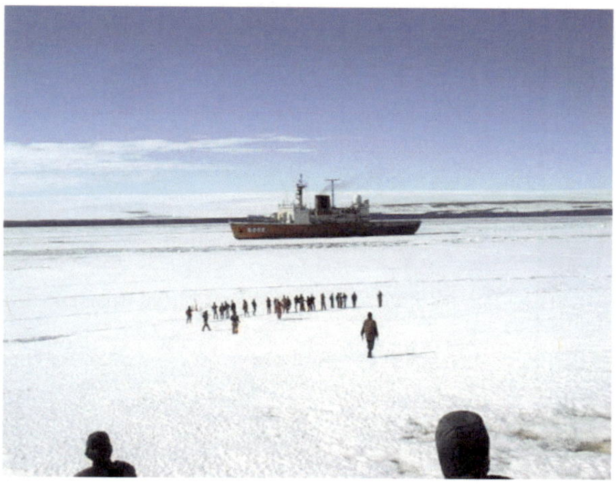

4. Antarctic doctors must treat every disease with limited medical equipment without paramedical staff

There are thirty or forty participants who undertake the winter-over every year with two doctors as part of the team. Every member must undergo medical examination to confirm that they are healthy enough to engage in Antarctic activity. Even with this level of screening however, participants need medical consultations four times on average during a single winter.

From 1956 to 2003, a total of 4932 medical consultations have been undertaken. Forty five percent of these are surgical and orthopaedic cases. Injuries, frostbite, sprain, lumbago and back pain, burns, fractures etc. are included. Internal disease comprises 23% of cases consisting of digestive diseases, respiratory ones, head-ache, hypertension, mountain sickness etc.. Dental problems account for 12% in third place. Others are made up from skin troubles 8%, eye problems 6%, ear, nose and throat 4%, mental problems 2%, and urinary disease. These proportions are preserved in recent survey (shown in the figure) and similar to other nations' stations.

Injuries increase in spring and summer as the frequency of field works increases. Frostbite is observed ordinarily in August, September and October or the coldest season. Another peak of frostbite is shown on April and May, the first period of wintering. People coming from Japan never experience the degree of cold present in Antarctica, so even at the warmest Antarctic season, they are not inured to cold injury.

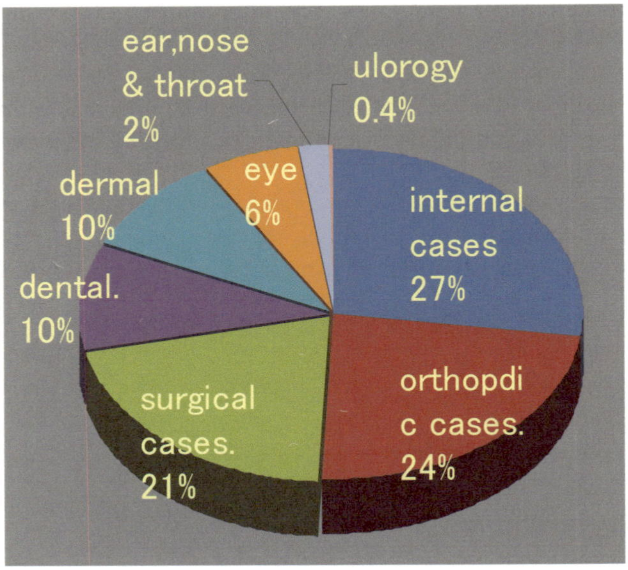

the proportion of 1942 medical consultations from 1997 to 2007

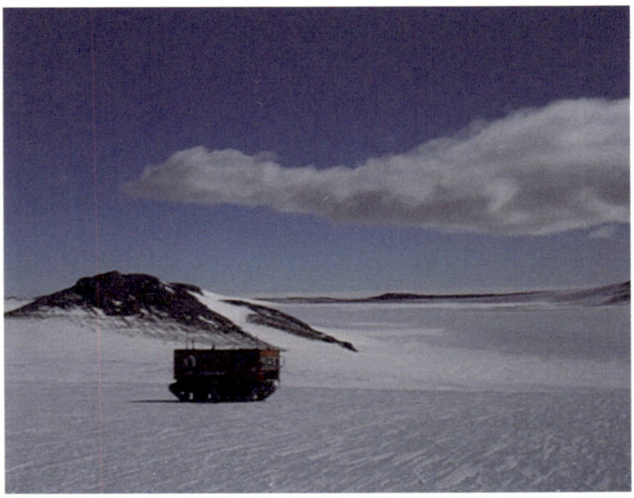

Mountain sickness is experienced with inland operation, especially Dome Fuji trip. Respiratory diseases is rare in winter period in Antarctica where there are no indigenous viruses and immunity to the prevailing one rapidly develops. These increase in summer when the ship with new members arrives station bringing with it a new population of virus. A common problem with teeth is crown dislocations. There is no dentist, so these have to be treated by medical doctors instead.

Some diseases are affected by Antarctic natural conditions such as dryness, strong ultraviolet ray and stiff breeze. For example, photo dermatitis, keratosis, snow blindness, foreign bodies in eyes and pharyngeal spaces are frequently seen. Mental disorders appear to be less of a problem in Japanese stations than in some others where significant depression and other problems have been reported. In Japanese stations the main problems are insomnia and some neuroses.

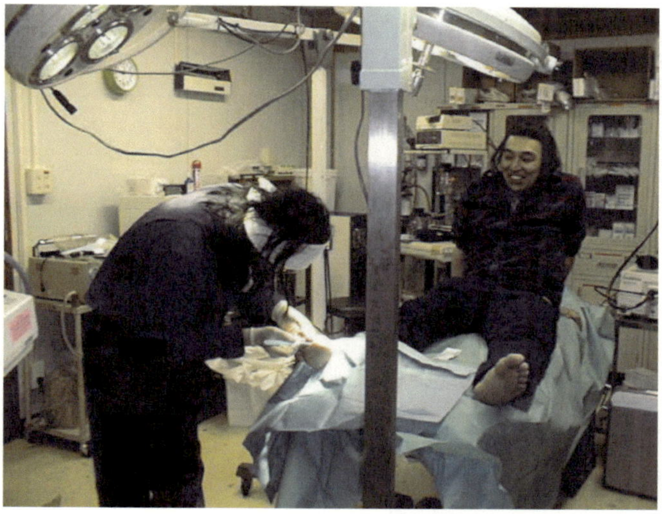

The operation theatre at Syowa Station

There is medical care unit at the station with electrocardiogram, ultrasonic diagnostic equipment, blood laboratory examinations, roentgenogram and fluoroscopy. Medical equipment is available and prepared to perform surgical operations under general anesthesia if needed. Most Antarctic stations have only one medical doctor, but there are two doctors at Syowa station. Usually one goes with field team in summer and the other stays at station. This makes it difficult to perform operations so that only two appendectomies have been done in fifty years.

The possibility of medical evacuation is restricted to summer, but four evacuations have been done. Three of them were with ship for a transcervical femoral fracture caused by falling in a crevasse, a pelvic fracture from a "traffic accident", acute renal failure secondary to prostatic hypertrophy. These three cases were in summer when the ship was near the station to pick up and send the patient to South Africa by ship then to Japan by air. The whole evacuation chain can take almost one month. The fourth case showing arrhythmia at Dome Fuji used air evacuation to shorten the journey time. First a local plane transported the patient to one station providing intercontinental connections. Then the patient was sent to Japan via South Africa. Seven days were needed for the operational evacuation.

In summary, it is necessary for the Antarctic doctor to manage a whole spectrum of diseases by himself with limited facilities, no medical or paramedical colleagues and no option of outgoing evacuation and incoming rescue for much of the year. The doctor is always a little anxious. Unexpected problems become part of ordinary life, and impossibility of rescue for severe cases creates concern.
It is just such a situation that makes telemedicine indispensable to Antarctic medical operation.

Medical evacuation by air from Dome Fuji toJapan.

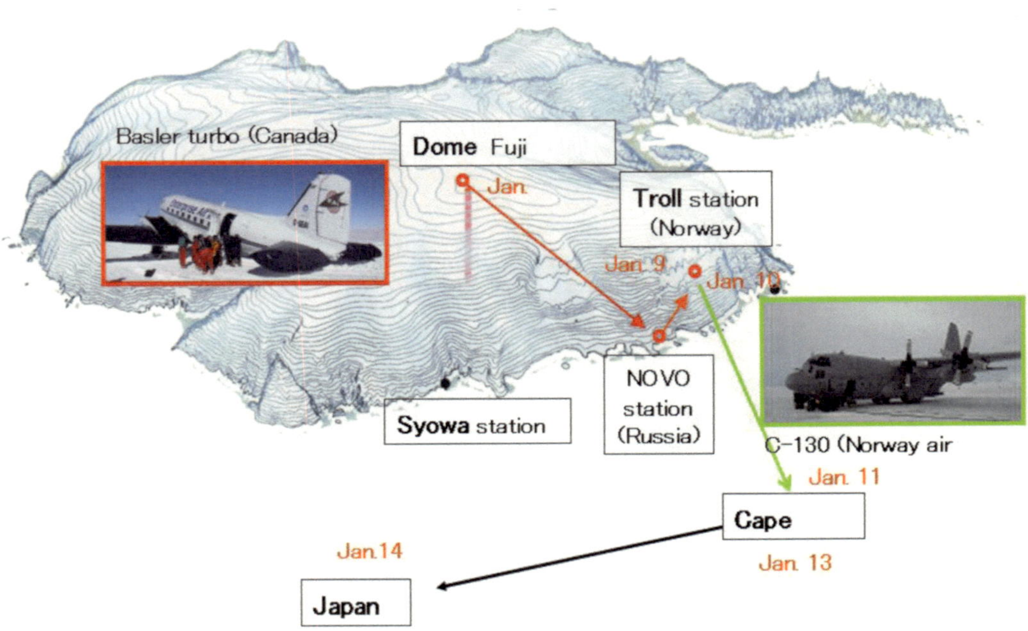

5. The isolated station needs telemedicine supports

Though the necessity of medical telecommunication has been recognized for a long time, the practical application stage had to wait for the development of tele-communication engineering.
For two decades after the expedition started in 1956, a radiotelegraph was the only method to communicate with Japan. It was impossible to use the device effectively for medical communications. In 1975, trials of sending electrocardiogram by radio facsimile were made and successfully introduced. Satellite radio-telephone and satellite radio facsimile (1981) was useful to consult directly but without the ability to transmit medical pictures. E-mail by Internationa Mobile Satellite Organization (INMALSAT) making connection every 2 hours and permitting only a maximum 100kb/mail.
In 2004, switching to International Telecommunications Satellite organization (INTELSAT) made connection constantly available, and increased the maximum to a 10Mb/mail making the transmission of still and moving pictures possible.
So INTELSAT makes practical medical telecommunication possible.

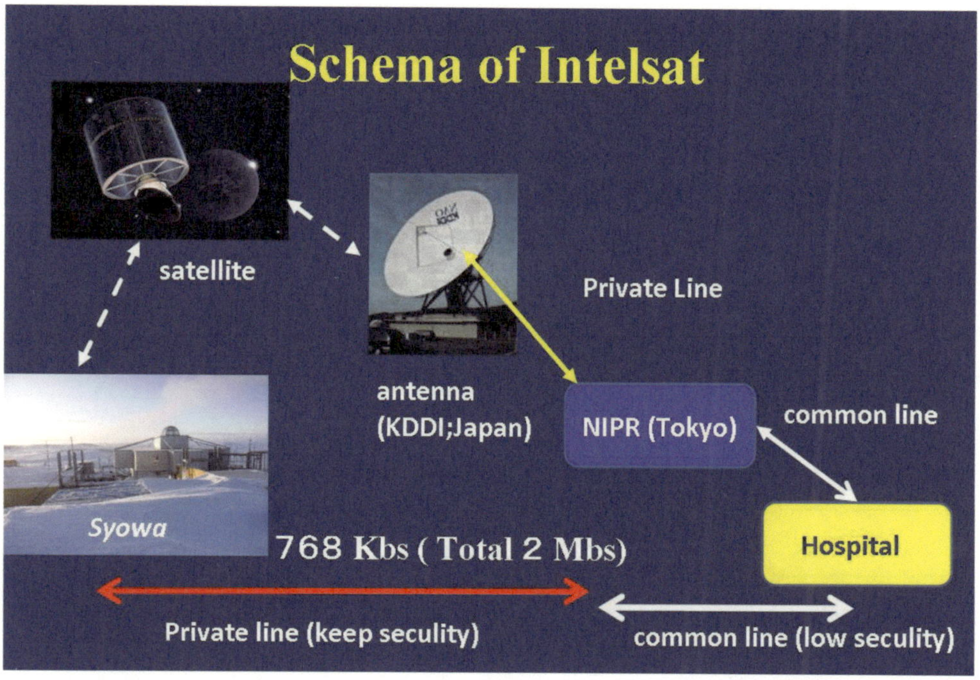

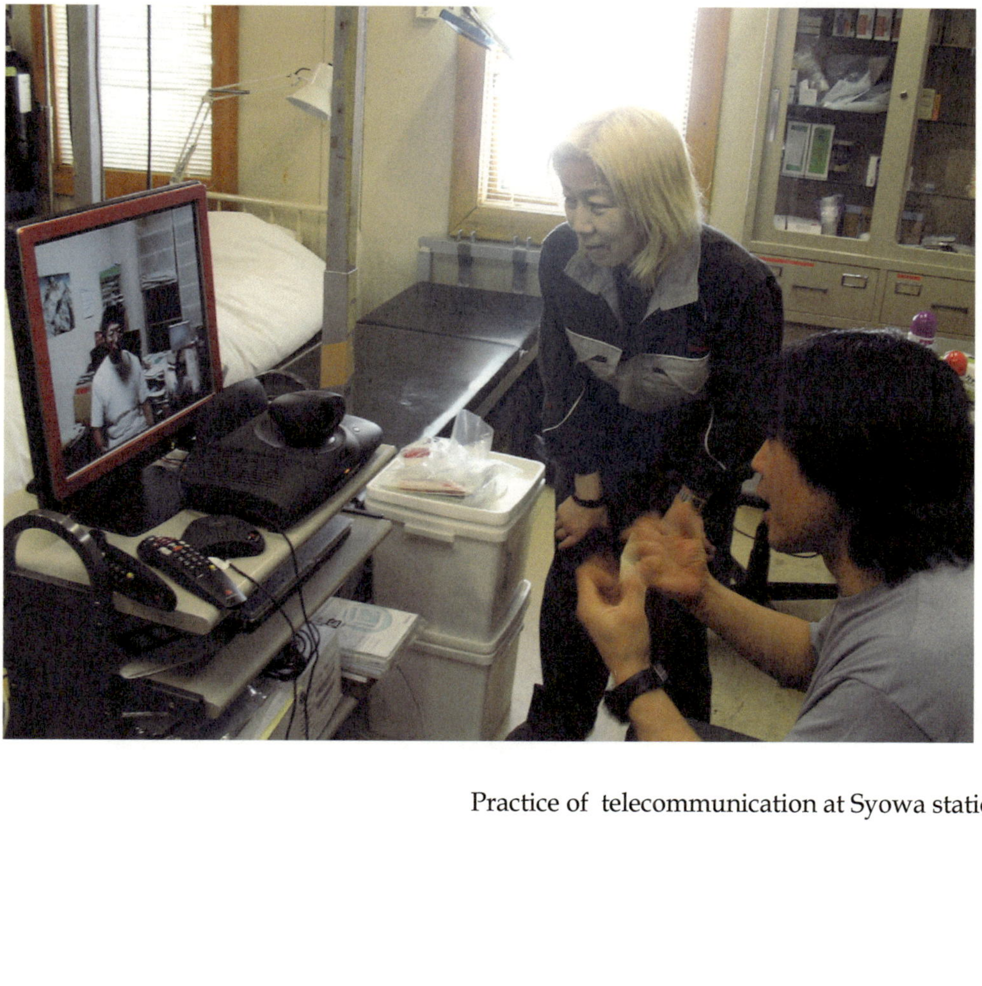

Practice of telecommunication at Syowa station

6. The regular scheduled consultation is performed monthly

The Antarctic doctor (Local doctor) sends some reports about patients' information and images to Japan in advance. A Japanese doctor (home doctor) prepares adequate specialist advice and information responding to this submitted report.

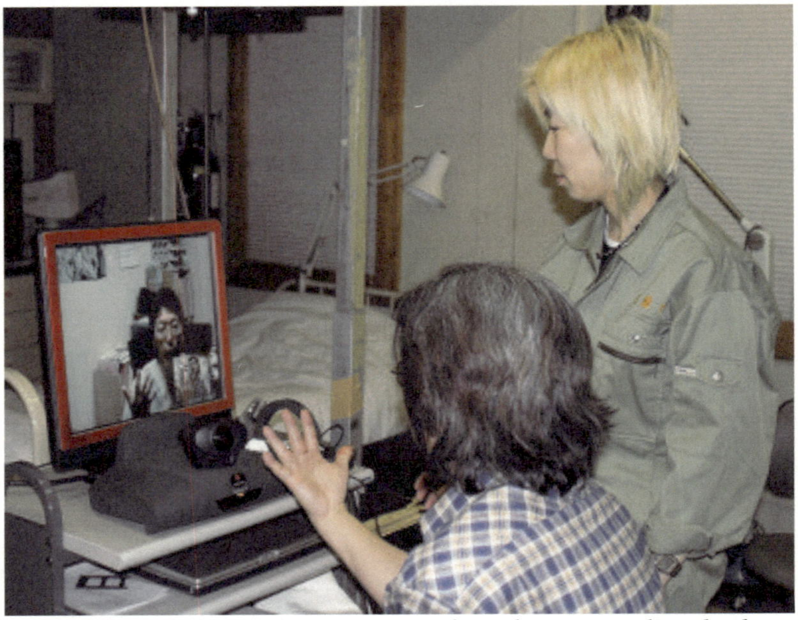

In the tele-communication, home doctor can speak to the patient directly through the TV. The patient also can explain to the doctor satisfactorily without technical terms. Doctor can watch and make an examination as he need in detail.

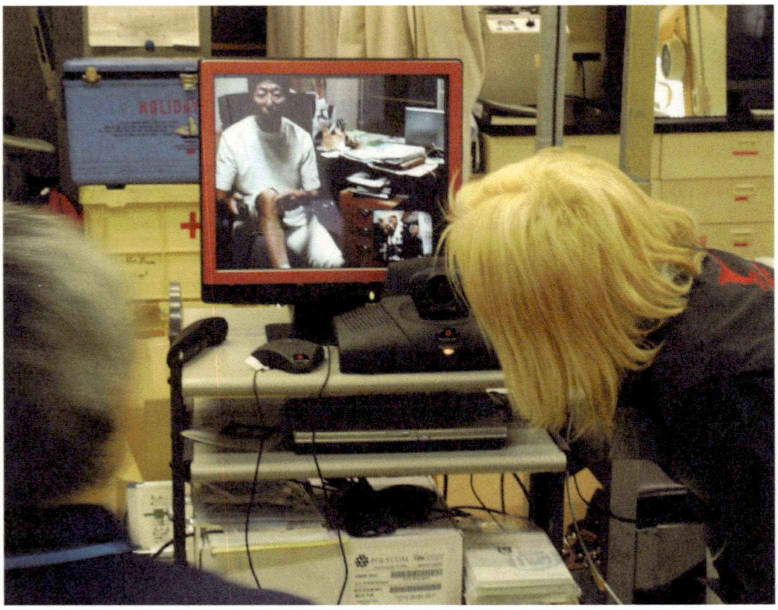

Instead of direct physical examination, home doctor asks the patient and local doctor to do while he watches the video. Thus, the findings through the TV give physical information and so direct interview and substitute physical examination is possible.
It is also possible to counsel on treatment. The home doctor can demonstrate what should be done to the local doctor and he advises and can in real time.

7. Emergency case

May 14, 20XX
Syowa Station local time (SLT). Sunrise 10:05 SLT, Sunset 14:31SLT, clear sky, temperature maximum -12.2°C, minimum -20.8°C.
11:45: (SLT) as 17:40 Japan local time (JLT).
An accident occurred. When one person was moving cargo with a crane, his leg got caught between one cargo and snow tractor.
12:04 SLT: The rescue team with medical doctor arrived on the scene.
12:43 SLT: The patient was admitted to the station. He was shivering and the doctor administered an antibiotic and analgesic agent.
13:25 SLT: The X-ray examination was performed to reveal a fracture of the fibula.
13:30 SLT.(19:30 JLT) First report was sent to National Institute of Polar Research (NIPR) in Japan.
20:00JLT NIPR made the initial call to the collaborating hospital in Japan.
14:30 SLT. Local doctor requested the consultation of specialist
20:30 JLT. Orthopedic surgeons were assembled.

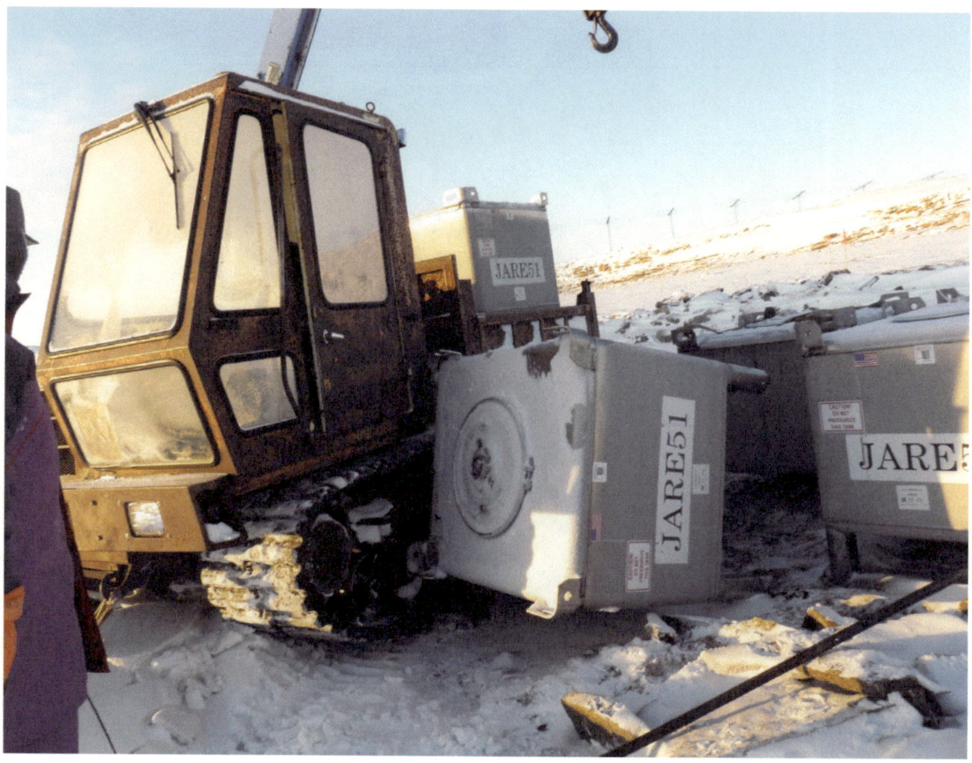

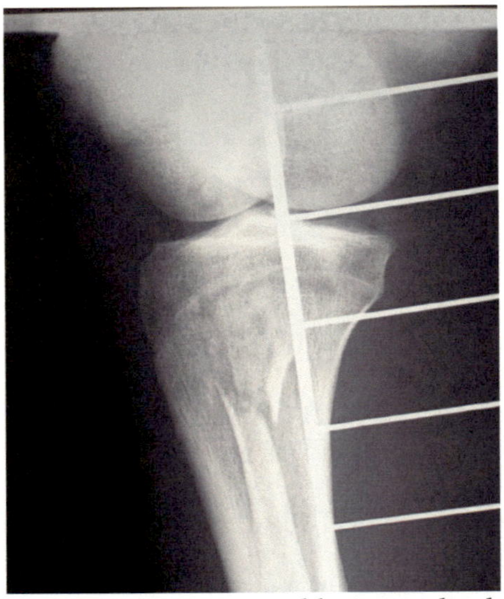

21:15 JLT (15:30 SLT) The consultation was started between the doctor at Syowa station and orthopedic surgeon with telephone and X-ray image sent by e-mail. Diagnosis of fracture was confirmed and therapeutic advice was indicated.
June 4, 20XX

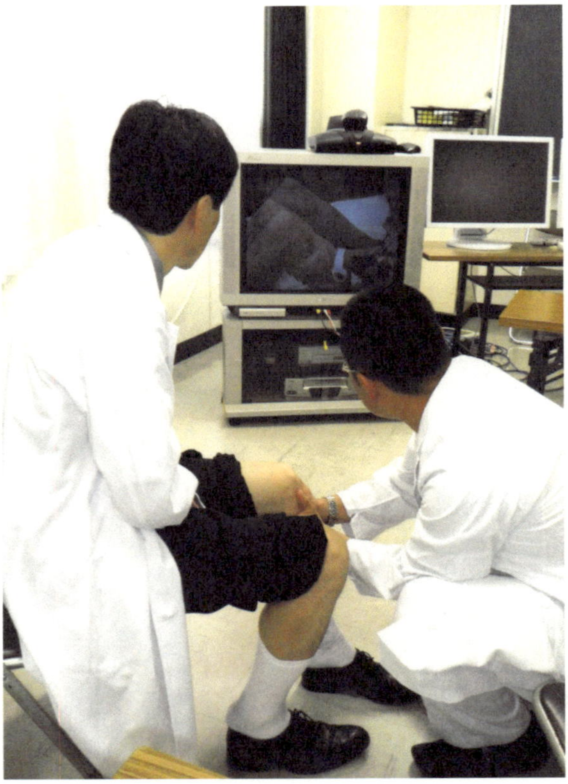

The actual state of telecommunication at hospital in Japan

Second consultation was performed with TV system. Orthopedic surgeon observed the patient directly and performed physical examination through local doctor. It showed a frontal slippage of knee joint suggesting the ligament injury of knee.
June 18, 20XX
In the third consultation, it was confirmed that the healing of bone was satisfactory. The orthopedic surgeon ordered rehabilitation demonstrating the method practically.
It was ten months after the accident when the patient returned Japan to visit the orthopedic doctor face to face.

8. The potential of telecommunication in medical operation.

During one wintering over (February 2004 to January 2005), there were 185 medical consultations. In this wintering team, there were two doctors, one surgeon and one internal physician. The proportion of diseases shows orthopaedic cases were most frequent followed by internal medical cases, surgical cases and skin troubles. Telemedicine consultations were performed for twenty two cases. The TV-system was used 29 times in 17 cases, and still images were sent by e-mail in 5 cases. It is distinctive that telemedicine support is used in many ways for orthopaedic cases and skin in diseases. And also it is interesting that in skin diseases and eye problems, still pictures are preferred to video. Real time communication makes it possible to convey information about mobility without the confusion of verbal descriptions and specific terms showing great advantage in treatment of orthopaedic diseases.
It is notable that the telecommunication system supplies the local doctors with something they are not experts in. Doctors tend to be selected from surgeon, because the surgical injury is frequent and it may be lethal without surgeon. On the other hand, it is difficult for one or two doctors treat all medical cases including those from out of their specialties, one of those areas is the dental problem. Most doctore now are specialists, Antarcticc practice requires the ultimate generalist.

Practical cases of Telemedicine
2005 Feb.~ 2006 January

	case	telemedicine	TV-system case(times)	email
total	185	22	17(29)	5
Internal med.	42	1	1 (3)	
Surgery	35	1	1 (3)	
Orthopedics	66	13	13(20)	
Ophthalmology	9	1		1
Dermatology	17	4	1 (1)	3
Otorhinaryngology	2			
Urology	1	1	1 (2)	
Dentistry	13	1		1

Some technical problems are still could be improved. It is a basic issue to establish a stable communication. At the first year, only 9 of 24 telecommunication trials were successful. The first five consecutive times failed and thereafter quite often repeated failure to connect voice or picture or both occurred. From the second year, it has made better but there is still a failure a few times each year.
It is necessary to connect directly between Antarctic station and collaborating hospital in an emergency. When the connection becomes required, it has in the past needed NIPR staff to relay, these people are not present in the middle of the night nor on holidays. In 2011, it becomes possible to make connection directly to the hospital without the relay.
There are some concerns about the security of information which is not encrypted or perfectly secure. This is being studied. There is a six-hour time difference between Syowa station and Japan. This can lead to some difficulties in providing arrangements of adequate consulting staff.
A high quality of movie image is desired for diagnosis.

9. Conclusions for telemedicine

1. Antarctic Telemedicine support system shows great advantages
2. Real time communication by TV / Video system makes effective medical interview, physical examination and therapeutic management especially in orthopedic cases.
3. High resolution images sent by e-mail are useful to understand the lesions precisely in eyes and skin.
4. Emergency consultation will be effective if adequate consulting staff are prepared and available in spite of time difference.
5 Further improvements in technology will make telemedicine more useful and indispensable.

10. References

[1] Grant IC: Telemedocone in the British Antarctic survey. Int J Circumpolar Health. 2004 Dec, 63(4): 356-64
[2] Giichiro Ohno, Takahiro Miyata: Morbidity of wintering-over participants in the First to the Thirty-ninth Japanese Antarctic Research Expeditions: Analysis of 4233 cases. Antarctic Record, Vol. 44, No.1, 1-13, 2000
[3] Giichiro Ohno, Takahiro Miyata: Comparision of medical service systems at Syowa Station with Antarctic stations: Medical staff, mortality and evacuation. Antarctic Record, Vol.44, No.1, 42-50, 2000
[4] Giichiro Ohno, Takahiro Miyata: Diseases due to ultraviolet radiation in Antarcticc wintering personnel: Analysis of geneses, seasonal change and annual variation. Antarctic Record, Vol.44, No.3, 239-248, 2000
[5] Giichiro Ohno, Kentaro Watanabe: We need a broad network of Antarctic medical research---- report of the Japanese workshop on Antarctic Medical Research and Medicine. Circumpolar Hearth Supplements / Proceedings of the 14th international congress on Circumpolar Health 2010(7), 564-567

22

Telestroke for the Long-term Management of Risk Factors in Stroke Survivors

Joubert J[2], Medeiros de Bustos E[1], Decavel P[3], Chopard JL[3], Joubert LB[4] and Moulin T[1]
[1]*University of Franche-Comte*
[2]*Royal Melbourne Hospital*
[3]*University Hospital of Besancon*
[4]*University of Melbourne*
[1,3]*France*
[2.4]*Australia*

1. Introduction

Stroke is a major public health issue worldwide and, being the largest cause of chronic disability in adults , places a significant burden on health care systems. According to the World Health Organisation (WHO), around 15 million people each year suffer a stroke, and 5 million are left with a permanent disability . Over the past two decades, stroke has become an increasingly treatable disease with the development of evidence-based treatments such as tissue plasminogen activator (rt-PA) for the treatment of acute ischemic stroke and admission of patients to stroke units. This has led to a decrease in stroke mortality in developed countries and an increase in the number of survivors with impairment or disability. Stroke is an example of a largely preventable disease that presents acutely, with a short time window within which damage to the brain can be reduced. There is a high risk for residual disability which impacts significantly on society, the patients and their families . Stroke recurrence can lead to a progressive decline into dependency, subsequently placing a significant financial burden on society. In 2008, the indirect and direct costs of stroke in the United States were calculated at $65.5 billion .

87% of strokes are caused by cerebral infarction and are therefore amenable to a number of pre-stroke preventive strategies as well as thrombolytic therapy or intravascular clot retrieval strategies in the acute phase . The second major subtype of stroke, i.e. intracerebral parenchymal haemorrhage, is largely preventable through pre-stroke blood pressure control.

In this chapter, we will primarily discuss the current data regarding prevention and limitation of acute brain damage resulting from cerebral infarction, but will also consider other expanding areas in stroke care where telemedicine has a potential role. We will therefore examine the use of telestroke in stroke survivors after discharge from hospital, with particular emphasis on developed models of care and their applicability.

2. The prevalence of recurrent stroke

In stroke survivors, the overall risk of recurrent stroke (fatal or nonfatal) is high (approximately 20%) at 5 years . A recent study carried out in Perth, Australia, which aimed to determine the absolute frequency of first recurrent stroke and disability, as well as the relative frequency of recurrent stroke, demonstrated that over a 10-year follow-up period, the risk of first recurrent stroke is 6 times higher than the risk of first-ever stroke in the general population of the same age and sex. In addition, almost one half of survivors remain disabled, and one seventh require institutional care. The burden of stroke will continue to be a significant healthcare problem unless the incidence of not only first-ever, but also recurrent stroke and its disabling sequelae are reduced.

2.1 Risk factor management

In 1970, a landmark paper showed that hypertension was a major risk factor for all types of stroke. It has since been confirmed in more recent studies that high blood pressure is indeed a powerful determinant of risk for both ischaemic stroke and intracranial haemorrhage .
Other major risk factors for stroke such as obesity, smoking, embolic heart disease and diabetes mellitus are well recognised .
The potential for recurrent stroke can be substantially reduced by effective management of these risk factors, and the development of systems that can enhance the prevention of stroke recurrence is an important priority and challenge in both the developed and developing worlds. The same few major risk factors account for many of the leading chronic health problems worldwide. Nevertheless they remain on the increase and are poorly managed in the majority of affected individuals. According to the WHO, the number of overweight people worldwide will increase to 2.3 billion by 2015, and more than 700 million will be obese . In parallel, more than 200 million people have diabetes and the WHO projects that the prevalence will double between 2005 and 2030 .

2.2 Importance of preventive strategies

The main challenge involves reducing the prevalence of recurrent stroke, particularly in remote and rural areas, through: i) effective strategies for the management of risk factors; and ii) educating the target population (essentially stroke victims and carers/family members) to increase awareness of risk factors and preventive strategies.
Prevention is the most effective way of reducing the burden of recurrent stroke on society . Although it has been shown that effective long-term risk factor management can reduce the risk of recurrent stroke by around 70-80% through the implementation of simple best practice recommendations , secondary prevention measures remain frequently sub-optimally implemented in stroke survivors . Indeed, in an editorial in the journal *Stroke*, Hachinski specified that despite the worldwide increase in stroke occurrence as a result of several well-known risk factors, these factors are often poorly managed. 'Therapeutic inertia' is common at primary care level and there is a high rate of medication discontinuation in stroke survivors after discharge . This was highlighted in a French urban study , which served to emphasise that there is currently a gap between recommendations and implementation of best practice management of risk factors, even in Western Europe. A large Swedish population-based cohort study involving 28,449 participants revealed an increased hypertension rate (79.4%) in people with a history of previous stroke 7.5 years after enrolment. Only half were taking anti-hypertensive medication and only 11.5%

achieved a blood pressure reading < 140/90 mm Hg. In addition, the majority of stroke survivors with hypercholesterolaemia were not prescribed lipid lowering medication, and only 38% received antithrombotics. One third of patients were still smoking, two thirds were obese and the overall calculated stroke risk was found to be significantly higher in stroke survivors than in people without stroke . A randomized controlled trial of an outreach nursing support programme for recently discharged stroke patients in the Netherlands showed that quality of life deteriorated significantly in the post-discharge period and that about 50% of stroke survivors were dissatisfied with the care provided after discharge. Canadian data suggests that although many hospitals have focused their attention on acute service provision, ongoing patient support related to secondary prevention has not been adequately addressed . Similarly, a review of hospital-based stroke services in North Carolina showed that, over a 5-year period, virtually no progress had been made in hospital programmes for stroke prevention .
All this would argue that secondary prevention and long-term management of risk factors is a neglected area that requires urgent attention and has clearly defied efforts, even in the developed world, for optimal implementation.

2.3 Barriers to effective risk factor management

Globally, the majority of strokes occur in rural areas where there is often a lack of stroke services. In these areas, stroke care is often fragmented and does not adhere to recommended guidelines . This, together with the geographical barriers that are associated with a general attenuation of access to healthcare resources and the paucity of stroke experts frequently leads to an inequitable distribution of resources and limited access to preventive strategies and evidence-based care. On a global scale it would seem that not only are vascular risk factors on the increase, but they are also not systematically recognised or diagnosed. The results of a recent longitudinal cohort study in the United States, for example, revealed high rates of undiagnosed hypertension and diabetes among stroke survivors .
The problem is further compounded by the lack of public awareness and knowledge of stroke risk factors and preventive strategies. A recent study of stroke survivors found that only 60.5 percent were able to identify one stroke risk factor and only 55.3% were able to identify one stroke warning sign . Similarly, a study of 286 consecutive patients who were attending a stroke outpatient clinic in Switzerland for the first time 3 months after being discharged from hospital for a first stroke, reported that despite an improvement in hospital treatment, cerebrovascular risk factor control was not optimal . This may have been partly related to the patients' awareness and knowledge. Older patients and patients with excellent recovery were at particular risk of recurrent stroke due to poor awareness of vascular risk factor control. Better strategies are clearly needed to help stroke survivors recognise and play a part in the control of vascular risk factors so as to improve the prevention rate of recurrent stroke.

3. Telemedicine and its potentials

3.1 Background to telemedicine and telestroke

Telemedicine has been defined, simply, as the delivery of healthcare services to the underserved, employing telecommunication . A more extensive definition is "the process by which electronic, visual and audio communications are used to provide diagnostic and consultation support to practitioners at distant sites, assist in or directly deliver medical care to patients at distant sites, and enhance the skills and knowledge of distant medical care providers . Telemedicine, as a distance communication tool, was first attempted in radiology 50 years ago and subsequently in psychiatry . Since 1999 there has been a gradual increase in the number of telemedicine programmes and more recently a growing interest in its use in stroke, mainly in facilitating thrombolysis , but also in establishing diagnoses and guiding treatment options .

"Telestroke" refers to the application of telemedicine to stroke care. This is a new application of existing technology in the care of stroke patients . Evidence suggests that telestroke is beneficial where immediate access to regular stroke expertise is not available . Thus it may help to provide stroke care to patients in remote regions and smaller urban hospitals without stroke expertise and to extend clinical research into a broader global community, thereby furthering the goal of establishing universal access to care at all levels, regardless of geographical location or hospital facilities .

Although telemedicine has until now mainly focused on the area of thrombolysis in the acute stage, it has the potential to address the remaining stages of the stroke victim's journey following discharge from hospital or in the rehabilitation setting . Attention at all these levels can substantially lower the net cost of recurrent stroke to society through reduction of lost productivity, nursing home costs and rehabilitation .

Demonstration projects have proven the feasibility of telestroke and suggested its potential to facilitate access to specialist stroke expertise in hospitals without access to specialist clinicians. In particular, the use of this technology may promote implementation of best practice management of vascular risk factors in stroke survivors after discharge . One of the main drivers has been technological advancement, such as the digitisation and compression of data permitting the rapid transfer of images . This can now be linked to systems of care that integrate person-to-person contact (which have already been developed in the areas of psychiatry and social work), thus providing a structure which delivers care to underserved areas by combining state-of-the-art technology providing the face-to-face contact that patients still need.

3.2 Review of the relevant literature on telestroke for stroke survivors

3.2.1 Methodology

In 2009 we reviewed evidence of telestroke support in stroke survivors discharged from hospital. The Canadian Agency for Drugs and Technologies in Health (CADTH) reported on a systematic review of 5 bibliographic databases examining telestroke from 1966 to December 2006. 863 citations were identified, and from these, 35 potentially relevant reports yielding 22 studies originating from the US, Germany, Canada, China, the Netherlands, Italy and Finland. Using this as a base, we further searched the literature which involved searching the relevant primary and secondary databases for all papers (peer-reviewed where possible) that covered stroke and telemedicine in stroke survivors. We combined MeSH searching with (relevant) 'words anywhere' searching. The results were examined via abstracts; if no abstracts were available, full text-versions were sighted. Selected papers were obtained in full-text version and additional relevant papers were searched and reviewed as needed from references cited in papers. The searches were limited to the period from 1998 to 2009 and no restriction was placed on study designs. Primary databases searched were Medline EMBASE, CINAHL, AMED and PsycInfo. We also searched the Cochrane databases. The main subject terms used were telemedicine, telephone, electronic mail, videoconferencing and stroke. Additional subject terms searched were patient discharge and hospitals, and other relevant terms searched were telestroke, telehealth, primary-secondary and post-acute, patient surveillance, patient monitoring, and risk assessment. From the primary sources we found 82 papers in total of which 72 were retained for examination. From Cochrane, one systematic review was found. The final studies included can be seen in Table 1. In 8 studies the telemedicine focus was not on rehabilitation; of these six were RCTs. Telerehabilitation was the focus of 12 other studies, only one being an RCT. A total of 28 studies evaluated a variety of measures in stroke patients.

Study Type	Reference	Telemedicine Intervention	Target Groups	Health Professional Involved
RCT	Mayo NE, et al, 2008	Telephone calls by nursing care coordinator over 6 weeks after discharge.	190 stroke patients n=96 intervention n=94 controls	Nurse Care Manager, Patient's Local Physician
RCT	Joubert 2008	Integrated model of care (ICARUSS) Risk factor management	91 stroke survivors and 95 controls	Care-Coordinator and Patient's General Practitioner
RCT	Joubert 2008	Integrated model of care (ICARUSS) Screening for depression (PHQ9)	91 stroke survivors and 95 controls	Care-Coordinator and Patient's General Practitioner
RCT	Grant JS et al, 2002	Telephone contact strategy for problem- solving therapy over 18 months.	74 Stroke Survivors and Caregivers in three groups: treatment, sham and control	Research Nurse
RCT	Boter H, 2004	Outreach care included 3 telephone calls and a home visit within 5 months of discharge.	Randomized 536 stroke patients; 263 (with 211 carers to standard care plus outreach care and 273 (with 230 carers) to standard care only.	13 Stroke nurses
Qualitative study	Pierce 2004	Internet based education and support	9 Caregivers of patients with stroke using Caring~Web	Nurse
Descriptive Study	Buckley KM, Tran BQ, Prandoni CM, 2004	Tele-health nurses use videophones to contact caregivers	21 family caregivers of stroke patients	Nurse Investigator

Table 1. Non-Rehabilitation Studies using Telestroke in Stroke Survivors

3.2.2 Post-discharge telestroke models

Of the non-rehabilitation telestroke studies involving stroke survivors, one was an Internet educational model, there was one passive case management model , one was a videophone-supported educational model, one was a nursing outreach telephone support model , one was an interactive telephone support model and one was a telephone/ Internet-based EDC integrated care model . Three involved caregivers only , one involved patients and general practitioners , one involved patients and caregivers , and one involved stroke specialists, patients, caregivers and primary care physicians . There were 21 studies (one being an RCT) describing the application of telestroke in rehabilitation. Most of the studies have described the use of technology solutions, principally to support rehabilitation activities .

The HESTIA Study Group instituted a programme of outreach care consisting of 3 telephone calls and one home visit by nursing staff within the 5 months after discharge . The target population was patients and carers, and the intervention was general support, education and advice. General practitioners were indirectly involved, in that nurses advised contact with the general practitioner where appropriate. Quality of life according to the Short Form 36 (SF 36) and dissatisfaction with care were assessed at 6 months. Apart from improved scores on the SF-36 domain 'Role Emotional' no difference was found between patients receiving outreach nursing stroke care and controls.

In the study by Pierce at al. an Internet-based education and support intervention was directed at rural caregivers. Outcomes in this qualitative study were satisfaction with the intervention and an exploration of caregivers' experience. Of the nine caregivers studied, all indicated satisfaction with the "Caring-Web" and eight agreed or strongly agreed that the tool was needed.

An RCT evaluating the effect of telephone intervention with family caregivers of stroke survivors, involving a social problem-solving therapy over a period of 18 months, yielded significantly positive results on a variety of measures such as problem-solving skills, social functioning, caregiver depression, measures of vitality, role limitations related to emotional issues and caregiver preparedness. The target population was caregivers, and intervention was weekly or bi-weekly telephone calls. The three groups were tested-intervention, sham and control.

In a descriptive study, targeting family caregivers of stroke patients, Buckley et al. used videophones to provide education and support and to assess patients and monitor progress. They studied the factors that influenced receptiveness for the use of this tool. The telehealth calls were made weekly and the duration of the intervention was 5 weeks.

Mayo et al. evaluated the effect of passive case management over a period of 6 weeks after discharge of stroke patients from hospital. The telestroke intervention was telephone contact and involved surveillance, information exchange, medication management, health system guidance, active listening, family support, teaching and risk identification. The target populations in this RCT was the stroke patients and their general practitioners. There was no difference between patients exposed to usual post-discharge management and this intervention regarding health-related quality of life, reduction of health services utilisation or stroke impact.

Moulin et al. have reported on the emergency neurology network in Franche-Comté (RUN-FC) , which monitors stroke victims over a five-year period following discharge. A nurse from the network maintains regular contact with the patients and organizes a consultation with a neurologist if a problem is detected. The patient's GP is also kept informed at all times. Since 2003, 2,600 stroke victims have been followed up within the network and 20%

have required action to be taken by the network at least once. The survival rate of discharged patients at 18 months has risen from 87% between 1987 and 1994, to 94% between 2003 and 2006. For patients in the network, the stroke recurrence rate at 18 months has also increased from 4.8% between 1998 and 2002, to 2.6% between 2003 and 2007 . RUN-FC illustrates the usefulness of telemedicine for stroke survivors and the need to develop it further throughout France. Furthermore, in the long-term, the network has significantly reduced the stroke mortality rate and the number of recurrences, and has considerably improved the quality of life of patients in the network.

Joubert et al. examined the effect of a telemedicine intervention on both vascular risk factor management and depressive symptoms in the ICARUSS study. In this RCT, the intervention was telephone contact with patients and carers, and bi-directional information sharing between coordinator, patient and general practitioner using telephone and facsimile, coupled with data management, surveillance and response through a web-based EDC. Telephone contact between stroke specialist and primary care physician was maintained by telephone. The target populations were patients, carers and general practitioners. In this study, the pilot results were supportive of this simple telestroke model in that there was a significant improvement in a variety of outcome measures, such as optimal management of risk factors, BMI, physical activity, and disability as measured by modified Rankin score (mRS) in patients exposed to the telestroke intervention compared to usual care. Moreover, depressive symptoms were significantly reduced in the telestroke group. The protocols for the ICARUSS model are diagrammatically depicted in figures 1 and 2. The initial results from the pilot study have resulted in the multicentre Australian Study using the adapted ICARUSS model of care in urban stroke patients. As a result of the experience accrued from the ICARUSS study, important role players in an effective telestroke model have been identified. Moreover, the implementation of telestroke at various stages of the stroke survivor's journey has been clarified.

3.2.3 Major role players in telestroke

i) Caregivers

About 80% of stroke survivors are reliant on family caregivers for emotional and physical support, ranging from assisting with activities of daily living to arranging and escorting to medical appointments. Caregivers are often elderly, and often frequently infirm themselves. Caregiver failure or collapse is more frequently a cause for stroke survivor institutionalisation than is commonly realised. If the carer can be 'enrolled' and supported as a member of the team, there is an increased likelihood that the stroke survivor will remain in the community.

The Internet-based support study by Pierce et al. highlights the need of caregivers for emotional and social support and the general acceptance of a telestroke support system. Pilot work had indicated that a major issue identified by caregivers was the low level of knowledge about stroke in general, which their Internet-based study attempted to rectify. Important issues of acceptance by caregivers was emphasised in the study of Buckley et al. who found that for some carers, a technological challenge constituted only an extra burden. Some caregivers only wanted simple telephone support. In this study, it was evident that the nurse's support was paramount.

Assessment of caregivers' needs and limitations is important. Their level of technical competence, fear of intrusion into their privacy and desire for inclusion into a telestroke system all need to be evaluated.

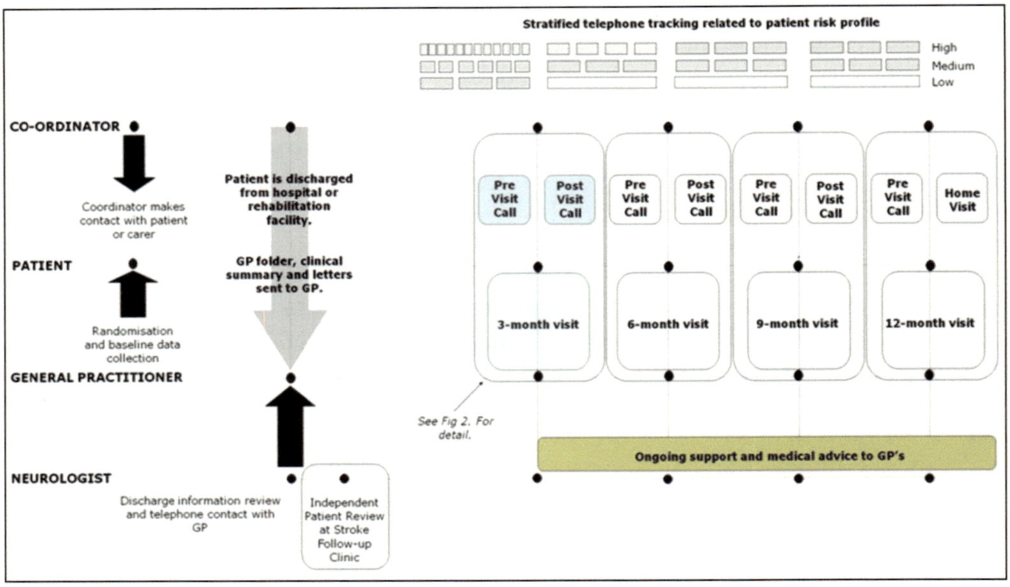

Fig. 1. Diagrammatic representation of telestroke process (ICARUSS protocol)

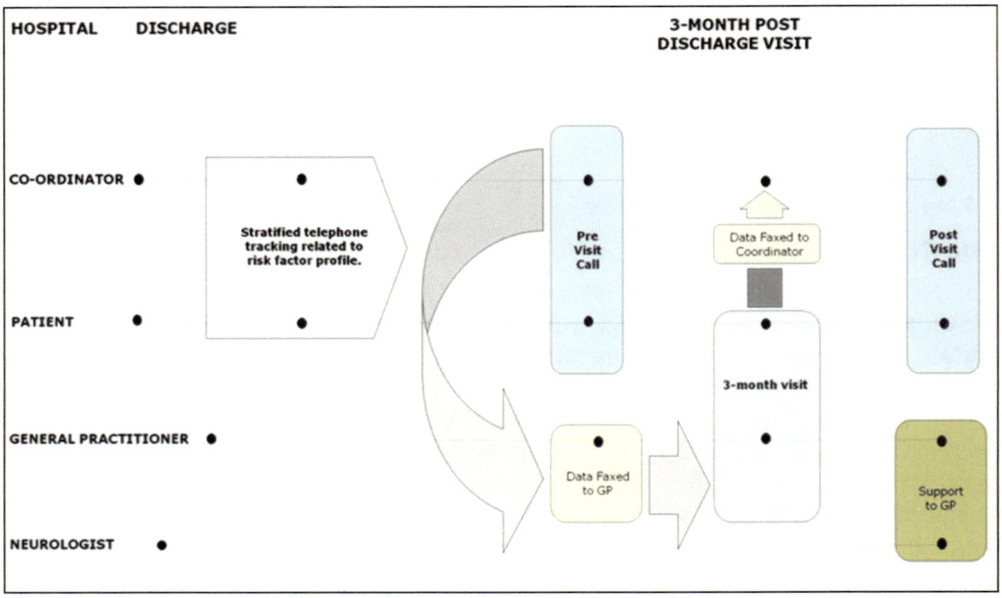

Fig. 2. Three-monthly Telestroke cycle of communication between coordinator, patient, caregiver and general primary care physician illustrating pre- and post general practice telecommunication (ICARUSS protocol)

Often overlooked issues include the functional ability of the caregiver, the amount of time able to be provided by the caregiver, the number of individuals sharing the burden, and involvement of the caregiver in management planning prior to discharge. The need for a flexible approach to telephone contact with caregivers has been emphasised in several

studies. These studies stress that there is an unmet need in caregivers, and that although the solution is probably not simple, further research is required in this area.
The multicentre RCT in the Netherlands did not show evidence of either improving quality of life or lessening dissatisfaction with care. However, the study was of short duration with a low level of intervention, and a deliberately passive, but supportive and advisory role. Thirteen stroke nurses were employed for intervention in 263 stroke survivors. The Australian study, ICARUSS, differed in that one nurse coordinator supported over 90 patients for a period of one year. Similar to the Dutch study, a negative result was obtained in the study by Mayo et al. where the intervention was deliberately passive case management. In the study by Grant et al. , the problem-solving partnership resulted in significant improvement over many domains, as in the ICARUSS study.

ii) Stroke survivors

There is now evidence from the ICARUSS study that an integrated telestroke model can result in significantly improved risk factor management , as well as decreased levels of post-stroke depressive symptoms . Despite the published importance of implementing best practice management principles, this is the only telestroke study that has addressed risk factor management directly and shown results in an RCT.

iii) Medical professionals

There are different roles to consider for primary care physicians and specialists in stroke services. In the study by Boter et al. , patients and carers were advised to seek help from primary care physicians when necessary. The contact and coordination with primary care physicians was more direct and active in the study by Mayo et al . Neither supported the general practitioner in risk factor management. In the Australian ICARUSS model, there is bi-directional information sharing regarding risk factor status of stroke survivors between the coordinator, specialist stroke services and primary care physician . Determined reaction to persistently abnormal values is an integral part of the model. The telephone support from the specialist physician to the primary care physician is part of the "shared care" component. In ICARUSS, screening for symptoms of depression is performed on a three-monthly basis and the results are faxed to the primary care physician. ICARUSS is an example of a telestroke model that maintains specialist involvement in the long-term. The immediate, real-time specialist support to the primary care physician provides the "contemporaneous sharing of responsibility" between primary care physicians and specialists, which is the element of shared care.

iv) Coordinators

The coordinator plays a key role in all the telestroke models for stroke survivors described above. In some, the role is passive , while in others the interaction is more active. The coordinator plays a part in problem-solving , education, surveillance and reaction , as well as psychological and social support. In the ICARUSS model, the coordinator provides the link between patient, caregiver, primary care physician and specialist stroke services.

3.2.4 Telestroke support management services

To date, the limited availability and acceptance of past Information and Communication Technology (ICT) possibilities has limited the possible support options. At this stage, it is now possible to explore what Telestroke Support Management Services are available and appropriate as an adjunct to human contact, and in combination with some of the current telemedicine services outlined in Table 2. Any new technology should viewed as an advance on existing systems and compared rigorously in terms of cost-effectiveness as well as efficacy .

i) Technology Options for Telestroke

Across the different studies, a range of technology options have been used including telephone, facsimile, email, videoconferencing, and internet-based communication, which may be generic or personalized. Simple telephone contact has been shown to be useful in different situations, such as giving practical problem-solving advice to caregivers. Moreover, the contact has been useful in reducing stress . Telephone interviews have been shown to be reliable in the application of a variety of assessment and measuring tools, such as the Stroke Impact Scale (SIS) and proven reliable for the evaluation of disability and cognitive function in community outpatients . Telephone administration of the Patient Health Questionnaire (PHQ9) has also been validated in stroke patients. This instrument has demonstrated reliability as a screening tool for Post Stroke Depression. There is a need to determine the best modality to achieve the requisite goal in stroke survivors. These goals may be risk factor modification, patient and carer education, detection and management of post-stroke depression, carer support, strategy implementation, rehabilitation or simple surveillance of health service usage. Different modalities may be appropriate for different goals; simple telephone calls may suffice for patient and carer education or support , whereas a tele-rehabilitation programme may require videoconferencing , as would a psychiatric intervention for depression.

TELESTROKE SERVICES					
Care Coordination and Secondary Stroke Prevention		Other Telemedicine Functions			Tele-Rehabilitation
Carer Support and Problem-Solving	Risk Factor Management	Emergency Response	Health Information and Education	Medication Compliance	Remote assessment and therapy

Table 2.Overview of Telestroke potential

It is unlikely and undesirable that single solutions for different scenarios can be developed to meet the above telestroke service needs. Functional requirements need to be analysed and all available options considered. Although the literature reveals an interest in experimenting with new ICT from video conferencing and Internet web-cams, to virtual reality haptic workbenches, most ICT studies have relied on the telephone to study post-acute stroke survivor needs. Many of the ongoing assessment tools could potentially be integrated into handheld devices where audio and visual evidence could be directly captured.

Some studies have indicated that technology choices are limited to those acceptable to the survivors and/or their carers. Perhaps more important is the fact that the spectrum of ICT options is expanding rapidly, while costs are decreasing. However, deployment of these options is not uniformly available across all geographical and demographic users. For example, fibre optic cable is not yet as ubiquitous as copper networks and 3G intelligent mobile phone networks do not have the same coverage as GSM.

ii) Care Coordinator Requirements

A missing systems requirement in the design of telestroke services is the functional requirement for implementation of the care coordinator role. Solutions adopted will depend on a number of factors such as the capture area of the services, remoteness of care and health provider locations, and the number of survivors involved - in other words, the caseload. It is expected that caseloads of over 80 stroke survivors would need a full time care coordinator, and their productivity would depend on the support systems available . The coordinator requirements are outlined in Table 3.

Telestroke Modality	**Costs**	**CC to CR/ICG Operational Issues**	**CC to GP / Specialist and/or Hospital ED**	**Special Issues**
Telephone contact	Inexpensive	Reliance on Phone contacting limits case load for CC. Ubiquitous and Saves Travel Validated for several assessments.	Generally effective Gives personal contact. Non-threatening to elderly	Note-taking of interactions
Facsimile	Inexpensive	Ubiquitous	Generally effective. Specified usage	Storage needed
Video-conferencing for visual contact	As for ICG; saves travel. Initial Setup can be costly and is time-consuming if used frequently.	Not readily available at home. Skype and webcam is possible.	Can be useful for case referral conferences	Effort required to arrange; visit may be more effective
Internet Contact	Medium to high costs to setup computer, modem and broadband services	Most efficient use of CC time for data collection, but not effective for human interaction. Elderly may have usage barrier	Can be useful for sharing electronic records and reports	Privacy and data security obligations
Web Page	Costly to set up and resources needed to maintain content	Provides a 24/7 resource to ICG/CR on more frequent types of info needs. Elderly may have usage barrier	Enables links to service provider organisations of relevance to users	Needs updating regularly to be relevant; users may need a secure log-on
Health Records [1]	Initial filling-in on paper is fast and low cost if well designed	An effective system is required that meets medical authority standards.	Need to be able to share with appropriate third parties	Security and privacy requirements; long-term storage
Contact Database [2]	Software is available for this function; desirable to integrate with EDS	Essential for efficient interactions	Essential for efficient interactions	Needs to portable

Electronic Documents System [3]	Can be expensive and needs tailoring for CC needs	Effective for data searching, studies and archiving.	Assists efficient support for hospitals, GPs and specialists	Secure archiving of data is essential

CC: Care Coordinator; CR: Care Receiver / Stroke Survivor; ICG: Informal Care Giver; GP: General Practitioner (of CR); ED: Emergency Department

[1] These may be proformas or other reports handled in paper form.

[2] For tracking client interactions - planned and completed.

[3] For managing all documents electronically - paper is scanned

Table 3. Technology Options for Care Coordinator (CC)

3.3 Further potential and possible limitations of telestroke for stroke survivors

Telestroke programmes should address the post-discharge management of stroke survivors and the needs of caregivers. They should facilitate risk factor and other areas of medical management by the primary care physician (traditional general practitioner or clinic-based physician). Telestroke should also counteract the effects of isolation and limited access to specialist services in rural areas.

3.3.1 Desirable functional requirements for a telestroke model

Ideally, in a comprehensive telemedicine model a variety of items related to medical management, process, quality control and outcomes should be measured. These are shown in the Box. Of particular importance is the monitoring of vascular risk factors for the reduction of recurrent vascular events, primarily stroke - e.g. blood pressure, cholesterol, anticoagulation and blood sugar. Compliance with medication and surveillance of laboratory tests can be readily coordinated in a telestroke model.

The literature has suggested that there are a range of telestroke services that should now be considered to meet the wider needs of post-acute stroke survivors and the integrated care requirements:

- Telestroke model should facilitate knowledge transfer, particularly in relation to education and best practice recommendations for risk factor management .
- The system should provide, support and monitor clear management plans for secondary stroke prevention .
- There should be regular survey methods applicable to telemedicine of patient, carer and health provider satisfaction .
- The model should facilitate the provision, as needed, for expert consultation related particularly to stroke prevention, but also home rehabilitation and addressing patient and carer problems .
- Telestroke should reduce the need for travel, particularly in remote areas .
- Ideally, a telestroke model should provide ongoing, updated guidelines for risk factor management to primary physicians in an accessible, user-friendly way .
- The system should be able to scientifically evaluate outcomes and cost, and to address the questions of effectiveness and economic implications .
- The system should be capable of 'flagging' patients at increased risk. This should be part of the bi-directional information feedback loop.
- Telestroke should allow for evaluation of health-related quality of life (HRQL) .

- There should be a standardised manner of reporting stroke outcome measures, risk outcome measures and resource utilisation across multiple telestroke systems to allow for comparison .
- The telestroke system should facilitate what is essentially case-management of stroke survivors in a bi- or multidirectional way (health provider to client and client to health provider).

In stroke survivors, the most appropriate and acceptable support for patients and their carers and families should take into account to the fact that most stroke patients are elderly, as are their carers, and the majority are not technologically proficient . This means that the model of telecommunication should be adaptable and appropriate to the needs of patients to ensure compliance and usage both in the short- and the long-term . It should be remembered that three role players need to be supported after discharge - i.e. patient, carer and primary care physician. Patients and care givers need psychological support, practical advice in addressing what is often a combination of risk factor management and adaptation to physical disability and social change. The primary care physician needs support and guidance in implementing the best practice guidelines for risk factors management and the treatment of post-stroke depression. An integrated care model should enhance the quality of care for stroke survivors by linking together domains such as education, surveillance, and detection of abnormalities. Such a telestroke model should contain discrete elements of intervention, so that depending on the social and economic setting, the appropriate intervention elements of the model can be selected.

- Risk factors
- Social support
- Mental health of patients
- Quality of Life
- Economic measures (utilization of services)
- Measurement of neurological impairment
- Measurement of disability and functioning
- Medication compliance
- Laboratory tests
- Recurrent stroke, vascular event or death
- Knowledge transfer

Box

3.3.2 Implications for future developments in post–acute telestroke models

A range of current telemedicine applications is potentially available for telestroke use. Many studies have shown the effectiveness of telemedicine for care management in a variety of chronic diseases such as for general health status monitoring (self-reported, or with home-based devices) with scheduled interventions such as nurse visit or GP consultation (video, telephone or physical attendance) ; medication compliance and modification, depending on symptoms and side-affects; and the early detection of deterioration of patients leading to 'just-in-time' interventions, preventing unnecessary admissions and healthcare costs . These are summarised in Table 3.

3.3.3 Significant implementation issues

Telemedicine studies have shown various drawbacks which need to be considered . Many telehealth projects are neither successfully implemented, nor accepted despite being medically appropriate and technically viable. Cho et al. recently analysed the theoretical framework underpinning the implementation of a telestroke service (REACH) and a Swedish teleradiology service as models of care. Barriers to implementation were identified as insufficient planning of IT infrastructure, lack of long-term vision for sustainability, lack of contextual perspective, and poor communication with a lack of early involvement of important role players. Financial barriers contributing to difficulties with the diffusion of the project, if not foreseen and accounted for from early on, can lead to limited or aborted important implementation issues. Existing work practices have to be acknowledged, as IT innovations do not occur *ex vacuo.*

Organisational structures and various public and insurance funding changes may be needed to accommodate a different care regime that includes outreach through telemedicine . The sharing of patient health records between public and private health providers, medical and care professionals, and hospital and community centre care coordinators, leads to security, privacy and liability issues that need solving . More efficient use of communication dialogue and methods are needed to efficiently manage each patient interaction - especially as coordinator and medical case loads increase with greater use of telemedicine links to patients and carers. For example, there may need to be a differentiation between problem-solving, education and motivational dialogue from structured rehabilitation management tasks . In addition, an improved human/technology interface functionality is needed to take into account individual patient disabilities, time limitations and the technical skills of the carer. A flexibility of technology solutions should be adopted that allows for rates of obsolescence, local availability of supply, and support of hardware and software, especially as such telemedicine options are extended to different regions, states and countries . The current pilot studies of home-telemedicine do not provide sufficient evidence for full deployment scaling using major public health funding, although some have produced projected business cases and others are studying world wide practices. Telehealth models vary in systems architecture from two-way to three or more ways, with various implied control modes - nursing care coordinator or clinician (agency, hospital or clinic) or community. This impacts on the cost-effectiveness of bandwidth and computing intensive solutions, even though the component costs appear to be falling. This complexity makes the difficulty of technology selection all the greater.

3.3.4 Economic evaluation of telestroke Implementations

Although a specific search strategy for this aspect was not undertaken in this review, we noted that the resource implications of telestroke had been raised as an issue in several studies. To date, most studies have been designed to provide evidence for the technical feasibility of using current (telephone, videoconferencing) or new (Internet, Virtual Environment) technologies. Many of these studies are project-funded to address efficacy issues and full economic costs have not published . The economic impact of these telestroke systems is a critical area in need of more research . Costs involved in telestroke may include both set-up and operating costs, which have seldom been quantified. Moreover, many reported cost studies are based on such diverse technical, organisational and cost contexts that it would be difficult to draw conclusions in order to undertake a comprehensive cost-effectiveness study . It has been noted that a lack of reimbursement for clinicians may be a major impediment to the use of telestroke. Such economic issues require further investigation .

The CADTH review was inconclusive as to whether telestroke was cost-effective and safe compared to face-to-face care . The authors highlighted the lack of standardised reporting that precluded comparisons between studies and best practice determination. This would also have implications for undertaking economic evaluation studies. Thus, the evidence related to costs and cost-effectiveness of telestroke appears limited. More recently, Ehlers et al reported that at one year, the net cost per patient treated with thrombolysis using telestroke compared to standard practice was $50,000 and that at 2 years the intervention would save costs by reducing care and rehabilitation costs. However, the authors noted that although there may be potentially large savings associated with thrombolysis with alteplase delivered by telemedicine, the long-term calculations were uncertain. In another study designed to assess the cost-effectiveness of pharmacists giving advice via telephone to patients receiving a new medicine for a chronic condition (including stroke), the intervention was less costly and more effective than standard practice .

In 2010, Nelson et al. analysed the trade-off between short-term costs and long-term outcomes of telestroke in the Western States Stroke Consortium (WSSC). They studied a systematic method of comparing 2 or more interventions by measuring their costs and consequences (health outcomes) where the consequences of each are measured in common units related to the clinical objective of the interventions (e.g., life-years gained or quality-adjusted life-years). They show that telestroke was still cost-effective compared to usual care in the lifetime horizon model but not in the 90-day horizon model. However, there were certain limitations to the study. Their model did not consider stroke mimics, for example, which may also be the object of telestroke intervention. There are potential cost savings of not transferring such patients to tertiary care centres. Two new Canadian programmes have also been designed to address the economic and resource implications for telestroke, which may contribute further evidence to the debate on cost-effectiveness . Clearly, studies with long-term follow-up and consistent methodology are needed in this area.

3.3.5 Need for well-designed studies

Hersh et al. found that there were only a small number of well-designed telestroke studies in general, particularly in rural settings. There is a need for well-designed RCTs and longitudinal observational studies of clinical outcomes to demonstrate the effective use of telemedicine in stroke survivors discharged from hospital . Rigorously designed studies, such as those that have been recommended for telestroke in the acute phase , are needed .

4. Conclusion

Future trends and recommendations

There is clearly an urgent need, particularly in rural and underserved areas, to develop long-term management systems in stroke survivors that are both integrated and sustainable, serving all sections of the population , and with particular emphasis on the sustained implementation of best practice risk factor management . In these more remote areas of the world, the implementation of telemedicine may fill the gap in health care provision created by the high demand on healthcare provider time, the critical shortage of professional health services and geographical distance thereby progressing the ideals of the WHO contained in the Helsingborg Declaration .

Ultimately, the long-term management of risk factors in stroke survivors rests with the primary care physician or other health practitioner acting as the final 'locus of control' for the patient. Unfortunately, despite the enormous calculated benefits flowing from the effective implementation of best practice recommendations , therapeutic inertia is common at primary care level . To address this, a combination of 'hub and spoke' case-management model (care coordinator, with multiple stroke survivors) and linear model (specialist, coordinator, carer, patient and primary care physician) could be advantageous. Telestroke may also minimise the inappropriate variations in medical practice . ICARUSS provides one telestroke model that is adaptable to various scenarios and integrates the roles of coordinator, primary care physician, specialist services and other telestroke support services in the care of both stroke survivor and caregiver. The model supports the implementation of secondary stroke prevention strategies and the detection of post-stroke depression. The focus is on providing care, support and specialist guidance to rural, remote or underserved areas in all fields related to the care of stroke survivors, in a model that continues to provide patients and carers with the face-to-face experience, but that also fully exploits the available modern technology options.

5. Acknowledgement

The RUN-FC network has been supported and funded by the French Health Ministry.
The ICARUSS study is supporte Ad by funding from the HCF HEALTH AND MEDICAL RESEARCH FOUNDATION. We would like to thank Melanie Cole for her editing assistance.

6. References

Adamson, J., A. Beswick, et al. (2004). "Is stroke the most common cause of disability?" Journal of stroke and cerebrovascular diseases : the official journal of National Stroke Association 13(4): 171-177.

AHA (2008). Heart Disease and stroke Statistics—2008 Update. Dallas, TX, American Heart Association.

Audebert, H. (2006). "Telestroke: effective networking." Lancet neurology 5(3): 279-282.

Boter, H. (2004). "Multicenter randomized controlled trial of an outreach nursing support program for recently discharged stroke patients." Stroke; a journal of cerebral circulation 35(12): 2867-2872.

Bouffard, K. (1997). "Telemedicine: who's in charge?" Michigan medicine 96(9): 10-15; 17-19.

Brenner, D. A., R. M. Zweifler, et al. (2010). "Awareness, treatment, and control of vascular risk factors among stroke survivors." Journal of stroke and cerebrovascular diseases : the official journal of National Stroke Association 19(4): 311-320.

Broens, T. H., R. M. Huis in't Veld, et al. (2007). "Determinants of successful telemedicine implementations: a literature study." Journal of telemedicine and telecare 13(6): 303-309.

Buckley, K. M., B. Q. Tran, et al. (2004). "Receptiveness, use and acceptance of telehealth by caregivers of stroke patients in the home." Online journal of issues in nursing 9(3): 9.

Bulik, R. J. (2008). "Human factors in primary care telemedicine encounters." Journal of telemedicine and telecare 14(4): 169-172.

Cadilhac, D. A., R. C. Carter, et al. (2007). "Why invest in a national public health program for stroke? An example using Australian data to estimate the potential benefits and cost implications." Health policy 83(2-3): 287-294.

Camilo, O. and L. B. Goldstein (2003). "Statewide assessment of hospital-based stroke prevention and treatment services in North Carolina: changes over the last 5 years." Stroke; a journal of cerebral circulation 34(12): 2945-2950.

Champonnois, L., E. de Bustos, et al. (2010). RUN-FC (Réseau des Urgences Neurologiques en Franche-Comté). Symposium HAS-BMJ.

Cherry, J. C., K. Dryden, et al. (2003). "Opening a window of opportunity through technology and coordination: a multisite case study." Telemedicine journal and e-health : the official journal of the American Telemedicine Association 9(3): 265-271.

Cho, S., E. V. Khasanshina, et al. (2007). "An analysis of business issues in a telestroke project." Journal of telemedicine and telecare 13(5): 257-262.

Croquelois, A. and J. Bogousslavsky (2006). "Risk awareness and knowledge of patients with stroke: results of a questionnaire survey 3 months after stroke." Journal of neurology, neurosurgery, and psychiatry 77(6): 726-728.

de Bustos, E., T. Moulin, et al. (2009). "Barriers, legal issues, limitations and ongoing questions in telemedicine applied to stroke." Cerebrovascular Diseases 27(Suppl 4): 36-39.

de Bustos, E. M., F. Vuillier, et al. (2009). "Telemedicine in stroke: organizing a network--rationale and baseline principles." Cerebrovascular Diseases 27(Suppl 4): 1-8.

Demaerschalk, B. M., H. M. Hwang, et al. (2010). "Cost analysis review of stroke centers, telestroke, and rt-PA." The American journal of managed care 16(7): 537-544.

Demiris, G., C. L. Shigaki, et al. (2005). "An evaluation framework for a rural home-based telerehabilitation network." Journal of medical systems 29(6): 595-603.

Dergalust, S., M. Rofail, et al. (2003). "The incidence of discontinuation of extended release dipyridamole/aspirin, clopidogrel and warfarin for the secondary prevention of stroke." Presented at the 55th American Academy of Neurology Annual Meeting; Honolulu, Hawaii. April 3.

Deshpande, A., S. Khoja, et al. (2010). "Telehealth for Acute Stroke Management (Telestroke): Systematic Review and Environmental Scan [Technology overview 37]." Ottawa: Canadian Agency for Drugs and Technologies in Health; 2008. 60(6): 991-999.

Dhamoon, M. S., R. R. Sciacca, et al. (2006). "Recurrent stroke and cardiac risks after first ischemic stroke: the Northern Manhattan Study." Neurology 66(5): 641-646.

Doze, S., J. Simpson, et al. (1999). "Evaluation of a telepsychiatry pilot project." Journal of telemedicine and telecare 5(1): 38-46.

Ehlers, L., W. M. Muskens, et al. (2008). "National use of thrombolysis with alteplase for acute ischaemic stroke via telemedicine in Denmark: a model of budgetary impact and cost effectiveness." CNS drugs 22(1): 73-81.

Elliott, R. A., N. Barber, et al. (2008). "The cost effectiveness of a telephone-based pharmacy advisory service to improve adherence to newly prescribed medicines." Pharmacy world & science : PWS 30(1): 17-23.

Goldstein, L. B. and P. M. Rothwell (2007). "Primary prevention and health services delivery." Stroke; a journal of cerebral circulation 38(2): 222-224.

Grant, J. S., T. R. Elliott, et al. (2002). "Telephone intervention with family caregivers of stroke survivors after rehabilitation." Stroke; a journal of cerebral circulation 33(8): 2060-2065.

Hachinski, V. (2002). "Stroke: the next 30 years." Stroke; a journal of cerebral circulation 33(1): 1-4.

Hachinski, V., G. A. Donnan, et al. (2010). "Stroke: working toward a prioritized world agenda." Stroke; a journal of cerebral circulation 41(6): 1084-1099.

Hailey, D. and B. Crowe (2003). "A profile of success and failure in telehealth--evidence and opinion from the Success and Failures in Telehealth conferences." Journal of telemedicine and telecare 9 Suppl 2: S22-24.

Hardie, K., G. J. Hankey, et al. (2004). "Ten-year risk of first recurrent stroke and disability after first-ever stroke in the Perth Community Stroke Study." Stroke; a journal of cerebral circulation 35(3): 731-735.

Hebert, M. A. and B. Korabek (2004). "Stakeholder readiness for telehomecare: implications for implementation." Telemedicine journal and e-health : the official journal of the American Telemedicine Association 10(1): 85-92.

Hersh, W. R., D. H. Hickam, et al. (2006). "Telemedicine for the medicare population: update." Evidence report/technology assessment(131): 1-41.

Hess, D. C., S. Wang, et al. (2005). "REACH: clinical feasibility of a rural telestroke network." Stroke; a journal of cerebral circulation 36(9): 2018-2020.

Hjelm, N. M. (2005). "Benefits and drawbacks of telemedicine." Journal of telemedicine and telecare 11(2): 60-70.

Hopp, F., P. Whitten, et al. (2006). "Perspectives from the Veterans Health Administration about opportunities and barriers in telemedicine." J Telemed Telecare 12: 404-409.

Jencks, S. F., T. Cuerdon, et al. (2000). "Quality of medical care delivered to Medicare beneficiaries: A profile at state and national levels." JAMA : the journal of the American Medical Association 284(13): 1670-1676.

Joubert, J., L. Joubert, et al. (2008). "The positive effect of integrated care on depressive symptoms in stroke survivors." Cerebrovascular diseases 26(2): 199-205.

Joubert, J., L. B. Joubert, et al. (2009). "Telestroke in stroke survivors." Cerebrovascular diseases 27 Suppl 4: 28-35.

Joubert, J., L. F. Prentice, et al. (2008). "Stroke in rural areas and small communities." Stroke; a journal of cerebral circulation 39(6): 1920-1928.

Joubert, J., C. Reid, et al. (2006). "Risk factor management and depression post-stroke: the value of an integrated model of care." Journal of clinical neuroscience : official journal of the Neurosurgical Society of Australasia 13(1): 84-90.

Jutras, A. (1959). "Teleroentgen diagnosis by means of video-tape recording." The American journal of roentgenology, radium therapy, and nuclear medicine 82: 1099-1102.

Kannel, W. B., P. A. Wolf, et al. (1970). "Epidemiologic assessment of the role of blood pressure in stroke. The Framingham study." JAMA : the journal of the American Medical Association 214(2): 301-310.

Kjellstrom, T., B. Norrving, et al. (2007). "Helsingborg Declaration 2006 on European stroke strategies." Cerebrovascular diseases 23(2-3): 231-241.

Kondalsamy-Chennakesavan, S., W. Hoy, et al. (2004). "Chronic disease surveillance and management in remote Aboriginal Australia: role of web-based applications." J Telemed Telecare 10: 101.

LaBresh, K. A., M. J. Reeves, et al. (2008). "Hospital treatment of patients with ischemic stroke or transient ischemic attack using the "Get With The Guidelines" program." Archives of internal medicine 168(4): 411-417.

LaMonte, M. P., M. N. Bahouth, et al. (2003). "Telemedicine for acute stroke: triumphs and pitfalls." Stroke; a journal of cerebral circulation 34(3): 725-728.

Lee, P. W., H. C. Schulberg, et al. (2007). "Concordance between the PHQ-9 and the HSCL-20 in depressed primary care patients." Journal of affective disorders 99(1-3): 139-145.

Levine, S. R. and M. Gorman (1999). ""Telestroke" : the application of telemedicine for stroke." Stroke; a journal of cerebral circulation 30(2): 464-469.

Levine, S. R. and K. M. McConnochie (2007). "Telemedicine for acute stroke: when virtual is as good as reality." Neurology 69(9): 819-820.

Lewis, M., J. Trypuc, et al. (2006). "Has Ontario's Stroke System really made a difference?" Healthcare quarterly 9(4): 50-59, 52.

Li, C., G. Engstrom, et al. (2008). "Long-term stroke prognosis in relation to medical prevention and lifestyle factors. A prospective population-based study." Cerebrovascular diseases 25(6): 526-532.

Lutz, B. J., N. R. Chumbler, et al. (2007). "Care coordination/home-telehealth for veterans with stroke and their caregivers: addressing an unmet need." Topics in stroke rehabilitation 14(2): 32-42.

Mackay, J. and G. A. Mensah (2004). "The atlas of heart disease and stroke." Geneva WHO.

Mayo, N. E., L. Nadeau, et al. (2008). "Bridging the gap: the effectiveness of teaming a stroke coordinator with patient's personal physician on the outcome of stroke." Age and ageing 37(1): 32-38.

Meade, B. J. and J. A. Dunbar (2004). "A virtual clinic: telemetric assessment and monitoring for rural and remote areas." Rural and remote health 4(3): 296.

Merino, J. G., S. U. Lattimore, et al. (2005). "Telephone assessment of stroke outcome is reliable." Stroke; a journal of cerebral circulation 36(2): 232-233.

Meschia, J. F., M. A. Lojacono, et al. (2004). "Reliability of the questionnaire for verifying stroke-free status." Cerebrovascular diseases 17(2-3): 218-223.

Miley, M. L., B. M. Demaerschalk, et al. (2009). "The state of emergency stroke resources and care in rural Arizona: a platform for telemedicine." Telemedicine journal and e-health : the official journal of the American Telemedicine Association 15(7): 691-699.

Misra, U. K., J. Kalita, et al. (2005). "Telemedicine in neurology: underutilized potential." Neurology India 53(1): 27-31.

Moulin, T., P. Decavel, et al. (2004). "Information technology (IT) support in the implementation of a stroke programme: the RUN-Stroke experiment." Cerebrovascular Diseases 17((supp 5)): 6.

Moulin, T., J. Joubert, et al. (2011). Telemedicine in Stroke: Potentials, Limitations and Ongoing Issues. Advances in Telemedicine: Applications in Various Medical Disciplines and Geographical Regions. Available from: http://www.intechopen.com/articles/show/title/telemedicine-in-stroke-potentials-limitations-and-ongoing-issues, InTech.

Nelson, R., G. Saltzman, et al. (2010). Cost-Effectiveness of Telestroke for Ischemic Stroke: A Literature-Based Decision-Analytic Model Poster session presented at: American Heart Association / American Stroke Association International Stroke Conference, San Antonio, TX.

Noel, H. C., D. C. Vogel, et al. (2004). "Home telehealth reduces healthcare costs." Telemedicine journal and e-health : the official journal of the American Telemedicine Association 10(2): 170-183.

Ovbiagele, B., O. Drogan, et al. (2008). "Outpatient practice patterns after stroke hospitalization among neurologists." Stroke; a journal of cerebral circulation 39(6): 1850-1854.

Park, S. and L. H. Schwamm (2008). "Organizing regional stroke systems of care." Current opinion in neurology 21(1): 43-55.

Pierce, L. L., V. Steiner, et al. (2004). "Internet-based support for rural caregivers of persons with stroke shows promise." Rehabilitation nursing : the official journal of the Association of Rehabilitation Nurses 29(3): 95-99, 103.

Puskin, D. S. (2001). "Telemedicine: follow the money modalities." Online journal of issues in nursing 6(3): 2.

Rahimi, B. and V. Vimarlund (2007). "Methods to evaluate health information systems in healthcare settings: a literature review." Journal of medical systems 31(5): 397-432.

Roine, R., A. Ohinmaa, et al. (2001). "Assessing telemedicine: a systematic review of the literature." CMAJ : Canadian Medical Association journal = journal de l'Association medicale canadienne 165(6): 765-771.

Rosamond, W., K. Flegal, et al. (2008). "Heart disease and stroke statistics--2008 update: a report from the American Heart Association Statistics Committee and Stroke Statistics Subcommittee." Circulation 117(4): e25-146.

Sato, S. and K. Ohta (1993). "[New network for emergency medical services of stroke with CT-picture teleradiology system]." Nippon rinsho. Japanese journal of clinical medicine 51 Suppl: 246-250.

Schneider, N. M. (2004). "Managing congestive heart failure using home telehealth." Home healthcare nurse 22(10): 719-722.

Schwamm, L. H., H. J. Audebert, et al. (2009). "Recommendations for the implementation of telemedicine within stroke systems of care: a policy statement from the American Heart Association." Stroke; a journal of cerebral circulation 40(7): 2635-2660.

Schwamm, L. H., R. G. Holloway, et al. (2009). "A review of the evidence for the use of telemedicine within stroke systems of care: a scientific statement from the American Heart Association/American Stroke Association." Stroke; a journal of cerebral circulation 40(7): 2616-2634.

Schwamm, L. H., A. Pancioli, et al. (2005). "Recommendations for the establishment of stroke systems of care: recommendations from the American Stroke Association's Task Force on the Development of Stroke Systems." Stroke; a journal of cerebral circulation 36(3): 690-703.

SOTPSS (2004). Southeastern Ontario Telestroke Proposal Stroke Strategy.

Susman, E. (1997). "Telemedicine to give rural stroke victims fair chance of recovery with new treatment." Telemedicine Virtual Reality 2: 1-2.

Swanepoel de, W. and J. W. Hall (2010). "A systematic review of telehealth applications in audiology." Telemedicine journal and e-health : the official journal of the American Telemedicine Association 16(2): 181-200.

Tatlisumak, T., S. Soinila, et al. (2009). "Telestroke networking offers multiple benefits beyond thrombolysis." Cerebrovascular diseases 27 Suppl 4: 21-27.

Taylor, D. and L. Capamagian (2007). "Experience with planned and coordinated care using telemedicine." J Telemed Telecare 13: 86-87.

Taylor, P. (2005). "Evaluating telemedicine systems and services." Journal of telemedicine and telecare 11(4): 167-177.

Touze, E., J. Coste, et al. (2008). "Importance of in-hospital initiation of therapies and therapeutic inertia in secondary stroke prevention: IMplementation of Prevention After a Cerebrovascular evenT (IMPACT) Study." Stroke; a journal of cerebral circulation 39(6): 1834-1843.

Tran, B. Q., K. M. Buckley, et al. (2002). "Selection & use of telehealth technology in support of homebound caregivers of stroke patients." Caring : National Association for Home Care magazine 21(3): 16-21.

Wang, D. Z. (2003). "Editorial comment-- telemedicine: the solution to provide rural stroke coverage and the answer to the shortage of stroke neurologists and radiologists." Stroke; a journal of cerebral circulation 34(12): 2957.

Webb, D. and P. Williams (2006). Telemedicine and the Digital Door Doctor. 4th Australian Information Security Management Conference, Edith Cowan University, Perth, W. Australia, School of Computer and Information Science, Edith Cowan University, Perth, Western Australia.

Whisnant, J. P. (1997). "Modeling of risk factors for ischemic stroke. The Willis Lecture." Stroke; a journal of cerebral circulation 28(9): 1840-1844.

Whitten, P. S., F. S. Mair, et al. (2002). "Systematic review of cost effectiveness studies of telemedicine interventions." BMJ 324(7351): 1434-1437.

WHO. (2011). "Fact Sheet N° 311, Obesity and Overweight." Retrieved 06 May, 2011, from http://www.who.int/mediacentre/factsheets/fs311/en/index.html.

WHO. (2011). "Fact Sheet N° 312, Diabetes." Retrieved 06 May, 2011, from http://www.who.int/mediacentre/factsheets/fs312/en/index.html.

Wiborg, A. and B. Widder (2003). "Teleneurology to improve stroke care in rural areas: The Telemedicine in Stroke in Swabia (TESS) Project." Stroke; a journal of cerebral circulation 34(12): 2951-2956.

Williams, L. S., E. J. Brizendine, et al. (2005). "Performance of the PHQ-9 as a screening tool for depression after stroke." Stroke; a journal of cerebral circulation 36(3): 635-638.

Winters, J. Telerehabilitation Applications. BIEN 167 Module 3 Telerehabilitation. Milwaukee, Wisconsin, Marquette University.

Wittson, C. L., D. C. Affleck, et al. (1961). "Two-way television in group therapy." Mental hospitals 12: 22-23.

Yusuf, S. (2002). "Two decades of progress in preventing vascular disease." Lancet 360(9326): 2-3.

Zerwic, J., S. Y. Hwang, et al. (2007). "Interpretation of symptoms and delay in seeking treatment by patients who have had a stroke: exploratory study." Heart & lung : the journal of critical care 36(1): 25-34.

23

The Role of Telemedicine in the Management of Acute Trauma Referrals to a Regional Plastic and Hand Surgery Unit in the South East of England

David Wallace[1] and Mark Pickford[2]
[1]*Queen Elizabeth Hospital, Edgbaston, Birmingham*
[2]*Queen Victoria Hospital, East Grinstead, West Sussex*
UK

1. Introduction

1.1 The Queen Victoria Hospital

The Queen Victoria Hospital (QVH) provides Burns and Plastic Surgery services, on a hub and spoke model, to the South East of England (4.5 million population), with a catchment area extending into the Southern aspect of greater London. Geographically the region is 50 by 70 miles; the transport links are primarily organised towards London, rather than East Grinstead where the QVH is situated, halfway between London and the coast. For some patients, travelling to the QVH can be time consuming and expensive.

The QVH receives about 400 acute trauma and burns referrals per month; our own audits demonstrate an increasing demand for trauma services each year. Hand injuries account for the majority of referrals to our service and the London and South East geographical region is under considerable capacity strain with 17% of hand surgery units being closed to referrals at any one time (Skillman et al. 2003).

1.2 Why we considered telemedicine

Telemedicine can be defined as "The practise of medicine at a distance"; it typically involves rapid access to remote medical expertise using telecommunication and information technologies. We had previous experience of many patients unnecessarily transferred to the QVH for specialist care after inadequate initial assessment, including some who had been transported at great expense by helicopter air ambulance. Besides cost implications there are clinical risks associated with inter-hospital transfer (Bledsoe & Smith 2004).

Numerous studies have shown that specialists improve the clinical assessment of hand (Nassab et al. 2007; Patel et al. 1998) and burn injuries (Collis et al. 1999; Hagstrom et al. 2003; Laing et al. 1991), our most frequent referrals. Therefore with a defined clinical need and available technology we believed that telemedicine could assist in the management of injured patients referred to the QVH from distant hospitals.

Telemedicine has been investigated since the 1970's (Murphy et al. 1972; Dunn et al. 1977) yet only from the late 1990's onwards do we see widespread pilot studies (Hailey et al. 2002;

Benger 2000). Numerous papers have reported Telemedicine technologies that have the potential to improve the accuracy of triage e.g. to correctly assess patients with burn injuries (Saffle et al. 2009; Saffle et al. 2004), patients who may be candidates for replantation surgery (Buntic et al. 1997), other soft tissue injuries (Pap et al. 2002; Wirthlin et al. 1998; Hsieh et al. 2004; Ong 2008) and also fractures (Ricci & Borrelli 2002; Jacobs et al. 2002). Guides to successful use of telemedicine suggest the clinical users are best placed to choose the type of telemedicine system for their requirement (Yellowlees 1997). The telemedicine team consisted of Consultants, Trainee surgeons, Nursing staff, Medical illustrators, Information Technology experts and audit personnel.

1.3 Store-and-forward or videoconferencing telemedicine?

The two main types of telemedicine were considered for applicability to our need, Store-and-forward and real-time videoconferencing. Videoconference systems had already been demonstrated for Minor Injury Units (Tachakra et al. 2002), major trauma management (Rogers et al. 2001), Dermatology (Loane et al. 2000; Wallace et al. 2002), Orthopaedics (Harno et al. 2001), Intensive care (Rosenfeld et al. 2000), Psychiatry (Elford et al. 2000) and for educational purposes (Kingsnorth et al. 2000; Ward et al. 2001). Educational benefits can include a reduction in referrals (Darkins et al. 1996).

We were concerned about limited availability of the necessary technology at the many referring hospitals in our catchment area if we were to use videoconferencing systems, the cost of triple ISDN (Integrated Services Digital Network) lines for adequate bandwidth and line charges for each use, when no extra revenue was expected. In contrast Store-and-forward systems could allow review at any computer in our hospital, use existing technology and without any discernible cost per referral. In addition, the accuracy for diagnosis compared to face-to-face consultation (concordance) appeared to favour a Store-and-forward system rather than videoconferencing.

Studies on the use of telemedicine in dermatology have revealed greater accuracy for Store-and-forward telemedicine (70 to 95%), rather than videoconferencing (51 to 80%), when compared to face-to-face consultation (Wootton et al. 2000; Lowitt et al. 1998; High et al. 2000; Krupinski et al. 1999; Gilmour et al. 1998; Oakley et al. 1997; Taylor et al. 2001). At the QVH we chose a Store-and-forward application to allow encrypted email image transfer. We planned to pilot this on a limited basis and to carry out a qualitative review of the system.

2. Pilot study 1: Telemedicine at the QVH

2.1 Overview of pilot

Referrals were taken as usual by telephone call, supplemented by the transmission of clinical images via email over the NHS intranet from three referring hospitals. Details of all referrals were recorded on small cards (8 x 14cm) to facilitate hand-over for clinicians and provide an audit trail (Figure 1, see below). Specialty advice over the phone can be poorly documented by referring clinicians (Cartmill & White 2001), therefore this also provided a medico legal record of any advice given.

We maintained confidentiality during the trial by not including any images that could identify the patient. We used Joint Professional Expert Group (JPEG) image compression, which did not appear to compromise image quality (Roa et al. 1999). We provided digital compact cameras and undertook training of the Emergency department personnel at the referring hospitals selected for inclusion in our pilot study.

Patient Address

Further Information

Appropriate referral? Y N

From the photo:

Any change in plan? (Tick as appropriate)

No change

Confirmation

Change in Advice/Treatment (Give details)

Change in Priority (Give details)

QVH TRAUMA PATIENT SUMMARY

Doctor On Call: Date: Time:

Patient Name: DOB:

Referring Unit / Hospital: Referring Doctor:

Referral Information:

RHD LHD

Smoker Y N

ψ Y N

Fit and well Y N

Occup.

Diagnosis / Management Plan

Action (More than one box may be Applicable)

Unable to accept	Assess in MIU	Admit (via MIU)
Day Surgery Unit	Advice	Photo requested received
Outlier	Dressing Clinic	Outpatients

Fig. 1. QVH trauma card to collect data on all referrals

We were referred a wide variety of injuries such as burns, facial lacerations, and hand injuries including fractures, tendon and nerve injuries during the study period. Consultants and trainees compared the clinical assessment and prioritisation of 150 consecutive patient images with the face-to-face consultation. Injuries were grouped as follows: i. skin only ii. closed fractures and nerve injuries iii. open fractures and flexor tendon injuries iv. uncertain vascularity v. devascularised tissue and burn injuries requiring formal resuscitation. Clinical priority was organised into five groups of immediate, urgent (<6 hours), very soon (<24 hours), soon (<48 hours) and later (>48 hours). The correlation coefficient was 0.78 to 0.81 for grading of the injury and 0.87 to 0.93 for priority of injury (Jones et al. 2004).

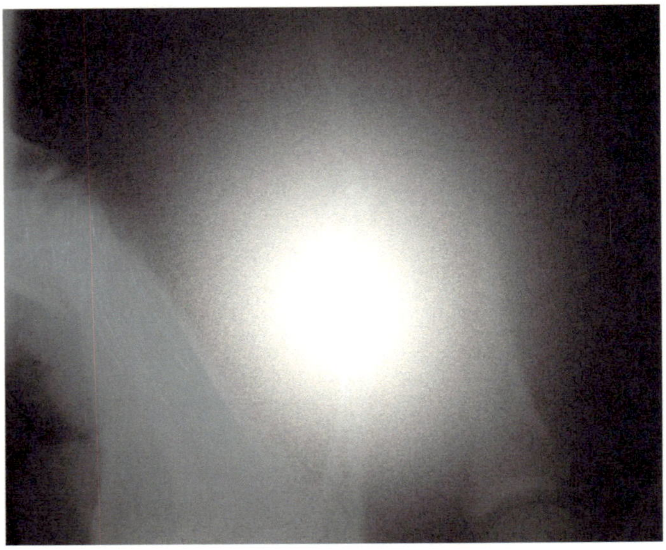

Fig. 2. Flash reflection in an image of an X-ray taken on a viewing box

2.2 Analysis of first QVH telemedicine Pilot study

The results of the pilot study were judged to be satisfactory enough to continue with our plan to establish a Store-and-forward type telemedicine system at the QVH. Although the clinical priority was more accurately validated (concordant) than injury severity, the telemedicine images were judged to provide the receiving clinicians with greater confidence in managing referrals.

Only 82 images were analyzed of the series of 150, as 20 were unusable and there was incomplete data on a further 48, which further demonstrated the need for education at referring hospitals to improve the quality of images (see figure 2). When the pilot study was carried out digital systems for X-ray did not exist and particular problems were encountered recording images of hard-copy X-ray films on viewing boxes; we therefore created guidelines for photographing radiographs, specifically omitting the use of flash.

Education needed to be a continuous program due to the turnover of junior medical staff in referring Emergency departments. We also found that technical problems were highly discouraging to both the referring and receiving clinicians and that they were often given a low priority by IT departments at referring hospitals; a software designer was therefore employed to provide a bespoke application for encrypted email image transfer. A plastic surgery trainee was employed to supervise and drive the project forward.

3. Store-and-forward encrypted telemedicine for acute plastic surgery

3.1 Transmission of images

Encryption software was installed at the QVH and several referring units (DISTAR Telemedicine; Digital Image ST-orage And Retrieval, and TM Client©). The software provided users with 5 simple screens to capture the appropriate images from digital cameras, check the images, allow demographic data entry, provide a record of patient consent, and initiate transmission (see figures 3 to 7). The file size was 500 to 700 KB, with 24-bit colour and 1600 x1200 pixel resolution. We provided an Olympus, C-3020 or a Nikon Coolpix 4500 (minimum 2048 x 1536 pixels) digital compact camera on our own site and at the units with the encryption software installed. These cameras were chosen for their reasonable cost (approximately £200 / $300), simple operation, easily replaceable AA batteries, and good image quality.

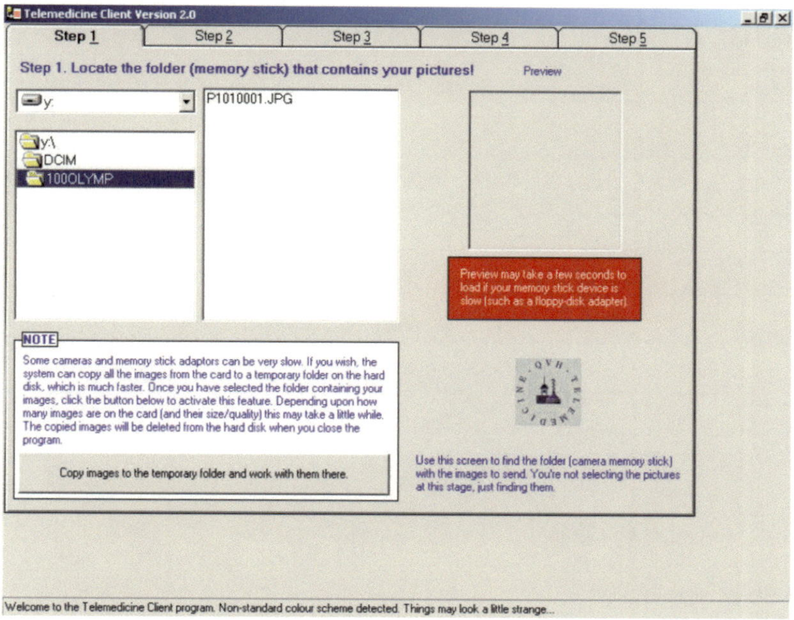

Fig. 3. Locating the images

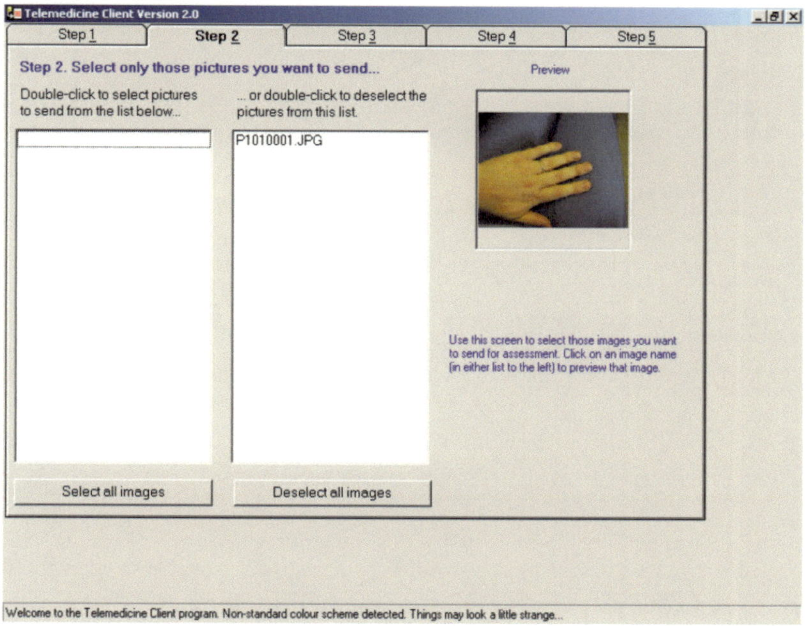

Fig. 4. Selecting the correct images

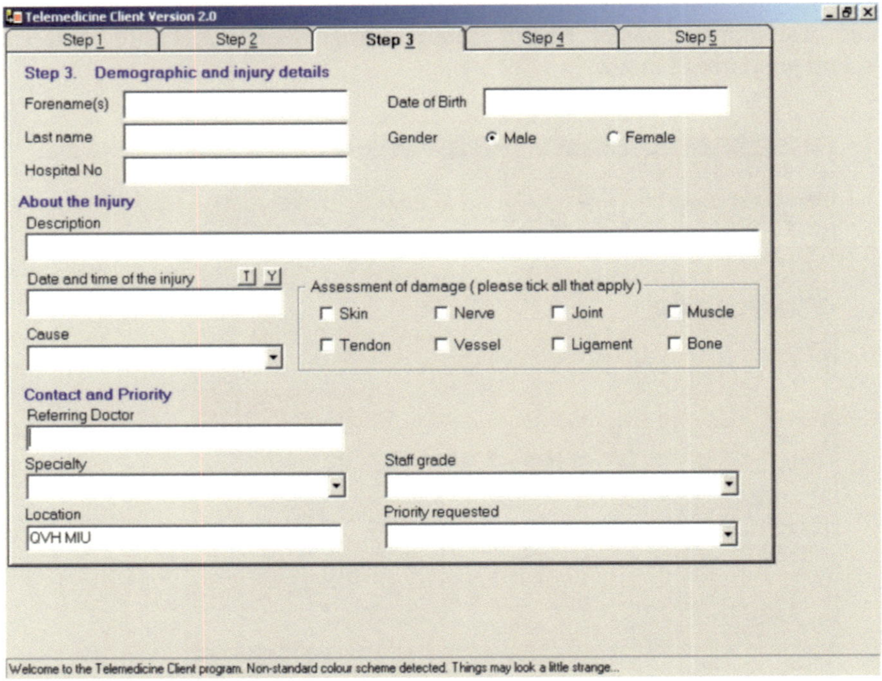

Fig. 5. Demographic data entry

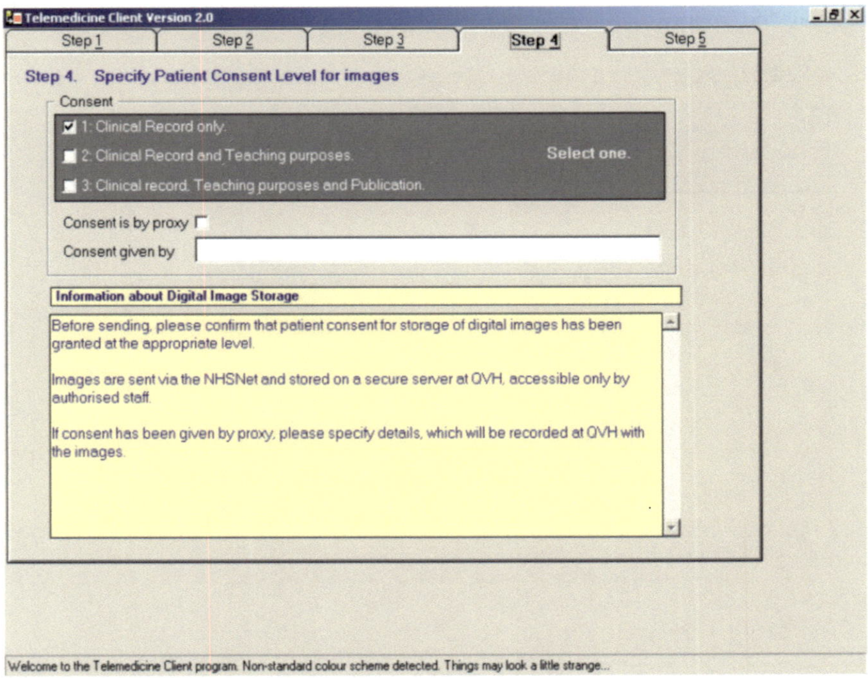

Fig. 6. Recording patient consent

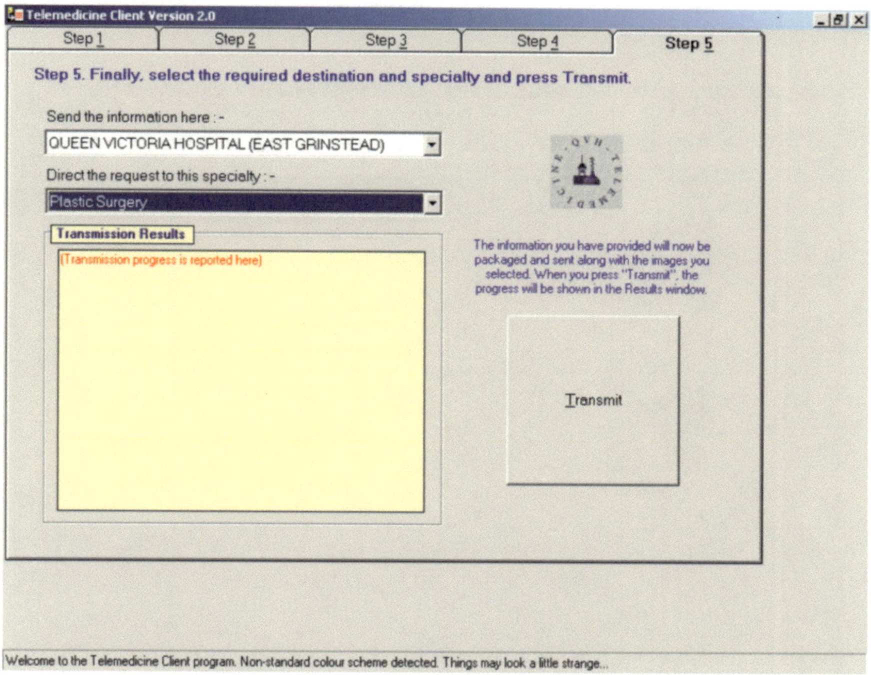

Fig. 7. Initiation of transmission

3.2 Received images

All encrypted email referrals from external units arrive at the QVH server (Pentium 4 256MB RAM and RAID-1 mirrored 14GB disks - these have been upgraded since 2002). Each email is decrypted by the software and is then available on any computer in the QVH to a logged on clinician (see figures 8 & 9). Every operating theatre at the QVH has a computer thus allowing a surgeon to remain scrubbed and view images during surgery. The hospital computers operated Windows NT and were a minimum of Pentium II, 64 RAM in 2002. These have now been upgraded to Windows XP professional and 2G RAM with Dual Core 3GB Pentium. Our monitors were routinely set to 800 x 600 pixels in 2002; now the minimum is 1024 x 768 pixels.

3.3 Pilot study 2: Ten week retrospective evaluation of the telemedicine system (DISTAR software)

We conducted a retrospective evaluation of the DISTAR encryption software. Over a ten-week study period we received 973 referrals (644 male and 329 female; 730 adults and 174 children). Telemedicine was used in 42% of referrals during the study period, according to protocols for trainee surgeons indicating when images should be requested. Telemedicine was available in three referring units and was also used at the QVH by the trainee surgeons to facilitate communication with other members of the on call team.

Qualitative feedback confirmed that the software was "user friendly" and facilitated the referral process. Following review of the second pilot study the telemedicine team were satisfied with our encryption software. We then supplied cameras, encryption software and training to further accident and emergency departments and minor injuries units in our catchment area.

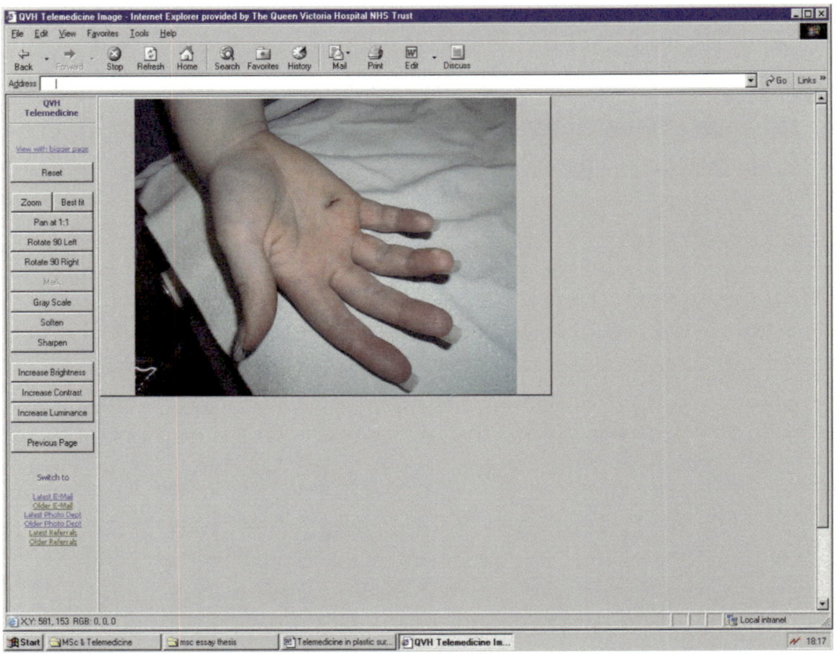

Fig. 8. Software for the receiving clinician at QVH

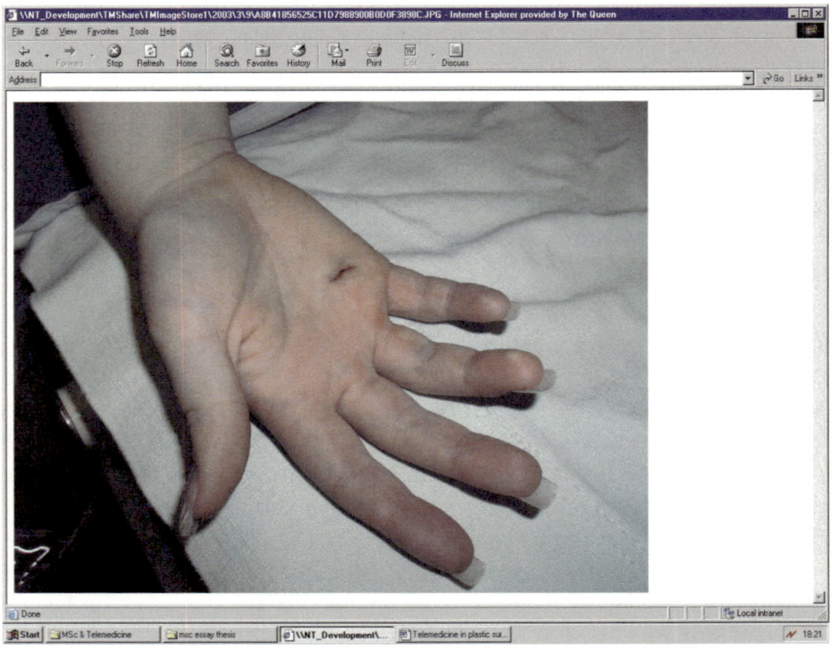

Fig. 9. Image can be enlarged to fill the screen

4. Pilot study 3: Twelve week prospective cohort study of the telemedicine system

4.1 Method

A prospective study was designed to determine the role of telemedicine in assessing different types of injury referred to the regional Plastic Surgery service at the QVH and to find out whether the information gained from telemedicine had any impact on the medical management, for example in prioritization of care. We classified injuries into 3 groups; closed, tidy and untidy. Closed injuries had no cutaneous wound e.g. closed hand fractures, dislocations or ligament injuries. Tidy injuries were defined as cuts and lacerations without loss of skin or subcutaneous tissue. Untidy 'injuries' included burns, wounds caused by crush or avulsion, wounds involving devascularization and infections. Management options included transfer to the QVH for review and treatment as an in- or out-patient/day-case, review at an out-patient/ dressing clinic (possibly at a peripheral hospital) or to decline the referral having giving appropriate advice on wound care/ further management.
Referrals assisted by telemedicine were compared to telephone only referrals with regards to initial clinical management for all trauma referrals to the Plastic Surgery service at the QVH during the study period. Further specific analysis was undertaken of burn injury and hand surgery patients provisionally scheduled for (day-care) surgery on the basis of the referral details alone. Results were analyzed with SPSS version 10.0.

4.2 Results

There were a total of 996 referrals to the Plastic Surgery service at the QVH (711 male and 285 female) during the twelve-week study period (March to May 2003), with established telemedicine links in eleven hospitals. The telemedicine system was used for 246 referrals, 63% of the 389 referrals for which the system was available. Due to a lack of ready access to a computer terminal at night 4% of telemedicine images were not reviewed immediately. We saw a significant difference (P 0.004) in the management of referrals overall, see figure 10 (Wallace et al. 2008). The Telemedicine group had fewer attendances for clinical review,

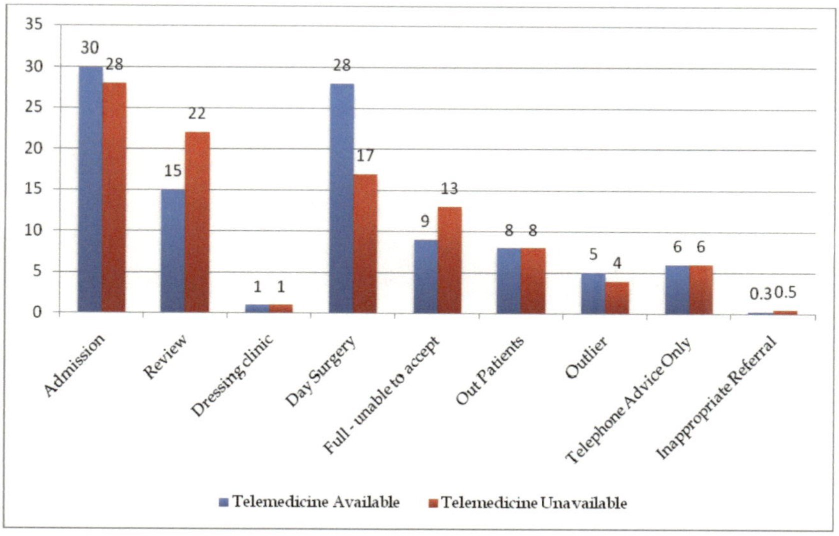

Fig. 10. Management choices of referrals with and without telemedicine availability (P0.004)

fewer referrals declined and increased use of day surgery. This significant difference was found in each of the three groups of closed, tidy and untidy injuries with the availability of telemedicine (Wallace et al. 2007).

Hand injury patients were triaged directly to Day Surgery with significantly greater accuracy, see figure 11. Upon arrival at the Day Surgery Unit 13% of telephone only referrals and 3% of telemedicine assisted referrals were redirected.

Figure 12 shows the significant difference (P 0.007) in the management of the 103 patients attending the Burns Unit who were expected to be managed by assessment, treatment and discharge, i.e. minor burns not requiring admission. All of the telemedicine referrals we were sent home, while 21% of the telephone-only referrals required unexpected admission.

Figure 13 gives the management choices of 121 burn referrals (given as percentages), which did not reach significance (P 0.11). As with the whole cohort there were fewer referral declined.

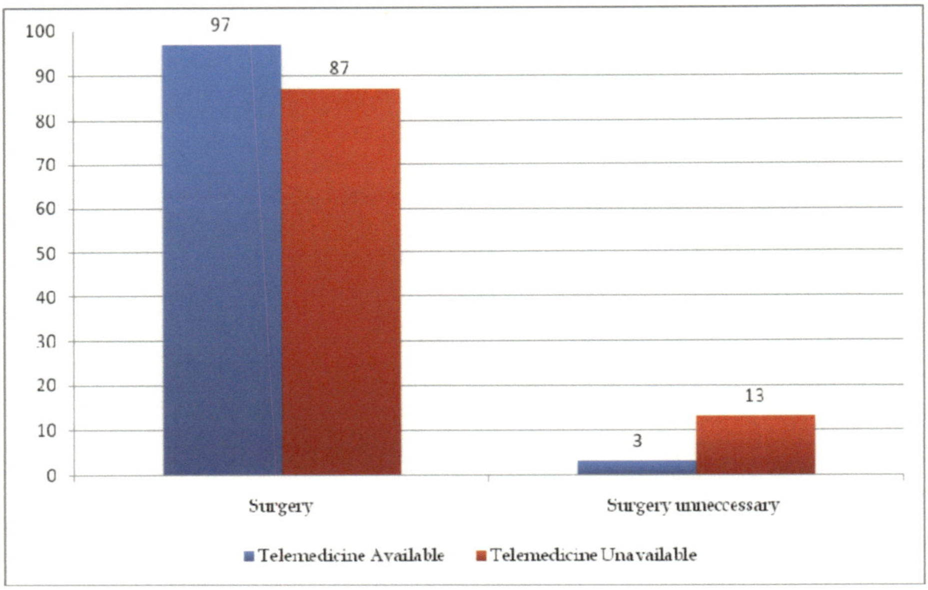

Fig. 11. Management of patients triaged to the Day Surgery Unit for definitive surgery (P 0.007)

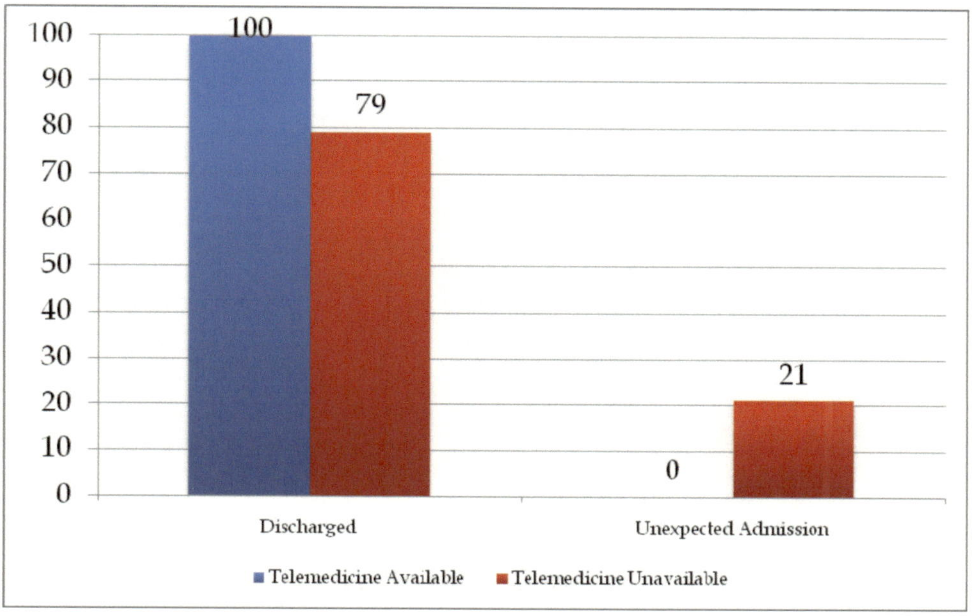

Fig. 12. Burn Injuries attending the Burns Unit for review (P0.007)

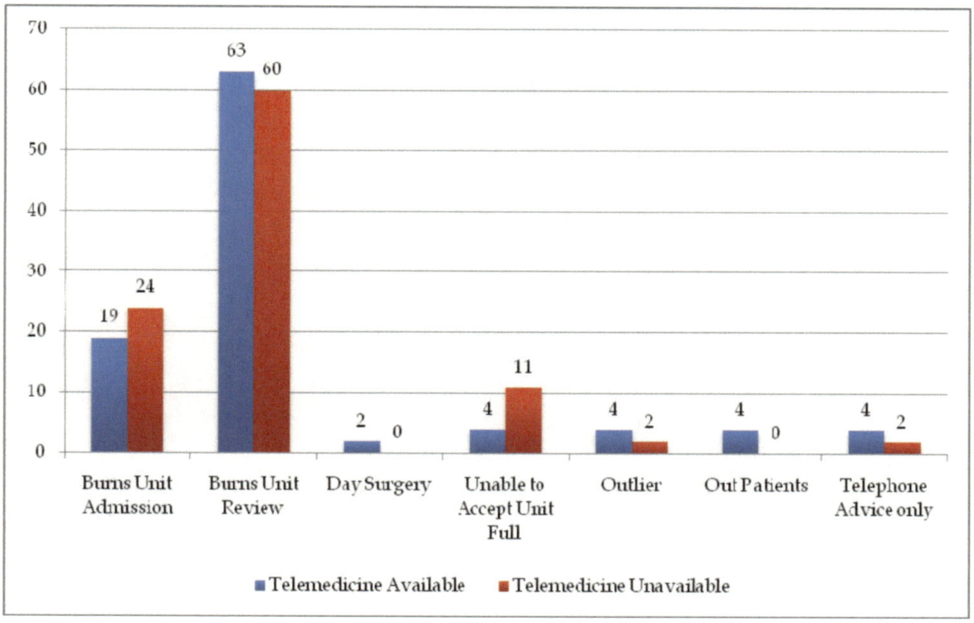

Fig. 13. Management of burn injuries with and without telemedicine availability

4.3 Illustrative case vignettes

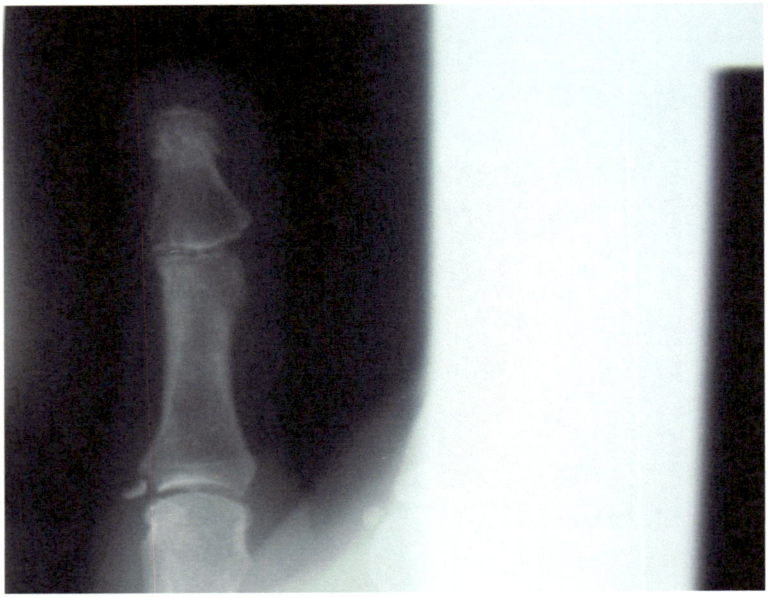

Fig. 14. Referring clinician had difficulty describing the radial avulsion fracture. Receiving clinician able to book directly into the Day Surgery Unit for a specific Hand Consultant.

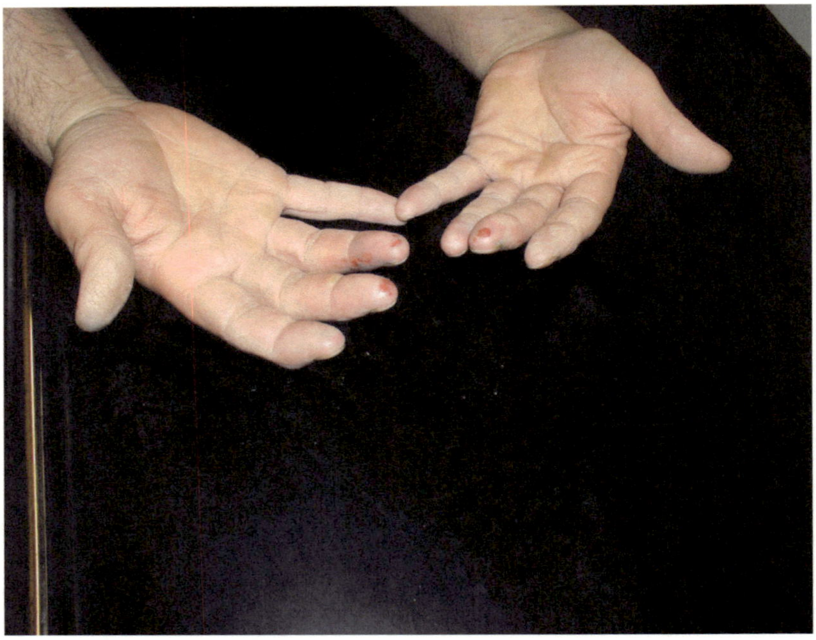

Fig. 15. Patient sustained a small chemical burn to the tips of several digits, thoroughly washed, and pH neutral. Referring clinician requested blue light transfer. On review of the images the receiving clinicians were able to down-grade of the urgency of transfer.

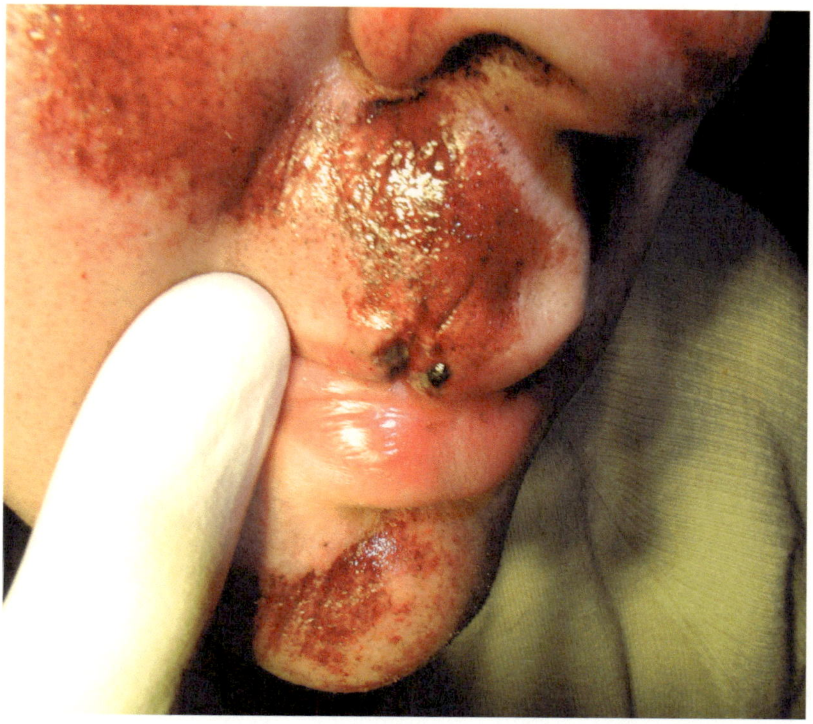

Fig. 16. Patient suffered facial abrasion and lip laceration after fall from bicycle. Abrasion not initially mentioned in telephone referral conversation. Referral priority upgraded to ensure urgent scrub to avoid gravel tattoo.

5. Discussion

5.1 What we have achieved?

We have developed a Store-and-forward encrypted telemedicine system to assist in the management of injured patients referred to the Plastic Surgery service at the QVH. Its use has increased over the last decade to become a routine part of the care pathway for the management of injured patients, see figure 22. We have published evidence of the change in management of our patients due to the system, with improved triage and efficiency of our acute services (Wallace et al. 2007; Wallace et al. 2008). Use of the telemedicine system has now become part of routine acute trauma management, see figure 17.

5.2 Why have been successful?

Changing clinician's behaviour can be challenging (Foy et al. 2001; Cabana et al. 1999; Grol & Grimshaw 2003), and requires a full appreciation of the potential problems associated with a change of practice. We were ultimately able to successfully introduce telemedicine to the QVH and to engage fellow clinicians at referral centres by starting with a limited number of collaborating units, i.e. few partners, then, by a process of evaluation involving the various pilot studies described we were able to iron-out technical and other problems and roll the program out to all key referrers in our catchment area. Also, we were strongly supported by QVH management because telemedicine allowed us to run a more efficient and cost effective service for injured patients.

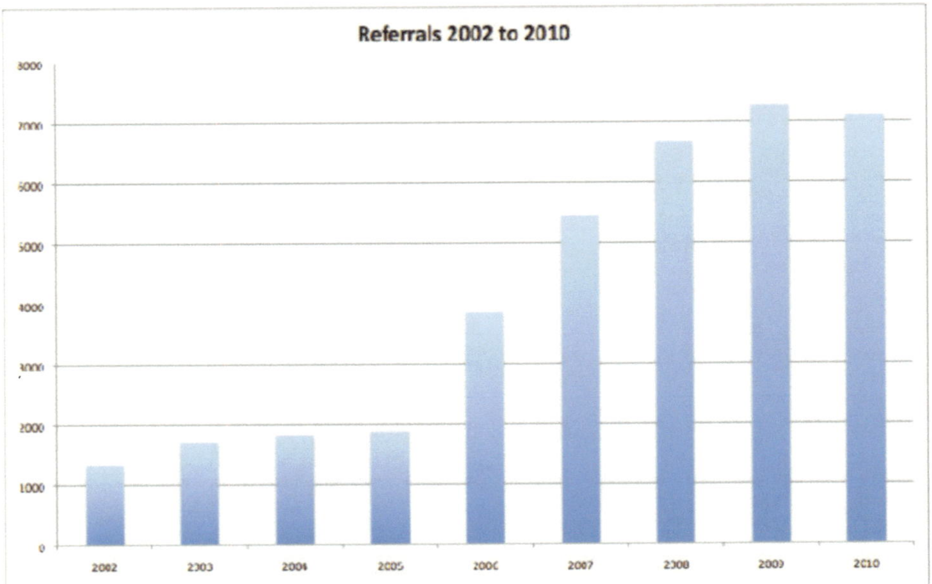

Fig. 17. Usage of Telemedicine system at QVH 2002-2010

5.2.1 Evidence base

An adequate evidence base is essential to demonstrate to clinicians that proposed changes offer benefit and are not detrimental to their patients (Yellowlees 2005; Tanriverdi & Iacono 1999; Stronge et al. 2008). Unfortunately throughout telemedicine (Roine et al. 2001; Whited 2006; Whitten et al. 2002), Burn injury management (Al-Benna et al. 2010) and Plastic surgery (Chung et al. 2002) numerous reviews bemoan the lack of high quality and randomised controlled trials. Our large prospective cohort study (pilot study 3) provides the current best level evidence for acute plastic surgery trauma management with a telemedicine system. Our studies combined with extrapolations from similar specialities (e.g. dermatology) have provided a useful evidence base (Levin & Warshaw 2009; Warshaw et al. 2009) to inform clinicians of the value of our system.

5.2.1.a Image resolution

Good quality images are vital in telemedicine; resolution must be adequate, perspective correct and focus sharp. Poor image quality can affect a clinician's ability to make a clear diagnosis (Briggs et al. 1998; Stutchfield et al. 2007); if necessary additional images should always be requested. Our own pilot study (pilot study 1) demonstrated 800 x 600 pixel resolution was adequate for diagnosis and grading of urgency of transfer (Jones et al. 2004). This concurs with other telemedicine studies of wound assessment (Wirthlin et al. 1998; Murphy et al. 2006) and dermatology (Eedy & Wootton 2001; Krupinski et al. 2008). Resolutions of greater than 1024 x 768 pixels does not appear to benefit the viewer for burn images (Jones et al. 2003), whilst limited file compression (JPEG) does not negatively affect confidence or accuracy (Jones et al. 2003; Roa et al. 1999). Lower resolution systems (mobile phone screens) can result in discordance between face-to-face management and telemedicine assisted referrals (Hsieh et al. 2004). We found no discordance for acute burn management (see figure 12) and a 3% discordance for hand injuries at 800 x 600 pixel resolution, see figure 11 (Wallace et al. 2007). Compact digital cameras have now surpassed this threshold, so that concerns over resolution obscuring subtle findings on computer screens are of historical relevance (Scott et al. 1993; Jacobs et al. 2002), although there may be a contemporary relevance if images are viewed on mobile phone displays.

Mobile phones were a relatively novel technology when we planned our system originally. Mobile phones are now ubiquitous, and restrictive use policies are being removed within the NHS (2009b). Therefore reports of mobile phones being used to view telemedicine images for neurosurgery (Waran et al. 2008), hand injuries (Hsieh et al. 2004) and burns (Shokrollahi et al. 2007) are of interest but at QVH we have no plans to use mobile phones for telemedicine purposes. Data protection cannot be safeguarded, nor can we keep patient information on the hospital computing system for audit purposes (Wallace & Durrant 2005).

5.2.1.b Legal & security concerns

Anonymising all data transferred by telemedicine can allay concerns over patient confidentiality, and has been used in early UK military telemedicine systems (Scerri & Vassallo 1999). In Plastic Surgery though, many images would be patient identifiable, e.g. facial images, and the volume of referrals we deal with would preclude such an anonymised system from having any practical value. We use the NHSnet, which is in effect a very large intranet for NHS hospitals; when combined with image encryption this meets legal requirements for data protection.

In the UK data protection compliance has been noted to be (woefully) inadequate (Webb 2002; Mole et al. 2006). Therefore ad hoc procedures and reliance on staff knowledge of data protection would be insufficient. Documentation of patient consent was made integral to the data entry with the QVH telemedicine system, which satisfied the requirements local Data protection.

5.2.2 Clinical ownership

At the start of the project we formed a telemedicine team that included clinicians who were involved in trauma management and who were users of the system. We have maintained their involvement to ensure that the system can be usefully changed, as demonstrated by our early recognition of the need for bespoke encryption software. We delivered both top-down and bottom-up pragmatic style management, rather than rigid idealism, to optimize change of clinical practice (Yellowlees 2005; Grol & Grimshaw 2003). We used plastic surgical trainees to lead the installation and education process since they were judged to be familiar with the demands of the acute service and could be seen to be assisting with rather imposing a new working practice upon colleagues that demanded extra work for the referring clinician.

5.2.3 User friendly systems

We considered whether to opt for a videoconferencing interactive system, or for a Store-and-forward system. Videoconferencing systems can provide good support for acute referrals needing expert review in the UK (Tachakra et al. 1998; Tachakra et al. 2002). Unfortunately videoconferencing systems usually require a designated room, and consultations can take substantially longer, often two to three fold longer (Benger et al. 2004; Tachakra & Rajani 2002). The flexibility of a Store-and-forward system is well suited to the multiple locations of the acute surgical team at the QVH. The receiving clinical team can be in different locations within the hospital, communicating by telephone, while viewing images on the nearest computer screen. This assists not only the patients at a distance from

QVH, but also those already on site to facilitate senior involvement in decision making, even if scrubbed in theatre. Recently we have begun to incorporate clinical images downloaded from our telemedicine database directly into patient's clinical records and we also include telemedicine images in power point presentations that form the basis of daily hand-over discussions for the duty trauma team. Furthermore, all images are stored in databases that are easily accessible for clinicians who wish to view them for clinical purposes and teaching. Clinicians have responsibility for ensuring the best care of their patients, and if the technology does not assist in this then one cannot expect it to be used (Yellowlees 2005). One early Store-and-forward system could only process twenty cases in an hour (Taylor et al. 2001), which is clearly inadequate. Technology projects are expected to give substantial benefits, occasionally even mortality reductions (Longhurst et al. 2010). However this is not always the case, with extra clinical work required (Jones 2003), or even adverse clinical outcomes (Han et al. 2005). Clinicians naturally seek solutions for technology that does not meet their needs (Andersen et al. 2009). We were very keen to install a simple system that could be easily used even without specialist training. We conducted a feedback survey, which demonstrated very high satisfaction amongst referring clinicians, with 33 of 34 happy to recommend the system to others.

On each occasion during the prospective cohort trial that a referring clinician reported that the telemedicine was faulty, the system was inspected on site either the following day or next working day. Technical faults were reported on 91 occasions, yet less than 10 were validated on inspection. These issues highlight the need of designing systems around the clinician (Yellowlees 2005).

5.2.4 Training & support

Initially we anticipated that once the telemedicine system was installed minimal support would be required, but where staff turnover is high the training needs to be continual (Blignault & Kennedy 1999; Krupinski et al. 2003). We also found, like others (Lian et al. 2003), a significant percentage of images inadequate for diagnostic needs ((20 of 150; e.g. bad views, poor focus). Guidance was needed for taking images (see figure 2); Plastic Surgery trainees taught both technical use of the system and clinical topics (such as burn and hand surgery management) at the referring hospitals. From both experience and the literature (Jakowenko 2009; Whitehouse 1999) we recommend cleaning the injured area thoroughly. Then, with the flash on, a general image for zoning the area and a close up of the injured part are routinely requested. When taking images of non-digital X-rays on a backlit screen the flash should be off. We distributed a handout of tips for good image acquisition and use of the telemedicine system.

We assumed that the referring clinicians would be the most useful personnel to teach in each referring department. However, experience suggested the entire clinical staff, including nurses, should become familiar with the system, thereby increasing the likelihood of a trained member of staff being on duty when the need arises. To retain the camera in a secure and accessible place we recommend the Controlled Drugs Cabinet; ideally with rechargeable batteries available.

One of the few drawbacks of our Store-and-forward system is the limited educational potential when compared to videoconferencing systems. In Minor Injury Unit support in the UK such systems can lead to decreased referral rates due to clinical education of the staff (Tachakra et al. 2000). When we evaluated the 996 referrals in the prospective study we determined only 1% to be inappropriate, therefore we do not expect to see a drop in referrals (see figure10).

5.2.5 Cost analysis

We received central government assistance with the capital outlay for the purchase and installation of computer equipment and cameras, network lines and software of £70 000 ($110 000). We continue to employ a clinical telemedicine officer at the QVH to ensure support, ongoing education and promotion of the system. We have not charged referring units for such telemedicine training. We believe this would be detrimental to encouraging the use of the system, which benefits the patient and our efficient use of resources, but does not assist the referring unit more than the standard phone call. We have shown an overall 10% decrease in the need for face-to-face review prior to treatment since the introduction of telemedicine at the QVH.

Cost savings have rarely been demonstrated from the use of telemedicine systems (Whitten & Buis 2007; Whitten et al. 2002) although reducing patient transportation costs may be possible (Saffle et al. 2004) and has been demonstrated by several telemedicine systems (Tsai et al. 2007; Goh et al. 1997). Typically only when the health care provider also pays for the transportation does this occur, i.e. in the military and prisons (McManus et al. 2008; Brunicardi 1998).

5.3 Why does telemedicine help?

There are several possible reasons why telemedicine images help in the referral process. Firstly the receiving clinician is able to validate any information already given over the phone. Secondly, there may be additional information from the images supplied. This may be important for non specialists referrers, whose lack of knowledge may lead to an incomplete or incorrect assessment (Kruger & Dunning 1999). In casualty departments the infrequency of burn injuries precludes the ability for most emergency clinicians to become confident in their burn-wound assessments (Chipp et al. 2008). Without adequate clinical experience expertise is difficult to gain (Ericsson 2008), and without feedback learning is very challenging (Croskerry 2000). Decisions are made in an environment that is vulnerable to error (Croskerry & Sinclair 2001). We know that Hand (Patel et al. 1998; Nassab et al. 2007) and Burn injury (Collis et al. 1999; Hagstrom et al. 2003; Laing et al. 1991; Irwin et al. 1993) assessment is suboptimal by non specialists, and the role of the referring clinician is to "sell the patient" to the receiving unit (Nugus et al. 2009).

Burn beds are such a precious resource in the UK that we have a national bed bureau that contacts all burn centres twice daily to update on capacity. This facilitates the management of the acutely injured burn patient if the nearest provider is unable to take the referral. We studied patients attending the QVH Burns unit for clinical review (fgure 12). These were patients who, on the basis of the referral information, we would anticipate to be treated and discharged home. All of the telemedicine assisted referrals were reviewed and discharged home; whereas 21% of the telephone only referrals could not be safely discharged home and required an unexpected admission (Wallace et al. 2007). We also noted a decrease in the proportion of referrals we were unable to accept, as the unit was full, though this did not reach signifcance.

Thirdly, with better quality communication, there should be fewer errors for clinicians involved in the process of referring injured patients for specialist care (Sexton et al. 2000; Foy et al. 2010; Coiera 2000). Finally, one of the unexpected but significant benefits of introducing telemedicine to the QVH has been the almost routine involvement of senior clinicians in key management decisions for trauma cases due to the ease of access to telemedicine images at computer terminals throughout the hospital, plus access via the

NHSnet to X-rays taken in referring hospitals. The involvement of senior medical staff in trauma management should, logically, be accompanied by improved standards of care and greater efficiency (Wyatt et al. 1999; Treasure 2007).

6. Future developments

In the UK provision for trauma care has been shown to be suboptimal (Anderson et al. 1988). Trauma networks are being introduced throughout the UK (Treasure 2007; 2009a; Celso et al. 2006). Telemedicine applications for ambulance crews to assist with cardiac patients have lead to mortality benefits (Bjorklund et al. 2006). For certain specific injuries that are attended by ambulance crews the possibility exists now for patients to be referred with telemedicine directly to the QVH without having to be taken to another hospital's accident department; it may be possible for advice to be given on treatment to paramedics attending injured patients, which, in turn, saves an unnecessary hospital attendance. With telemedicine, ambulance crews can take injured patients to the most appropriate facility, rather than the nearest.

7. Conclusion

We introduced a secure encrypted email telemedicine system to our unit, having identified a need for increasing objective information to assist in the management of acute burn and plastic surgery injuries. We maintained clinical ownership by convening a group of clinical users and information technology experts to assess the requirements, specify the type and design, and assess the clinical impact of the system. The systematic and staged evaluation allowed clinical confidence to grow and encouraged the involvement of all users of the system. We have demonstrated significant improvements in clinical management with the use of the system. This has led to the successful integration into routine practise for acute plastic surgery referrals. As technological applications continue to develop we look to move forward by involving the pre hospital personnel in improving the initial triage by direct contact with ourselves, facilitating expert and senior guidance at the pre hospital site.

8. Acknowledgements

We would like to thank Scott Reynolds from Godalming Computer Products for the development of the telemedicine software and the IT department of QVH (in particular Nasir Rafiq and Ted Balk) for their knowledge and support from inception to the present day. We also thank Sophie Jones, the first telemedicine officer, and Gary Taylor the current telemedicine officer. These individuals were instrumental in the introduction of the system and moving the system from a project to an integral part of acute trauma care, respectively.

9. References

2009a. Using mobile phones in NHS hospitals. Department of Health - Estates and Facilities Division, Leeds.

2009b. Regional trauma systems: interim guidance for commissioners. The intercollegiate group on trauma standards.

Al-Benna, S., D. Alzoubaidi, and Y. Al-Ajam. 2010. Evidence-based burn care--An assessment of the methodological quality of research published in burn care journals from 1982 to 2008. Burns 36:1190-5.

Andersen, P., A.M. Lindgaard, M. Prgomet, N. Creswick, and J.I. Westbrook. 2009. Mobile and fixed computer use by doctors and nurses on hospital wards: multi-method study on the relationships between clinician role, clinical task, and device choice. J Med Internet Res 11:e32.

Anderson, I.D., M. Woodford, F.T. de Dombal, and M. Irving. 1988. Retrospective study of 1000 deaths from injury in England and Wales. Br Med J (Clin Res Ed) 296:1305-8.

Benger, J. 2000. A review of telemedicine in accident and emergency: the story so far. J.Accid.Emerg.Med. 17:157-164.

Benger, J.R., S.M. Noble, J. Coast, and J.M. Kendall. 2004. The safety and effectiveness of minor injuries telemedicine. Emerg Med J 21:438-45.

Bjorklund, E., U. Stenestrand, J. Lindback, L. Svensson, L. Wallentin, and B. Lindahl. 2006. Pre-hospital thrombolysis delivered by paramedics is associated with reduced time delay and mortality in ambulance-transported real-life patients with ST-elevation myocardial infarction. Eur Heart J 27:1146-52.

Bledsoe, B.E., and M.G. Smith. 2004. Medical helicopter accidents in the United States: a 10-year review. J Trauma 56:1325-8; discussion 1328-9.

Blignault, I., and C. Kennedy. 1999. Training for telemedicine. J.Telemed.Telecare. 5 Suppl 1:S112-S114.

Briggs, R., J.E. Bailey, C. Eddy, and I. Sun. 1998. A methodologic issue for ophthalmic telemedicine: image quality and its effect on diagnostic accuracy and confidence. J.Am.Optom.Assoc. 69:601-605.

Brunicardi, B.O. 1998. Financial analysis of savings from telemedicine in Ohio's prison system. Telemed.J. 4:49-54.

Buntic, R.F., P.P. Siko, G.M. Buncke, D. Ruebeck, G.M. Kind, and H.J. Buncke. 1997. Using the Internet for rapid exchange of photographs and X-ray images to evaluate potential extremity replantation candidates. J.Trauma 43:342-344.

Cabana, M.D., C.S. Rand, N.R. Powe, A.W. Wu, M.H. Wilson, P.A. Abboud, and H.R. Rubin. 1999. Why don't physicians follow clinical practice guidelines? A framework for improvement. JAMA 282:1458-1465.

Cartmill, M., and B.D. White. 2001. Telephone advice for neurosurgical referrals. Who assumes duty of care? Br.J.Neurosurg. 15:453-455.

Celso, B., J. Tepas, B. Langland-Orban, E. Pracht, L. Papa, L. Lottenberg, and L. Flint. 2006. A systematic review and meta-analysis comparing outcome of severely injured patients treated in trauma centers following the establishment of trauma systems. J Trauma 60:371-8; discussion 378.

Chipp, E., J. Walton, D.F. Gorman, and N.S. Moiemen. 2008. A 1 year study of burn injuries in a British Emergency Department. Burns 34:516-20.

Chung, K.C., L.K. Kalliainen, S.V. Spilson, M.R. Walters, and H.M. Kim. 2002. The prevalence of negative studies with inadequate statistical power: an analysis of the plastic surgery literature. Plast.Reconstr.Surg. 109:1-6.

Coiera, E. 2000. When conversation is better than computation. J Am Med Inform Assoc 7:277-86.

Collis, N., G. Smith, and O.M. Fenton. 1999. Accuracy of burn size estimation and subsequent fluid resuscitation prior to arrival at the Yorkshire Regional Burns Unit. A three year retrospective study. Burns 25:345-351.

Croskerry, P. 2000. The feedback sanction. Academic Emergency Medicine 7 1232-1238.

Croskerry, P., and D. Sinclair. 2001. Emergency medicine: A practice prone to error? CJEM 3:271-6.

Darkins, A., C.H. Dearden, L.G. Rocke, J.B. Martin, L. Sibson, and R. Wootton. 1996. An evaluation of telemedical support for a minor treatment centre. J.Telemed.Telecare. 2:93-99.

Dunn, E.V., D.W. Conrath, W.G. Bloor, and B. Tranquada. 1977. An evaluation of four telemedicine systems for primary care. Health Serv.Res. 12:19-29.

Eedy, D.J., and R. Wootton. 2001. Teledermatology: a review. Br.J.Dermatol. 144:696-707.

Elford, R., H. White, R. Bowering, A. Ghandi, B. Maddiggan, K. St John, M. House, J. Harnett, R. West, and A. Battcock. 2000. A randomized, controlled trial of child psychiatric assessments conducted using videoconferencing. J.Telemed.Telecare. 6:73-82.

Ericsson, K.A. 2008. Deliberate practice and acquisition of expert performance: a general overview. Acad Emerg Med 15:988-94.

Foy, R., A. Walker, and G. Penney. 2001. Barriers to clinical guidelines: the need for concerted action. British Journal of Clinical Governance 6 166-174.

Foy, R., S. Hempel, L. Rubenstein, M. Suttorp, M. Seelig, R. Shanman, and P.G. Shekelle. 2010. Meta-analysis: effect of interactive communication between collaborating primary care physicians and specialists. Ann Intern Med 152:247-58.

Gilmour, E., S.M. Campbell, M.A. Loane, A. Esmail, C.E. Griffiths, M.O. Roland, E.J. Parry, R.O. Corbett, D. Eedy, H.E. Gore, C. Mathews, K. Steel, and R. Wootton. 1998. Comparison of teleconsultations and face-to-face consultations: preliminary results of a United Kingdom multicentre teledermatology study. Br.J.Dermatol. 139:81-87.

Goh, K.Y., C.K. Lam, and W.S. Poon. 1997. The impact of teleradiology on the inter-hospital transfer of neurosurgical patients. Br.J.Neurosurg. 11:52-56.

Grol, R., and J. Grimshaw. 2003. From best evidence to best practice: effective implementation of change in patients' care. Lancet 362:1225-30.

Hagstrom, M., G.A. Wirth, G.R. Evans, and C.J. Ikeda. 2003. A review of emergency department fluid resuscitation of burn patients transferred to a regional, verified burn center. Ann.Plast Surg 51:173-176.

Hailey, D., R. Roine, and A. Ohinmaa. 2002. Systematic review of evidence for the benefits of telemedicine. J.Telemed.Telecare. 8 Suppl 1:1-30.

Han, Y.Y., J.A. Carcillo, S.T. Venkataraman, R.S. Clark, R.S. Watson, T.C. Nguyen, H. Bayir, and R.A. Orr. 2005. Unexpected increased mortality after implementation of a commercially sold computerized physician order entry system. Pediatrics 116:1506-12.

Harno, K., E. Arajarvi, T. Paavola, C. Carlson, and P. Viikinkoski. 2001. Clinical effectiveness and cost analysis of patient referral by videoconferencing in orthopaedics. J.Telemed.Telecare. 7:219-225.

High, W.A., M.S. Houston, S.D. Calobrisi, L.A. Drage, and M.T. McEvoy. 2000. Assessment of the accuracy of low-cost store-and-forward teledermatology consultation. J Am Acad Dermatol 42:776-83.

Hsieh, C.H., H.H. Tsai, J.W. Yin, C.Y. Chen, J.C. Yang, and S.F. Jeng. 2004. Teleconsultation with the mobile camera-phone in digital soft-tissue injury: a feasibility study. Plast Reconstr.Surg 114:1776-1782.

Irwin, L.R., C.A. Reid, and N.R. McLean. 1993. Burns in children: do casualty officers get it right? Injury 24:187-188.

Jacobs, M.J., M.J. Edmondson, and J.C. Lowry. 2002. Accuracy of diagnosis of fractures by maxillofacial and accident and emergency doctors using plain radiography compared with a telemedicine system: a prospective study. Br.J.Oral Maxillofac.Surg. 40:156-162.

Jakowenko, J. 2009. Clinical photography. J Telemed Telecare 15:7-22.

Jones, M.R. 2003. "Computers can land people on Mars, why can't they get them to work in a hospital?" Implementation of an Electronic Patient Record System in a UK Hospital. Methods Inf.Med. 42:410-415.

Jones, O.C., D.I. Wilson, and S. Andrews. 2003. The reliability of digital images when used to assess burn wounds. J Telemed Telecare 9 Suppl 1:S22-4.

Jones, S.M., C. Milroy, and M.A. Pickford. 2004. Telemedicine in acute plastic surgical trauma and burns. Ann.R.Coll.Surg Engl. 86:239-242.

Kingsnorth, A., A. Vranch, and J. Campbell. 2000. Training for surgeons using digital satellite television and videoconferencing. J.Telemed.Telecare. 6 Suppl 1:S29-S31.

Kruger, J., and D. Dunning. 1999. Unskilled and unaware of it: how difficulties in recognizing one's own incompetence lead to inflated self-assessments. J Pers Soc Psychol 77:1121-34.

Krupinski, E., A. Burdick, H. Pak, J. Bocachica, L. Earles, K. Edison, M. Goldyne, T. Hirota, J. Kvedar, K. McKoy, D. Oh, D. Siegel, N. Antoniotti, I. Camacho, L. Carnahan, P. Boynton, R. Bakalar, R. Evans, A. Kinel, P. Kuzmak, B.C. Madden, S. Peters, L. Rosenthal, S. Simmons, J. Bernard, and J. Linkous. 2008. American Telemedicine Association's Practice Guidelines for Teledermatology. Telemed J E Health 14:289-302.

Krupinski, E.A., A.M. Hughes, G.P. Barker, A.M. Lopez, and R.S. Weinstein. 2003. Fluctuations in telemedicine case volume: correlation with personnel turnover rates. Telemed J E Health 9:369-73.

Krupinski, E.A., B. LeSueur, L. Ellsworth, N. Levine, R. Hansen, N. Silvis, P. Sarantopoulos, P. Hite, J. Wurzel, R.S. Weinstein, and A.M. Lopez. 1999. Diagnostic accuracy and image quality using a digital camera for teledermatology. Telemed.J. 5:257-263.

Laing, J.H., B.D. Morgan, and R. Sanders. 1991. Assessment of burn injury in the accident and emergency department: a review of 100 referrals to a regional burns unit. Ann.R.Coll.Surg Engl. 73:329-331.

Levin, Y.S., and E.M. Warshaw. 2009. Teledermatology: a review of reliability and accuracy of diagnosis and management. Dermatol Clin 27:163-76, vii.

Lian, P., K. Chong, X. Zhai, and Y. Ning. 2003. The quality of medical records in teleconsultation. J Telemed.Telecare. 9:35-41.

Loane, M.A., S.E. Bloomer, R. Corbett, D.J. Eedy, N. Hicks, H.E. Lotery, C. Mathews, J. Paisley, K. Steele, and R. Wootton. 2000. A comparison of real-time and store-and-forward teledermatology: a cost-benefit study. Br.J.Dermatol. 143:1241-1247.

Longhurst, C.A., L. Parast, C.I. Sandborg, E. Widen, J. Sullivan, J.S. Hahn, C.G. Dawes, and P.J. Sharek. 2010. Decrease in hospital-wide mortality rate after implementation of a commercially sold computerized physician order entry system. Pediatrics 126:14-21.

Lowitt, M.H., I.I. Kessler, C.L. Kauffman, F.J. Hooper, E. Siegel, and J.W. Burnett. 1998. Teledermatology and in-person examinations: a comparison of patient and physician perceptions and diagnostic agreement. Arch.Dermatol. 134:471-476.

McManus, J., J. Salinas, M. Morton, C. Lappan, and R. Poropatich. 2008. Teleconsultation program for deployed soldiers and healthcare professionals in remote and austere environments. Prehosp Disaster Med 23:210-6; discussion 217.

Murphy, R.L., Jr., T.B. Fitzpatrick, H.A. Haynes, K.T. Bird, and T.B. Sheridan. 1972. Accuracy of dermatologic diagnosis by television. Arch Dermatol 105:833-5.

Murphy, R.X., Jr., M.A. Bain, T.E. Wasser, E. Wilson, and W.J. Okunski. 2006. The reliability of digital imaging in the remote assessment of wounds: defining a standard. Ann Plast Surg 56:431-6.

Nassab, R., K. Kok, J. Constantinides, and V. Rajaratnam. 2007. The diagnostic accuracy of clinical examination in hand lacerations. Int J Surg 5:105-8.

Nugus, P., J. Bridges, and J. Braithwaite. 2009. Selling patients. BMJ 339:b5201.

Oakley, A.M., D.R. Astwood, M. Loane, M.B. Duffill, M. Rademaker, and R. Wootton. 1997. Diagnostic accuracy of teledermatology: results of a preliminary study in New Zealand. N.Z.Med.J. 110:51-53.

Ong, C.A. 2008. Telemedicine and wound care. Stud Health Technol Inform 131:211-25.

Pap, S.A., E. Lach, and J. Upton. 2002. Telemedicine in plastic surgery: E-consult the attending surgeon. Plast.Reconstr.Surg. 110:452-456.

Patel, J., R. Couli, P.A. Harris, and N.J. Percival. 1998. Hand lacerations. An audit of clinical examination. J Hand Surg Br 23:482-4.

Ricci, W.M., and J. Borrelli. 2002. Teleradiology in orthopaedic surgery: impact on clinical decision making for acute fracture management. J.Orthop.Trauma 16:1-6.

Roa, L., T. Gomez-Cia, B. Acha, and C. Serrano. 1999. Digital imaging in remote diagnosis of burns. Burns 25:617-23.

Rogers, F.B., M. Ricci, M. Caputo, S. Shackford, K. Sartorelli, P. Callas, J. Dewell, and S. Daye. 2001. The use of telemedicine for real-time video consultation between trauma center and community hospital in a rural setting improves early trauma care: preliminary results. J.Trauma 51:1037-1041.

Roine, R., A. Ohinmaa, and D. Hailey. 2001. Assessing telemedicine: a systematic review of the literature. CMAJ. 165:765-771.

Rosenfeld, B.A., T. Dorman, M.J. Breslow, P. Pronovost, M. Jenckes, N. Zhang, G. Anderson, and H. Rubin. 2000. Intensive care unit telemedicine: alternate paradigm for providing continuous intensivist care. Crit Care Med. 28:3925-3931.

Saffle, J.R., L. Edelman, and S.E. Morris. 2004. Regional air transport of burn patients: a case for telemedicine? J Trauma 57:57-64.

Saffle, J.R., L. Edelman, L. Theurer, S.E. Morris, and A. Cochran. 2009. Telemedicine evaluation of acute burns is accurate and cost-effective. J Trauma 67:358-65.

Scerri, G.V., and D.J. Vassallo. 1999. Initial plastic surgery experience with the first telemedicine links for the British Forces. Br J Plast Surg 52:294-298.

Scott, W.W., Jr., J.E. Rosenbaum, S.J. Ackerman, R.L. Reichle, D. Magid, J.C. Weller, and J.N. Gitlin. 1993. Subtle orthopedic fractures: teleradiology workstation versus film interpretation. Radiology 187:811-815.

Sexton, J.B., E.J. Thomas, and R.L. Helmreich. 2000. Error, stress, and teamwork in medicine and aviation: cross sectional surveys. BMJ 320:745-749.

Shokrollahi, K., M. Sayed, W. Dickson, and T. Potokar. 2007. Mobile phones for the assessment of burns: we have the technology. Emerg.Med.J 24:753-755.

Skillman, J.M., D. Dewar, H. Davies, M. McCabe, A. Fleming, and D. Gateley. 2003. Audit of pattern of closures to acute hand services in Pan Thames area. J Hand Surg [Br] 28:381-383.

Stronge, A.J., T. Nichols, W.A. Rogers, and A.D. Fisk. 2008. Systematic human factors evaluation of a teledermatology system within the U.S. military. Telemed J E Health 14:25-34.

Stutchfield, B.M., R. Jagilly, and B.R. Tulloh. 2007. Second opinions in remote surgical practice using email and digital photography. ANZ J Surg 77:1009-12.

Tachakra, S., and R. Rajani. 2002. Social presence in telemedicine. J.Telemed.Telecare. 8:226-230.

Tachakra, S., U.C. Uko, and A. Stinson. 2002. Four years' experience of telemedicine support of a minor accident and treatment service. J.Telemed.Telecare. 8 Suppl 2:87-89.

Tachakra, S., C. Wiley, M. Dawood, A. Sivakumar, D. Dutton, and J. Hayes. 1998. Evaluation of telemedical support to a free-standing minor accident and treatment service. J.Telemed.Telecare. 4:140-145.

Tachakra, S., D. Dutton, R. Newson, J. Hayes, A. Sivakumar, P. Jaye, and J. Bak. 2000. How do teleconsultations for remote trauma management change over a period of time? J.Telemed.Telecare. 6 Suppl 1:S12-S15.

Tanriverdi, H., and C.S. Iacono. 1999. Diffusion of telemedicine: a knowledge barrier perspective. Telemed.J. 5:223-244.

Taylor, P., P. Goldsmith, K. Murray, D. Harris, and A. Barkley. 2001. Evaluating a telemedicine system to assist in the management of dermatology referrals. Br.J.Dermatol. 144:328-333.

Treasure, T. 2007. Trauma: Who cares? NCEPOD.

Tsai, S.H., J. Kraus, H.R. Wu, W.L. Chen, M.F. Chiang, L.H. Lu, C.E. Chang, and W.T. Chiu. 2007. The effectiveness of video-telemedicine for screening of patients requesting emergency air medical transport (EAMT). J Trauma 62:504-11.

Wallace, D., and C. Durrant. 2005. Mobile messaging: emergency image transfer. Ann R Coll Surg Engl 87:72-3.

Wallace, D.L., R.W. Smith, and M.A. Pickford. 2007. A cohort study of acute plastic surgery trauma and burn referrals using telemedicine. J Telemed.Telecare. 13:282-287.

Wallace, D.L., S.M. Jones, C. Milroy, and M.A. Pickford. 2008. Telemedicine for acute plastic surgical trauma and burns. J Plast Reconstr Aesthet Surg 61:31-6.

Wallace, P., A. Haines, R. Harrison, J. Barber, S. Thompson, P. Jacklin, J. Roberts, L. Lewis, and P. Wainwright. 2002. Joint teleconsultations (virtual outreach) versus standard outpatient appointments for pateints referred by their general practioner for a specialist opinion: a randomised trial. Lancet 359 1961-1968.

Waran, V., B.M. Selladurai, N.F. Bahuri, G.J. George, G.P. Lim, and M. Khine. 2008. Teleconferencing using multimedia messaging service (MMS) for long-range consultation of patients with neurosurgical problems in an acute situation. J Trauma 64:362-5; discussion 365.

Ward, J.P., J. Gordon, M.J. Field, and H.P. Lehmann. 2001. Communication and information technology in medical education. Lancet 357:792-796.

Warshaw, E.M., F.A. Lederle, J.P. Grill, A.A. Gravely, A.K. Bangerter, L.A. Fortier, K.A. Bohjanen, K. Chen, P.K. Lee, H.S. Rabinovitz, R.H. Johr, V.N. Kaye, S. Bowers, R. Wenner, S.K. Askari, D.A. Kedrowski, and D.B. Nelson. 2009. Accuracy of teledermatology for pigmented neoplasms. J Am Acad Dermatol 61:753-65.

Whited, J.D. 2006. The quality of telemedicine research. J Telemed.Telecare. 12:271-273.

Whitehouse, R.W. 1999. Use of digital cameras for radiographs: how to get the best pictures. J R.Soc.Med. 92:178-182.

Whitten, P., and L. Buis. 2007. Private payer reimbursement for telemedicine services in the United States. Telemed.J E.Health 13:15-23.

Whitten, P.S., F.S. Mair, A. Haycox, C.R. May, T.L. Williams, and S. Hellmich. 2002. Systematic review of cost effectiveness studies of telemedicine interventions. BMJ 324:1434-1437.

Wirthlin, D.J., S. Buradagunta, R.A. Edwards, D.C. Brewster, R.P. Cambria, J.P. Gertler, G.M. LaMuraglia, D.E. Jordan, J.C. Kvedar, and W.M. Abbott. 1998. Telemedicine in vascular surgery: feasibility of digital imaging for remote management of wounds. J.Vasc.Surg. 27:1089-1099.

Wootton, R., S.E. Bloomer, R. Corbett, D.J. Eedy, N. Hicks, H.E. Lotery, C. Mathews, J. Paisley, K. Steele, and M.A. Loane. 2000. Multicentre randomised control trial comparing real time teledermatology with conventional outpatient dermatological care: societal cost-benefit analysis. BMJ 320:1252-1256.

Wyatt, J.P., J. Henry, and D. Beard. 1999. The association between seniority of Accident and Emergency doctor and outcome following trauma. Injury 30:165-168.

Yellowlees, P. 1997. Successful development of telemedicine systems--seven core principles. J.Telemed.Telecare. 3:215-222.

Yellowlees, P.M. 2005. Successfully developing a telemedicine system. J Telemed.Telecare. 11:331-335.